Cellular Mechanisms for
Calcium Transfer and Homeostasis

Cellular Mechanisms for Calcium Transfer and Homeostasis

Edited by GEORGE NICHOLS, Jr.

*Cancer Research Institute
New England Deaconess Hospital
Boston, Massachusetts*

R. H. WASSERMAN

*Department of Physical Biology
New York State Veterinary College
Cornell University
Ithaca, New York*

 *1971*

ACADEMIC PRESS   New York and London

COPYRIGHT © 1971, BY ACADEMIC PRESS, INC.
ALL RIGHTS RESERVED
NO PART OF THIS BOOK MAY BE REPRODUCED IN ANY FORM,
BY PHOTOSTAT, MICROFILM, RETRIEVAL SYSTEM, OR ANY
OTHER MEANS, WITHOUT WRITTEN PERMISSION FROM
THE PUBLISHERS.

ACADEMIC PRESS, INC.
111 Fifth Avenue, New York, New York 10003

United Kingdom Edition published by
ACADEMIC PRESS, INC. (LONDON) LTD.
24/28 Oval Road, London NW1 7DD

LIBRARY OF CONGRESS CATALOG CARD NUMBER: 76-154382

PRINTED IN THE UNITED STATES OF AMERICA

CONTENTS

List of Contributors   xvii
Preface   xxv
Credits   xxix
Acknowledgments   xxxi
Franklin Chambers McLean and the State of Calcium in Body Fluids   xxxiii
   by A. Baird Hastings

I. THE STATE OF CALCIUM IN BODY FLUIDS

The Structure, Properties, and Formation of Calcium Phosphates in Hard Tissue

Aaron S. Posner

Introduction	3
Hydroxyapatite Structure	5
Carbonate Apatites	8
Bone Apatite	9
Amorphous Calcium Phosphate in Bone Mineral	12
Tissue Mineralization	15
Conclusions	20
References	21
Discussion	23

Differentiation Processes in Calcified Tissues
Leon J. Richelle

Introduction	25
Development as a General Process	26
Development in Bone and Dental Tissues	30
Conclusion	36
References	37
Discussion	39

The Binding of Calcium with Nucleic Acids and Phospholipids
Charles W. Carr and Kim Yong Chang

General Procedures	41
Nucleic Acids	42
Phospholipids	51
Conclusions and Summary	58
References	60
Discussion	61

Chemical Structure of Bone Sialoprotein and a Preliminary Study of Its Calcium-Binding Properties
G. M. Herring, A. T. deB. Andrews, and A. R. Chipperfield

Isolation of Bone Sialoprotein	64
Composition of BSP	65
Physical Properties of BSP	68
Binding of Radioelements to BSP	68
Calcium Binding and Inhibition of Calcium Phosphate Precipitation	69
Conclusion	70
References	71
Discussion	72

II. ROLE OF CALCIUM IN MEMBRANE STRUCTURE AND INTEGRITY

The Biionic Action Potential and Indispensability of Divalent Cations in the External Medium for Nerve Excitation
Akira Watanabe and Ichiji Tasaki

Introduction	77
Intracellular Perfusion of the Squid Giant Axon	78

Effects of Calcium Ions Inside the Axon	79
The Biionic Action Potential	80
Ionic Mechanism of Nerve Excitation	88
Change in the Hydrophobicity of the Membrane Macromolecules during Nerve Excitation	89
Conclusions	96
References	97
Discussion	98

The Calcium Homeostatic System as a Physiological Regulator of Cell Proliferation in Mammalian Tissues

A. D. Perris

Introduction	101
Basic Phenomena	102
Mechanism	103
Physiological Significance	105
Summary	118
References	124
Discussion	126

III. CALCIUM TRANSFER ACROSS CELL AND SUBCELLULAR MEMBRANES

A Calcium Pump in Red Cell Membranes

Frank F. Vincenzi

Text	135
References	146
Discussion	148

Calcium Transport in Kidney Cells and Its Regulation

André B. Borle

Calcium Pools	153
Calcium Fluxes	162
A Model for Cellular Calcium Metabolism	170
References	171
Discussion	171

Recent Observations on the Mechanism of Ca^{2+} Transport by Fragmented Sarcoplasmic Reticulum Membranes

A. Martonosi, A. G. Pucell, and R. A Halpin

Introduction	175
Role of Phospholipids in ATPase Activity and Calcium Transport	176
Protein Composition of Sarcoplasmic Reticulum Membranes	183
Isolation of a Phosphopeptide from Microsomal Membranes Labeled with AT^{32}P or Acetyl-^{32}P	188
References	191
Discussion	191

IV. CELL MECHANISMS IN MINERALIZED TISSUES

The Concept of a Bone Membrane: Some Implications

William F. Neuman and Warren K. Ramp

Text	197
References	206
Discussion	206

Bone Cells, Calcification, and Calcium Homeostasis

George Nichols, Jr., Peter Hirschmann, and Peggy Rogers

Text	211
References	235
Discussion	236

The Role of Mitochondria in Intracellular Calcium Regulation

J. L. Matthews, J. H. Martin, C. Arsenis, R. Eisenstein, and K. Kuettner

Experimental Protocol	240
Method	241
Results	243

Contents

Summary	249
References	251
Discussion	253

Bone Formation and Resorption by Osteocytes

D. Baylink and J. Wergedal

Introduction	257
Methods	258
Results	266
Discussion	282
Conclusions	285
References	285
Discussion	286

V. CALCIUM TRANSFER ACROSS EPITHELIAL TISSUES

Intestinal Calcium Absorption, Vitamin D, Adaptation, and the Calcium-Binding Protein

R. H. Wasserman, R. A. Corradino, A. N. Taylor, and R. L. Morrissey

A Dual Effect of Vitamin D?	294
Adaptation	298
Synthesis of CaBP in Organ Culture	305
Concluding Remarks	307
Summary	308
References	309
Discussion	310

Vagaries in the Use of Isolated Intestinal Mucosal Cell Preparations with Particular Emphasis on Calcium Uptake

Richard C. Bray and Irwin Clark

Introduction	313
Materials and Methods	317
Results	319
Summary and Conclusions	334
References	335
Discussion	335

Active Transport of Calcium across Placenta and Mammary Gland Measured *in Vivo*

D. S. Kronfeld, C. F. Ramberg, Jr., and Maria Delivoria-Papadopoulos

Introduction	339
Placental Calcium Transport	340
Mammary Calcium Transport	344
References	347
Discussion	348

Calcium Transfer across the Avian Shell Gland

Harald Schraer and Rosemary Schraer

Introduction	351
Anatomical Considerations	352
Autoradiographic Localization of Calcium	357
Calcium Transport Studies	358
Mitochondria and Metal Ion Translocation	363
References	368
Discussion	369

Active Transcellular Transport of Calcium by Embryonic Chick Chorioallantoic Membrane

A. Raymond Terepka, James R. Coleman, James C. Garrison, and Robert F. Spataro

Electron Probe Investigations	375
Oxygen Consumption and Active Calcium Transport	379
Sulfhydryl Groups and Calcium Transport	382
Concluding Remarks	385
References	386
Discussion	386

VI. SITES AND MODES OF ACTION OF HUMORAL FACTORS

Chemistry of Parathyroid Hormone

J. T. Potts, Jr., H. D. Niall, H. T. Keutmann, G. W. Tregear, R. Sauer, M. L. Hogan, B. Dawson, and G. D. Aurbach

Isolation	394
Sequence Analysis	395

Contents

Synthesis: Properties of the Synthetic Peptide	397
Conclusion	397
References	399
Discussion	399

Physiological Importance of Thyrocalcitonin

Paul L. Munson, Cary W. Cooper, T. Kenney Gray, James D. Hundley, and Ahmed M. Mahgoub

Text	403
References	416
Discussion	417

Metabolism and Mechanism of Action of 25-Hydroxycholecalciferol

H. F. DeLuca

Physiological Actions of Vitamin D	421
Metabolism of Vitamin D	423
Metabolism of 25-HCC	432
Mechanism of Action of Vitamin D	437
References	438
Discussion	439

Induction of Bone Resorption in Tissue Culture: Interaction of Humoral Agents and Ions

Lawrence G. Raisz and Clarence L. Trummel

Induction Model	442
Role of RNA Synthesis	443
Role of Cyclic Adenosine 3′,5′-Monophosphate (cAMP)	444
Synergism between PTH and 25-HCC	446
Effect of Thyrocalcitonin	447
Effect of Calcium on Induction	447
Conclusion	449
References	450
Discussion	451

ABSTRACTS OF SUBMITTED PAPERS

I. Calcification

Time Study of *in Vivo* Incorporation of ^{32}P-Orthophosphate into Phospholipids of Chicken Epiphyseal Tissues
    E. Eisenberg and R. Wuthier   457

Metabolic Activity at the Cement Line of Bone
    Josef Eschberger   458
Calcification of the Cartilage Formed on Avian Bones
    Brian K. Hall   458
Evidences of a Direct Effect of Vitamin D_3 or 25-Hydroxycholecalciferol upon Human Adult Bone Mineralization
    P. Bordier, L. Miravet, S. Tun Chot, and D. Hioco   459
Role of Protein–Polysaccharide Aggregates as a Biological Inhibitor of Mineral Growth
    David S. Howell, Julio C. Pita, Juan F. Madruga, and Francisco J. Muller   460
Calcification of Cartilage by Means of Mineralized Spherules
    Herbert K. Kashiwa   461
Decalcified Bone Implants under Hormonal Influence
    Erkki V. S. Koskinen, Soini A. Ryöppy, and T. Sam Lindholm   462
Mechanism of Calcification
    Fred Leonard, Clarence W. R. Wade, and Andrew F. Hegyeli   463
Biological Role of Heterologous Antibodies against Cartilage Protein Polysaccharide Complex Light Fraction (PP-L)
    Tawfik Y. Sabet and Charles E. Hawley   464
Isolation of Membrane-Bounded Extracellular Particles Associated with Calcification in Cartilage Matrix
    Stanley W. Sajdera, Margaret Whelan, H. Clarke Anderson, and S. Yousuf Ali   465
Electron Microscope Measurements of Alkaline Earth Transport
    Elizabeth Lloyd   466
Calcium Transport and Calcification Studies by Microperfusion
    Marshall R. Urist, H. Peter Meyer, and Karen S. Merickel   467

II. Calcitonin: Calcium Ion Activity and Pharmacological Action: Tooth Formation

^{47}Ca Turnover of a Readily Exchangeable Calcium Pool in Pregnant and Lactating Cows
    J. J. B. Anderson and W. C. Crackel   147
Metabolic Clearance Rate of Radioiodinated Human Calcitonin in Man
    Raymond Ardaillou, Pierre Sizonenko, Alain Meyrier, and Gabreil Vallèe   472
Extraosseous Actions of Calcitonin
    Gerard A. Charbon and Elisabeth E. M. Pieper   473
Crystal-Matrix Relationship in Amelogenesis
    Jay D. Decker   474

Contents

Different Isozymes of Acid Phosphatase in Bone and Developing Teeth
    Lars E. Hammarstrom, Jacob S. Hanker, and Svein U. Toverud   475

Provisional Calcification of Cartilage in Tissue Culture
    Uriel S. Barzel   476

Bone Cell Response to Serum Calcium-Altering Drugs
    Barbara G. Mills, P. Holst, A. Haroutinian, and L. A. Bavetta   476

Calcium Ion Activity in Plasma: Effects of Metabolic and Respiratory Acid-Base Changes
    I. C. Radde, B. Hoeffken, and D. K. Parkinson   477

A Calcium Concentration Dependent Hypocalcemic Effect of Calcitonin in the Perfused Dog Limb
    G. A. Rodan, U. A. Liberman, and M. Anbar   478

Natriuric Effect of Calcitonin in Man
    Olav Bijvoet and Jaap van der Sluys Veer   479

Remissions in Paget's Disease Produced by Human Synthetic Calcitonin (Calcitonin M)
    N. J. Y. Woodhouse, M. Reiner, D. N. Kalu, L. Galante, G. F. Joplin, and I. MacIntyre   480

Relationship between Alkaline Phosphatase, Inorganic Pyrophosphatase, and L-Ascorbic Acid in Calcifying Hamster Molars
    J. H. M. Wöllgens, S. L. Bonting, and Olav Bijvoet   481

III. Diphosphonates; Bone Resorption; Osteoporosis

Mechanical Effects on Cell Mechanisms in Bone
    Göran C. H. Bauer and Tomihisa Koshino   485

Canalicular and Interstitial Changes in Osteocytic Osteolysis
    Leonard F. Bélanger, S. S. Jande, and J. D. Cipera   486

Effect of Calcium Deficiency on Healing of Experimental Fractures in the Avian Tarsus as Determined by the Fracture Repair Ratio
    John R. Beljan   487

Effect of Phosphonates on Bone Tissue: Studies in Man and Animals
    M. E. Cabanela and J. Jowsey   488

Sites and Modes of an Estrogen–Gestagen Combination on Calcium and Phosphate Metabolism in Senile Osteoporosis
    Angelo Caniggia and Carlo Gennari   489

Resorption of Bone Collagen by Multinucleated Giant Cells
    James T. Irving and John D. Heeley   490

Effect of Disodium Ethane-1-hydroxy-1,1-diphosphonate on Bone Formation in Animals
    W. R. King, M. D. Francis, and W. R. Michael   491

Effectiveness of Diphosphonates in Preventing Osteoporosis of Disuse in the Rat
    W. R. Michael, W. R. King, and M. D. Francis   492

Osteoporosis and Parathyroid Glands: The Effect of Prolonged Calcium Deficiency on Thyroparathyroidectomized Adult Rats
    J. A. Sevastikoglou   493

Role of a Lipoprotein in the Intracellular Hydroxyapatite Formation in *Bacterionema Matruchotii*
    J. J. Vogel and J. Ennever   494

Hormonal Effects on Calcium Transport in Liver
    S. Wallach, A. B. Chausmer, and B. S. Sherman   494

IV. Intestinal Absorption of Calcium and Bone Metabolism

Osteocyte as a Bone Pump
    James S. Arnold and Harold M. Frost   499

25-Hydroxycholecalciferol (25-HCC): Effects in Deficiency Rickets and Vitamin D-Resistant Rickets
    Sonia Balsan   500

Induction of Calcium-Binding Protein (CaBP) Biosynthesis by Vitamin D_3 and 25-Hydroxycholecalciferol (25-HCC)
    Ronal R. MacGregor, David V. Cohn, and James W. Hamilton   501

Effect of Cortisol on Calcium-Binding Protein in Rat Duodenum
    G. Eilon, E. Mor, H. Karaman, and J. Menczel   501

A Study of Nephron Permeability to Calcium by Microinjection Technique
    M. Gagnan-Brunette and M. Aras   502

A Study of Calcium-Binding Proteins in Human Animal Small Bowel Mucosa
    A. J. W. Hitchman, J. M. Finlay, and Joan E. Harrison   503

A Method for Studying the Configuration, Dimensions, and Distribution of Remodeling Centers on the Endosteal, Cortical, and Trabecular Surfaces
    Z. F. Jaworski and H. M. Frost   504

Transport of Iodoantipyrine-^{125}I (I-Ap) In Cortical Bone
    P. J. Kelly, Tada Yipintsoi, and James B. Bassingthwaighte   505

Ca^{2+} Sensitive ATPase In Duodenal Mucosa: Localization in Basal Membranes
    D. K. Parkinson and I. C. Radde   506

Refractive Index of Newly Forming Bone Tissue
    W. L. Past   506

Bovine Serum Albumin (BSA) Calcium-Binding Studies with a Calcium-Selective Liquid Membrane Electrode
    C. E. Sachs and A. M. Bourdeau   507

Contents

Passage of Calcium and Strontium across the Intestine in Man
    Herta Spencer, Janet Warren, and Joseph Samachson   508

Concept of Electropositive Crystal Bond Based on Ossification and Other Phenomena
    Tomasz Cieszyński   509

SUBJECT INDEX   511

LIST OF CONTRIBUTORS

Numbers in parentheses indicate the pages on which the authors' contributions begin.

S. YOUSUF ALI (465), *The Institute of Orthopaedics, University of London, London, England*

M. ANBAR (478), *Stanford Research Institute, Palo Alto, California*

H. CLARKE ANDERSON (465), *The Rockefeller University, New York, New York*

J. J. B. ANDERSON (471), *College of Veterinary Medicine, University of Illinois, Urbana, Illinois*

M. ARAS (502), *Maisonneuve Hospital, University of Montreal, Montreal, Canada*

RAYMOND ARDAILLOU (472), *Groupe de Recherches de Nephrologie Normale, et Pathologique de l'I.N.S.E.R.M., Hôpital Tenon, Paris, France*

JAMES S. ARNOLD (499), *University of Missouri Medical Center, Kansas City, Missouri*

C. ARSENIS (239), *Department of Microscopic Anatomy, Baylor University, College of Dentistry, Dallas, Texas*

G. D. AURBACH (393), *Section on Mineral Metabolism, National Institute of Arthritis and Metabolic Diseases, National Institutes of Health, Bethesda, Maryland*

SONIA BALSAN (500), *Centre d'Etudes des Maladies du Métabolisme de l'Enfant, Hôpital des Enfants-Malades, Paris, France*

URIEL S. BARZEL (476), *Montefiore Hospital and Medical Center, Metabolic Endocrine Laboratory, Bronx, New York*

JAMES B. BASSINGTHWAIGHTE (505), *Department of Orthopedic Surgery, Mayo Clinic, Rochester, Minnesota*

GÖRAN C. H. BAUER (485), *Department of Orthopaedic Surgery, Lund University Hospital, Lund, Sweden*

L. A. BAVETTA (476), *Department of Biochemistry, School of Dentistry, University of Southern California, Los Angeles, California*

D. BAYLINK (257), *Veterans Administration Hospital, Seattle, Washington*

LEONARD F. BÉLANGER (486), *University of Ottawa, Ottawa, Canada*

JOHN R. BELJAN (487), *Bioastronautics Laboratory, School of Medicine, University of California, Davis, California*

OLAV BIJVOET (479, 481), *Department of Biochemistry and Internal Medicine, University of Nijmegen, Nijmegen, Netherlands*

S. L. BONTING (481), *Department of Biochemistry and Internal Medicine, University of Nijmegen, Nijmegen, Netherlands*

P. BORDIER (459), *Unité de Recherche sur le Métabolisme Phospho-Calcique, Hôpital Lariboisière, Paris, France*

ANDRÉ B. BORLE (151), *Department of Physiology, University of Pittsburgh School of Medicine, Pittsburgh, Pennsylvania*

A. M. BOURDEAU (507), *Centre d'Etudes des Maldies du Métabolisme de l'Enfant, Hôpital des Enfants-Malades, Paris, France*

RICHARD C. BRAY (313), *Departments of Orthopedic Surgery and Biochemistry, College of Physicians and Surgeons, Columbia University, New York, New York*

M. E. CABANELA (488), *Department of Orthopedic Research, Mayo Clinic, Rochester, Minnesota*

ANGELO CANIGGIA (489), *Istituto di Semeiotica Medica, Dell'Universita di Siena, Italy*

CHARLES W. CARR (41), *Department of Biochemistry, University of Minnesota, Minneapolis, Minnesota*

KIM YONG CHANG (41), *Departments of Pharmacology and Therapeutics, McGill University, Montreal, Quebec, Canada*

GERARD A. CHARBON (473), *Department of Cardiovascular Surgery, Rudolf Magnus Institute for Pharmacology, University of Utrecht, Utrecht, The Netherlands*

A. B. CHAUSMER (494), *State University of New York, Downstate Medical Center, Brooklyn, New York*

A. R. CHIPPERFIELD[1] (63), *Department of Biophysics, Institute of Cancer Research, Sutton, Surrey, England*

S. TUN CHOT (459), *Unité de Recherche sur le Métabolisme Phospho-Calcique, Hôpital Lariboisière, Paris, France*

TOMASZ CIESZYŃSKI (509), *Second Surgical Clinic of the Medical Academy in Wroclaw, Wroclaw, Poland*

J. D. CIPERA (486), *Animal Research Institute, Canada Department of Agriculture, Ottawa, Canada*

IRWIN CLARK[2] (313), *Departments of Orthopedic Surgery and Biochemistry, College of Physicians and Surgeons, Columbia University, New York, New York*

DAVID V. COHN (501), *Calcium Research Laboratory, Veterans Administration Hospital, Kansas City, Missouri*

JAMES R. COLEMAN (371), *Department of Radiation Biology and Biophysics, University of Rochester, School of Medicine and Dentistry, Rochester, New York*

---

[1] Present address: Department of Physiology, The University, Leicester, England
[2] Present address: Department of Orthopaedic Surgery and Biochemistry, University of North Carolina, School of Medicine, Chapel Hill, North Carolina

List of Contributors

CARY W. COOPER (403), *Department of Pharmacology, School of Medicine, University of North Carolina, Chapel Hill, North Carolina*

R. A. CORRADINO (293), *Department of Physical Biology, New York State Veterinary College, Cornell University, Ithaca, New York*

W. C. CRACKEL (471), *College of Veterinary Medicine, University of Illinois, Urbana, Illinois*

B. DAWSON (393), *Endocrine Unit, Department of Medicine, Massachusetts General Hospital, Boston, Massachusetts*

A. T. DEB. ANDREWS[3] (63), *Medical Research Council, External Scientific Staff, Bone Research Laboratory, Churchill Hospital, Headington, Oxford, England*

JAY D. DECKER (474), *Department of Orthodontics, University of Washington, Seattle, Washington*

MARIA DELIVORIA-PAPADOPOULOS (339), *Department of Clinical Studies, School of Veterinary Medicine and Department of Physiology, School of Medicine, University of Pennsylvania, Philadelphia, Pennsylvania*

H. F. DELUCA (421), *Department of Biochemistry, University of Wisconsin, Madison, Wisconsin*

G. EILON (501), *Department of Medicine, Shaare Zedek Hospital, Jerusalem, Israel*

E. EISENBERG (457), *University of California Service, San Francisco General Hospital, San Francisco, California*

R. EISENSTEIN (239), *Department of Microscopic Anatomy, Baylor University, Dallas, Texas*

J. ENNEVER (494), *University of Texas, Houston, Texas*

JOSEF ESCHBERGER (458), *Facharzt für Unfallchirurgie, Kuirinagasse, Vienna, Austria*

J. M. FINLAY (503), *Department of Medicine, University of Toronto, Toronto, Canada*

M. D. FRANCIS (491, 492), *The Procter and Gamble Company, Miami Valley Laboratories, Cincinnati, Ohio*

HAROLD M. FROST (499, 504), *Department of Orthopaedic Surgery, Henry Ford Hospital, Detroit, Michigan*

M. GAGNAN-BRUNETTE (502), *Maisonneuve Hospital, University of Montreal, Montreal, Quebec, Canada*

L. GALANTE (480), *Wellcome Unit of Endocrinology, Royal Postgraduate Medical School, Ducane Road, London, England*

JAMES C. GARRISON (371), *Department of Radiation Biology and Biophysics, University of Rochester, School of Medicine and Dentistry, Rochester, New York*

CARLO GENNARI (489), *Istituto di Semeiotica Medica, Dell'Universita di Siena, Italy*

T. KENNEY GRAY (403), *Department of Pharmacology, School of Medicine, University of North Carolina, Chapel Hill, North Carolina*

BRIAN K. HALL (458), *Department of Biology, Dalhousie University, Halifax, Nova Scotia, Canada*

R. A. HALPIN (175), *Department of Biochemistry, St. Louis University School of Medicine, St. Louis, Missouri*

[3] Present address: National Institute for Research in Dairying, Shinfield, Reading Berkshire, England

List of Contributors

James W. Hamilton (501), *Calcium Research Laboratory, Veterans Administration Hospital, Kansas City, Missouri*

Lars E. Hammarstrom[4] (475), *Dental Research Center, University of North Carolina, Chapel Hill, North Carolina*

Jacob S. Hanker (475), *Dental Research Center, University of North Carolina, Chapel Hill, North Carolina*

A. Haroutinian (476), *Department of Dental Biochemistry, University of Southern California, Los Angeles, California*

Joan E. Harrison (503), *Department of Medicine, University of Toronto, Toronto, Canada*

Charles E. Hawley (464), *University of Illinois College of Dentistry, Chicago, Illinois*

John D. Heeley (490), *Forsyth Dental Center, Boston, Massachusetts*

Andrew F. Hegyeli (463), *U. S. Army Medical Biomechanical Research Laboratory, Walter Reed Army Medical Center, Washington, D.C.*

G. M. Herring (63), *Medical Research Council External Scientific Staff, Bone Research Laboratory, Churchill Hospital, Headington Oxford, England*

D. Hioco (459), *Unité de Recherche sur le Metabolisme Phospho-Calcique Hôpital Lariboisiere, Paris, France*

Peter Hirschmann[5] (211), *Cancer Research Institute, New England Deaconess Hospital, Boston, Massachusetts*

A. J. W. Hitchman (503), *Department of Medicine, University of Toronto, Toronto, Canada*

B. Hoeffken (477), *Research Institute, Hospital Sick Children, Toronto, Canada*

M. L. Hogan (393), *Endocrine Unit, Department of Medicine, Massachusetts General Hospital, Boston, Massachusetts*

P. Holst (476), *University of Southern California, Department of Biochemistry, Los Angeles, California*

David S. Howell (460), *University of Miami School of Medicine, Miami, Florida*

James D. Hundley (403), *Department of Pharmacology, School of Medicine, University of North Carolina, Chapel Hill, North Carolina*

James T. Irving (490), *Forsyth Dental Center, Boston, Massachusetts*

S. S. Jande (486), *University of Ottawa, Ottawa, Canada*

Z. F. Jaworski (504), *Department of Medicine, Ottawa General Hospital, University of Ottawa, Ottawa, Canada*

G. F. Joplin (480), *Wellcome Unit of Endocrinology, Royal Postgraduate Medical School, Ducane Road, London*

J. Jowsey (488), *Department of Orthopedic Research, Mayo Clinic, Rochester, Minnesota*

D. N. Kalu (480), *Wellcome Unit of Endocrinology, Royal Postgraduate Medical School, Duncane Road, London, England*

H. Karaman (501), *Department of Medicine, Shaare Zedek Hospital, Jerusalem, Israel*

Herbert K. Kashiwa (461), *University of Washington School of Medicine, Seattle, Washington*

P. J. Kelly (505), *Department of Orthopedic Surgery, Mayo Clinic, Rochester, Minnesota*

[4] Present address: Department of Oral Histopathology, Faculty of Dentistry, Karolinska Institutet, Stockholm, Sweden

[5] Present address: University of Manchester, Turner Dental School, Manchester, England

List of Contributors

H. T. KEUTMANN (393), *Endocrine Unit, Department of Medicine, Massachusetts General Hospital, Boston, Massachusetts*

W. R. KING (491, 492), *The Procter and Gamble Company, Miami Valley Laboratories, Cincinnati, Ohio*

TOMIHISA KOSHINO (485), *Hospital for Special Surgery, New York, New York*

ERKKI V. S. KOSKINEN (462), *Clinic for Orthopaedics and Traumatology, University of Helsinki, Helsinki, Finland*

D. S. KRONFELD (339), *Department of Clinical Studies, School of Veterinary Medicine and Department of Physiology, School of Medicine, University of Pennsylvania, Philadelphia, Pennsylvania*

K. KUETTNER (239), *Department of Microscopic Anatomy, Baylor University, Dallas, Texas*

FRED LEONARD (463), *U. S. Army Medical Biomechanical Research Laboratory, Walter Reed Army Medical Center, Washington, D.C.*

U. A. LIBERMAN (478), *Beilinson Hospital, Petah Tikwa, Israel*

T. SAM LINDHOLM[6] (462), *The Orthopaedic Hospital of the Invalid Foundation, Helsinki, Finland*

ELIZABETH LLOYD (466), *U.S. Atomic Commission, Radiological Physics Division, Argonne National Laboratory, Argonne, Illinois*

RONAL R. MACGREGOR (501), *Calcium Research Laboratory, Veterans Administration Hospital, Kansas City, Missouri*

I. MACINTYRE (480), *Wellcome Unit of Endocrinology, Royal Postgraduate Medical School, London, England*

JUAN F. MADRUGA (460), *University of Miami, School of Medicine, Miami, Florida*

AHMED M. MAHGOUB (403), *Department of Pharmacology, School of Medicine, University of North Carolina, Chapel Hill, North Carolina*

J. H. MARTIN (239), *Department of Microscopic Anatomy, Baylor University, College of Dentistry, Dallas, Texas*

A. MARTONOSI (175), *Department of Biochemistry, St. Louis University School of Medicine, St. Louis, Missouri*

J. L. MATTHEWS (239), *Department of Microscopic Anatomy, Baylor University, College of Dentistry, Dallas, Texas*

J. MENCZEL (501), *Department of Medicine, Shaare Zedek Hospital, Jerusalem, Israel*

KAREN S. MERICKEL (467), *UCLA Bone Research Laboratory, Los Angeles, California*

H. PETER MEYER (467), *UCLA Bone Research Laboratory, Los Angeles, California*

ALAIN MEYRIER (472), *Groupe de Recherches de Nephrologie Normale, et Pathologique de l'I.N.S.E.R.M., Hôpital Tenon, Paris, France*

W. R. MICHAEL (491, 492), *The Procter and Gamble Company, Miami Valley Laboratories, Cincinnati, Ohio*

BARBARA G. MILLS (476), *Department of Dental Biochemistry, University of Southern California, Los Angeles, California*

L. MIRAVET (459), *Unité de Recherche sur le Métabolisme Phospho-Calcique, Hôpital Lariboisiére, Paris, France*

E. MOR (501), *Department of Medicine, Shaare Zedek Hospital, Jerusalem, Israel*

R. L. MORRISSEY (293), *Department of Physical Biology, New York State Veterinary College, Cornell University, Ithaca, New York*

[6] Present address: The Orthopaedic Hospital of the Invalid Foundation, Tenalav/gen 10, Helsingfors 28, Finland

FRANCISCO J. MULLER (460), *University of Miami School of Medicine, Miami, Florida*

PAUL L. MUNSON (403), *Department of Pharmacology, School of Medicine, University of North Carolina, Chapel Hill, North Carolina*

WILLIAM F. NEUMAN (197), *Department of Radiation Biology and Biophysics, School of Medicine and Dentistry, University of Rochester, Rochester, New York*

H. D. NIALL (393), *Endocrine Unit, Department of Medicine, Massachusetts General Hospital, Boston, Massachusetts*

GEORGE NICHOLS, JR. (211), *Cancer Research Institute, New England Deaconess Hospital, Boston, Massachusetts*

D. K. PARKINSON (477, 506), *Research Institute, Hospital Sick Children, Toronto, Canada*

W. L. PAST (506), *Department of Pathology, University of Louisville School of Medicine, Louisville, Kentucky*

A. D. PERRIS[7] (101), *Division of Biology, National Research Council of Canada, Ottawa, Canada*

ELISABETH E. M. PIEPER (473), *Department of Cardiovascular Surgery and Rudolf Magnus Institute of Pharmacology, University of Utrecht, Utrecht, The Netherlands*

JULIO C. PITA (460), *University of Miami School of Medicine, Miami, Florida*

AARON S. POSNER (3), *Hospital for Special Surgery, Cornell University Medical College, New York, New York*

J. T. POTTS, JR., (393), *Endocrine Unit, Department of Medicine, Massachusetts General Hospital, Boston, Massachusetts*

A. G. PUCELL (175), *Department of Biochemistry, St. Louis University School of Medicine, St. Louis, Missouri*

I. C. RADDE (477, 506), *Research Institute, Hospital for Sick Children, Toronto, Canada*

LAWRENCE G. RAISZ (441), *Department of Pharmacology and Toxicology, Medicine and Dentistry and Dental Research, University of Rochester, School of Medicine and Dentistry, Rochester, New York*

C. F. RAMBERG, JR., (339), *Department of Clinical Studies, School of Veterinary Medicine and Department of Physiology, School of Medicine, University of Pennsylvania, Philadelphia, Pennsylvania*

WARREN K. RAMP (197), *Department of Radiation Biology and Dentistry, University of Rochester, Rochester, New York*

M. REINER (480), *Wellcome Unit of Endocrinology, Royal Postgraduate Medical School, Ducane Road, London, England*

LEON J. RICHELLE (25), *School of Dental Medicine and Institute of Materials Science, University of Connecticut, Storrs, Connecticut*

G. A. RODAN (478), *Weizmann Institute of Science, Rehovot, Israel*

PEGGY ROGERS (211), *Cancer Research Institute, New England Deaconess Hospital, Boston, Massachusetts*

SOINI A. RYÖPPY[8] (462), *Department of Orthopaedies and Traumatology, University Central Hospital, Helsinki, Finland*

TAWFIK Y. SABET (464), *Department of Histology, University of Illinois at the Medical Center, Chicago, Illinois*

[7] Present address: Department of Biological Sciences, The University of Aston in Birmingham, Birmingham, England
[8] Present address: Uudenmaank 14C, Helsinki, Finland

List of Contributors

C. E. Sachs (507), *Centre d'Etudes des Maladies du Métabolisme de l'Enfant, Hôpital des Enfants-Malades, Paris, France*

Stanley W. Sajdera (465), *State University of New York, Downstate Medical Center, Brooklyn, New York*

Joseph Samachson (508), *Metabolic Section, Veterans Administration Hospital, Hines, Illinois*

R. Sauer (393), *Endocrine Unit, Department of Medicine, Massachusetts General Hospital, Boston, Massachusetts*

Harald Schraer (351), *Department of Biochemistry, The Pennsylvania State University, University Park, Pennsylvania*

Rosemary Schraer (351), *Department of Biochemistry, The Pennsylvania State University, University Park, Pennsylvania*

J. A. Sevastikoglou (493), *Umea University, Umea, Sweden*

B. S. Sherman (494), *State University of New York, Downstate Medical Center, Brooklyn, New York*

Pierre Sizonenko (472), *Clinique Universitaire de Pédiatrie, Hôpital Cantonal, Geneva, Switzerland*

Robert F. Spataro (371), *Department of Radiation Biology and Biophysics, University of Rochester, School of Medicine and Dentistry, Rochester, New York*

Herta Spencer (508), *Metabolic Section, Veterans Administration Hospital, Hines, Illinois*

Ichiji Tasaki (77), *Laboratory of Neurobiology, National Institute of Mental Health, Bethesda, Maryland*

A. N. Taylor (293), *Department of Physical Biology, New York State Veterinary College, Cornell University, Ithaca, New York*

A. Raymond Terepka (371), *Department of Radiation Biology and Biophysics, University of Rochester School of Medicine and Dentistry, Rochester, New York*

Svein U. Toverud (475), *Dental Research Center, University of North Carolina, Chapel Hill, North Carolina*

G. W. Tregear (393), *Endocrine Unit, Department of Medicine, Massachusetts General Hospital, Boston, Massachusetts*

Clarence L. Trummel (441), *Department of Pharmacology and Toxicology, Medicine and Dentistry and Dental Research, University of Rochester School of Medicine and Dentistry, Rochester, New York*

Marshall R. Uriet (467), *UCLA Bone Research Laboratory, Los Angeles, California*

Gabreil Vallèe (472), *Laboratoire des Isotopes, Hôpital Necker, Paris, France*

Jaap van der Sluys Veer (479), *University Hospital, Leiden, The Netherlands*

Frank F. Vincenzi (135), *Department of Pharmacology, School of Medicine, University of Washington, Seattle, Washington*

J. J. Vogel (494), *University of Texas, Houston, Texas*

Clarence W. R. Wade (463), *U. S. Army Medical Biomechanical Research Laboratory, Walter Reed Army Medical Center, Washington, D.C.*

S. Wallach (494), *State University of New York, Downstate Medical Center, Brooklyn, New York*

JANET WARREN[9] (508), *Metabolic Section, Veterans Administration Hospital, Hines, Illinois*

R. H. WASSERMAN (293), *Department of Physical Biology, New York State Veterinary College, Cornell University, Ithaca, New York*

AKIRA WATANABE (77), *Laboratory of Neurobiology, National Institute of Mental Health, Bethesda, Maryland*

J. WERGEDAL (257), *University of Washington School of Medicine, Veterans Administration Hospital, Seattle, Washington*

MARGARET WHELAN (465), *State University of New York, Downstate Medical Center, Brooklyn, New York*

J. H. M. WÖLTGENS (481), *Department of Biochemistry and Internal Medicine, University of Nijmegen, Nijmegen, The Netherlands*

N. J. Y. WOODHOUSE (480), *Wellcome Unit of Endocrinology, Royal Postgraduate Medical School, Ducane Road, London, England*

R. WUTHIER (457), *Department of Orthopaedic Surgery, University of Vermont School of Medicine, Burlington, Vermont*

TADA YIPINTSOI (505), *Department of Orthopedic Surgery, Mayo Clinic, Rochester, Minnesota*

[9] Present address: Regional Department of Clinical Physics and Bio-Engineering, Glasgow, Scotland

PREFACE

Several factors led to the organization of the Workshop Conference on Cell Mechanisms for Calcium Transfer and Homeostasis held at Wentworth-by-the-Sea in Portsmouth, New Hampshire, September 13–16, 1970, the proceedings of which are reported in this volume. Extensive recent progress in understanding the critical role of calcium in the structure and function of a wide variety of biological systems, in delineating the mechanisms of transport of calcium across cells and cellular membranes, and in elucidating the role of cells in the deposition and removal of calcium salts in calcified tissues had not been covered systematically since 1962, and the assembling of individuals responsible for many of these advances was deemed to be long overdue. As well as permanently recording the newer data and views of these workers, this book, by reporting the discussion which followed each contribution, indicates the current views of other representatives of the many disciplines now involved in studies in which calcium plays a central role. The exchange of points of view which these discussions reflect help to pinpoint unsolved problems, specific aspects wherein conceptual differences lie, and areas for future investigation.

This type of conference, in a prior year, would have found Dr. Franklin C. McLean (1888–1968) among the conferees, and all would have benefitted from his presence. It was fitting, then, that a further reason for this volume and the Conference was to commemorate Dr. McLean who, through his original research, personal encouragement of others, extensive writing, and capacity to grasp and interpret new facts and ideas, represented a dynamic force in inspiring excellence in this field.

The contents of this volume reflect the ubiquity of the involvement of calcium in the structure and function of biological systems and present a number of new ideas about calcium metabolism and its control. The contributions have been grouped in successive sections, each bearing upon a specific area. These have been arranged to progress from fundamental physicochemical aspects through influences of calcium on membrane structure and function, to studies of calcium transfer across subcellular membranes, across cells of mineralizing and nonmineralizing tissues, and across epithelial membranes, such as intestine and placenta. Control of these mechanisms by humoral factors is discussed only in the final section, reflecting an emphasis on calcium metabolism per se in contradistinction to other recent symposia focused on the calcium-regulating hormones. The discussion recorded after each formal presentation has been included as nearly verbatim as possible after each chapter.

In addition to the formal presentations, four sessions of the conference were devoted to a series of submitted scientific papers of shorter length. This part of the program was developed to reflect Franklin McLean's deep interest in newly launched investigations and investigators. Although space precludes the publication in this volume of the texts of these short talks *in extenso* or the discussion which they evoked, short abstracts of the forty-eight papers presented under the headings beneath which they appeared in the program have been assembled in the latter part of this book.

A number of new concepts and ideas are recorded here and many older notions are enlarged and strengthened. These include the suggestion of major roles for calcium not only as a component of bone mineral, but in the control of cell replication and growth, the structural organization of the nerve cell membrane and, through it, in the initiation and propagation of the nerve impulse. New data regarding calcium transport across cellular and subcellular membranes are presented which indicate that a transport mechanism aimed at the active extrusion of calcium from the intracellular compartment may be present in all cells. Recent concepts regarding the involvement of cells and cellular mechanisms in the deposition and removal of calcium stores in mineralizing tissues are strengthened with new data by several contributors, and exciting new evidence regarding the ways in which calcium is translocated across several cellular epithelial structures including the gut, the avian shell gland, and the chorioallantoic membrane of the chick is revealed for the first time. In addition, important information regarding new developments in the fields of parathyroid hormone and vitamin D chemistry and the modes of action of both these agents and calcitonin in the control of calcium metabolism discussed in the final conference session are included. Thus, the contents of this volume will be of interest to workers in many fields of biology and medicine whose investigations may lead them, perhaps unexpectedly, to the necessity of considering the role of calcium or some other divalent cation in the organization of the system which they are studying.

G. NICHOLS, JR.
R. H. WASSERMAN

CREDITS

Many deserve credit for this book. Especially valuable were the contributions to the conference of the members of the secretariat, especially Miss Barbara Deisroth and Mrs. Dorothy Werner. The encouragement and advice of Dr. Pacita Pronove, Executive Secretary, General Medicine B Study Section, proved invaluable. Special appreciation is due to the Chairmen of the various sessions, Drs. Wallace D. Armstrong, Cyril L. Comar, D. Harold Copp, Paul Goldhaber, Harold E. Harrison, Gerald Mechanic, William F. Neuman, Robert E. Rowland, Roy V. Talmage, and Marshall R. Urist, whose brief introductions to the topics to be covered and skillful management of the discussion were so important to the smooth running of the proceedings.

Thanks are due also to Miss Shirley Graham and Mrs. Santina Turner of Boston and Mrs. Norma Jayne and Mrs. Janetta McCoy of Ithaca for their secretarial and technical assistance in preparing manuscripts and discussion for the publisher and to Mr. Stanley Rudbarg, Academic and Scientific Reporting Co., who capably recorded the conference discussions. We are especially grateful to our fellow members of the organizing committee, Drs. Paul L. Munson, Paul Goldhaber, and Marshall R. Urist, without whose contributions the conference and this book could not have materialized. We owe special thanks to Dr. Urist for his untiring efforts in the collection, selection, and arrangement of the submitted scientific papers.

Finally, we wish to express for the committee our thanks to the speakers for the excellent quality of their presentations and to all the participants for their spirited discussion of the formal contributions, both of which contributed so importantly to the success of this entire venture.

ACKNOWLEDGMENTS

The generous financial support of the following which made both this volume and the Conference possible is gratefully acknowledged:

The National Institutes of Health General Medicine B Study Section
The National Institutes of Health Dental Study Section
The United States Atomic Energy Commission
The Easter Seal Foundation

FRANKLIN CHAMBERS McLEAN AND THE STATE OF CALCIUM IN BODY FLUIDS

"Cellular Mechanisms for Calcium Transfer and Homeostasis" is indeed a comprehensive title for this work. The important words in our title are calcium and cells. If we can understand them, I have no fear for mechanisms, transfer, or homeostasis.

Just how did so many of us in this century derive pleasure and puzzlement through asking the question: "What is the state of calcium in biological fluids?" In my case, I did so on three different occasions for three entirely different reasons. The first time was in 1919 when Henry Alexander Murray enlisted my interest in following the serum calcium of dogs after removal of their parathyroids; the second time was in 1924 when C.D. Murray (Harry's younger brother) got Sendroy and myself to tackle the question of how much of serum calcium is ionic by studying equilibria between serum and bone salts; the third time was in the early thirties with Franklin McLean. The story of how this came about will comprise the bulk of what I shall subsequently say.

The ramifications of calcium and its many roles in the body's economy is to be the subject of this book. It all seemed so simple and straightforward fifty years ago. In our naivete, all we needed, we thought, were accurate analytical methods and the sound application of established

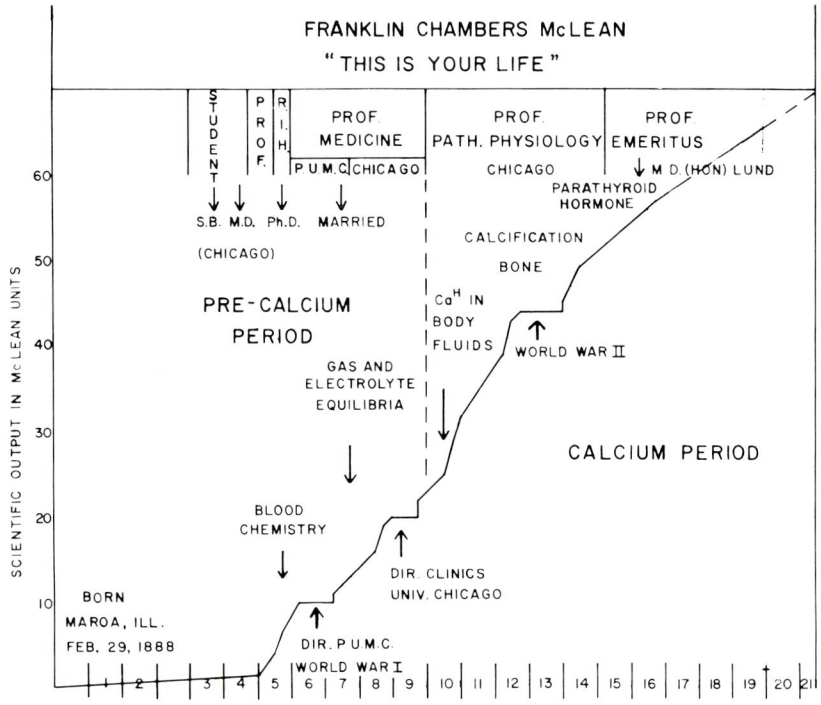

Fig. 1. Modified from figure on page 5 of "The Parathyroids" (Hastings, 1961).

physicochemical laws to describe the biological behavior of calcium. Little did we think that our calcium problems instead of being solved would be multiplied in number and in complexity. And the kindest wish I can have for you who are beginning your own half century with calcium is that a complete understanding of the roles of this ancient element will be as elusive to you as it has been to me.

I shall now discuss calcium ions and Franklin McLean, as I remember them.

To begin with, I can do no better than refer to the lifeline of Franklin McLean which I prepared ten years ago on the occasion of a Symposium on Parathyroid Research Trends (Hastings, 1961). To our sorrow, this lifeline has now been terminated. Those of you who have seen it before will recall that he had the good fortune to have been born on February 29, so that his birthdays were less than one-fourth those of yours and mine. That he was precocious is attested by his having received his M.D. at 22 and a professorship of pharmacology at 23. That he was wise is evidenced by his restarting his career as a resident at the hospital of the Rockefeller Institute at 26. That he was productive is evidenced by the line of his cumulative publications, which plateaued only during war times, and his administrative periods. However, he had a hard time continuing as a scientist because his talents included a flair for administration which received early recognition. He was appointed Director of the newly formed Peiping Union Medical College at 28, where he stayed until 1923 when he went to the University of Chicago as Professor of Medicine at 35, and subsequently served as Director of University Clinics.

What is remarkable to me is that in spite of these administrative interruptions in his life he continued to produce significant scientific work—first in biochemical methodology and its application to clinical problems and then with L. J. Henderson and D. D. Van Slyke and their colleagues on the study of blood as a physicochemical system.

How calcium and bone physiology became his primary concern beginning at age 43 occurred while I was at the University of Chicago. It is a good example of what a deciding role serendipity can play.

But before I relate these events, let me recall some of our uncertainties about the state of calcium in body fluids in the early thirties. As early as 1913, Rona and Takahashi had proposed that nondiffusible calcium of blood serum was combined with serum proteins. In 1923, Salvesen and Linder (1923–1924) obtained evidence substantiating this conclusion. In 1926, Marrack and Thacker, in an extensive and thorough paper entitled "The State of Calcium in Body Fluids," showed that serum calcium is present partially in combination with serum proteins and partially as diffusible calcium, which they assumed to be calcium ions.

As it turned out, they were approximately correct, but at the time there was grave question as to whether all diffusible calcium was ionic or not. Several investigators, including those in our laboratory, had tried to measure calcium ion activities in body fluids directly. Methods such as calcium–amalgam electrodes, zinc second-order electrodes, the solubility of difficultly soluble calcium salts, and the minimum oxalate required for calcium oxalate precipitation were employed. They pointed to some nonionic, diffusible calcium of varying amount, but the results were inconsistent or, in retrospect, invalid. At all events, there was a feeling at the time that only a portion of diffusible calcium was ionic and the rest was in combination with some diffusible anion such as citrate, which combined reversibly with calcium. This also turned out to be true, but to only about 10% of the ionic calcium.

So much for the background of the state of calcium in biological fluids in the 1930's and McLean's entry into the subject.

Franklin and I had become acquainted through Donald Van Slyke at the hospital of the Rockefeller Institute, and I had joined him at the University of Chicago in the Fall of 1926 as a Professor of Physiological Chemistry. He was then Professor of Medicine. In 1928 he engineered my transfer to the Department of Medicine where I would engage in fulltime research on degenerative diseases under the newly established Lasker Foundation for Medical Research at the University of Chicago and occupy the laboratory suite originally designed for him.

In 1928, Franklin had become Director of University Clinics. As an administrator Franklin was as effective and efficient as he was a scientist. For him to recognize that some action needed to be taken was for him to take it at once, and explain later. Most people in academic circles are not accustomed to being deprived of the time-consuming custom of lengthy committee meetings, and the Chicago medical faculty was no exception. Thus, Franklin's habit of immediate action created problems for him.

Since I was a Ph.D. and not dependent on department funds, I was a friend of all factions, and became aware of Franklin's precarious situation as an administrator before he did. This led me to want to help this good friend for whom I had great admiration and affection. My solution was to get him out from behind his Director's desk and into the laboratory where decisions are not made by committees.

To do this I enlisted the assistance of Dr. Lillian Eichelberger, with whom I was working on muscle electrolytes and edema. It occurred to me that we might study this subject in the perfused rabbit heart, *in vitro*; but to do this, we needed to set up a heart perfusion system according to Loewi. We set up our apparatus as far as we could alone and then I went into Franklin's office and said: "Franklin, you once worked in Otto Loewi's lab. Won't you please come out in the lab and help Lil and me set up a heart perfusion apparatus so that we can get on with our study of edema." With that he followed me, I helped him into a lab coat, and he, figuratively speaking, never took it off again. That was in 1932.

We soon found that the Loewi closed system perfusion method which recirculated the fluid was not going to meet our purposes, so we undertook to continuously perfuse rabbit hearts through their coronaries without recirculation of the perfusion fluids and record their mechanical work and electrocardiograms. Our immediate objective was to find the optimal ionic perfusion fluid. This was all carried out in a 38° constant temperature room that adjoined my laboratory in the Department of Medicine. We soon found that minute variations from normal in the calcium ion concentration of our perfusion fluids instantly and measurably changed the force of contraction, whereas comparable small changes in potassium ion concen-

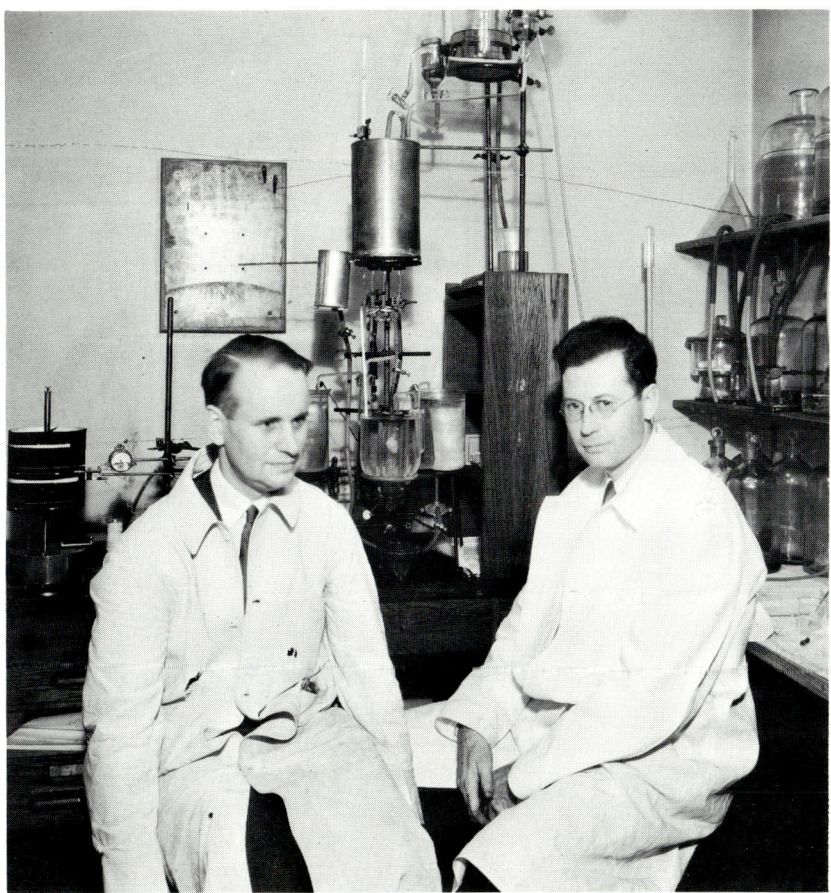

Fig. 2. F. C. McLean and A. B. Hastings perfusing a rabbit heart (center) in 38°C laboratory of Department of Medicine, University of Chicago, 1932.

tration primarily modified the EKG. One day we were hard at work studying these ion effects in detail when I got a call from the Dean's office. It was certainly not the most propitious moment for me to call on the Dean. I was hot, sweaty, and dehydrated from several hours work in our 38° room which was, of course, saturated with water vapor. To my utter astonishment, I learned from the Dean that a condition of acceptance by the incoming Chairman of Medicine was that McLean was not to work anywhere within the precincts of the Department of Medicine, which included my laboratory. Even today, I cannot recall this incident without my blood "boiling," as it did then. What irritated me still more at the time was the equanimity with which Franklin accepted the decision. His only response was silence. I found myself getting mad at him because he wouldn't get mad. Then, shortly after, A. J. Carlson, that great Viking physiologist, saved the day by inviting Franklin to be a Professor of Pathological Physiology in his department. This meant transferring our experimental work across the court, but the rub was that the physiology department had no 38° incubator room so continuing our work with rabbit hearts was out! "Why not see what we can do with frog hearts in the open laboratory if we can't use rabbit hearts?" suggested Franklin. So that's how it came about that the frog heart assay for quantitative measurement of calcium ion concentrations in biological fluids was born, how this method was used to demonstrate the mass law applicability to the reaction between calcium ions and plasma proteins, and how it resulted in the widely used nomogram for estimating calcium ion concentration in plasma from calcium and protein concentrations (McLean and Hastings, 1934, 1935).

Lest you think that the frog heart assay for calcium ion concentration in biological fluids was born full blown, I must disillusion you. There were not only the problems of standardizing our perfusion technique and of recording sensitively the force of contraction, but the convincing of ourselves that the hearts were uniquely sensitive to changes in calcium ion concentration. (Several others since the time of Straub in 1912 had shown the frog heart to be sensitive to the calcium concentration of nutrient fluids, but its documentation as a quantitative indicator of calcium ions in biological fluids had not hitherto been done.)

At the beginning, we analyzed bulk samples of serum and cerebrospinal fluid for their inorganic constituents, particularly potassium, calcium, magnesium, pH, and CO_2. We then made up an array of standard solutions identical with the biological solutions so far as their inorganic composition was concerned except with respect to calcium ion concentrations. The calcium was varied from 0.8 to 1.5 millimoles per liter at 0.1 mM intervals—all other ions being held constant. A difference of 0.1 mM in calcium concentration was easily recognizable on our kymograph. Later we found that it took a change of minus 1 mM of potassium or plus 1 mM of magnesium ion concentration to cause a change in contraction of the heart equal to that produced by 0.1 mM of calcium. This made it possible to prepare standard solutions usually suitable for use with serum and other biological fluids without previously carrying out an analysis of their inorganic constituents.

A more serious problem was the uncertainty that existed as to whether the frog heart responded to both ionic and nonionic calcium. This was attacked in the following way. Solutions containing various concentrations of calcium and citrate were equilibrated with calcium carbonate and, after equilibration, analyzed for pH, CO_2, calcium, and citrate. From these data, we calculated the calcium ion concentration and finally the ionization pK of calcium citrate and found it to be 3.31. In a parallel series of experiments with citrate-containing solutions in which the frog heart was used for direct assay of calcium ion concentration, the calcium citrate pK was found to be 3.21, essentially agreeing with the independently found value. Since the nonionic calcium in these experiments varied over threefold, it was apparent that the frog heart was only responding to the ionic calcium, otherwise the two pK values would not have agreed so closely. However, this did not necessarily mean that the frog heart was insensitive to nonionic calcium when it was present as calcium proteinate. Nevertheless, McLean proceeded with this assumption with the result that we found the ionization of calcium proteinate could be described by the Mass Law Equation

$$pCa^{2+} + pPROT^{2-} - pCaPROT = pK = 2.22$$

The next year, Dr. E. G. Weir and I used the $CaCO_3$ equilibration technique in serum protein-containing solutions to independently estimate the ionization constant of calcium proteinates. We found a pK of 2.29, which, as in the case of calcium citrate, gave strong support to the insensitivity of the frog heart to nonionic calcium when present as calcium proteinate (Weir and Hastings, 1936).

Other related studies followed, such as the determination of the ionization constants of strontium citrate and magnesium citrate as well as *in vivo* studies of calcium ions of plasma in hyper- and hypoparathormone states, in hypoproteinemia, and in rickets.

I shall not continue to list many things Franklin thought of for us to do before we were sufficiently convinced to publish. Suffice it to say that it consumed about two years, and the only comment we got when we sent our paper in was: "Will the authors in the future please be less discursive and more concrete?" It isn't easy for chemists to acknowledge that frog hearts can do something better than potentiometers.

Thus was Franklin McLean launched—age 43—on his productive subsequent life work on calcium metabolism and the physiology of bone.

The story of McLean's subsequent studies on calcium and bone physiology with William Bloom, Marshall Urist, Ann Budy, and numerous other associates is known to you all. Especially stimulating to research was the contribution he made to the mode of action of the parathyroid hormone and the searching questions that he asked all of us who tried to describe bone formation and absorption in physicochemical terms. Three outstanding books on bone were published by Franklin and his associates during his lifetime. In each case they are notable for the questions they ask quite as much as for the information they contain.

Franklin McLean's life was long and productive. He never seemed to age in spirit, enthusiasm, or the ability to take definitive action. To identify a question to be answered, a wrong righted, a goal worth attaining was to him a challenge for immediate action. His stream of accomplishments in biochemistry, physiology, medicine, education, administration, government service, and society is his legacy to this century.

To those of us who had the privilege of knowing him as a colleague in bone physiology, there will always remain the example of his inspiring leadership. He served calcium and American medicine unselfishly and well.

But the most important act in Franklin McLean's life was his marriage to Helen Vincent in 1923 when they were both at the Peking Union Medical College. She is a graduate of Mount Holyoke and The Johns Hopkins Medical College. For 40 years, she has been an outstanding practicing psychiatrist and member of the staff of the Institute for Psychoanalysis in Chicago. To Franklin she brought affection, unfailing support, and a gracious home where friends found warm welcome whether home was in Chicago or Vermont. Helen's contribution to Franklin made Franklin's contribution to calcium possible.

A. BAIRD HASTINGS
University of California, San Diego

REFERENCES

Hastings, A. B. (1961). *In* "The Parathyroids" (R. O. Greep and R. V. Talmage, eds.), pp. 5–6. Thomas, Springfield, Illinois.
McLean, F. C., and Hastings, A. B. (1934). *J. Biol. Chem.* **107,** 337.
McLean, F. C., and Hastings, A. B. (1935). *J. Biol. Chem.* **108,** 285.
Marrack, J., and Thacker, G. (1926). *Biochem. J.* **20,** 580.
Rona, P., and Takahashi, D. (1913). *Biochem. Z.* **49,** 370.
Salvesen, H. A., and Linder, G. C. (1923–1924). *J. Biol. Chem.* **58,** 617.
Weir, E. G., and Hastings, A. B. (1936). *J. Biol. Chem.* **114,** 397.

Cellular Mechanisms for
Calcium Transfer and Homeostasis

I. The State of Calcium in Body Fluids

THE STRUCTURE, PROPERTIES, AND FORMATION OF CALCIUM PHOSPHATES IN HARD TISSUE*

Aaron S. Posner

Introduction

The mineral in the human skeleton is part of a calcium phosphate cycle which ranges throughout the earth's biosphere (Fig. 1). Originally, all of the minerals of the world, including calcium phosphate, were present in igneous rock. In time, the extended leaching of these primary rocks by the earth's water circulated calcium and phosphate (and other ions, of course), making them available all over the earth for biological or mineralogical redeposition. The oceans, rivers, and lakes provide the transportation for calcium phosphate throughout the earth's body just as the blood system in man brings mineral in solution to the locus of tissue mineralization.

Calcium, in passing through the marine cycle, enters the skeletons of some sea life in the form of calcium carbonate, while it appears as calcium phosphate in other species. The calcium carbonate and calcium phosphate skeletons which are not reabsorbed into the carniverous sea life cycle settle, after death, into the deepwater bottom to form sedimentary mineral deposits. Deepwater calcium phosphate deposits are also believed to form

* Publication No. 69 of the Laboratory of Ultrastructural Biochemistry. The original work in this paper was supported by PHS Grant DE-01945 from the National Institute of Dental Research.

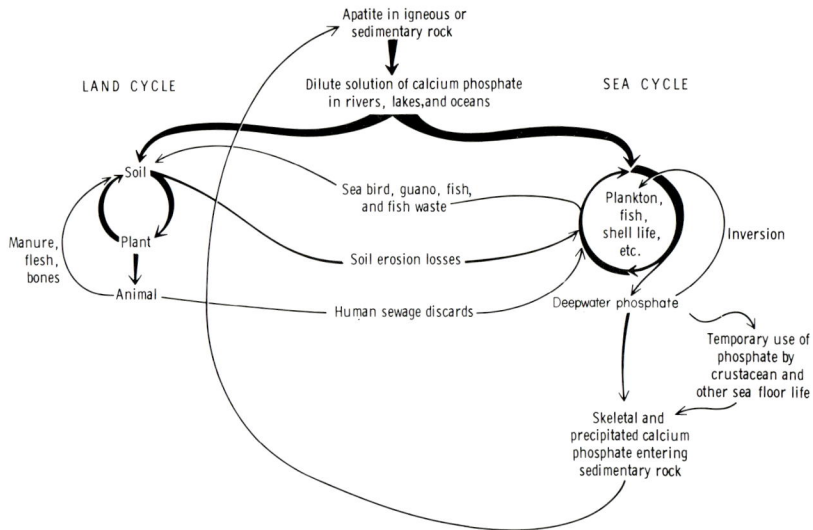

FIG. 1. Calcium phosphate cycle in the biosphere.

by a process of direct precipitation. In addition, some, but not all, of the calcium carbonate skeletal deposits are converted to calcium phosphate by reaction with dissolved phosphate.

Our concern here is with a very small part of these cycles. This paper will deal with the structure and the mechanism of deposition of the mineral portion of hard tissue in higher animals. The largest portion of mature bone mineral consists of a basic calcium phosphate, which resembles the mineral hydroxyapatite, $Ca_5(PO_4)_3OH$. Thus, historically, the study of bone mineral has been closely linked to the study of hydroxyapatite and the apatites in general. Since almost all calcium phosphate deposits throughout the world are apatitic, there is a broad interest in many fields of science in the apatite minerals. Analyses of the properties of mineral and synthetic apatites have taught us much about the nature of hard tissue mineral.

Recent studies (Harper and Posner, 1966; Eanes *et al.*, 1967b) on synthetic calcium phosphate systems have led us to the view that bone mineral is composed of at least two chemically and physically distinct calcium phosphate salts. The well-known, poorly crystallized bone apatite predominates in mature bone, while about 35% of the mineral by weight is a noncrystalline, or amorphous, calcium phosphate (Harper and Posner, 1966). In the following sections there will be a discussion of the apatite and amorphous components of the mineral in calcified tissue and of the synthetic mineral prototypes of these phases.

Hydroxyapatite Structure

A description of the atomic structure and properties of hydroxyapatite is fundamental to an understanding of bone mineral. De Jong (1926) was the first to observe the similarity between the x-ray diffraction patterns of bone powder with that of the basic calcium phosphate mineral hydroxyapatite. It was not until much later (Harper and Posner, 1966) that it was realized that a noncrystalline calcium phosphate was also present in bone.

The latest refinement of the spatial arrangement of the calcium, phosphate, and hydroxyl ions in the hydroxyapatite structure has been given by Kay *et al.* (1964) from neutron diffraction studies on geological samples. The unit cell (i.e., the imaginary parallelepiped containing the basic unit of ions which is repeated in space by symmetry operations to produce the crystal structure) for hydroxyapatite is a right, rhombic prism with a length along each edge of the basal plane of the cell of $a = 9.432$ Å, and a height of $c = 6.881$ Å (Posner *et al.*, 1958). The atomic contents of the cell are given by the formula $Ca_{10}(PO_4)_6(OH)_2$. The hexagonal spatial symmetry of the structure cannot be completely specified with less than this number of atoms, and thus one often sees the formula for hydroxyapatite written this way instead of as the simplest chemical formula, $Ca_5(PO_4)_3OH$. Both are correct.

The arrangement of these constituent atoms as projected along the c-axis onto the basal plane of the unit cell is shown in Fig. 2. As seen, the hydroxyl ions lie, in projection, at the corners of the rhombic base of the unit cell. Actually, the hydroxyls occur at equidistant intervals one-half the height of the cell (3.44 Å) along columns perpendicular to the basal plane and parallel to the c-axis. Six of ten calcium ions in the unit cell are associated with the hydroxyls in these columns, where they form equilateral triangles centered on and perpendicular to the axis of the hydroxyl ions. Successive calcium triangles rotated 60° about this axis are in like manner spaced one-half a unit cell distance apart (see Fig. 3). The other four calciums of the unit cell lie along two separate columns parallel to the c-axis and at heights halfway between the "hydroxyl-associated" calcium triangles. These "columnar" calcium ions are coordinated entirely by oxygens from the orthophosphate tetrahedra which occupy the bulk of the space between the calcium ions in the structure.

It was shown by Kay *et al.* (1964) that the asymmetric hydroxyl ions on the sixfold axis do not lie in the center of the triangular planes defined by the calcium ions as thought previously (Posner *et al.*, 1958). In fact, the oxygen center of each hydroxyl ion was shown to be displaced by about 0.3 Å from the center of the nearest triangle of calciums. The hydroxyl ion is always

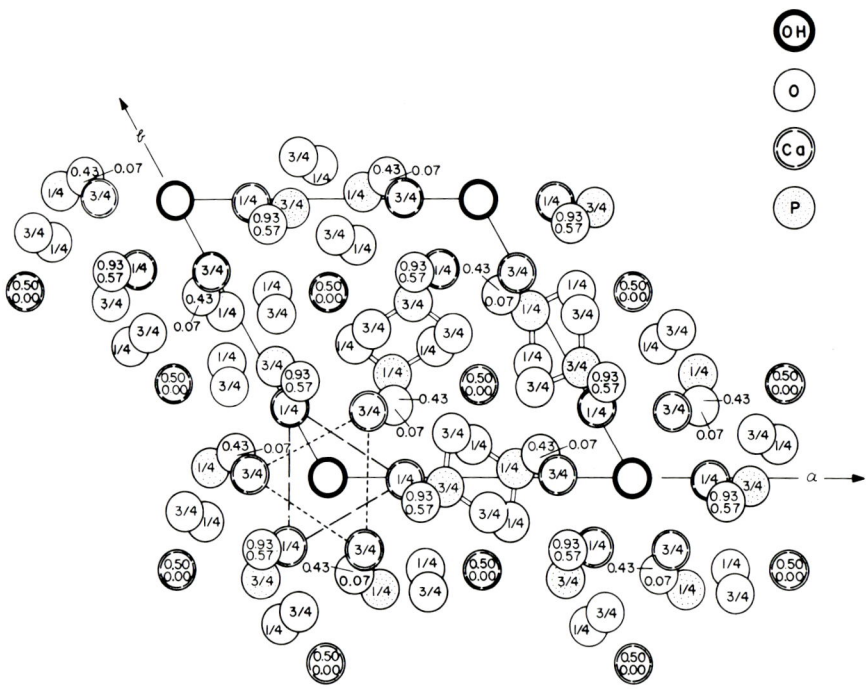

FIG. 2. Hydroxyapatite structure projected down the c-axis onto the basal plane. The a- and b-axes, intersecting at 120°, are perpendicular to the c-axis. These three axes make up the unit cell volume which contains the formula $Ca_{10}(PO_4)_6(OH)_2$. The numbers in the atoms are the c-axis (z) parameters. In the hydroxyl group, the oxygen is at $z=0.20$ or 0.30 and at $z=0.70$ or 0.80; H is at $z=0.06$ or 0.55 and at $z=0.56$ or 0.94. The dashed and dotted lines outline the calcium triangles at $z=\frac{1}{4}$ and $z=\frac{3}{4}$, respectively (see Fig. 3). Two of the oxygens in each phosphate tetrahedron are superimposed and partially overlap the phosphorus in this projection. In some of the tetrahedra the two remaining P–O bonds are indicated by connecting parallel lines (Young and Elliott, 1966).

oriented perpendicular to the nearest plane of calciums, with the hydrogen ion facing away from this plane in such a way that the O–H bond never cuts across the plane. However, the fluoride ions, when partially substituted for hydroxyl in hydroxyapatite (and fully substituted for hydroxyl in fluorapatite), do, in fact, lie in the center of the triangular calcium planes and are bisected by these planes (Young and Elliott, 1966) (Fig. 3). The closer coordination of the fluoride as compared to the hydroxyl by the nearest calciums accounts, in part, for the greater chemical stability of fluoride-substituted hydroxyapatite when compared to hydroxyapatite (Young and

Elliott, 1966), as in resistance to dental caries. Finally, unless a given column of hydroxyl ions in hydroxyapatite has ions missing or some fluoride is present, all of the hydroxyl dipoles must face in the same direction.

When chloride is substituted for hydroxyl in apatite, as in chlorapatite, $Ca_5(PO_4)_3Cl$, the chlorine is even further from the calcium triangles than the hydroxyl ion (Young, 1967). Thus the chlorine structure is less stable than the hydroxyl structure. This explains in part why biological apatites formed in the presence of so much chloride contain so few of these ions substituted for hydroxyl.

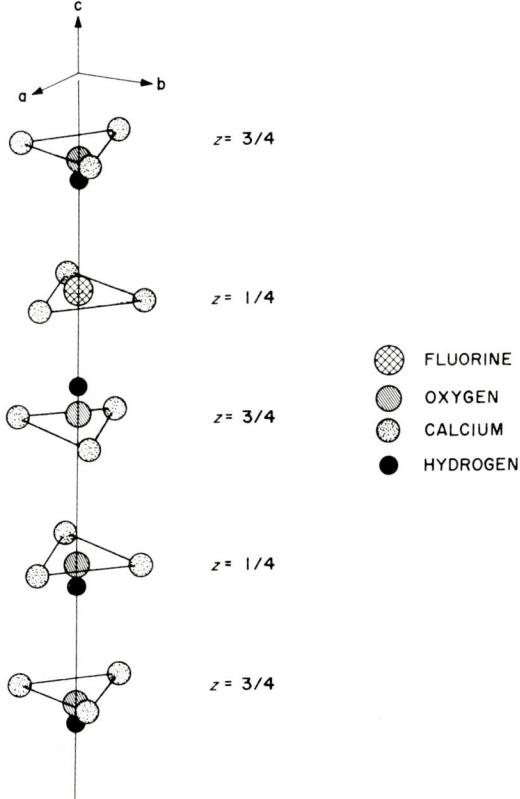

FIG. 3. Perspective drawing illustrating the placement of hydroxyl and fluorine in the calcium triangles of the screw axis in hydroxyapatite. The fluoride ion lies symmetrically in the plane, while the hydroxyl lies above or below. In chlorapatite, the chloride lies on this axis, not quite at the center line between the two calcium triangles (Young and Elliott, 1966).

As seen, the hydroxyapatite structure is subject to isomorphous substitution. It is well known that strontium, lead, and sodium (the last with the proper charge adjustment) can be substituted for calcium in the calcium positions. Similarly, the anions fluoride and chloride, as noted above, can replace hydroxyl ions under the proper conditions. Most substitutions in bone apatite, such as iron, copper, lead, manganese, tin, aluminum, strontium, and boron (Eastoe, 1961), appear as traces. Carbonate, however, is the third most abundant ion in bone mineral and in the apatites in general. Its role should be discussed in detail.

Carbonate Apatites

The fluorapatite mineral francolite contains 3.30 weight percent of carbonate calculated as carbon dioxide (Montel, 1968). Well crystallized hydroxyapatites have been synthesized with as much as 7% carbon dioxide (LeGeros et al., 1967). Since bone mineral contains carbonate in the same order of magnitude as francolite, it is useful to understand the structural role of carbonate in well crystallized as well as poorly crystallized apatite systems. There seems to be general agreement that the carbonate in apatites of large crystal size is present in the lattice as carbonate ions substituting in some manner either for phosphate and/or the hydroxyl ions (LeGeros et al., 1967; Montel, 1968; Elliott, 1964; Bonel and Montel, 1965). The exact mode of substitution and the method of achieving electrical neutrality with such suggested substitutions remains to be shown. Definitive diffraction experiments are yet to be published which show the exact location of the carbonate ions in these well crystallized apatites.

The problem is quite different in dealing with the carbonate content of finely divided hydroxyapatites, which have average particle sizes in the 100–500 Å region, similar to bone apatite. Here the surface area per unit volume is large and there is ample room to accommodate most if not all of the carbonate on crystal surfaces. In fact, Neuman and Mulryan (1967) showed by exchange experiments on apatites of small crystal size that 40% of the carbonate was exchangeable and presumably on the crystal surface, while the remainder was probably in the crystal. Earlier studies (Ames, 1959; Elliott, 1965) took the view that the majority of the carbonate in hydroxyapatite precipitated from solution was on crystal surfaces, while only a maximum of 10% was substituted in the lattice. Whatever the exact percentage on the surface, certainly it is safe to say that a large proportion of the carbonate in finely divided apatites is surface bound. The view that carbonate (as bicarbonate) on the bone crystal surface is available as

Bone Apatite

The poor resulution of the x-ray diffraction pattern of bone apatite results from the fact that the crystals in this tissue are well below 1000 Å in average diameter (Fig. 4). In an x-ray diffraction line broadening study, Carlström (1955) calculated that the largest dimension of bone crystallites was no greater than 230 ± 20 Å. From an analysis of the shape of the diffraction lines, Posner et al. (1963) estimated that this dimension may be as small as 96 ± 10 Å, while the other crystal dimensions were estimated to be one-half to one-third of that size.

Some electron microscopists have reported that bone crystals are needle-like, while others claim they are platelike in shape. In general, the needles are thought to be 30–60 Å in width and 400–1000 Å in length (Wolpers, 1949; Molnar, 1960; Ascenzi and Bonucci, 1966). Fernandez-Moran and Engström (1957), as well as Durning (1958), agree with reported needle widths but observe no lengths greater than 300 Å. Platelike bone crystals were reported to have dimensions in the range of about 400 × 300 × 50 Å (Robinson and Watson, 1952, 1955; Johansen and Parks, 1960).

Both the electron microscope and x-ray diffraction studies show that the smallest dimension of the bone apatite crystal is about 50 Å. Although considerable variation in crystal length appears to exist, the values reported from electron microscopy are consistently higher than those obtained from x-ray studies. A possible explanation for this discrepancy may be found in the frequently reported observation that bone crystals appear to be subdivided in the direction of elongation (Molnar, 1960; Ascenzi and Bonucci, 1966). It has been suggested (Eanes and Posner, 1970) that a fusion of smaller crystals to form bone particles would account for the variability in reported lengths and also may account for the divergent views on shape, if one assumes that a lateral fusion of microcrystals could occur as well. The x-ray diffraction study (Posner et al., 1963) which reports that the largest dimension is probably less than 100 Å is consistent with the view that a bone apatite particle as seen in the electron microscope is a mosaic of microcrystals rather than a continuously uniform single crystal.

Bone apatite is similar in size to the crystals of hydroxyapatite prepared by precipitation from aqueous solutions. From this evidence some have assumed that the same physicochemical factors (e.g., low solubility, high nucleation rate) which limit the size of the precipitated apatites control the size of bone apatite. However, there is considerable data showing that

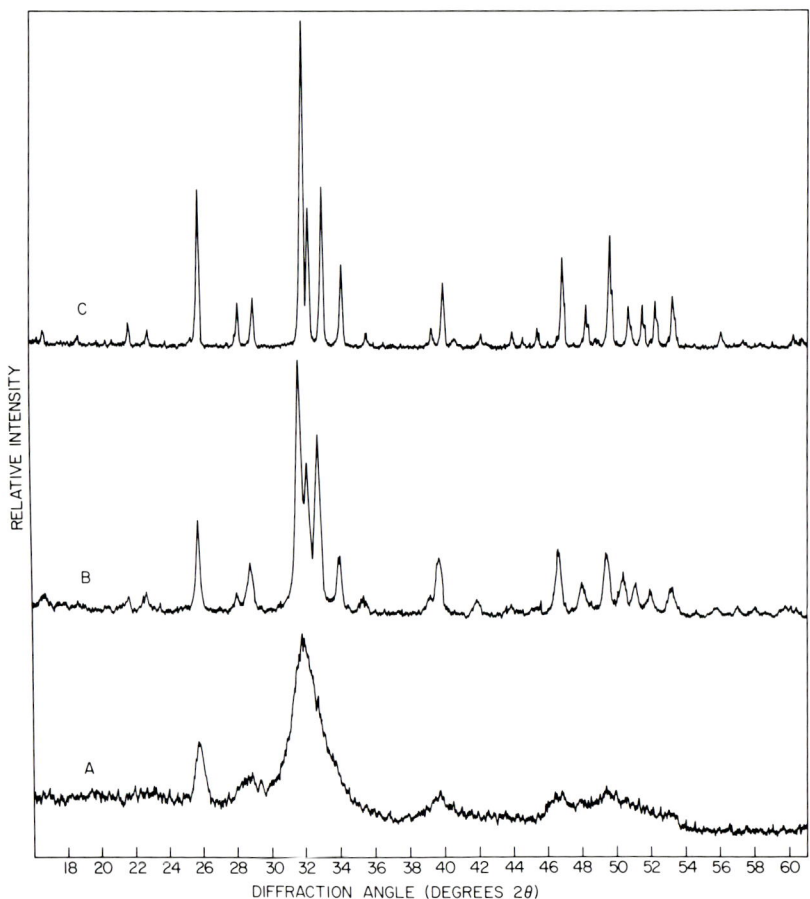

Fig. 4. Three x-ray diffraction patterns of synthetic hydroxyapatites of different crystal size. The poorly resolved pattern (A) was obtained from a finely divided specimen with an average crystal size of only a few hundred angstroms. The well-resolved pattern (C) is from a specimen with an average crystal size in excess of 5 μ. (Here the broadening of the x-ray maxima is due to the instrument alone.) The other pattern (B) is from hydroxyapatite with an average size of the order of 1000–2000 Å. This figure illustrates the progressive broadening of x-ray maxima as crystal size decreases. Under proper conditions, this broadening can be used to calculate crystal size. (Copper K-α radiation.)

biological factors are also important in establishing the size, shape, and orientation of bone crystals. Engström and Zetterström (1951) were able to show from x-ray diffraction studies on ossified bird tendon that the direction of the c-axis of the apatite crystallites was parallel to the collagen fibers. Further, in a low-angle x-ray diffraction study on compact bone, Finean and Engström (1953) reported that the c-axis of bone apatite was parallel to the largest crystallite dimension and that this dimension, in turn, was a multiple of the collagen fiber axis. Similar evidence has also been obtained from electron diffraction of parietal bones of young mice (Molnar, 1959). Electron microscopy has shown, too, that a parallel orientation exists between bone crystallite and collagen fibers (Robinson and Watson, 1955; Fitton-Jackson and Randall, 1956).

The results of an x-ray diffraction study (Posner *et al.*, 1963; Eanes *et al.*, 1965) on the effects of fluoride on human bone apatite lend further support to the fact that the collagenous matrix may govern the length that bone apatite crystals can attain parallel to the c-axis. A rise in fluoride content was accompanied by an increase in bone crystal size only in directions perpendicular to the c-axis, while the mean crystal size parallel to this axis remained constant regardless of the fluoride content. From information discussed above, we know that the c-axes of bone crystals grow parallel to the collagen fiber axes. These fluoride results then suggest that the length of a bone apatite crystal in the c direction is in some way limited by the length of the fundamental collagen period along this axis. In synthetic experiments where no organic matrix is involved, fluoride-induced growth of hydroxyapatite is seen in all crystallographic directions.

Bone apatite crystal size is not static but varies from species to species, between bone types in a given species, and with changes in age, disease, and diet (Posner, 1970). The mean crystal size of rat bone apatite was shown to increase in the early growth period of the animal, leveling off at maturity (Menczel *et al.*, 1965). Vitamin D deficiency, as well as other rachitic diets, appears to retard normal crystal maturity, producing a small crystal size for a given animal age (Muller *et al.*, 1966). It is well to keep in mind that crystal size is a parameter related to chemical reactivity in that smaller crystals have larger surfaces per unit weight available for reaction.

From an analogy with synthetic systems, it is believed that the apatite of bone mineral is essentially a nonstoichiometric, or calcium-deficient, hydroxyapatite. Basic calcium phosphates precipitated from aqueous solutions have x-ray diffraction patterns similar to that of hydroxyapatite but often are low in Ca/P molar ratio when analyzed chemically. Surface exchange studies showed that there was no excess phosphate on crystal surfaces to account for the low ratio, and thus some explanation involving missing calciums was sought. A number of workers (Posner and Perloff, 1957; Winand, 1965; Berry and Leach, 1966, 1967; Berry, 1967) suggested slightly varying pictures of an apatite structure, generally about 10% deficient in calcium, to explain the calcium deficiency. X-ray diffraction results indicate that the calcium deficiencies are found randomly in the columnar calciums, and it is possible to have a deficiency up to almost two calciums in ten per unit cell (Posner and Perloff, 1957). The charge differential caused by the missing ions is made up by some combination of hydrogen bonds (between phosphate groups clustered around the calcium holes) and missing hydroxyl ions (Posner et al., 1960; Stutman et al., 1962; Berry and Leach, 1967).

Synthetic and biological apatites improve in stoichiometry when left in contact with calcium solutions (Likins et al., 1958). In fact, there is reduction in (a) radiocalcium uptake and (b) solubility in mild acid of these apatites with the increase in Ca/P resulting from this calcium treatment. As the apatite approaches the ideal stoichiometry, it becomes more stable. In this light, it has been shown that the apatite fraction in bone mineral is perfecting chemically (higher Ca/P) as well as crystallographically (larger crystal size) with age (Menczel et al., 1965).

Amorphous Calcium Phosphate in Bone Mineral

The earliest evidence that not all of the mineral in bone was apatitic came from electron microscope studies (Fitton-Jackson and Randall, 1956; Molnar, 1959; Robinson and Watson, 1955). These reports described early mineral deposits in bone as noncrystalline in appearance yielding electron diffraction patterns characteristic of amorphous materials. Recent work on amorphous calcium phosphate as a precursor in the precipitation of hydroxyapatite led to measurement of the amorphous content of bone mineral. It is well to introduce the synthetic studies first for a better understanding of the bone studies.

X-ray diffraction studies have shown that the precipitation, which forms immediately upon the mixing of basic aqueous solutions of calcium and phosphate, is invariably noncrystalline in nature (Eanes et al., 1965a). The x-ray pattern obtained from this material is similar to one which might be obtained from noncrystalline materials such as liquids and glasses (Fig. 5). This noncrystalline precipitation, invariably a tricalcium phosphate (even though the preparative solution contained a Ca/P above or below 3:2), converts spontaneously into crystalline hydroxyapatite in a matter of hours if left in contact with water (Eanes and Posner, 1965; Eanes et al., 1967a). However, the conversion can be slowed down or completely stopped by the

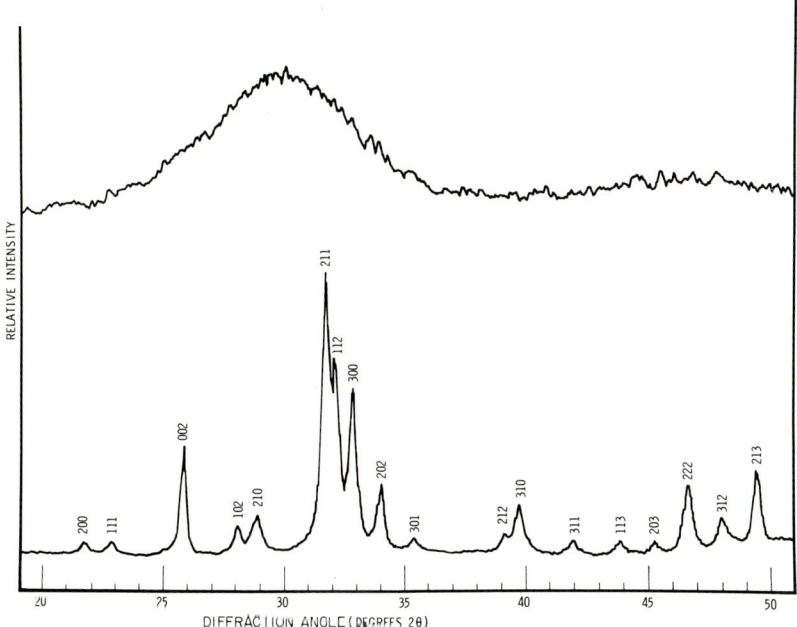

FIG. 5. A comparison of the x-ray diffraction patterns of amorphous tricalcium phosphate (top) and well-crystallized hydroxyapatite (bottom). The latter has its peaks indexed. (Copper K-α radiation.) (Bienenstock and Posner, 1968.)

presence of certain ions (e.g., Mg^{2+}, CO_3^{2-}) in the reaction solution (Bachra, 1963; Bachra et al., 1965). Removing water by freeze-drying also keeps the amorphous calcium phosphate from converting to apatite.

The synthetic amorphous precursor is a separate physical and chemical compound when compared to the hydroxyapatite it yields. Electron microscopy (Weber et al., 1967) has shown that this amorphous material is composed of spherical particles about 300 Å in diameter, thus differing from the final apatite crystals, which are much smaller in size and needlelike in appearance. Since amorphous calcium phosphate has a Ca/P ratio similar to calcium-deficient hydroxyapatite, some have suggested that it is in fact composed of deficient apatite crystals so small as to make the x-ray pattern appear amorphous. A recent radial distribution study (Harper and Posner, 1970) and x-ray diffraction calculations by Bienenstock and Posner (1968) have shown that the amorphous calcium phosphate is different in atomic structure from the apatites and therefore is not an apatite.

A word may be in order about the nature of amorphous substances, which unlike crystalline substances, have no long range, three-dimensional order of the constituent atoms. This does not mean that a local ordering of atoms does not exist in amorphous compounds in general or in amorphous calcium phosphate in particular. In fact, the presence of a few broad interference (diffraction) maxima in the pattern (Fig. 5) is indicative of a certain amount of local arrangement. One can assume that the phosphate tetrahedra (PO_4) are intact but that their placement in space with regard to one another and to the calcium ions in the structure is not rigorously periodic as it is in crystalline apatite.

X-ray diffraction studies showed that an amorphous calcium phosphate phase represented 30–40% of the mineral in adult bone (Harper and Posner, 1966; Termine and Posner, 1966, 1967). The presence of this amorphous phase in bone was demonstrated by showing that the x-ray intensity due to the crystallite portions of the bone diffraction pattern alone could not account for the total amount of calcium phosphate present in bone. Concomitant infrared and electron spin resonance spectroscopy studies showed the same amorphous content in bone (Termine and Posner, 1966; Eanes et al., 1967b). It is interesting to note that Molnar (1959) using electron microscopy reported seeing amorphous particles in mouse parietal bone which have the same appearance and size as the synthetic particles of amorphous calcium phosphate.

The percent crystallinity of bone mineral (i.e., the percent by weight of the total mineral which is apatitic and not amorphous) is another important physical parameter of this tissue. Like bone apatite crystal size, mentioned above, this parameter varies with age, with disease, and with diet. Many studies suggest that younger, less calcified bones contain more amorphous mineral than do more mature bones (Termine and Posner, 1966; Quinaux and Richelle, 1967). Even within a given bone, the calcification front is richer in amorphous content than the more mature portion. In this regard, the epiphyseal region of a chick femur is considerably lower in percent crystallinity than is the metaphysis of the same limb (Termine and Posner, 1967). A higher amorphous content in bone accompanies certain nutritional deficiencies, including various forms of rickets, resulting in what might be termed a less mature bone mineral for a given animal age (Termine and Posner, 1967). On the other hand, bone loss due to disease (e.g., lathyrism and osteoporosis) did not affect the amorphous crystalline composition.

Physiologically, it is significant that the amorphous calcium phosphate persists in bone at high levels throughout life. Reasoning from the synthetic experiments, part of the amorphous phase of bone acts as a precursor of the crystalline phase, but part of the amorphous phase is stabilized in some way and remains unchanged. Upon death of the tissue, the stabilization of much of the amorphous phase is lost and the percent crystallinity of excised bone rises on standing (Harper and Posner, 1966). This may explain why it has been difficult to see the amorphous phase in the electron microscope, since the ultrathin tissue slices employed in this method are usually treated in various aqueous solutions where the unstabilized amorphous phase may convert to apatite. In fact, in the work mentioned above, Molnar (1959) did not use fixing methods employing aqueous solutions in her electron microscopic observation of the amorphous phase.

Tissue Mineralization

Tissue mineralization is generally considered to be the last step in bone formation following cellular differentiation and matrix formation. The mineral salts of bone are assumed to be predominantly calcium phosphates with the crystalline apatite as the thermodynamically stable phase. Blood plasma is considered supersaturated in calcium and phosphate ions with respect to the bone apatite (Strates and Neuman, 1958), but apparently undersaturated with respect to the actual concentrations needed in its formation (Fleisch, 1964). Finally, the formation of the sparingly soluble bone salts from body fluids involves the process of nucleation (i.e., the formation of the minimum grouping of ions capable of survival and growth) as the first and rate-determining step in mineralization. However, the various theories of mineral formation differ as to whether the nucleation can be considered homogeneous (primary) or heterogeneous (secondary). The theories also differ as to whether the soft tissue is involved in the nucleation of bone salts.

Tissue calcification theories can be divided into three classes: (a) those which propose mechanisms that would raise the [Ca] $\times$ [PO$_4$] solution product locally to levels at which mineral would precipitate spontaneously; (b) those which propose mechanisms that would create nucleating sites, or remove barriers to these sites, at local calcifying areas (these sites would lower the energy barrier to precipitation so that bone apatite could form readily from normal serum levels of calcium and phosphate); and (c) those theories which propose that apatite does not precipitate directly from serum, but that a less basic calcium phosphate salt is formed initially which then hydrolyzes in some way into apatite.

Robison (1923) was the first to propose a possible mechanism to elevate locally the [Ca] $\times$ [PO$_4$] solution product to a point where apatite could spontaneously precipitate. He proposed that the enzyme, alkaline phosphatase, hydrolyzed phosphate esters to produce an excess of free inorganic phosphate at calcification centers. According to this view, the local rise in phosphate concentration would temporarily produce the necessary increase in the supersaturation of tissue fluid to precipitate the apatite. The involvement of organic matrix fibers was not directly implicated in Robison's theory. Also, there was no concomitant elevation in the concentration of free calcium ions postulated, for the rise in phosphate concentration was presumed to be sufficient to effect mineral deposition as a result of raised $[Ca] \times [PO_4]$ product.

Several objections to the theory have been raised. On purely physicochemical grounds, Neuman and Neuman (1958) considered it improbable that the phosphate concentration could be increased locally to the three times the normal serum level which they considered necessary for spontaneous precipitation of apatites. Another argument against the Robison theory was that there appeared to be insufficient substrate upon which the enzyme could act. To circumvent this weakness in his original theory, Robison *et al.* (1930) proposed that another enzyme might be responsible for the production of the required phosphate ester substrate. Harris (1932) suggested, however, that the necessary organic phosphate could be obtained from the breakdown of glycogen. In support of this, Gutman and Yu (1950) demonstrated that calcification was stopped by enzyme inhibition of the glycolytic cycle and postulated that the necessary phosphate esters were produced by glycolysis. In opposition to this view, Sobel and his colleagues (1957) showed that cartilage would calcify *in vitro* in the absence of glycolysis. Finally, the most serious drawback to Robison's theory is the obvious fact that alkaline phosphatase is present in tissues that do not normally calcify.

In light of all of these objections to the Robison theory, attention was gradually drawn away from the general idea that a local increase in solution calcium and phosphate ions was responsible for initiating the precipitation of bone mineral. Instead, interest was centered on the possibility that the organic matrix was in some way involved in the calcification process. It seemed clear that the major barrier to mineralization was the step leading to the formation of the apatite nucleus. This process would then be followed by the spontaneous growth of this nucleus into a mature bone crystal at normal serum levels. Thus, efforts were centered on elucidating factors in the organic components of bone tissue that could effectively induce the formation of such nuclei from normal body fluids.

Collagen, the major organic component of bone, is considered by many as principally responsible for the nucleation of bone mineral. Electron microscopy studies, as noted before, show a close morphological relationship between bone crystals and collagen fibrils in developing bone (Robinson and Watson, 1955; Fitton-Jackson and Randall, 1956; Molnar, 1960). The inference from such observations as these is that sites exists in and/or on the fibrils of collagen which act as foci for the inception of crystallization. Glimcher (1959) has demonstrated that only native collagen showing the 640 Å periodicity in the fibril direction (as opposed to other forms of collagen) will calcify *in vitro*. Further, he suggested that the creation of these sites depends upon the specific organization of collagen macromolecules into fibers rather than upon the stereochemical configuration of the tropocollagen molecule per se. However, other investigators have noted that specific amino acids may be important in defining these sites. Robinson and Watson (1955) found apatite crystals near the cross-bands of collagen where basic and acidic amino acids are thought to be more concentrated. Solomons and Irving (1958) obtained evidence to suggest that the ε-amino groups of lysine and hydroxylysine may be involved in the process of crystal seeding. It was suggested that the ε-amino groups may be the site for the bonding of phosphate to the collagen. In fact, the phosphorylation of collagen is considered by some as a possible first step in the calcification of the matrix (Weidmann, 1963). There is some evidence to suggest that collagen alone is not the critical factor in initiating calcification. Histochemical studies on the changes in the organic matrix just prior to calcification indicate that components of the ground substance, such as protein polysaccharides and phospholipids, may be involved in mineralization (Nylen and Scott, 1960; Dziewiatkowski *et al.*, 1957).

The organic components of bone tissue are also found in connective tissues that do not normally calcify. No conclusive evidence is available to suggest that there exist subtle chemical or conformational differences between mineralizing and nonmineralizing connective tissue that may explain the ability of the former to calcify. Fleisch (1964) has pointed out that the nonmineralizing collagen will calcify under *in vitro* conditions at which bone collagens will not. He further postulated that all 640 Å native collagen is probably calcificable *in vivo* and that systemic factors are present which normally prevent such calcification from occurring. Fleisch further suggested that organic pyrophosphate acts as such a protective factor by blocking nucleating sites on collagen by bonding to the fibers via basic side chains. He intimated that in areas of calcification this pyrophosphate inhibitor is destroyed by the enzyme pyrophosphatase. The defect in this idea is the same one that plagues most of the other theories; that is, the enzyme pyrophosphatase occurs in all tissue, both mineralizing and nonmineralizing.

The third general class of theories on tissue mineralization does not attempt to circumvent the difficulties inherent in the other hypotheses, but instead emphasizes the fact that there is an initial precipitation of a less basic calcium phosphate phase than apatite which subsequently converts by hydrolysis into the latter. A less basic calcium phosphate, even though more soluble, could by virtue of its lower surface tension have a lower free energy barrier to nucleation, and therefore form first in preference to apatite. Experimental support for a precursor to apatite comes partially from studies on the solubility behavior of bone salt in aqueous solutions. These studies indicate that solution calcium and phosphate levels in serum are in equilibrium with neutral or possible acidic calcium phosphates rather than with crystalline apatite (MacGregor, 1966). Brushite, $CaHPO_4 \cdot H_2O$ (Neuman and Neuman, 1958), and octacalcium phosphate, $Ca_4H(PO_4)_6 \cdot 2\frac{1}{2}H_2O$ (Brown, 1965, 1966), have been suggested as the possible initial mineral phase in bone formation, but no direct evidence (say, by x-ray diffraction) as to their existence in bone has been obtained (Glimcher, 1968). Amorphous calcium phosphate, on the other hand, is apparently present in bone to a considerable extent and it appears to possess many of the properties expected of a mineral intermediate to apatite which is less basic than apatite. As discussed in a previous section, this material is the first phase seen by electron microscopy in developing bone. Its synthetic counterpart has the lower surface free energy expected of less basic calcium phosphates as evidenced by the preferential precipitation of this phase under conditions favoring the formation of apatite and by its subsequent hydrolysis into apatite. In addition, this nonreversible hydrolysis readily occurs in aqueous media at physiological pH values (Fleisch, 1964; Termine, 1970).

Amorphous calcium phosphate apparently forms only under conditions favoring spontaneous precipitation of calcium phosphate salts. As Fleisch (1964) has pointed out, the minimum levels of calcium and phosphate necessary for such spontaneous precipitation at physiological pH, temperature, and ionic strength are considerably higher than normal serum levels for these ions. It is most probably then that body fluids are very much more undersaturated in calcium and phosphate ions with respect to the formation of amorphous calcium phosphate than with respect to the precipitation of crystalline apatite. Therefore, to account for the *in vivo* formation of amorphous calcium phosphate, it appears that a local increase in the concentration of ionic calcium and/or phosphate must be postulated. Robison's original alkaline phosphatase model for effecting a local increase in solution phosphate is probably not correct, but the possibility of a local elevation of precipitating ions need not depend specifically on the action of this particular enzyme. The difficulty in past models may be in the emphasis placed on the notion that extracellular factors alone were involved in the deposition of mineral salts in osseous tissue. The cells, even though oviously responsible for the elaboration of a calcificable matrix, were not assumed to have an explicit role in the mineralization of this matrix. It seems unlikely, however, that extracellular mechanisms alone could rapidly generate the required degree of supersaturation needed for a spontaneous *in vivo* separation of the amorphous phase.

Several reasons can be given for assuming that the cell plays a direct role in the calcification process. Cells generally surround and cover the areas that are being mineralized. If the chemical components of bone salts must be concentrated by the bone cells for deposition at the mineralization front, then the overall serum levels of calcium and phosphate need not reflect the concentrations of these ions at the sites of calcification. Pautard (1966) gives an example of intracellular calcification by demonstrating the presence of intracellular deposits of apatite in the baleen of the sei whale. In addition, it has been shown that in tissue that normally does not calcify, subcellular structures such as mitochondria can concentrate calcium and phosphate to form granules of amorphous calcium phosphate (Greenawalt *et al.*, 1964). Bernard and Pease (1969) reported that the initial bone calcification locus appears to be a cellularly derived globule apparently originating from an osteoblastic Golgi vesicle. Anderson (1969) showed a similar effect in the calcification of cartilage. Further support of this view was given by Matthews (Matthews *et al.*, 1968) when he showed the presence of inorganic (probably calcium phosphate) particles in the interior of actively calcifying cartilage cells. Finally, Nichols and his co-workers (1969) have shown a much higher concentration of calcium in the bone cells than in the surrounding extracellular fluid or in any kind of soft tissue cells. In fact, bone cell fractions (prepared by Hirschmann and Nichols) have been found to contain calcium phosphate mineral by this writer.

It seems reasonable from what we know at present that bone cells are involved in the calcification process. It has been suggested that the production of amorphous calcium phosphate is a product of cellular activity (Eanes *et al.*, 1967b; Eanes and Posner, 1970). It could be postulated that through a cellularly controlled pumping mechanism, the calcium and phosphate ion product is raised to the needed level of supersaturation to precipitate amorphous calcium phosphate. It is not completely clear whether the precipitation occurs intracellularly with subsequent movement of mineral to the extracellular areas or whether, in fact, the actual precipitation takes place extracellularly but close to the cell itself. Taves (1965) in this regard has suggested the possibility of secretion via the osteoblast Golgi apparatus of a calcium phosphoprotein complex. This complex when excreted from the cell reacts, according to Taves, with extracellular phosphatase freeing the phosphate to combine at elevated concentrations with calcium, resulting in precipitation of the amorphous calcium phosphate.

The amorphous salt, once formed, can now become the controlling source of ions for the precipitation of bone apatite crystals. Since it is more soluble than apatite, the amorphous material through dissolution provides the fluid levels of calcium and phosphate needed for extracellular formation of apatite. Bone collagen might still provide the preferential sites for the primary heterogeneous nucleation of the first apatite crystals. Secondary nucleation using apatite itself as a substrate may also be important in the formation of crystals not directly associated with collagen, such as those which fill the intercollagenous space. In this model, the primary factor responsible for limiting the formation of apatite crystals to those areas that normally calcify is not alkaline phosphatase or a pyrophosphatase, but a cellularly derived amorphous calcium phosphate. In this proposal, the cell ultimately governs the entire calcification process.

Conclusions

It has been shown that bone mineral consists of two calcium phosphate pools; a noncrystalline (amorphous) calcium phosphate and a crystalline (apatite) phase. The two phases are chemically and physically distinct. Reasoning from the results on synthetic systems, one may speculate that the amorphous phase is a tricalcium phosphate stabilized in some manner yet unknown. In the formation of bone mineral, it seems that the amorphous phase is laid down first by some active process of the bone cell. Subsequently, some of the phase is stabilized to remain noncrystalline, while a larger portion is transformed, via solubilization, to the crystalline form. Thus, the percent crystallinity of the bone (i.e., the percent by weight of the total mineral which is apatitic and not amorphous) is another important physical parameter of this tissue. Like the bone apatite crystal size mentioned above, this parameter varies with bone age, with disease, and with diet. It should be added that mature human dentin contained the same proportions of amorphous and crystalline calcium phosphate as bone mineral (Termine and Posner, 1966). The same study showed that mature human enamel contained only a crystalline phase. Whether developing enamel contains an amorphous phase (as we would predict from our synthetic and developing bone studies) remains to be determined.

The crystalline portion of bone mineral is some finely divided form of apatite. It seems clear that certain bone-seeking ions, such as strontium and fluoride, can be substituted in the interior of these crystals. Present evidence suggests some carbonate substitution, but certainly at least half of this ion is present as a surface component. Finally, it is reasonable to assume that the bone crystal is a calcium-deficient apatite tending toward stoichiometric perfection with age but probably never reaching the true perfection of perfect hydroxyapatite.

The exact distribution of ions which are not calcium and phosphate (e.g., carbonate) between the two mineral pools is yet to be determined. Since magnesium stabilizes the amorphous phase, one wonders whether this ion, for example, is not found exclusively with this noncrystalline phosphate. In addition, the mechanism by which the amorphous phase is stabilized *in vivo* is still under investigation.

REFERENCES

Ames, L. L., Jr. (1959). *Econ. Geol.* **54**, 829–841.
Anderson, H. C. (1969). *J. Cell. Biol.* **41**, 59–72.
Ascenzi, A., and Bonucci, E. (1966). *Calcif. Tissues 1965, Proc. Eur. Symp., 3rd, 1965*
Bachra, B. N. (1963). *Ann. N. Y. Acad. Sci.* **109**, 251–255.
Bachra, B. N., Trautz, O. R., and Simon, S. L. (1965). *Arch. Oral Biol.* **10**, 731–738.
Bernard, G. W., and Pease, D. C. (1969). *Amer. J. Anat.* **125**, 271–290.
Berry, E. E. (1967). *J. Inorg. Nucl. Chem.* **29**, 317–327.
Berry, E. E., and Leach, S. A. (1966). *Eur. Symp. Calcif. Tissues, 4th, 1900* pp. 6–8.
Berry, E. E., and Leach, S. A. (1967). *Arch. Oral Biol.* **12**, 171–174.
Bienenstock, A., and Posner, A. S. (1968). *Arch. Biochem. Biophys.* **124**, 604–607.
Bonel, G., and Montel, (1965). *In* "Reactivity of Solids" (G. M. Schwab, ed.), Elsevier, Amsterdam.
Brown, W. E. (1965). *In* "Tooth Enamel" (M. V. Stack and R. W. Fearnhead, eds.), pp. 11–14. John Wright, Bristol, England.
Brown, W. E. (1966). *Clin. Orthop. Related Res.* **44**, 205–220.
Carlström, D. (1955). *Acta Radiol. Supp. 121.*
de Jong, W. F. (1926). *Rec. Trav. Chim. Pays-Bas* **45**, 445–448.
Durning, W. C. (1958). *J. Ultrastruct. Res.* **2**, 245–260.
Dziewiatkowski, D. D., Diferrante, N., Bronner, F., and Okinaka, G. J. (1957). *J. Exp. Med.* **106**, 509–524.
Eanes, E. D., and Posner, A. S. (1965). *Trans. N. Y. Acad. Sci.* [2] **28**, 233–241.
Eanes, E. D., and Posner, A. S. (1970). *In* "Biological Calcification: Cellular and Molecular Aspects" (H. Schraer, ed.), Appleton, New York.
Eanes, E. D., Gillessen, I. H., and Posner, A. S. (1965a). *Nature (London)* **208**, 365–367.
Eanes, E. D., Zipkin, I., Harper, R. A., and Posner, A. S. (1965b). *Arch. Oral Biol.* **10**, 161–173.
Eanes, E. D., Gillessen, I. H., and Posner, A. S. (1967a). *In* "Crystal Growth" (H. S. Peiser, ed.), pp. 373–376. Pergamon Press, Oxford.
Eanes, E. D., Termine, J. D., and Posner, A. S. (1967b). *Clin. Orthop. Related Res.* **53**, 223–235.
Eastoe, J. E. (1961). *In* "Biochemists' Handbook" (C. Long, ed.), pp. 715–720. Van Nostrand, Princeton, New Jersey.
Elliott, J. C. (1964). Thesis, London Hospital Medical College, London.
Elliott, J. C. (1965). *In* "Tooth Enamel" (M. V. Stack and R. W. Fearnhead, eds.), pp. 20–22. John Wright, Bristol, England.

Engström, A., and Zetterström, R. (1951). *Exp. Cell Res.* **2**, 268–274.
Fernandez-Moran, J., and Engström, A. (1957). *Biochim. Biophys. Acta* **23**, 260–264.
Finean, J. B., and Engström, A. (1953). *Biochim. Biophys. Acta* **11**, 178–189.
Fitton-Jackson, S., and Randall, J. T. (1956). *Bone Struct. Metab. Ciba Found. Symp., 1955* pp. 47–64.
Fleisch, H. (1964). *Clin. Orthop. Related Res.* **32**, 170–180.
Glimcher, M. J. (1959). *Rev. Mod. Phys.* **31**, 359.
Glimcher, M. J. (1968). *Calcif. Tissue Res.* **2**, Suppl., 1.
Greenawalt, J. W., Rossi, C. S., and Lehninger, A. L. (1964). *J. Cell Biol.* **23**, 21–38.
Gutman, A. B., and Yu, T. F. (1950). *Conf. Metab. Interrelations, Trans.* **2**, 167–190.
Harper, R. A., and Posner, A. S. (1966). *Proc. Soc. Exp. Biol. Med.* **122**, 137–142.
Harper, R. A., and Posner, A. S. (1970). *Materials Res. Bull.* **5**, 129–136.
Harris, H. A. (1932). *Nature (London)* **130**, 996–997.
Johansen, E., and Parks, H. F. (1960). *J. Biophys. Biochem. Cytol.* **7**, 743–746.
Kay, M. I., Young, R. A., and Posner, A. S. (1964). *Nature (London)* **204**, 1050–1052.
LeGeros, R. Z., Trautz, O. R., LeGeros, J. P., and Klein, E. (1967). *Colloq. Int. Phosphates Mineraux Solides, 1967* pp. 66–72.
Likins, R. C., Posner, A. S., and Steere, A. C. (1958). *J. Amer. Dent. Ass.* **57**, 335.
MacGregor, J. (1966). *Calcif. Tissues 1965, Proc. Eur. Symp., 3rd, 1965* pp. 138–142.
Matthews, J. L., Martin, J. H., Lynn, J. A., and Collins, E. J. (1968). *Calcif. Tissue Res.* **1**, 330–336.
Menczel, J., Posner, A. S., and Harper, R. A. (1965). *Isr. J. Med. Sci.* **1**, 251–252.
Molnar, Z. (1959). *J. Ultrastruct. Res.* **3**, 39–45.
Molnar, Z. (1960). *Clin. Orthop.* **17**, 38–42.
Montel, G. (1968). *Bull. Soc. Chim. Fr. Spec. No.*, pp. 1693–1700.
Muller, S. A., Posner, A. S., and Firschein, J. E. (1966). *Proc. Soc. Exp. Biol. Med.* **121**, 844.
Neuman, W. F., and Mulryan, B. J. (1967). *Calcif. Tissue Res.* **1**, 94–104.
Neuman, W. F., and Neuman, M. W. (1958). "The Chemical Dynamics of Bone Mineral." Univ. of Chicago Press, Chicago, Illinois.
Nichols, G., Flanagan, B., and Sluys Veer, J. (1969). *Arch. Intern. Med.* **124**, 530–538.
Nylen, M. U., and Scott, D. B. (1960). *J. Dent. Med.* **15**, 80–84.
Pautard, F. G. E. (1966). *Calcif. Tissues 1965, Proc. Eur. Symp., 3rd, 1965* pp. 108–122.
Posner, A. S. (1970). In "Osteoporosis" (U. S. Barzel, ed.), Grune & Stratton, New York.
Posner, A. S., and Perloff, A. (1957). *J. Res. Nat. Bur. Stand.* **58**, 279–286.
Posner, A. S., Perloff, A., and Diorio, A. F. (1958). *Acta Cryst.* **11**, 308–309.
Posner, A. S., Stutman, J. M., and Lippincott, E. R. (1960). *Nature (London)* **188**, 485.
Posner, A. S., Eanes, E. D., Harper, R. A., and Zipkin, I. (1963). *Arch. Oral Biol.* **8**, 549–570.
Quinaux, N., and Richelle, L. J. (1967). *Isr. J. Med. Sci.* **3**, 667–690.
Robinson, R. A., and Watson, M. L. (1952). *Anat. Rec.* **114**, 383–410.
Robinson, R. A., and Watson, M. L. (1955). *Ann. N. Y. Acad. Sci.* **60**, 596–628.
Robison, R. (1923). *Biochem. J.* **17**, 286–293.
Robison, R., McLeod, M., and Rosenheim, A. H. (1930). *Biochem. J.* **24**, 1927–1941.
Sobel, A. E., Burger, M., Deane, B. C., Albaum, H. G., and Cost, K. (1957). *Proc. Soc. Exp. Biol. Med.* **96**, 32–39.
Solomons, C. C., and Irving, J. T. (1958). *Biochem. J.* **68**, 499–503.
Strates, B., and Neuman, W. F. (1958). *Proc. Soc. Exp. Biol. Med.* **97**, 688–691.
Stutman, J. M., Posner, A. S., and Lippincott, E. R. (1962). *Nature (London)* **193**, 368.

Taves, D. R. (1965). *Clin. Orthop. Related Res.* **42**, 207–220.
Termine, J. D. (1970). Unpublished results.
Termine, J. D., and Posner, A. S. (1966). *Science* **153**, 1523–1525.
Termine, J. D., and Posner, A. S. (1967). *Calcif. Tissue Res.* **1**, 8–23.
Weber, J. C., Eanes, E. D., and Gerdes, R. J. (1967). *Arch. Biochem. Biophys.* **120**, 723–724.
Weidmann, S. M. (1963). *Int. Rev. Connect. Tissue Res.* **1**, 339–377.
Winand, L. (1965). *In* "Tooth Enamel." (M. V. Stack and R. W. Fearnhead, eds.), pp. 15–19. John Wright, Bristol, England.
Wolpers, C. (1949). *Grenzgeb. Med.* **2**, 527.
Young, R. A. (1967). *Trans. N. Y. Acad. Sci.* [2] **29**, 949–959.
Young, R. A., and Elliott, J. C. (1966). *Arch. Oral Biol.* **11**, 699–707.

Discussion

Dr. Armstrong: With regard to the amorphous calcium phosphate, this is a matter of definition, isn't it? If it doesn't reveal its crystallinity, it is therefore amorphous? Can you give us any information, perhaps speculative, as to the chemical constitution of the amorphous calcium phosphate, wherein it may or may not differ from that calcium phosphate in bone which you recognize to be crystalline and call apatite? Is there a difference in chemical composition between the crystalline and amorphous forms of calcium phosphate, and are their surface areas different? As you mentioned, the reactivity should also vary between these two species of calcium phosphate. What I am getting at is, is there any possibility of separation of these two forms of calcium phosphate, thereby furnishing indubitable proof of your theories?

Dr. Posner: We define synthetic amorphous calcium phosphate as "amorphous" to x-ray diffraction. Such a compound resembles a liquid in that it contains short-range atomic order (e.g., the phosphate tetrahedra are intact) but not long-range order as in the crystalline state. An x-ray diffraction pattern with only a few broad maxima tells us that a material is noncrystalline, or amorphous. A crystalline material, because of the three-dimensional order throughout each constituent crystal, gives an x-ray diffraction pattern with many well-defined maxima. In the synthetic state, the amorphous compound (a hydrated tricalcium phosphate) differs chemically and physically from hydroxyapatite, $Ca_{10}(PO_4)_6(OH)_2$. We have not been able to separate the amorphous and apatitic phases in bone mineral, so we cannot state for certain the chemical identity of each of these phases. By analogy with the synthetic systems, we are assuming that the amorphous phase is a compound of lower Ca/P than hydroxyapatite, is different physically from apatite, and is stabilized in some way to prevent its conversion to apatite.

The question as to whether these two calcium pools are metabolically different remains to be answered. Our work on laboratory rats with bone loss induced by cortisone or immobilization showed that there was no preferential resorption of either phase. On the other hand, a recent study on the resorption of eel vertebrae (by hormone injection) showed that the amorphous phase was mobilized more rapidly that the crystalline [E. Lopez, H. S. Lee, and C. A. Baud, *C.R. Acad. Sci.* **270**, 2015 (1970)].

A final area which needs attention is the partition of certain ions (e.g., carbonate) between the two mineral phases. Can we assume equal distribution? Probably not, but this remains to be investigated.

Dr. H. M. Myers: In your discussion on the presence of chloride in chlorapatite, you indicated that the exclusion of chloride from apatite was largely due to mass law considerations. Doesn't it seem improbable that you could keep the chloride level depressed that far by mass law when there is so much chloride present in body fluid? Furthermore, wouldn't you expect to find relatively more chloride in the amorphous phase if it were formed first and was going to be dissolved anyway?

Dr. Posner: The entry of chloride as compared to hydroxyl in the bone apatite at the time of bone mineralization is much lower than you would expect by reasoning from the mass action law. There is very little chloride in bone mineral, even though this ion is plentiful in body fluids. It is reasonable to assume that this differentiation is due in great part to the fact that hydroxyl is more tightly held in the apatite structure than is chloride.

Dr. Irving: How do you explain the gradual increase in hydroxyapatite and a decrease in amorphous calcium phosphate as the bone gets older?

Dr. Posner: We think that all bone apatite must go through the amorphous precursor state. Some of the amorphous calcium is stabilized, while the greater part is transformed into bone apatite. One can speculate that newly formed bone is richer in amorphous calcium, because the partial transformation to apatite has not yet taken place.

Dr. Mechanic: Wouldn't the resorbing bone be made up mainly of the amorphous calcium phosphate because it is in a higher energy state?

Dr. Posner: Yes, if the amorphous phase were not stabilized in such a way as to make it equal to bone apatite in resistance to resorption. As I noted in my answer to Dr. Armstrong's question, we are not certain whether these two bone mineral phases are metabolically different. In fact, the amorphous phase in young bone may be stabilized in a different manner from the same phase in older bone. After all, collagen has different intramolecular bonds in older bone when compared with new bone. In summary, much remains to be done in this field.

Dr. Howell: The quantitation of the amorphous phase in bone is based on the area under the curve and shape of the deflection of the x-ray diffraction pattern. What is the precision of the method for this quantitation of amorphous phase in the presence of organic matrix?

Dr. Posner: We have found the maximum relative error of measurement of percent crystallinity to be $\pm 5\%$.

Dr. Howell: Thus, you mean that you can add collagen to a mineral phase up to, as an example, 40% and this would not interfere with the quantitation?

Dr. Posner: We can correct for the presence of that much nonmineral substance and obtain the above precision.

DIFFERENTIATION PROCESSES IN CALCIFIED TISSUES

Leon J. Richelle

Introduction

Even though much work has been done on certain specific aspects of the development of bone and dental tissues, little is known that could be related to the concepts of molecular biology that have led in recent years to spectacular progress in understanding the regulation of protein biosynthesis and that of other fundamental biological processes.

It is now widely accepted that the phenomenological observations of many biological disciplines must be reduced to the concepts of molecular biology. Within such concepts, mineralization is the only developmental process specific to hard tissues. The molecular structure of apatitic calcium phosphates, as well as that of the one or more mineral phases present in bone and teeth, have been the subject of many studies. These studies have recently been reviewed in considerable detail (Elliott, 1969; Posner, 1969; Richelle and Onkelinx, 1969). Similarly, the structure and properties of the macromolecules that represent the major constituents of the organic phase of bone and dental tissues have been described, and hence, theories linking mineralization to the stereospecificity of the macromolecular arrangements have been offered and were recently reviewed (Miller and Martin, 1968; Glimcher and Krane, 1968). The minor organic constituents have lately begun to attract considerable attention in that respect (Herring, 1970).

Development as an overall process has not been described at the molecular level either in calcified tissues or, for that matter, in any other complex or even relatively simple tissue or organism. The aim of this paper is to evaluate the concepts now at hand, to discuss their possible application to calcified tissues, and to examine past work in the light of these relatively new ideas. In so doing we are aware that much of what will be discussed is familiar to the informed reader.

Development as a General Process

In biology many definitions have been proposed over the years for the general term "development." It has been elegantly defined by Sussman (1965) as a programmed sequence of phenotypic changes under temporal, spatial, and quantitative control, irreversible or difficultly reversible under normal circumstances, the sum total of these modifications constituting the life cycle of the organism.

Viewed in those terms, processes that can be termed developmental extend to the life cycle of single cells, be they independently existing microorganisms or specialized cells in multicellular forms. The progression in the life cycle of the organism or in the development of the biological system under study most frequently implies going from the relatively small and simple to the relatively large and complex. Growth represents the small-to-large component of development. Simple-to-complex, or the order-increasing component, as Grobstein (1964) puts it, is referred to as differentiation. It includes increased levels of order together with increased levels of heterogeneity, manifested by an increase in the number of kinds of things, be it molecules, organelles, cells, tissues, and so on. Cytodifferentiation represents increase in the number of cellular types. The hypothesis that cytodifferentiation is determined by regulated patterns of protein biosynthesis, as described by Jacob and Monod in bacteria (1961), has been accepted for some years by most workers in the field, maybe because of its "considerable heuristic value" (Grobstein, 1963). No comparable conceptual breakthrough has yet been recorded for tissue differentiation, or, in better words, tissue organization. Indeed, even if one assumes a solution to the problem of cytodifferentiation in terms of macromolecular biosynthesis, it will not necessarily provide for an understanding of phenomena observed at the next level of organization, such as orientation and organization of structural elements as fibrous proteins or lipoproteins lamellae (Gross et al., 1963). Similarly, a series of operationally defined developmental phenomena cannot, as yet, be accounted for by concepts widely accepted in molecular biology. This includes, for instance, tissue interaction or induction in experimental embryology, and cell recognition in tissue culture.

Cytodifferentiation and Macromolecular Synthesis—A Useful Hypothesis

A number of years ago various authors (Spiegelman, 1948; Markert, 1956, 1960) suggested that differentiation of cells is fundamentally a switching of biosynthetic activity leading to the appearance of new macromolecular species whose accumulation or export is manifested as specialized structure or activity (Grobstein, 1963). Very early (Ebert, 1955), questions were raised as to whether or not this was the whole story, but the hypothesis gained considerable ground when (a) the concept of the genetic code was established, with the amino acid sequence in proteins being determined by the nucleotide sequence in DNA (Nirenberg and Matthaei, 1961; Speyer *et al.*, 1962); and (b) provision for regulation without sacrifice of the nucleotide sequence in the genome was made in the operon model of Jacob and Monod (1963) in which control of biosynthetic activities through regulator genes results from the switching on and off of structural genes. This was one particularly elegant solution to the socalled "dilemma of differentiation," viz., how do supposedly equivalent genomes in nuclei control cells as different as a chondrocyte or an ameloblast.

The following statement was then proposed (Jacob and Monod, 1963): "Two cells are differentiated with respect to each other if, while harboring the same genome, the pattern of proteins which they synthesize is different." The standard of genomic equivalence and the limitation to protein synthesis are important in this definition. It has been rephrased in more general terms (Grobstein, 1963) to extend it to more complex differentiating systems. There is a class of phenomena involving change of stability in the cellular pattern of protein synthesis without known changes in the replicative properties of the genome. The class includes phenomena like bacterial induction and repression and embryonic cytodifferentiation that have mechanisms in common. Within this conceptual framework, one chooses to emphasize the similarities rather than the differences by considering all these phenomena as variation on a common theme, namely differentiation.

Limitations to the Usefulness of the Hypothesis

There are obvious limitations to the usefulness of the hypothesis described above, especially when dealing with eucaryotic rather than procaryotic cells, and even more when dealing with multicellular tissues and organisms. For the sake of clarity one can distinguish three categories.

Theoretical Limitations

It is easy, and Monod and Jacob (1961) made it quite explicit, to design at the molecular level regulatory circuits capable of locking differentiation after transient contact with an inducer, or capable of oscillating between two differentiated states, etc. These circuits, though imaginary, are built of elements known to operate in bacteria (regulator genes, operator, repressors, etc.) They ignore, however, a number of facts of considerable importance.

Compared with cells in higher organisms, bacterial cells are very simple indeed: no other nuclear structure than its one chromosome, and sometimes, an episome; as a rule, no intracellular organelles except mesosomes. In bacteria, the whole cell is per force the only meaningful unit of organization. In more highly developed cells, and *a fortiori* in tissues, there exists a higher level of heterogeneity together with a higher level of order and organization. This has been expressed by saying that the cell or a cellular population may be represented as a succession of concentric domains with different levels of control acting on any of a series of progressively more peripheral circuits. For example, the fact that not only enzyme biosynthesis but also enzyme activities are regulated provides a clear-cut illustration that there exist various "shells" in the cell within which feedback regulatory circuits operate. Some authors go further and argue that the multiplicity of causes and controls is an essential aspect of differentiation, necessary for the stability, for instance, of morphogenesis. Using as an example cell wall biosynthesis in a cellular slime mold, Wright (1966) argues that sucessful development, in this case, appears to be dependent on multiple limiting factors and on a series of competing biochemical reactions, without direct relationship to a single trigger mechanism at the genetic level. Although the potential for all enzymes is to be found at the genetic level, at the moment differentiation occurs the message and the control it implies may have been transmitted to the RNA level, as in amphibians, or to the enzyme level, as in the slime mold.

Many analogous discussions can be found in the literature—necessity for control mechanism in time, but also in space and in magnitude (Sussman, 1965; Gross *et al.*, 1963); existence of multivalent repression and of multiple effectors and inhibitors of enzyme activity (Freundlich *et al.*, 1962; Garfinkle, 1966). These discussions may be taken as various representations of one theoretical problem that has been called the problem of multiple entities in development. Order, disorder, complexity, information, and communication are concepts that have been examined by theoretical biologists. Their relationships with the concepts of molecular biology are yet to be studied in depth. Interested readers might want to consult, in that respect such authors as Hommes and Zillikan (1962), Apter (1966), Sugita (1966), Arbib (1967), and Rosen (1967).

Limitations of the Molecular Models

It has been demonstrated that, given a defined primary structure (i.e., a defined sequence of amino acids in the peptide chain), polypeptides fold into a three-dimensional structure characteristic for that protein. Various proteins, including enzymes, have indeed been shown to refold spontaneously after they have been unfolded. This is true, for instance, of ribonuclease (Sela *et al.*, 1957) and myoglobin (Rosi-Fanelli *et al.*, 1964). Furthermore, it appears that association of more than a single peptide chains occurs via similar physicochemical forces. Complexes of several enzymes needed to carry out sequential reactions (Mukherjee *et al.*, 1965) are formed in the same way. Koshland and Kirtley (1966) have proposed to extrapolate the idea to the whole of cellular organization. Even though protein chemistry cannot presently describe in detail the processes involved, they argue that all we need to understand cellular differentiation is, apart from physical chemistry, a knowledge of the genetic code and of its regulated transcription and translation into amino acid sequences. The possibility of assembling *in vitro* gene products to form a morphologically perfect T4 phage appears as a striking demonstration of the point (Wood, 1968).

As pointed out by the physical chemist himself (Koshland and Kirtley, 1966), it is, however, highly improbable that a cell could be disaggregated, that its proteins could be unfolded, and that the whole could then be reconstituted in the test tube by physical forces alone. As already discussed in the previous paragraph, the acknowledged inability to account for a cell in those terms comes partly from the fact that biological systems are not simply mixtures, but really systems of interacting molecules, i.e., a collection of elements that do not exist independently but, on the contrary, are linked, in a defined geometry, through a network of communications that can be represented by transfers of matter or energy that carry information. Beyond the molecular models, the geometrical and temporal complexity of the system must be taken into account when what one attempts to describe is that very differentiation.

Experimental Limitations

In trying to relate Jacob and Monod's definition of differentiation to the problems faced by the embryologist, Lash (1963) remarks not without irony, that "... biological definitions are most satisfactory when they possess a certain degree of operational feasibility." In view of the relative uselessness of the concepts offered by the molecular biologists as far as experimentation in embryology is concerned, Lash (1963) chooses to be less specific and, for instance, defines "induction" operationally as "the interaction between two tissues that results in the acquisition of specific metabolic patterns" rather than, in the stricter terms of molecular biology, as "the control of the expression of genetic information." As he recalls, experimental embryologists, as many other biologists, have little or no access to the genetic material of their cells. Very elegant *in vitro* experiments dealing with the interaction in the differentiation of pancreatic cells have been realized by Grobstein (1959) and are, by now, classic in the field. Many experiments of the same type have been realized on various tissues, including bone (Crelin and Koch, 1966, 1967) and teeth (Koch, 1967).

There are in the literature multitudinous examples of experimental work dealing with systems as yet irreducible to the concepts of molecular biology. In most cases, even when using the techniques of biochemistry and biophysics, the experimentalists use operational definitions of biological phenomena. As we shall see in the next paragraphs this is generally the case in calcified tissues research.

Development in Bone and Dental Tissues

In the preceding paragraph we have attempted to evaluate the concepts now available to developmental biologists. Are they applicable to calcified tissues? What can be gained from examining past work in their light? These questions can now be envisaged.

At the Molecular Level

In bone, one structural protein produced by the osteoblast, namely collagen, has been assigned by Glimcher and his colleagues the role of the specific macromolecular structure capable of inducing nucleation of apatitic crystals (for a review, see Glimcher and Krane, 1968). One feature of this proposal lies in the fact that the structural requirement for the nucleation of apatitic crystals by collagen depends not only upon the integrity of the molecular structure but also upon a specific packing of the molecules into native type collagen fibrils. In addition to a number of more or less specific interactions between the organic phase and mineral ions, protein-bound organic phosphorus is assumed to play an important part in the formation of the mineral phase.

Both soft tissues collagen and bone collagen exist in the form of native fibrils; both contain protein-bound organic phosphorus in approximately the same amount. Differentiated fibroblasts and osteoblasts have also been shown (Green *et al.*, 1966) to produce, in tissue culture, the same relative amount of protein in the form of collagen, i.e., 10%. If we follow Jacob and Monod's strict definition of cytodifferentiation, fibroblasts and osteoblasts would appear, with respect to each other, to be undifferentiated cells both qualitatively and quantitatively. Collagen would not be the specific differentiating protein to be looked for. One must, however, be careful. Beyond the controversies that exist in the literature (Miller *et al.*, 1967; Katz *et al.*, 1969), it is possible that differences do exist between collagens of various origins.

The argument according to which differentiation in calcified tissues can be accounted for in terms of specific structural proteins, has more value if one considers the various molecular species present in the organic matrix of bone and dentin, accepting that collagen is a necessary but not a sufficient factor. For instance, when dentinal collagen is demineralized by EDTA, the organic residue contains a greater amount of phosphorus per collagen molecule than skin or bone collagen (Veis and Schlueter, 1964). This organic phosphorus is, however, largely confined to a peptide of about 38,000 molecular weight which has been isolated and showed to have an amino acid composition quite different from that of collagen (Veis and Perry, 1967). Similarly, specific stereochemical configurations resulting from the interaction between collagen and protein-polysaccharide complexes have been considered to be either promoting crystal formation in cartilage (Sobel *et al.*, 1960) or, conversely, inhibiting mineralization in noncalcified tissues (Glimcher, 1959). One of bone glycoproteins—the bone sialoprotein, or BSP—has also been studied in detail. It is a typical glycoprotein of molecular weight 25,000 (Andrews *et al.*, 1967, 1969). It is highly acidic and has, therefore, cation-binding properties (Williams and Peacock, 1967).

In enamel, there are also variations in the molecular heterogeneity of the organic phase at various stages of development. One must distinguish between the inter- and intraprismatic organic matrix, which is lost upon mineralization, and the material of the prism sheaths that remain uncalcified (Glimcher *et al.*, 1965). The neutral and acid-soluble protein of embryonic enamel, as well as the proteins of adult enamel differ from collagen in their amino acid composition. They also contain considerable amounts of protein-bound organic phosphorus to which a role similar to that of collagen-bound organic phosphorus has been assigned in the mineralization of enamel (Levine and Glimcher, 1965; Glimcher and Levine, 1966; Levine *et al.*, 1967).

Differentiation between fibroblasts and osteoblasts could also be supported by other, enzymic proteins. The old theories of Robison (1923) have been revived in altered form and Fleisch and his colleagues (Fleisch and Russell, 1970) have recently proposed that one or more specific pyrophosphatases are key enzymes in the regulation of mineral deposition in or release from bone tissues. Similarly, much work has also been done on hydrolytic enzymes present in lysosomes and presumably involved in bone or cartilage resorption (Vaes, 1966; Sledge, 1966). If these proposals are correct, bone cells differentiation would represent one particular case of a general phenomenon somehow comparable to enzymic induction in bacteria and the regulation, albeit not necessarily the mechanism, of mineralization would essentially be a cell-mediated event, with little or no role for collagen or other structural proteins.

At the Phenomenological Level

In this section, we would like to briefly describe classes of studies which, as will be obvious to the reader, fall under one or more of the categories of limitations we have proposed above. These studies range from simple qualitative morphological analyses to complex mathematical analyses, based on biochemical and biophysical measurements. Most of them have in common a conceptual content that can be reexpressed in the language of molecular biology. At the experimental level, however, such reexpression presently appears to be out of reach.

In Bone

Based essentially on morphological analyses a first class of developmental studies describe both *in vitro* and *in vivo* the genesis of skeletal pieces. Among others, the classic tissue culture work of Fell (for a review, see Fell, 1956) indicated that undifferentiated fragments of tissue from limb buds can grow into recognizable cartilaginous rudiments of specific bones (Fell, 1932; Fell and Canti, 1934). At later developmental stages, the organotypic cultures of Gaillard (1961) are another example. Because diaphyseal bone growing in a cartilage model can be made to alter its morphology under the influence of mechanical stresses (Glucksmann, 1942), Fell (1956) summarized what was at the time a general consensus: " . . . while the general shape of the cartilaginous skeleton may develop in response to intrinsic factors, extrinsic influences are concerned with providing the right conditions for the normal expression of inherent potencies and for maintaining the normal structure once it has developed." *In vivo*, other and more recent studies have used transplantation techniques. Chalmers

(1965), for instance, has grown femurs after transplantation in the spleen as isografts. Their morphology is maintained even in the absence of mechanical stresses normally present *in situ*. Experiments have also been conducted in which mesenchyme cells are removed from the pelvic region of mouse embryos. These develop into typical pubic joints in culture and can then be transplanted into young female mice where they grow and function normally (Crelin and Koch, 1966).

The influence of many factors acting as external signals to modify the expression of the genome have been studied, as for instance, oxygen tension (Goldhaber, 1958) and mechanical stresses (Bassett and Hermann, 1961; Bassett, 1962). In particular, the importance of mechanical stresses in maintaining the architecture of skeletal pieces has led to a detailed study of bone material as a piezoelectric generator (Bassett and Becker, 1962; Lavine and Shamos, 1963). In a review of this work, Bassett (1966) proposes a regulatory circuit built partly of electronic transducers. Notwithstanding the validity and the interest of this work, it is difficult presently to see how it could be related to the cell machinery for differentiation, as proposed by molecular biologists.

Specific events in the differentiation of bone cells have been studied with the aid of autoradiography. For instance, the length of the S period in the cell cycle, the period of DNA synthesis, has been determined through the uptake of tritium-labeled thymidine (Tonna, 1961; Young, 1962). Young (1963a,b,c) has made quantitative studies of cytodifferentiation in the metaphysis and Owen (Owen and MacPherson, 1963; Owen, 1963, 1965) has done the same for the periosteum. Young's studies suggest that specialized cells in bone are derived from a common precursor, the osteoprogenitor cell and that precursor and specialized cells represent different functional stages of the same cell. Owen suggests that the osteoprogenitor cell may be part of the larger pool of mesenchymal cells and that "bone cells" represent only one of their many possible specializations. Both authors refer to the model of Jacob and Monod as a possible explanation of their observations, but Owen (1965) concludes carefully, "However, as yet, there is little understanding of these mechanisms at a molecular biological level." Further work by Owen concerns the synthesis of RNA in growing bone (1966a) and the inhibition of bone collagen synthesis by actinomycin D (1966b).

In our experimental work on bone growth and mineralization, we have attempted to develop a formal mathematical analysis based on biochemical and biophysical measurements (Richelle *et al.*, 1966, 1967; Richelle, 1967). While it takes into account the molecular heterogeneity of bone tissue, the analysis defines series of time functions that are obviously simplified expressions of the underlying processes of cellular activity. The analysis, therefore, cannot be related to the regulation of differentiation at the molecular level. On the basis of the observations of Deakins (1942) and Robinson (1960) that in a constant volume of calcified tissue, the amount of organic material does not change, water being replaced by mineral, bone was considered to be made up of a heterogeneous population of elementary volumes. The evolution of the system with time was considered to result from three fundamental events: (a) appearance of new volumes, (b) subsequent mineralization, and (c) destruction. Such a model allows defining time functions which express the number of volumes formed, destroyed, or present at a given time during the growth of the animal. Taken together with the data resulting from separation of bone samples into specific gravity fractions, these functions allow deriving functions of time for the kinetics of events taking place in any elementary volume of the population, and in particular, a function of mineralization which describes how an elementary volume calcifies as it ages. Once the biological significance of a sample of given specific gravity had thus been established, x-ray diffraction and infrared spectrometry were used to study the various specific gravity fractions (Quinaux and Richelle, 1967; Quinaux, 1968). As the specific gravity increases, we observed that the mineral phase, first deposited as a noncrystalline material—as described by Posner and his group (Posner, 1969)—is transformed into a crystalline precipitate. The crystalline precipitate is a calcium-deficient apatite which progressively matures into hydroxyapatite.

In Dental Tissues

The development and morphogenesis of the tooth has been reviewed by Gaunt and Miles (1967) in a relatively recent treatise on the "Structural and Chemical Organization of Teeth." It appears from that review that, often, the concepts used in tooth development research are somewhat outdated. Specifically, concepts such as "field" and "gradient," rejected by modern developmental biologists (Grobstein, 1963), are still thought fundamental for the analysis of the material reviewed in that and other papers. Without attempting more than an illustration of this statement, we will briefly describe a few examples found in the literature of past and recent years.

The developmental organization of the embryo, as studied by classic embryologists, reveals that dental tissues derive partly from the *neural crests*. These structures derive themselves from the margins of the neural plate: they are not incorporated into the neural tube upon its formation, but are left on its dorsolateral surfaces to form a projecting ridge on each side. The cells composing the neural crests are called ectomesenchymal cells, because if their origin is thought to be the ectoderm, they behave like mesenchymal cells. In particular, they can migrate easily from one region to another in the embryo. Experimental embryologists, by extirpation and grafting experiments in amphibians have been able (a) to locate with precision the position of tooth formative neural crest, distinguishing the zones for upper and lower teeth; and (b) to show that, if the cells of the neural crests have the potential to form teeth, the endoderm and ectoderm of the mouth are necessary to bring the process to completion. The only information which is reported (Gaunt and Miles, 1967) concerning the molecular events underlying these processes is the histochemical demonstration of an increase in RNA content in regions of tooth development. The presence of high amounts of alkaline phosphatase and glycogen is also mentioned.

Transplantation and tissue culture techniques have also been used to study the development of teeth. Classic experiments in transplantation (Huggins *et al.*, 1934) showed that if one transplants the enamel organ or the dental papilla alone, no development can be observed. The simultaneous transplantation of both the enamel organ and the dental papilla lead to the development of a tooth, with adequate cytodifferentiation and proper morphogenesis. Fleming (1952) has also studied histologically the development of tooth germs transplanted to various sites, including the transplantation of well-differentiated tooth germs in the anterior chamber of the eye. Glasstone (1954) has also used, with success, the chorioallantoic membrane of the developing chick to grow germs of molars of rats, mice, and hamsters. More recently, Hoffman (1960) transplanted subcutaneously developing hamster molars prior to the formation of periodontal tissues. Though the transplants included no bone, they developed periodontal ligaments and alveolar bone, provided they were adequately vascularized by the host tissue. Orientation of the fibers in the nonfunctioning ligaments and the necessity of a "stimulus" to form osteoblasts (the origin of which is not known) are noted and discussed in terms of concepts such as "organizer," "wholeness," "competence," etc. In further work (Hoffman and Gillette, 1964), the mitosis patterns in the same system are studied with the aid of thymine-^{3}H and are discussed in terms of growth centers. The interactions between bone and dental tissues have also been studied by transplanting molars in femurs (Hoffman, 1966). Experiments of a similar type have also been performed in tissue culture. All authors acknowledge the relative difficulty of the technique. In a short review published in 1967, Glasstone explains one of the goals of growing tooth germs was "... to determine whether a morphogenetic field is present within the tooth itself or whether it is dependent on extrinsic factors." The concepts referred to are those of "fields," "gradients," etc., as expressed by Huxley and DeBeer in 1934. Glasstone notes that in appropriate media, it is found that teeth do indeed continue to grow *in vitro*. Odontoblasts differentiate and form dentine. Ameloblasts also differentiate and sometimes form enamel. More recently, Koch (1965) studied the development of embryonic mouse mandibular tooth rudiments excised from the host and placed *in vitro* on a glass–plasma clot interface to find that cells migrating from the clot invaded and destroyed the explant. Successful development took place when the rudiments were placed on artificial filter membranes such as Millipore. Using histological techniques, the author concludes that these rudiments grow and differentiate *in vitro*. No major deviation is reported from the *in vivo* histogenesis. Mitoses are observed, and later odontoblasts and ameloblasts do deposit extracellular matrices. In a second paper, published in 1967, Koch studied the interaction between the epithelial covering and the inner mesenchyme papilla, using the classical transfilter interaction technique of Grobstein (1959). Each separated tissue failed to differentiate when grown singly *in vitro*. When cultivated on opposite sides of a Millipore filter, the tissues differentiated, and this differentiation led to the deposition of characteristic extracellular matrices. The analysis is essentially histological. As to the nature of the transfiltered factor, it is said that few studies exist in mammalian tissues to suggest the nature of the material; "one study showed the passage of both large and small proteinaceous materials" (Koch and Grobstein, 1963).

Conclusion

In this paper we have tried to evaluate the possible impact of the advances of molecular biology on the understanding of differentiation in calcified tissues. It is apparent that a considerable gap still exists between the limited concepts now available to developmental biologists and the problems raised by experimenting with tissues as complex as bone and teeth. Numerous points of convergence, however, have emerged from this analysis of the literature. They suggest that experimental progress along this line is not unlikely.

Studying development in hard tissues may be a better choice than one might judge at first sight. Bone, and more especially teeth, retain in their molecular structure permanent marks of their biological history. This, at least, has allowed in the past and will allow in the future bringing to bear on the problem of their differentiation the sophisticated tools of structural analysis.

ACKNOWLEDGMENTS

This work has received the support of the U.S. Public Health Service, National Institute of Dental Research, Grant DE-02953. It was also supported by the University of Connecticut Research Foundation.

REFERENCES

Andrews, A. T. de B., Herring, G. M., and Kent, P. W. (1967). *Biochem. J.* **104,** 705.
Andrews, A. T. de B., Herring, G. M., and Kent, P. W. (1969). *Biochem. J.* **111,** 621.
Apter, M. J. (1966). "Cybernetics and Development." Pergamon Press, Oxford.
Arbib, M. A. (1967). *J. Theor. Biol.* **14,** 131.
Bassett, C. A. L. (1962). *J. Bone Joint Surg., Amer. Vol.* **44,** 1217.
Bassett, C. A. L. (1966). *Calcif. Tissues 1965, Proc. Eur. Symp., 3rd, 1965* p. 78.
Bassett, C. A. L., and Becker, R. O. (1962). *Science* **137,** 1063.
Bassett, C. A. L., and Hermann, I. (1961). *Nature (London)* **190,** 460.
Chalmers, J. (1965). *In* "Calcified Tissues" (L. J. Richelle and M. J. Dallemagne, eds.), p. 177. Coll. Univ. of Liège, Liège, Belgium.
Crelin, E. S., and Koch, W. E. (1966). *Anat. Rec.* **153,** 161.
Crelin, E. S., and Koch, W. E. (1967). *Anat. Rec.* **158,** 473.
Deakins, M. (1942). *J. Dent. Res.* **21,** 429.
Ebert, J. D. (1955). *In* "Aspects of Synthesis and Order in Growth" (D. Rudnick, ed.), p. 69. Princeton Univ. Press, Princeton, New Jersey.
Elliott, J. C. (1969). *Calcif. Tissue Res.* **3,** 293.
Fell, H. B. (1932). *J. Anat.* **66,** 157.
Fell, H. B. (1956). *In* "The Biochemistry and Physiology of Bone" (G. H. Bourne, ed.), p. 401. Academic Press, New York.
Fell, H. B., and Canti, R. G. (1934). *Proc. Roy. Soc., Ser. B* **116,** 316.
Fleisch, H., and Russell, R. G. G. *In* "International Encyclopedia of Pharmacology and Therapeutics" (H. Rassmussen, ed.), Sect. 51. Pergamon Press, Oxford. (In press.)
Fleming, H. S. (1952). *J. Dent. Res.* **31,** 166.
Freundlich, M., Burnes, R. O., and Umbarger, H. E. (1962). *Proc. Nat. Acad. Sci. U.S.* **48,** 1804.
Gaillard, P. J. (1961). *In* "The Parathyroids" (R. O. Greep and R. V. Talmage, eds.), p. 20. Thomas, Springfield, Illinois.
Garfkinkle, D. (1966). *J. Biol. Chem.* **241,** 286.
Gaunt, W. A., and Miles, A. E. W. (1967). *In* "Structural and Chemical Organization of Teeth" (A. E. W. Miles, ed.), Vol. 1, p. 151. Academic Press, New York.
Glasstone, S. (1954). *J. Anat.* **88,** 392.
Glasstone, S. (1967). *J. Dent. Res.* **46,** 858.
Glimcher, M. J. (1959). *Rev. Mod. Phys.* **31,** 359.
Glimcher, M. J., and Krane, S. (1968). *In* "Treatise on Collagen" (G. N. Ramanchandran, ed.), Vol. 2, Part B, p. 67. Academic Press, New York.
Glimcher, M. J., and Levine, P. T. (1966). *Biochem. J.* **98,** 742.
Glimcher, M. J., Daniel, E. J., Travis, D. F., and Kamhi, S. (1965). *J. Ultrastruct. Res. Supp.* 7.
Glucksmann, A. (1942). *J. Anat.* **76,** 231.
Goldhaber, P. (1958). *AMA Arch. Pathol.* **66,** 635.
Green, H., Ephrussi, B., Yoshida, M., and Hamerman, D. (1966). *Proc. Nat. Acad. Sci.* **55,** 41.

Grobstein, C. (1959). *In* "The Cell" (J. Brachet and A. E. Mirsky, eds.), Vol. 1, p. 437. Academic Press, New York.
Grobstein, C. (1963). *In* "Cytodifferentiation and Macromolecular Synthesis" (M. Locke, ed.), p. 1. Academic Press, New York.
Grobstein, C. (1964). *Science* **143**, 643.
Gross, J., Lapiere, C., and Tanzer, M. (1963). *In* "Cytodifferentiation and Macromolecular Synthesis" (M. Locke, ed.), p. 175. Academic Press, New York.
Herring, G. M. (1970). *Calcif. Tissue Res.* **4**, Suppl., p. 17.
Hoffman, R. L. (1960). *J. Dent. Res.* **39**, 781.
Hoffman, R. L. (1966). *Amer. J. Anat.* **118**, 91.
Hoffman, R. L., and Gillette, R. J. (1964). *Amer. J. Anat.* **114**, 321.
Hommes, I. F. A., and Zillikan, F. W. (1962). *Bull. Math. Biophys.* **24**, 71.
Huggins, C. B., McCarrol, H. R., and Dahlberg, A. A. (1934). *J. Exp. Med.* **60**, 199.
Huxley, J. S., and DeBeer, G. R. (1934). "The Elements of Experimental Embryology." Cambridge Univ. Press, London and New York.
Jacob, F., and Monod, J. (1961). *J. Mol. Biol.* **3**, 318.
Jacob, R., and Monod, J. (1963). *In* "Cytodifferentiation and Macromolecular Synthesis" (M. Locke, ed.), p. 30. Academic Press, New York.
Katz, E. P., Francois, C. J., and Glimcher, M. J. (1969). *Biochemistry* **8**, 2609.
Koch, W. E. (1965). *Anat. Rec.* **152**, 513.
Koch, W. E. (1967). *J. Exp. Zool.* **165**, 155.
Koch, W. E., and Grobstein, C. (1963). *Develop. Biol.* **7**, 303.
Koshland, D. E., and Kirtley, M. E. (1966). *In* "Major Problems in Developmental Biology" (M. Locke, ed.), p. 217. Academic Press, New York.
Lash, J. W. (1963). *In* "Cytodifferentiation and Macromolecular Synthesis" (M. Locke, ed.), p. 235. Academic Press, New York.
Lavine, L. S., and Shamos, M. I. (1963). *Nature (London)* **197**, 81.
Levine, P. T., and Glimcher, M. J. (1965). *Arch. Oral Biol.* **10**, 753.
Levine, P. T., Glimcher, M. J., and Krane, S. M. (1967). *Arch. Oral. Biol.* **12**, 311.
Markert, C. L. (1956). *Cold Spring Harbor Symp. Quant. Biol.* **21**, 339.
Markert, C. L. (1960). *Nat. Cancer. Inst., Monogr.* **2**, 3.
Miller, E. J., and Martin, G. R. (1968). *Clin. Orthop. Related Res.* **59**, 195.
Miller, E. J., Martin, G. R., Piez, K. A., and Powers, M. J. (1967). *J. Biol. Chem.* **242**, 5481.
Monod, J., and Jacob, F. (1961). *Cold Spring Harbor Symp. Quant. Biol.* **26**, 389.
Mukherjee, B. B., Matthews, J., Horney, D. L., and Reed, L. J. (1965). *J. Biol. Chem.* **13**, 669.
Nirenberg, N. W., and Matthaei, J. H. (1961). *Proc. Nat. Acad. Sci. U.S.* **47**, 1588.
Owen, M. (1963). *J. Cell Biol.* **19**, 19.
Owen, M. (1965). *In* "Calcified Tissues" (L. J. Richelle and M. J. Dallemagne, eds.), p. 11. Coll. Univ. of Liège, Liège, Belgium.
Owen, M. (1966a). *Calcif. Tissues 1965, Proc. Eur. Symp., 3rd, 1965* p. 36.
Owen, M. (1966b). *Proc. Eur. Symp. Calcif. Tissues, 4th, 1966* p. 83.
Owen, M., and MacPherson, S. (1963). *J. Cell Biol.* **19**, 33.
Posner, A. S. (1969). *Physiol. Rev.* **49**, 760.
Quinaux, N. (1968). Ph.D. Thesis, University of Liège, Liège, Belgium.
Quinaux, N., and Richelle, L. J. (1967). *Isr. J. Med. Sci.* **3**, 677.
Richelle, L. J. (1967). Ph.D. Thesis, University of Liège, Liège, Belgium.
Richelle, L. J., and Onkelinx, C. (1969). *In* "Mineral Metabolism" (C. L. Comar and F. Bronner, eds.), Vol. 3, p. 123. Academic Press, New York.

Richelle, L. J., Onkelinx, C., and Aubert, J-P. (1966). *Calcif. Tissues 1965*, *Proc. Eur. Symp., 3rd, 1965* p. 123.
Richelle, L. J., Onkelinx, C., and Aubert, J-P. (1967). *In* "L'Ostéomalacie" (D. Hioco, ed.), p. 171. Masson, Paris.
Robinson, R. A. (1960). *In* "Bone as a Tissue" (K. Rodahl, ed.), p. 186. McGraw-Hill, New York.
Robison, R. (1923). *Biochem. J.* **17**, 286.
Rosen, R. (1967). *J. Theor. Biol.* **15**, 282.
Rosi-Fanelli, A., Antonini, E., and Caputo, A. (1964). *Advan. Protein Chem.* **19**, 73.
Sela, M., White, F. H., and Anfinsen, C. B. (1957). *Science* **123**, 848.
Sledge, C. (1966). *Calcif. Tissues 1965*, *Proc. Eur. Symp., 3rd, 1965* p. 52.
Sobel, A. E., Burger, M., and Nobel, S. (1960). *Clin. Orthop.* **17**, 103.
Speyer, J. F., Lengyel, P., Basilio, C., and Ochoa, S. (1962). *Proc. Nat. Acad. Sci. U.S.* **48**, 441.
Spiegelman, S. (1948). *Symp. Soc. Exp. Biol.* **2**, 286.
Sugita, M. (1966). *J. Theor. Biol.* **13**, 330.
Sussman, M. (1965). *Annu. Rev. Microbiol.* p. 59.
Tonna, E. A. (1961). *J. Biophys. Biochem. Cytol.* **9**, 813.
Vaes, G. (1966). "La résorption osseuse et l'hormone parathyroïdienne." Gauthier-Villars, Paris.
Veis, A., and Perry, A. (1967). *Biochemistry* **6**, 2409.
Veis, A., and Schlueter, R. J. (1964). *Biochemistry* **3**, 1650.
Williams, P. A., and Peacock, A. R. (1967). *Biochem. J.* **105**, 1177.
Wood, W. (1968). *In* "The Molecular Basis of Life" (R. H. Haynes and P. E. Hanawalt, eds.), p. 153. Freeman, San Francisco, California.
Wright, B. (1966). *Science* **153**, 830.
Young, R. W. (1962). *Exp. Cell Res.* **26**, 252.
Young, R. W. (1963a). *In* "Bone Biodynamics" (H. Frost, ed.), p. 117. Thomas, Springfield, Illinois.
Young, R. W. (1963b). *Clin. Orthop. Related Res.* **26**, 147.
Young, R. W. (1963c). *In* "Mechanisms of Hard Tissue Destruction," Publ. No. 75, p. 471. Am. Assoc. Advance. Sci., Washington, D.C.

Discussion

Dr. Mechanic: Recently, Elton Katz in the *Biochim. Biophys. Acta* article on the *in vitro* nucleation and mineralization of collagen fibrils [Katz, E. P. (1969). *Biochim. Biophys. Acta* **194**, 121.] states that the nucleation phenomenon is an enzyme-mediated reaction. Why can't collagen, as it is laid down in the body, have sufficient minute subtleties to act as its own regulatory enzyme?

Dr. Richelle: This may be a question of semantics in the sense that when I refer to structural proteins I am essentially thinking of extracellular proteins as found in matrices. Whatever way they act, it has to be through some catalytic action. If you want to call them enzymes, that is perfectly alright. When I refer to the enzyme capability of the cell, I am referring to nonstructural, generally intracellular, enzymes. This is the difference that I was trying to emphasize.

Dr. Hastings: I am living among oceanographers, and they are not concerned with how apatite comes from collagen. But I think they are concerned with how the collagen comes from the apatite. The inorganic world was there a long time before the first cell, so how about having our template for our key polypeptides being there first?

Dr. Richelle: Obviously, as you well know, any set of concepts that are being used at any time are not universal. What I was merely trying to do here was to show that concepts that have been derived from bacterial work have some use in understanding more complex systems. But both new and old concepts are still very narrow and certainly do not pretend to go as far back as the origin of life.

Dr. Posner: Do you mean that collagen may not be involved in the nucleation of bone mineral because there are some cells which produce collagen which are not found in calcified tissue?

Dr. Richelle: No, I tried to point out, Aaron, that if you involve the cell, you are going to bring into play various enzymes presumably active in the process of mineralization. It does not necessarily mean that collagen is not involved in the mechanisms by which the mineral phase is brought about. Glimcher and Krane [M. J. Glimcher and S. Krane, *in* "Treatise on Collagen" (G. N. Ramanchandran, ed.), Vol. 2, Part B, p. 67. Academic Press, New York, 1968] make this point when they state that collagen may be a necessary but not a sufficient factor.

Dr. Goldhaber: What makes the cell put down collagen in the first place? I don't care whether you are talking about osteoblasts or fibroblasts, but what about that step?

Dr. Richelle: Molecular biologists would answer you that the appropriate DNA sequence in the genome has been derepressed.

Dr. Goldhaber: Isn't differentiation the place we have to start, rather than talking about it being calcifiable?

Dr. Richelle: No, what I said is that you are going to consider two cells as differentiated from one another when they produce different patterns of protein synthesis. If both cells produce the same proteins in the same amount, for all practical purposes, you have to consider them undifferentiated and look for something else.

Dr. Goldhaber: Why do you call them undifferentiated if they are already producing a product?

Dr. Richelle: Undifferentiated as far as the production of collagen is concerned, but osteoblasts and fibroblasts are obviously differentiated in other respects.

THE BINDING OF CALCIUM WITH NUCLEIC ACIDS AND PHOSPHOLIPIDS

Charles W. Carr and Kim Yong Chang

The study of the interaction of small ions with biological macroions has been carried out by countless investigators. It is one of several physicochemical techniques that is capable of yielding useful information about both the structure and function of these important polyelectrolytes. Probably the most thoroughly studied small ion has been the divalent cation calcium. Its interactions with just about all of the biological macroanions has been investigated at one time or another, nucleic acids and phospholipids being two groups of these substances that have received considerable attention. These two substances are major components of cellular structures, and the interaction of calcium with them is without question very important in the overall functioning of the cell.

Some time ago the authors undertook an investigation of the binding of calcium and other cations by deoxyribonucleic acids (DNA) and DNA–protein complexes (Chang and Carr, 1961, 1962, 1968). The work was later extended to ribonucleic acids (RNA), phospholipids, and their protein complexes (Choi and Carr, 1967; Joos and Carr, 1967, 1969). The present report is a summary of the data and conclusions resulting from this work.

General Procedure

The procedure that has been used for our work is that of equilibrium dialysis. Solutions of the substances to be tested for Ca^{2+}-binding were prepared in 1 mM NaCl and then adjusted to the desired pH by the addition of acid or base. A known volume of the test solution was placed inside a dialysis membrane, and an equal volume of calcium chloride or other chloride salt of known concentration was placed outside. The resulting system was then shaken for at least 8 hours, preliminary experiments showing that equilibrium was always attained in that time. The two compartments were then analyzed for their various constitutents. As a check, control systems were run from time to time in which the inside compartment contained water and the outside contained the salt solution under investigation. Calcium was determined by titration with ethylenediaminetetraacetic acid according to the method of Sobel and Hanok (1951). The phosphorus content of each solution tested was determined by the method of Fiske and SubbaRow (1929).

To determine the Donnan distribution factor for the counter ions, a measurement of the membrane potential was made with two saturated calomel electrodes which were connected to the two solutions inside and outside the membrane through saturated potassium chloride bridges. There was an appreciable Donnan correction only in experiments in which the Ca^{2+}-binding was measured at low concentration (<2 mM), i.e., those experiments in which the effect of free calcium concentration on the degree of binding was measured. For nearly all of the data presented here, the conditions were such that the negatively charged binding sites were saturated with bound calcium or other bound cations so that there was no detectable Donnan effect.

The binding of calcium was calculated to be the difference between the total concentration of calcium in the inside compartment and the free calcium concentration, which, in the absence of an appreciable Donnan effect, was assumed to be the same as the concentration measured in the outside compartment. The results were then expressed in terms of the ratio of the moles of calcium bound to the moles of phosphorus in the sample (Ca/P).

Nucleic Acids

Because nucleic acids are highly charged anionic polyelectrolytes at neutral pH, they readily form stable complexes with small cations, especially those that are di- or trivalent. Many investigators using a variety of techniques have shown both qualitatively and quantitatively that the binding of cations is correlated directly with the anionic charge of nucleic acids (Shack et al., 1953; Lawley, 1956; Wiberg and Neuman, 1957; Felsenfeld, 1962; Banerjee and Perkins, 1962; Lyons and Kotin, 1964).

Further, it has been shown that di- and multivalent small cations stabilize the double helix of DNA against heat denaturation (Tabor, 1962; Eichhorn, 1962; Mahler and Mehrota, 1962; Mandel, 1962). Both the cation-binding and stabilizing effect are considered to be the result of ion pair formation between the small cation and the multiple phosphate groups of the DNA backbone; studies with several physicochemical techniques have firmly established this idea (Lyons and Kotin, 1965; Feldman and Keil, 1965; Hoppe and Morales, 1966).

DEOXYRIBONUCLEIC ACIDS

The effect of calcium concentration on its binding with DNA is such that saturation of the monovalent phosphate groups occurs at about 4 mM free calcium (Fig. 1). The Ca/P ratio approaches the expected value of 0.5 at this concentration and remains constant up to a concentration of at least 50 mM. The effect of concentration below 4 mM is quite unusual because Ca/P drops to 0.35 at 1 mM and then tends to level off, dropping only to 0.30 at 0.3 mM. This behavior suggests the possibility of two modes of binding: (a) At a low concentration of calcium (0.5 mM), one cation is bound at a site which consists of a triangle of three anionic charges on the surface of the double helix of DNA (Ca/P = 0.33). The formation constant for this interaction would be of the order of 2×10^4. At a higher concentration (5 mM), the remaining phosphate charge becomes saturated

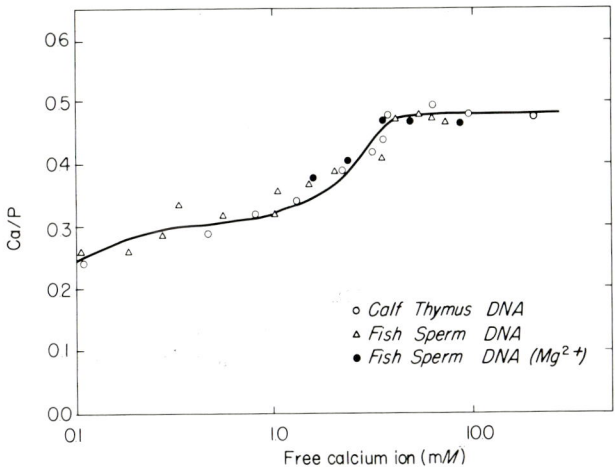

FIG. 1. The binding of Ca^{2+} by DNA as a function of Ca^{2+} concentration at pH 6.5.

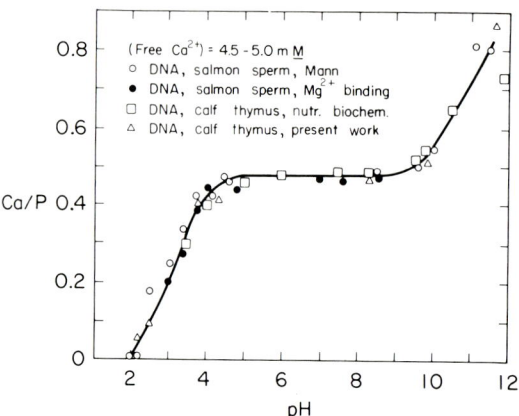

FIG. 2. The maximum binding of Ca^{2+} and Mg^{2+} by various DNA samples as a function of pH [*Biochim. Biophys. Acta* **157**, 130 (1968)].

with more weakly bound calcium, the formation constant being of the order of 500.

Titration curves for DNA clearly show that in the pH range 5–10, the anionic charge is entirely the result of diester phosphate ionization ($pK <$ 2.0) (Cox and Peacocke, 1956; Jordan, 1960). At pH values below 5.0, protonization of nitrogen bases takes place resulting in a decrease in the net negative charge of DNA. At pH values above 10.0, enol groups of guanine and thymine become ionized, and the negative charge increases by about 50% at pH 12. The results which we obtained for the effect of pH on the binding of calcium with DNA are in close agreement with the hydrogen ion titration curves (Fig. 2). Ca/P is 0.26 at pH 3.0, whereas the value predicted from titration data is 0.25. At high pH, 2.0 equivalents/4P of enol groups would be available for binding, which would mean that the upper limit for Ca/P would be about 0.75. The values we obtained at pH 11.5–12.0 are 0.70–0.80.

Several investigators have shown that sodium ion competes with calcium for binding with DNA (Shack *et al.*, 1953; Wiberg and Neuman, 1957; Felsenfeld and Huang, 1959, 1960). We have confirmed this, and in addition, have determined the competition for Ca^{2+}-binding with di-, tri-, and tetravalent cations (Figs. 3 and 4). When the ratio of the concentration of sodium chloride to calcium chloride is 20:1, the binding of calcium is decreased by one half (Ca/P = 0.25), and when the ratio is 50:1, the binding of calcium approaches zero. The divalent organic cations compete on almost an equal basis with calcium, for when the ratio of

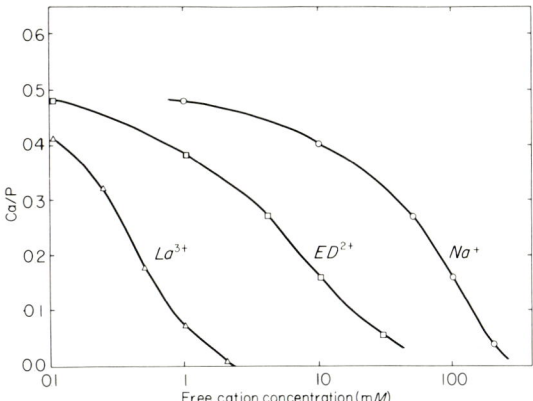

Fig. 3. The binding of Ca^{2+} by DNA in the presence of Na^+ (pH 7.0), ethylenediamine (pH 6.0), and La^{3+} (pH 4.5).

ethylenediamine (ED^{2+}) to calcium is just a little greater than 1, Ca/P = 0.25. The trivalent lanthanum and spermidine compete very strongly with calcium. According to the results in Fig. 3, when La^{3+}/Ca^{2+} is 0.06, Ca/P is 0.25. In Fig. 4 it is seen that La^{3+} and spermidine [3+] have about the same competitive effect as each other, and Th^{4+} and spermine [4+] also have about the same effect as each other but compete somewhat more strongly than the trivalent cations. Thus, these data on competitive

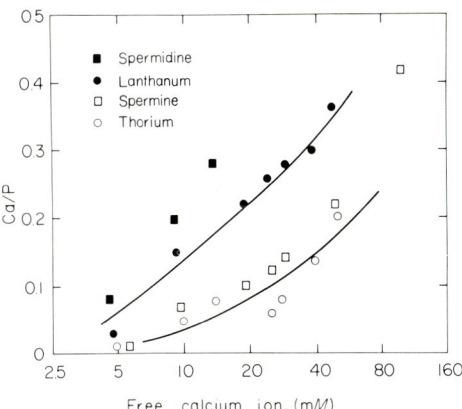

Fig. 4. The binding of Ca^{2+} by DNA in the presence of trivalent and tetravalent cations, pH 4.5 [*Biochim. Biophys. Acta* **157**, 133 (1968)].

binding with calcium reinforce the idea that the binding of small cations is primarily a coulombic interaction with the anionic groups of DNA.

In view of our results on the competitive binding of calcium with polyvalent amines, it became of interest to study the interaction of DNA with proteins by means of Ca^{2+}-binding measurements. The manner by which nucleic acids and proteins are held together in the nucleus has for a long time been attributed primarily to an electrostatic interaction between positively charged proteins and negatively charged nucleic acids (Mitchell, 1960; Bonner and Ts'o, 1964). Thus, it seemed likely that measurements of the binding of calcium by nucleic acid–protein complexes would yield some information about these complexes.

Our first experiments were carried out with DNA and protamine, and the results are shown in Fig. 5. From the pronounced decrease in Ca/P, it is easily seen that protamine masks the sites for binding of calcium with DNA. A quantitative evaluation of the decrease in Ca/P in the pH range 6–9 shows that the calcium which is displaced is equivalent to the amount of positive charge added in the form of protamine when 0.05% protamine is used. When higher concentrations are used, there is a further decrease in Ca/P, but it is less than equivalent to the amount of protamine added. This is most likely caused by a steric effect such that after 50–60% of the DNA phosphate groups are covered by protamine, the remaining areas for protamine binding are too small to accommodate whole molecules. Some of the positive groups of the protamine combine with phosphate groups, leaving the remainder of the protamine molecule unreacted with nucleic acid. Thus, it requires more than a stoichiometric amount of protamine to reduce Ca/P to 0.02–0.03.

Similar experiments were carried out with thymus histone, lysozyme,

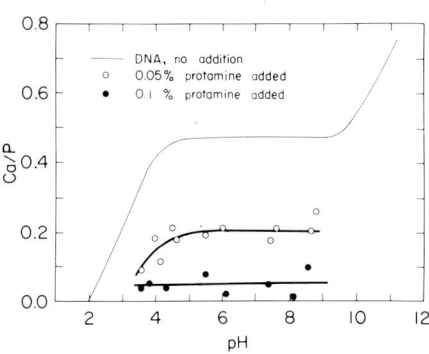

FIG. 5. The binding of Ca^{2+} by DNA–protamine complexes at various pH values, $[Ca^{2+}]$ 5.0 mM [*Biochim. Biophys. Acta* **157,** 133 (1968)].

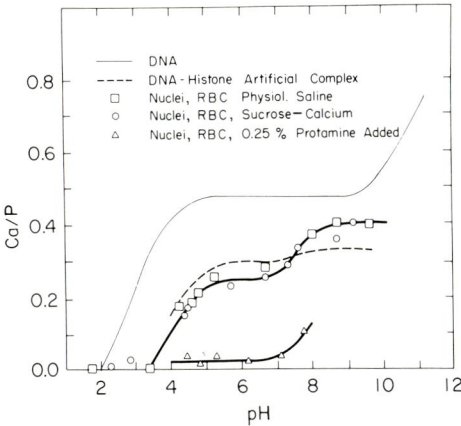

Fig. 6. The binding of Ca^{2+} by chicken erythrocyte (RBC) nuclei at various pH values. [Ca^{2+}] 5.0 mM [*Biochim. Biophys. Acta* **157**, 136 (1968)].

and serum albumin. For all these proteins in the pH range where they are positively charged, they masked Ca^{2+}-binding sites to the extent that was equivalent to the concentration of positive charges in the added protein.

Next, we turned to natural DNA–protein complexes, cell nuclei that have been isolated from various sources. Because of the ease of isolation and availability, most of our data were obtained with chicken erythrocyte nuclei and fish sperm nuclei. Results of some of these experiments are shown in Figs. 6 and 7.

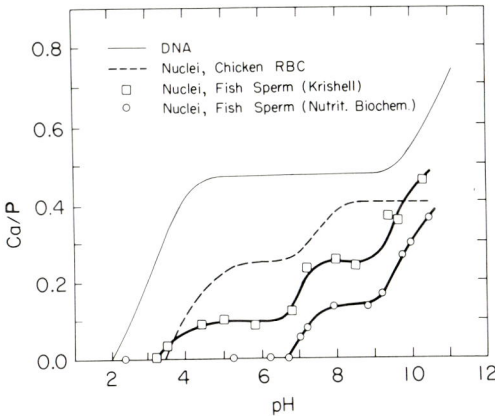

Fig. 7. The binding of Ca^{2+} by fish sperm nuclei at various pH values. [Ca^{2+}] 5.0 mM [*Biochim. Biophys. Acta* **157**, 136 (1968)].

The effect of pH on the binding of calcium to nuclei is very similar to that obtained with an artifical DNA–histone complex. In the pH range 3.0–6.5, there is a lowering of Ca/P which seems to be almost certainly due to the blocking of sites by protein. For the chicken erythrocyte nuclei, this decrease in Ca/P is about 50%, and for fish sperm nuclei it is 80–100%. This latter figure agrees with the data of Vendrely et al. (1960), which shows equivalence between the arginine content and phosphate content of fish sperm nuclei. Addition of protamine to chicken erythrocyte nuclei masks the remaining free DNA just as in the experiments with DNA–protamine complexes.

In the pH range 6.5–8.0, there is a further increase in binding which is similar to that observed with artifical histone and lysozyme complexes with DNA. It is surmised that this increased binding is caused by interaction with anionic binding sites in the nuclear protein.

Thus, for these two types of nuclei, the value of Ca/P at pH 5.0–6.5 appears to represent DNA phosphate groups not combined with strongly binding substances such as cationic proteins and polyamines. Variations in the increase of Ca/P above pH 6.5 apparently reflect differences in types of proteins that are present in the nucleus. With erythrocyte nuclei, a single rise is obtained, indicating that a single type of protein is the principal nonnucleic acid component. For fish sperm nuclei, two characteristic breaks are obtained, suggesting that there are two different types of binding substances present.

RIBONUCLEIC ACIDS

Studies of the binding of calcium and other divalent cations with ribonucleic acids show that for the most part RNA behaves like DNA. The

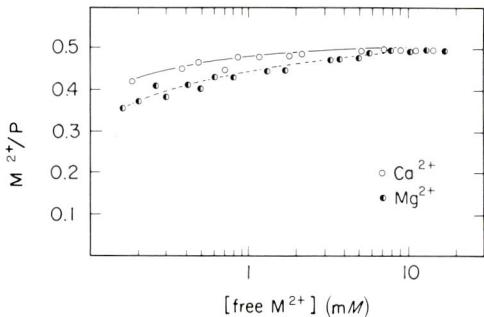

FIG. 8. The effect of cation concentration on the binding of Ca^{2+} and Mg^{2+} with RNA (pH 7.4, dog liver RNA).

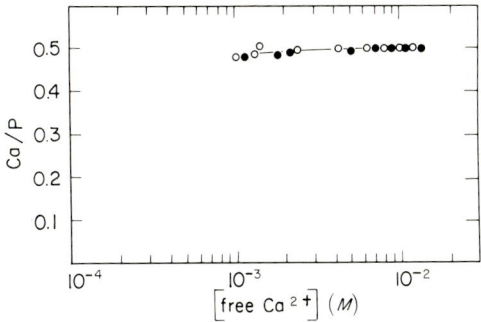

FIG. 9. Effect of Ca^{2+} concentration on Ca^{2+} binding to *Escherichia coli* ribosomes and ribosomal RNA in the presence of 5×10^{-3} M tris buffer (pH 7.4). (●) Ribosomes; (○) ribosomal RNA. [*J. Mol. Biol.* **25**, 341 (1967).]

effect of calcium concentration on the saturation of phosphate binding sites is very similar to that of DNA, except that saturation occurs in a somewhat lower concentration of free calcium (Fig. 8). It is also seen that magnesium is bound a little more weakly than calcium. The pH effect is almost the same as for DNA, except for a small difference in the acid region (pH 3–5). This is a reflection of the somewhat different pK_a values for the nitrogen bases as revealed by hydrogen ion titration curves (Cox et al., 1956; Cox and Littauer, 1963).

The addition of cationic proteins such as protamine and lysozyme to RNA decreases the binding of divalent cations exactly as with DNA. Further, competitive effects of monovalent cations (Na^+, K^+, NH_4^+) and polyamines (spermidine $^{3+}$, spermine $^{4+}$) are the same as for DNA (Choi and Carr, 1967).

One set of results that was quite different from that for DNA was the binding pattern with the naturally occurring RNA–protein complex, *Escherichia coli* ribosomes. Although these particles are about one-half protein, they retain their full capacity to bind small cations; i.e., at 5 mM free calcium, Ca/P = 0.5 (Fig. 9). The phosphate-binding sites remain accessible to all of the small cations, with the ribosomes behaving like cation exchange particles with a capacity equivalent to the RNA–phosphate. Thus, it is concluded that the electrostatic interaction of RNA–phosphate with basic amino acids of protein is not essential for the formation of the ribonucleoprotein complex of *E. coli* ribosomes.

Because *E. coli* ribosomes require magnesium for their optimal biological function, most of our data were obtained with that cation. However, it was shown that calcium will exchange completely with magnesium and that when this exchange takes place, there is a change in the organization of the ribosomal structure. Figures 10 and 11 show the ultracentrifugal patterns for Mg^{2+}–ribosomes and for Ca^{2+}–ribosomes. In the presence of 10 mM calcium there is an extra peak in addition to 70 S and 100 S which appeared to be 85–90 S. When the concentration of calcium was lowered to 2×10^{-2} mM, Ca^{2+}–ribosomes again exhibited an extra peak sedimenting between 30 S and 50 S. It has been shown by others (Abdul-Nour and Webster, 1960; Tissieres *et al.*, 1960) that Ca^{2+}–ribosomes are generally not as biologically active as Mg^{2+}–ribosomes. Thus, it appears that the association of these particles in the presence of magnesium is not simply a random aggregation of the subunits, but that the subunits associate in some meaningful fashion that is quite specific for magnesium over calcium.

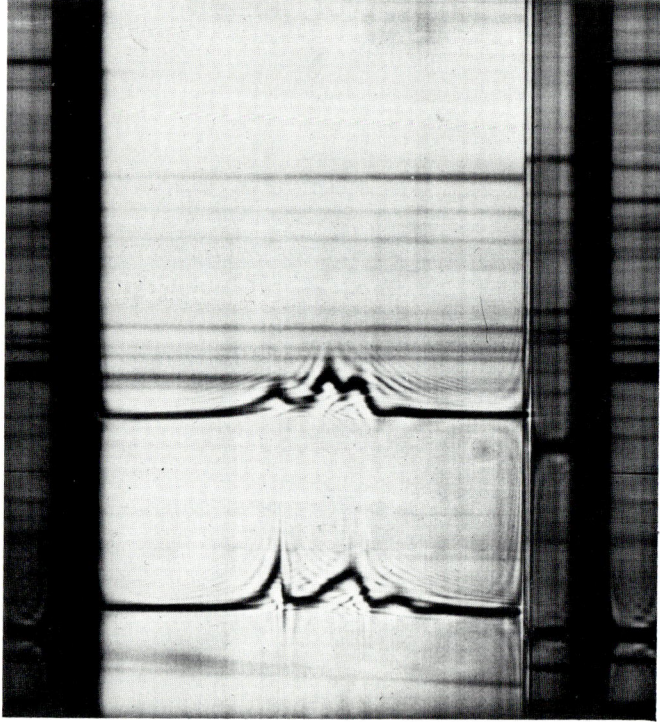

Fig. 10. Analytical ultracentrifuge pattern of *E. coli* ribosomes showing the changes of ribosomes when Mg^{2+} was completely displaced by Ca^{2+}. Schlieren plate was taken 16 minutes after the centrifuge had reached 29,500 rpm. The lower pattern represents the 50 S, 70 S, and 100 S ribosomes in 10^{-2} M tris buffer (pH 7.4) containing 10^{-2} M Mg^{2+}. The upper pattern represents the picture of Ca–ribosomes in 10^{-2} M tris buffer (pH 7.4) containing 10^{-2} M Ca^{2+}. [*J. Mol. Biol.* **25**, 340 (1967).]

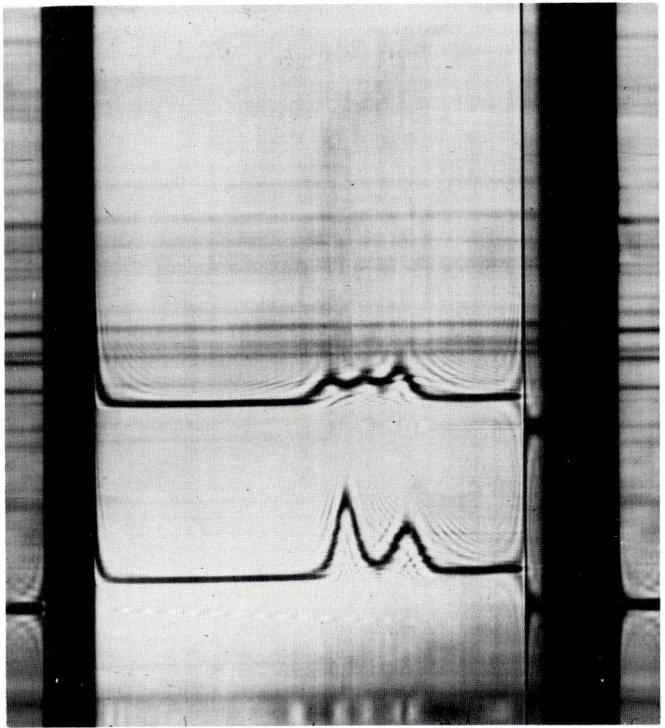

Fig. 11. Analytical ultracentrifuge pattern of *E. coli* ribosomes showing the changes of ribosomes when Mg^{2+} was completely displaced by Ca^{2+}. Schlieren plate was taken 32 minutes after the centrifuge had reached 29,500 rpm. The lower pattern represents the 30 S and 50 S ribosomes in 10^{-2} M tris buffer (pH 7.4) containing 5×10^{-5} M Mg^{2+}. The upper pattern represents the picture of Ca–ribosomes in 10^{-2} M tris buffer (pH 7.4) containing 5×10^{-5} M Ca^{2+}. [*J. Mol. Biol.* **25,** 340 (1967).]

Phospholipids

In the past decade, there has been a considerable interest in the binding of calcium with phospholipids. This interest has no doubt been generated to a large extent by certain findings concerning the role of phospholipids in membrane structure and function, by the effects of small cations on membrane permeability, and by new techniques for the separation of the various types of phospholipids in relatively purified form. The various types of phospholipids have anionic groups that act as binding sites for small cations. Some of the phospholipids also have cationic groups, with the result that in certain pH ranges, zwitterion formation occurs removing the capacity for interaction with counter ions. The numerous studies that have been made, including hydrogen ion titration curves, have indeed shown that the binding of small cations with phospholipids is correlated very closely with the chemical structures of the phospholipids (Abramson et al., 1964; Hendrickson and Fullington, 1965; Rojas and Tobias, 1965; Shah and Schulman, 1965).

PURIFIED PREPARATIONS

In our first experiments with phospholipids, it was found that their affinity for calcium is such that saturation of the binding sites occurs at about 3–5 mM free calcium, the same range as for nucleic acids. In some recent experiments we have also found that at low calcium concentration, considerable binding is observed in the range of 10^{-6}–10^{-4} M (Carr, 1970). Thus, the formation constant is indicated to be 10^4 or greater. Abramson and co-workers (1966) have reported values of 2×10^4 for calcium phos-

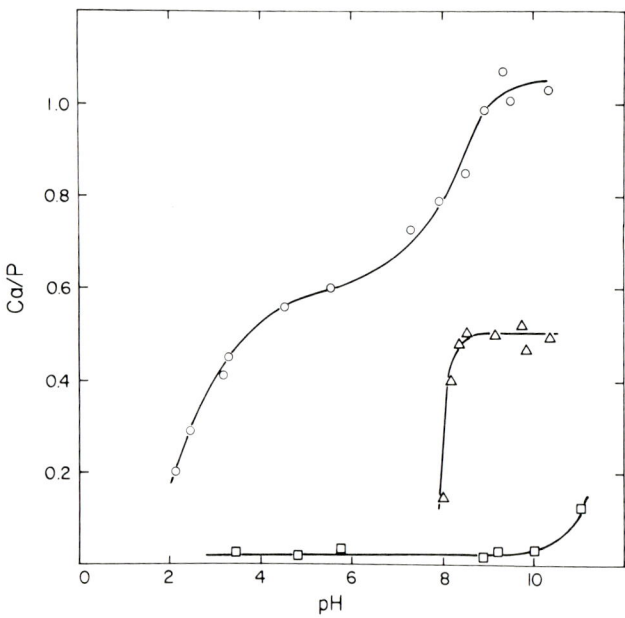

FIG. 12. Binding of Ca^{2+} with purified phospholipid preparations; ○ = phosphatidylserine (4.3 mM phosphate); △ = phosphatidylethanolamine (1.3 mM phosphate); □-phosphatidylcholine (4.1 mM phosphate) [*Proc. Soc. Exp. Biol. Med.* **124**, 1270 (1967)].

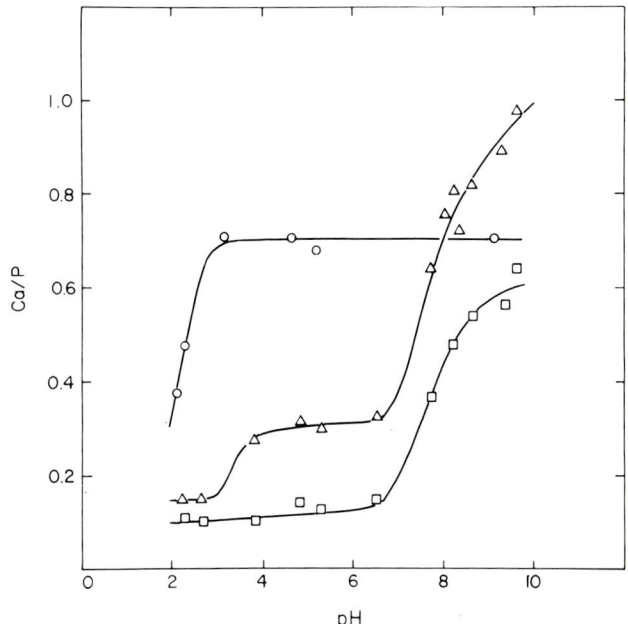

FIG. 13. Binding of Ca^{2+} with purified phospholipid preparations. ○ = monophosphoinositide (0.5 mM phosphate); △ = commercial inositol phosphatide (3.6 mM phosphorus); □ = calculated curve, triphosphoinositide; assumption that inositol phosphatide contains 25% phosphatidylserine. [*Proc. Soc. Exp. Biol. Med.* **124,** 1270 (1967).]

phatidic acid, and for triphosphoinositide, Hendrickson (1969) indicates that K_f is 10^5 for calcium.

The results that we have obtained for the saturation binding of calcium with phosphatidylcholine, phosphatidylethanolamine, and phosphatidylserine are shown in Fig. 12. There is no significant binding to phosphatidylcholine below pH 10.0 because of the zwitterion formation between the choline group and phosphate group. With phosphatidylethanolamine, maximum binding with Ca/P = 0.5 occurs at pH values above 8.5. The weakly basic ethanolamine group becomes uncharged above pH 8.5, and the phosphate group is free to bind calcium. With phosphatidylserine, as the carboxyl group becomes ionized ($pK_a = 3.0$), the net charge becomes -1, and Ca/P reaches 0.5 at pH 4.5. When the serine amino group loses its charge ($pK_a = 8$), the anionic charge of the phospholipid becomes -2 and Ca/P reaches 1.0.

The results with two phosphoinositide preparations are shown in Fig. 13.

The monophosphoinositide prepared as originally described by Hanahan and Olley (1958) binds calcium at low pH with Ca/P = 0.7. This value agrees with the equivalent cation composition of this purified fraction as reported by Hanahan and Olley; it is larger than would be expected for stoichiometric binding with pure monophosphoinositide (Ca/P = 0.5). Thin layer chromatography revealed that there are two components in this preparation (Joos and Carr, 1967), and in view of the binding data which indicated binding in only one pH region, as well as a report of major contamination of phosphoinositides by organic sulfates (Dittmer, 1965), it might be possible that the extra binding is due to a sulfate group.

The middle curve in Fig. 13 was obtained with a commercial inositol phosphatide preparation. Thin-layer chromatography and phosphorus analysis indicated that the substance was 75% triphosphoinositide and 25% phosphatidylserine. By using the Ca^{2+}-binding data presented in Fig. 12, the middle curve in Fig. 13 can be corrected for the contribution of 25% phosphatidylserine. This corrected curve, which is the curve indicated by squares in Fig. 13, would then represent the binding of triphosphoinositide in a phospholipid mixture in which it contributes 75% of the phosphorus. This curve is consistent with an equivalent Ca^{2+}-binding to the diesterified phosphate in the molecule at pH 2 in a manner like that for monophosphoinositide. The binding in the pH range 6.5–8.5 is just what would be predicted for the two monoesterified phosphates on the inositol ring. Thus, it appears that monoesterified phosphate in the molecule will bind calcium only when both protons are dissociated. The observation that monoesterified phosphate will not bind calcium at pH values below the anticipated ionization of the second proton has been reported previously for the phosphoprotein, casein (Carr, 1953; Zittle et al., 1958).

Our results with purified phospholipids are consistent with the anticipated stoichiometric combination of calcium with the net negative charge of the phospholipids. The net charge is a function of the acid dissociation constant for the binding group and the dissociation constant of the cationic partner of a phospholipid zwitterion. On the basis of these results, we have shown that it is possible to identify the individual components in a mixture of phospholipids from the pH–Ca^{2+}-binding profile (Joos and Carr, 1967). In the order of increasing pH, the groups that are responsible for Ca^{2+}-binding are (1) diesterified phosphate in phosphoinositides, (2) phosphatidylserine carboxyl (Abramson et al., 1964), (3) free fatty acid carboxyl, (4) phosphatidylserine phosphate and monoesterified phosphate in phosphoinositides, and phosphatidylethanolamine phosphate. If it is assumed that the magnitude of the binding in a given pH range is a reflection of the stoichiometric combination of calcium with a particular group, these interpretations are also consistent with the proportions of these substances found in the mixtures by means of silicic acid chromatography.

Although phospholipids are monomeric compounds, it is well known that in aqueous systems they exist as large micellar aggregates. The tendency for micelle formation is so great that estimations of their micellar weights and critical micelle concentration are quite uncertain. The micellar weights are at least 10^6, and the critical micelle concentrations are so low as to be undetectable (Robinson, 1960; Abramson et al., 1964). Not very much is known about the structure of these micelles, although there is evidence of a lipid bilayer type of structure in electron micrographs (Bangham and Horne, 1964). We would like to mention at this point that ion-binding data are consistent, at least, with a bilayer structure. Both the hydrogen ion titration curves and other cation-binding results show that all of the charged groups of the phospholipids are readily accessible to the bulk solution for ion exchange. For a minimum micellar weight of 10^6, there must be more than a thousand phospholipid molecules in one micelle. Such a micelle in which all of the charged groups can readily exchange with the medium must have a very open structure. Further, the strength of the divalent cation binding ($K_f \geq 10^4$) indicates a cooperative effect of neighboring charged groups that is similar to that observed with typical polyelectrolytes. Individual phosphate ester groups, even when monoesterified (R—O—PO_3^{2-}) have constants of the order of 10^2 or less with calcium (Schwarzenbach and Anderegg, 1957). Thus, the binding data alone indicate some kind of regular structure with the charged groups near each other and which have easy access to the bulk aqueous phase.

Some data that we have obtained recently indicate that sodium and ethylenediamine compete with calcium for phospholipid binding sites in a manner similar to that for nucleic acids (Carr, 1970). For example, in the presence of 100 mM NaCl, Ca/P for cephalin is reduced from 0.98 to 0.62 when the free calcium is 2.0 mM, and in the presence of 1.5 mM ethylenediamine, Ca/P is reduced from 0.95 to 0.61 when the free calcium is 1.0 mM.

B. Phospholipid–Protein Complexes

Because it has been shown that Ca^{2+}-binding is a sensitive indicator of the electrostatic binding capacity of phospholipids for cations, we considered that the possibility of proteins masking Ca^{2+}-binding sites might provide a method for quantitative studies of the interactions of proteins with phospholipids. Consequently, we have carried out some determinations of the binding of calcium by phospholipid–protein complexes. The results demonstrate the reversible stoichiometric binding of phospholipids with proteins caused by electrostatic interaction of positively charged proteins with negatively charged phospholipids. The strength of the interaction suggests that electrostatic bonding should occur in most lipoproteins.

In Fig. 14 is shown the effect of pH on Ca^{2+}-binding to cephalin and to a cephalin–protamine complex. The complex binding curve seen with cephalin alone reflects stoichiometric binding of calcium to the various charged groups in this phospholipid mixture (Joos and Carr, 1967). The results in Fig. 14 indicate that protamine represses Ca^{2+}-binding to cephalin in the pH range from 2 to 11. The Ca^{2+}-binding competition by protamine is essentially a stoichiometric displacement of calcium by the positive arginine residues in protamine. There is no Ca^{2+} binding to protamine alone over this extensive range of pH.

A similar experiment with a lysozyme–cephalin complex produced similar results. The pH effect is somewhat different in the alkaline range for two reasons. At pH values above 7.0, lysozyme alone binds calcium, and above the isoelectric point of lysozyme (pH 10.5), the masking effect becomes zero.

The competition of lysozyme and protamine for Ca^{2+}-binding with cephalin is shown to be a linear function of protein concentration in Fig.

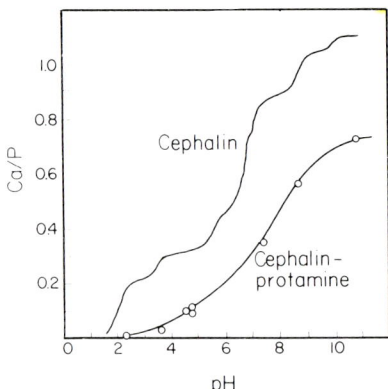

Fig. 14. Binding of Ca^{2+} with animal cephalin in the presence and absence of protamine; 2.6 mM cephalin phosphate, 2.4 meq protamine, 5 mM acetate, and ammonium buffers [*Proc. Soc. Exp. Biol. Med.* **132**, 866 (1969)].

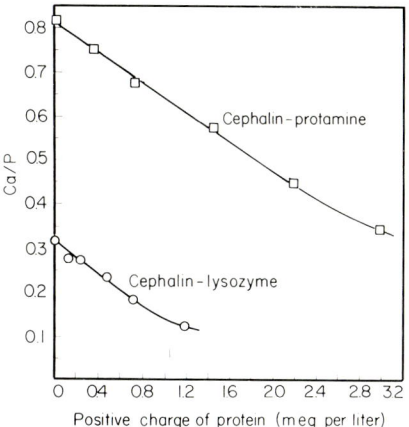

FIG. 15. Competition of increasing amounts of lysozyme and protamine for Ca^{2+} binding sites on phospholipids; □ = protamine, pH 8.8, 2.45 mM cephalin phosphate, 5 mM ammonia buffer; ○ = lysozyme, pH 4.6, 2.6 mM cephalin phosphate [*Proc. Soc. Exp. Biol. Med.* **132**, 867 (1969)].

15. A straight line indicates a porportional displacement of calcium by the proteins. When calculated on the basis of net positive charge on the proteins, the competition is stoichiometric at pH 8.8 for protamine and at pH 4.6 for lysozyme. At higher protein concentrations, there is less than stoichiometric displacement of calcium, which indicates that steric factors hinder protein competition. The results suggest that the net positive charges of the protein will bind stoichiometrically to phospholipids at proper pH and ionic environment when there is an excess of phospholipid anionic groups. Similarly, all negative charges of the phospholipid would be bound to proteins in the presence of a sufficient excess of proteins.

The ability of higher concentrations of free calcium to compete with protamine for cephalin binding sites is shown in Fig. 16. At concentrations below 16 mM free calcium there is a stoichiometric displacement of calcium by the added protamine. However, above 16 mM calcium, protamine is displaced by calcium. Competition studies of this kind enable comparison between the relative binding affinities of various substances. These data indicate a thirtyfold higher concentration of calcium is needed to displace protamine completely from cephalin than is needed to bind maximally to phospholipid alone.

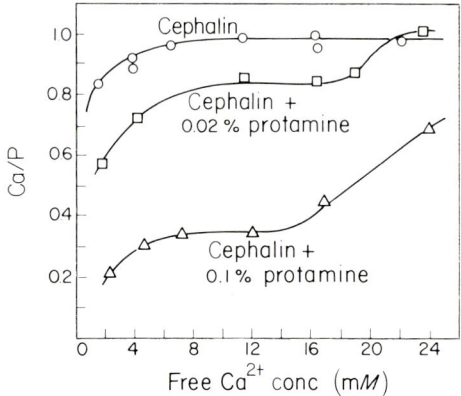

Fig. 16. Effect of Ca^{2+} concentration on protamine binding with cephalin; 2.3 mM cephalin phosphate [*Proc. Soc. Exp. Biol. Med.* **132**, 867 (1969)].

Conclusions and Summary

It is quite evident from studies of Ca^{2+}-binding with nucleic acids and phospholipids that these substances have a high capacity for calcium and a high affinity for calcium. The capacity to bind calcium has been shown to be equivalent to the net anionic charge of these substances. For nucleic acids in the pH range 5.5–9.5, this results in the binding of one calcium for every two nucleotides or two monovalent phosphate groups (Ca/P = 0.5). For phospholipids, the situation varies because there are several types of chemical structures present. Phosphatidylcholine does not bind calcium because its diester phosphate group is neutralized internally by the strongly basic choline group. The phosphatidylethanolamine diester phosphate group will bind calcium above pH 8 when the weakly basic ethanolamine becomes deprotonized. At saturation, Ca/P reaches 0.5. Phosphatidylserine binds one equivalent of calcium above pH 5.0 when the carboxyl group becomes ionized and binds another equivalent above pH 8.5 when the amino group is deprotonized. For this phospholipid, Ca/P = 1.0. Monophosphoinositide binds one equivalent of calcium per molecule because of its diester phosphate group. Triphosphoinositide binds five equivalents per molecule because in addition to a diester phosphate it has 2 monoesterified phosphate groups (Ca/P = 0.83). Thus, for phospholipids, with Ca/P varying from 0.0 to 1.0, the capacity for cation-binding in a phospholipid mixture will depend markedly on the specific composition of the mixture.

The affinity of calcium for nucleic acids and phospholipids is such that when the free calcium is 3–4 mM, there is saturation of the binding sites. Because of competitive effects with other cations, however, saturation of binding sites with calcium is not likely to occur in biological systems, even under the most favorable circumstances. For example, in mammalian extracellular fluid, free calcium is about 1.25 mM, sodium is 140 mM, and magnesium is 0.75 mM. When phospholipids are exposed to such a medium, it can be estimated that the binding of calcium will not be more than about 25% of capacity.

It has been suggested that both the capacity and affinity of the Ca^{2+}-binding process may be involved in certain physiological mechanisms. For example, Kai and Hawthorne (1969) have proposed that hydrolysis of phosphate groups from triphosphoinositide may be a means of controlling sodium and potassium transport across the nerve cell membrane. They suggest that on the hydrolysis of triphosphoinositide by a phosphomonoesterase, calcium is released from the membrane with a resultant increase is permeability. In this instance it is a change in the capacity of the binding agent that would be involved in the regulatory process.

It has also been indicated many times that the relative cation concentrations at the cell membrane may be one of the key factors in regulating the function of the cell membranes (Danielli, 1950; Schoffeniels, 1967). For example, a fixed ratio of $Na^+:Ca^{2+}$ in the extracellular fluid appears to be essential for normal function of the plasma membrane. Competitive binding data show that the level of Ca^{2+}-binding with components of membrane structure is directly affected by changes in the sodium concentration. The affinity for binding is involved in this type of regulatory process, i.e., the effect of concentration changes of small cations in the presence of a binding agent of fixed composition.

The studies of the competitive effects of the polyamines on Ca^{2+}-binding seem to be more pertinent than originally expected. Recently, there has been an increasing awareness of the importance of putrescine (butanediamine), spermidine, and spermine in many biological systems. They have been shown to play a role in growth processes in such diverse systems as bacteria and regenerating liver (Kremzner, 1970). Because of the well recognized affinity of polyamines for nucleic acids, it has been speculated that this type of interaction in particular may be the primary mechanism by which they exert their effects. We would make the further speculation that for such a mechanism, calcium and magnesium will also be involved through their competition for binding sites.

The study of Ca^{2+}-binding with polymeric complexes appears to be a useful approach to studying the structure of such complexes. With isolated nuclei, it has been shown that a quantitative coulombic interaction between nucleic acid phosphate and protein amino groups is a major factor involved in nuclear stability. On the other hand, in *E. coli* ribosomes, stability and biological function are maintained in the absence of such coulombic interactions.

With phospholipids, the binding data indicate that their micellar structure is such that all of the anionic groups are readily accessible to the bulk solution. The binding affinity also indicates that these groups are close together in an orderly arrangement allowing a considerably enhanced electrostatic effect. A structure of bimolecular layers which is seen in electron micrographs of phospholipids is consistent with the binding data.

Finally, our data indicate that lipoprotein complexes do involve coulombic interactions between negative phospholipids and positive proteins, although other types of interaction are also involved. The data for the competitive binding of calcium and protein with phospholipids suggest that one or more biological functions may be controlled by coupling of changes in pH and calcium concentration.

ACKNOWLEDGMENTS

The work of the authors was supported by research grants HE 01618, GM 08412, and 1RO1-AM-133300 from the National Institutes of Health, U.S. Public Health Service. The authors wish to acknowledge the permission of the editors and publishers of *Biochimica et Biophysica Acta, Journal of Molecular Biology*, and *Proceedings of the Society for Experimental Biology and Medicine* to reproduce figures 2, and 4–16 which appear in original articles in those journals.

REFERENCES

Abdul-Nour, B., and Webster, G. C. (1960). *Exp. Cell Res.* **20,** 226.
Abramson, M. B., Katzman, R., and Gregor, H. P. (1964). *J. Biol. Chem.* **239,** 70.
Abramson, M. B., Katzman, R., Gregor, H. P., and Curci, R. (1966). *Biochemistry* **5,** 2207.
Banerjee, K. C., and Perkins, D. J. (1962). *Biochim. Biophys. Acta* **61,** 1.
Bangham, A. D., and Horne, R. W. (1964). *J. Mol. Biol.* **8,** 660.
Bonner, J., and Ts'o, P. (1964). "Nucleohistones," Holden-Day, San Francisco, California, 1964.
Carr, C. W. (1953). *Arch. Biochem. Biophys.* **46,** 424.
Carr, C. W. (1970). Unpublished results.
Chang, K. Y., and Carr, C. W. (1961). *Abstr. Pap. 1st Meet., Amer. Soc. Cell Biol.* p. 30.
Chang, K. Y., and Carr, C. W. (1962). *Abstr. Pap., 2nd Meet., Amer. Soc. Cell Biol.* p. 31.
Chang, K. Y., and Carr, C. W. (1968). *Biochim. Biophys. Acta* **157,** 127.
Choi, Y. S., and Carr, C. W. (1967). *J. Mol. Biol.* **25,** 331.
Cox, R. A., and Littauer, U. Z. (1963). *Biochim. Biophys. Acta* **72,** 188.

Cox, R. A., and Peacocke, A. R. (1956). *J. Chem. Soc., London* p. 2499.
Cox, R. A., Jones, A. S., Marsh, G. E., and Peacocke, A. R. (1956). *Biochim. Biophys. Acta* **21**, 576.
Danielli, J. F. (1950). "Cell Physiology and Pharmacology," Elsevier, Amsterdam.
Dittmer, J. (1965). *Biochim. Biophys. Acta* **106**, 425.
Eichhorn, G. L. (1962). *Nature London* **194**, 474.
Feldman, I., and Keil, E. (1965). *J. Amer. Chem. Soc.* **87**, 3281.
Felsenfeld, G. (1962). "The Molecular Basis of Neoplasia," p. 104. Univ. of Texas Press, Austin.
Felsenfeld, G., and Huang, S. (1959). *Biochim. Biophys. Acta* **34**, 234.
Felsenfeld, G., and Huang, S. (1960). *Biochim. Biophys. Acta* **370** 425.
Fiske, C. H., and SubbaRow, Y. (1929). *J. Biol. Chem.* **81**, 629.
Hanahan, D. J., and Olley, J. M. (1958). *J. Biol. Chem.* **231**, 813.
Hendrickson, H. S. (1969). *Ann. N.Y. Acad. Sci.* **165**, 668.
Hendrickson, H. S., and Fullington, J. G. (1965). *Biochemistry* **4**, 1599.
Hoppe, J. A., and Morales, M. (1966). *J. Amer. Chem. Soc.* **88**, 2077.
Joos, R. W., and Carr, C. W. (1967). *Proc. Soc. Exp. Biol. Med.* **124**, 1268.
Joos, R. W., and Carr, C. W. (1969). *Proc. Soc. Exp. Biol. Med.* **132**, 865.
Jordan, D. O. (1960). "The Chemistry of Nucleic Acids," Butterworth, London.
Kai, M., and Hawthorne, J. N. (1969). *Ann. N.Y. Acad. Sci.* **165**, 761.
Kremzner, L. (1970). *Fed. Proc., Fed. Amer. Soc. Exp. Biol.* **29**, 1560.
Lawley, P. D. (1956). *Biochim. Biophys. Acta* **21**, 481.
Lyons, J. W., and Kotin, L. (1964). *J. Amer. Chem. Soc.* **86**, 3634.
Lyons, J. W., and Kotin, L. (1965). *J. Amer. Chem. Soc.* **87**, 1781.
Mahler, H. R., and Mehrota, B. D. (1962). *Biochim. Biophys. Acta* **55**, 252.
Mandel, M. (1962). *J. Mol. Biol.* **5**, 435.
Mitchell, J. S. (1960). "The Cell Nucleus," Butterworth, London.
Robinson, N. (1960). *Trans. Faraday Soc.* **56**, 1260.
Rojas, E., and Tobias, J. M. (1965). *Biochim. Biophys. Acta* **94**, 394.
Schoffeniels, E. (1967). "Cellular Aspects of Membrane Permeability," Chapter 7. Pergamon, Oxford.
Schwarzenbach, G., and Anderegg, G. (1957). *Helv. Chim. Acta* **40**, 1229.
Shack, J., Jenkins, R. J., and Thompsett, J. M. (1953). *J. Biol. Chem.* **203**, 373.
Shah, D. O., and Schulman, J. H. (1965). *J. Lipid Res.* **6**, 341.
Sobel, A. E., and Hanok, A. (1951). *Proc. Soc. Exp. Biol. Med.* **77**, 737.
Tabor, H. (1962). *Biochemistry* **1**, 496.
Tissieres, A., Schlessinger, D., and Gros, F. (1960). *Proc. Nat. Acad. Sci. U.S.* **46**, 1450.
Vendrely, R., Knoblauch-Mazen, A., and Vendrely, C. (1960). *In* "The Cell Nucleus," (J. S. Mitchell, ed.), p. 200. Butterworth, London.
Wiberg, J. S., and Newman, W. F. (1957). *Arch. Biochem. Biophys.* **72**, 66.
Zittle, C. A., Della Monica, E. S., Rudd, R. K., and Custer, J. H. (1958). *Arch. Biochem. Biophys.* **76**, 342 (1958).

Discussion

Dr. Martonosi: The titration curve of phosphatidylcholine was reasonably normal in character in the region of pH 8. On the other hand, with phosphatidylethanolamine there was a sharp rise from practically zero at pH 7.9 to a maximum value of around 8. Why the difference?

Second, several reports in the literature on the condensing effects of calcium on lecithin monolayers indicate calcium binding. Dr. Carr, I wonder what is the reason that, by your direct measurements, calcium binding is not apparent, contrary to the studies with monolayers.

Dr. Carr: Phosphatidylethanolamine, in the presence of calcium, forms a coagulum. We think this yields the steep curve, as compared with the smoother curve in a completely dispersed system.

With regard to the question about comparing monolayers with the equilibrium dialysis data, I do not have a good explanation for the difference.

Dr. Wuthier: I was wondering if you had studied competition between magnesium and calcium in the phospholipid binding studies.

Dr. Carr: No. We have done competitive binding studies with sodium, and the data are similar to those obtained with nucleic acid.

Dr. Cotmore: We found that magnesium ions would compete with calcium ions for binding sites on phospholipid molecules when the magnesium concentration was in excess of physiological values. Calcium ions (1 mM) in the presence of 0.1 M KCl or NaCl bound to certain purified phosphoglycerides, but not to lecithin. Dervichian [D. G. Dervichian, *in* "Biochemical Problems of Lipids" (G. Popjak and E. Le Breton, eds.), pp. 3–13. Wiley (Interscience), New York, 1956] and Kimizuka *et al.* [H. Kimizuka, T. Nakahara, H. Uejō, and A. Yamauchi, *Biochim. Biophys. Acta* **137**, 549 (1967)] have described this type of binding in detail.

Dr. Vincenzi: I was a little surprised at your use of extracellular fluid as a model. I might have expected you to use intracellular fluid, where free calcium is probably less than 10^{-5} M. Could you comment on the significance of your binding data, Dr. Carr, to intracellular events?

Dr. Carr: We don't know intracellular concentrations sufficiently well to even make an estimate of what the competitive effects would be. We must certainly look more closely, not only at concentrations, but at the activities of the ions in intracellular fluid.

Dr. Nichols: Dr. Carr, the question that intrigued me about your binding studies was whether you can displace proteins with calcium, as you do calcium with protein? There are some people who are beginning to think this could be a mechanism for the action of some hormones, particularly parathyroid hormone.

Dr. Carr: I am not familiar with those particular theories, but we have speculated that such competition could very well be a normal physiological mechanism where, not only calcium, but pH and calcium together would contribute to such a regulatory mechanism.

Dr. H. M. Myers: In your work with the undenatured DNA, is it possible that the reason that the positively charged molecules had an effect on calcium binding was that there was a denaturing effect on DNA that resulted in a change in its configuration and therefore its capacity to bind calcium?

Dr. Carr: Are you implying that the denatured DNA does not bind calcium?

Dr. H. M. Myers: If there were a change in configuration, the required spatial arrangement, which you mentioned as being a triangle, would not be present.

Dr. Carr: Other studies by us with denatured DNA, which are not published, show that it still has a similar capacity for calcium binding. With regard to polyvalent cations denaturing DNA, the work that has been done in this area indicates that at least divalent cations stabilize DNA, rather than cause its unwinding. With respect to the highly cationic materials, we cannot explain their effect.

CHEMICAL STRUCTURE OF BONE SIALOPROTEIN AND A PRELIMINARY STUDY OF ITS CALCIUM-BINDING PROPERTIES

*G. M. Herring, A. T. deB. Andrews, and A. R. Chipperfield**

The isolation and composition of bone sialoprotein (BSP) were first reported by Herring and Kent in 1961. Since then, a number of papers concerning its chemical and physical properties have been published. BSP was the first of the bone glycoproteins to be prepared as a homogeneous component in the investigations of the noncollagenous organic constitutents which began about 12 years ago. The purpose of these studies was to find substances which might be responsible for the binding of radioactive isotopes such as yttrium-90, plutonium, and americium in bone, where their distribution does not follow normal calcification patterns. The histochemical finding of a positive reaction to the periodic acid–Schiff technique in these sites of uptake pointed to the possible presence of glycoproteins (Vaughan, 1956; Jowsey *et al.*, 1956; Williamson and Vaughan, 1964). These ions do not, of course, occur normally in the body, and it might be expected that there should be a more physiological role for glycoproteins in bone. For this reason, calcium-binding studies have recently been undertaken.

* Supported by the U. K. Atomic Energy Authority under contract No. EMR 1926.

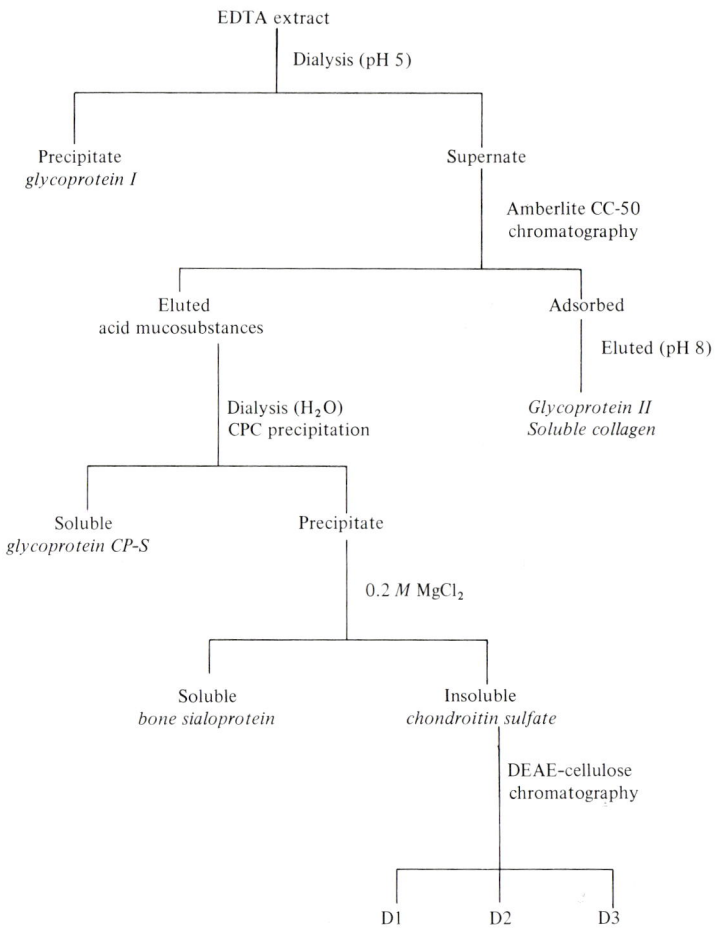

FIG. 1. The isolation of soluble macromolecules from bovine cortical bone; CPC = cetylpyridinium chloride.

Isolation of Bone Sialoprotein

Bovine cortical bone has been used in these studies, since it is a readily available material, it has a relatively low vascular and cellular content, and it can be easily freed from extraneous tissues. Full details of the extraction fractionation procedures have been published (Herring, 1964a, 1968), but a brief description is given here (Fig. 1). In order to achieve efficient decalcification, it was found essential to pulverize the bone to a powder, this being achieved in a liquid nitrogen-cooled mill. The resulting material was treated with a solution of the sodium salts of ethylenediaminetetraacetic acid (EDTA) at pH 7.5. Besides demineralizing the bone, the EDTA solubilizes 4–6% of the organic phase. From earlier studies it was clear that these extracts contained a complex mixture of macromolecules. Dialysis of the extract at pH 5 to remove calcium, phosphate, and EDTA resulted in a precipitate designated glycoprotein I. The supernate was subjected to chromatography on a column of Amberlite CG–50 ion exchange resin which retained soluble collagen and the glycoprotein II fraction. The more acidic substances were eluted at pH 5 and could be separated by cetylpyridinium chloride (CPC) fractionation (Scott, 1960) into three distinct components: (1) protein-bound chondroitin sulfate, (2) the acidic glycoprotein bone sialoprotein (BSP), and (3) another acidic glycoprotein (CP-S) which was soluble in 1% CPC. After repeated precipitations with CPC under the same conditions, as shown in Fig. 1, homogeneous BSP was obtained on electrophoresis and ultracentrifugation.

Composition of BSP

In several respects, BSP is unusual as a glycoprotein, particularly in its high content of sialic acid, the presence of both glucosamine and galactosamine, and the large number of acidic amino acids (Herring and Kent, 1963; Herring, 1964a; Andrews et al., 1967). About 40% of the molecule consists of carbohydrate residues (Table I) of which sialic acid predominates. The content of this sugar has varied considerably in different preparations from 14.3 to 20.5% by weight of BSP. However, most of the structural studies described here were performed on a preparation with the highest sialic acid content, and a fraction obtained by phosphate extraction at pH 8, which was studied at the same time, was closely similar in analytical composition (Andrews and Herring, 1965). Both N-acetyl- and N-glycollylneuraminic acid were identified after liberation by mild acid hydrolysis or by treatment with neuraminidase; therefore, these are probably located terminally on the molecule. Liberation of 82% of the fucose, but only 16% of the hexose, by hydrolysis in 0.1 N H_2SO_4 at 100°C for 8 hours suggested that fucose also occupies a terminal position. When BSP was treated with 0.2 N NaOH at 100°C for 2 hours, the recovery of nondiffusible hexose was 87.4%, which indicated that the linkage between carbohydrate and protein was most likely of the glycosylamine type.

Further information on the structure of the carbohydrate moiety was obtained from periodate oxidation studies (Andrews et al., 1969). The terminal positions of sialic acid and fucose were confirmed, and it was found

TABLE I

Composition of Bone Sialoprotein (BSP)[a]

Component	Composition	
	Percent by weight[a]	Mole per mole BSP
N-Acetylneuraminic acid	18.4	13.7
N-Glycollylneuraminic acid	2.1	1.5
Galactose	8.2	10.5
Mannose	2.5	3.1
Fucose	0.7	1.0
Glucosamine	4.6	5.9
Galactosamine	4.6	5.9
Phosphate	1.4	3.4
Lysine	1.59	2.52
Histidine	0.74	1.07
Arginine	0.76	1.04
Cysteic acid	0.81	1.10
Aspartic acid	8.80	15.20
Threonine	5.02	9.70
Serine	3.20	7.00
Glutamic acid	12.80	20.09
Proline	2.15	4.27
Glycine	3.49	10.71
Alanine	1.36	3.51
Valine	1.38	2.71
Isoleucine	1.25	2.19
Leucine	1.43	2.53
Phenylalanine	0.72	1.00
Tyrosine	1.54	1.95
Tryptophan	0.87	0.98
Ammonia	0.93	12.55

[a] Percentages are expressed in terms of dry weight of BSP [precipitated as the zinc salt (1.4% Zn)], the molecular weight of which is taken to be 23,000.

that one mannose and nine of the ten galactose residues were next in sequence. At the next degradation stage, one mannose, three glucosamine, and six galactosamine units were destroyed, leaving an inner core of one galactose, one mannose, and three glucosamine residues. Further oxidation steps left only glucosamine, which probably links the carbohydrate moiety to the peptide chain through a glycosylamine bond to asparagine. The conclusion that all the carbohydrate is contained in a single highly branched group with one linkage to the protein chain, was supported by studies using pronase digestion of BSP, in which glycopeptides containing most of the carbohydrate but only a few amino acids were produced. A tentative structure indicated by these results is shown in Fig. 2.

The polypeptide chain of BSP is unusual in containing over 40% (thirty-five out of eighty-nine residues) of the acidic amino acids. Glycine, serine, and threonine are also present in relatively large amounts, but the twelve other amino acids account for only a further twenty-six residues. Only seven of the acidic amino acid carboxyl side chains appeared to be blocked by amide groups (Peacocke and Williams, 1967). The presence of this large proportion of free carboxyl groups on the polypeptide chain accounts for the acidic nature of the molecule, even when the sialic acid residues are removed. No free N-terminal amino group could be detected by the usual procedures, but glycopeptides obtained by proteolytic digestion of BSP did react with fluorodinitrobenzene. This indicated that carbohydrate substitution of the N-terminal residue was very unlikely. The phosphate groups which amounted to 2.2–3.8 moles per mole of BSP (Andrews and Herring, 1965) are thought to occur as the esters of serine.

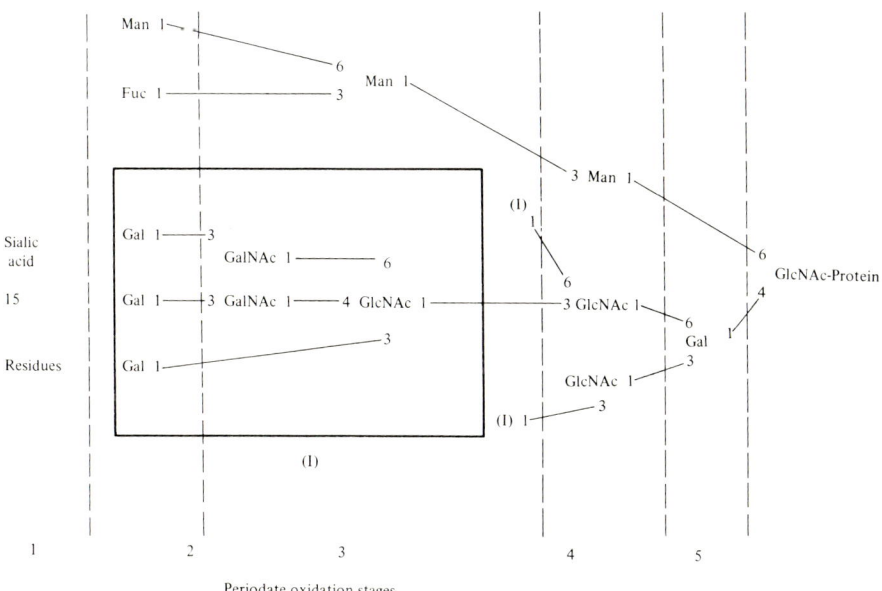

Fig. 2. Possible structure of the carbohydrate prosthetic group of BSP, as suggested from the results of the Smith periodate degradation procedure.

TABLE II

Values of Formation Constants (K_f) and Affinity or Exchange Parameters (K_p) for Calcium Complexes

Calcium complex	K_f	K_p
Bone sialoprotein	82.5 ± 22.2	2.26 ± 0.68
Bone chondroitin sulfate	26.8 ± 7.3	0.65 ± 0.18
Shark chondroitin sulfate	36.8 ± 6.1	0.88 ± 0.14
Polyglutamic acid	79.7 ± 26.5	1.69 ± 0.71

The inhibition of calcium phosphate precipitation was studied using the method of DiSalvo and Schubert (1967). Solutions containing varying amounts (0–1 mg/ml) of BSP or chondroitin sulfate fraction were mixed with solutions of calcium chloride and potassium dihydrogen phosphate buffered at pH 7.8, and the mixture allowed to stand for 20 hours at 25°C. The solution was centrifuged at 700 g for 10 minutes to give a calcium phosphate precipitate, R1, and the supernate was then centrifuged at 100,000 g for 30 minutes to give a further precipitate, R2. The reduction in the amount of phosphate in R1 was used as a measure of inhibition of precipitation. A 50% reduction in precipitation was obtained with 0.43 ± 0.04 mg/ml of BSP (mean value of seven experiments), and in the case of the bone chondroitin sulfate–protein complex, this value was 0.59 ± 0.08 mg/ml (eight experiments). Bone chondroitin sulfate which had all protein removed by alkaline hydrolysis, on the other hand, showed no inhibition up to a concentration of 0.91 mg/ml, whereas inhibition was virtually total in the presence of the other two fractions at this concentration. A finding of some interest was that at low concentrations (0.18–0.36 mg/ml) the BSP was largely in the R1 precipitate, and at higher concentrations (0.54–0.73 mg/ml) was distributed between R2 and the final supernate, S. This contrasts with the bone chondroitin sulfate–protein complex, most of which remained in S, as was found for the cartilage protein–polysaccharide by DiSalvo and Schubert (1967), and suggests that there may be some specific association between BSP and the microcrystals of calcium phosphate, under these conditions.

Conclusion

At present, any suggestions concerning the function of bone sialoprotein are very speculative. It would be difficult to prove conclusively that BSP is a specific component of bone and not found in any other tissues. However, we have been unable to detect it in the serum proteins (Herring, 1964a) or in tendon (Herring, 1969). A similar substance is the sialoglycoprotein isolated from dentin, another calcified tissue (Zamoscianyk and Veis, 1966).

It has been suggested by Eylar (1965) that since most glycoproteins are extracellular, the function of the bound carbohydrate may be to act as a chemical label which facilitates the passage of the protein through the cell membrane. Marsden (1969) has proposed that secretion of glycoproteins and acid mucopolysaccharides involves essentially the movement of highly negatively charged molecules from the cell. To maintain overall neutrality, cations must leave the cell simultaneously, and the type of cation will depend upon the function of the cell. The presence of carbohydrate may also enhance the solubility of the protein. This might be important in the case of metal-binding proteins where substitution of the majority of the ionizable groups could cause precipitation. These properties, together with the high capacity for metal ion binding of BSP, would seem to fit it well for a role in the transport of calcium ions from the cell. Alternatively, from the inhibition studies it appears that in the presence of BSP, calcium, and phosphate could move simultaneously from the cell without aggregation of the microcrystalline or amorphous calcium phosphate taking place prematurely. It may be supposed that the removal of BSP at a later time would then facilitate crystal growth. Recent results of Pugliarello et al. (1970) are perhaps relevant here. Their results can be interpreted as demonstrating that the noncollagenous protein, which is apparently present in large amounts in osteoid, disappears progressively as mineral is being laid down. BSP would not necessarily be specific among the other glycoproteins which would be taking part in this hypothetical process.

There are, of course, other possible functions for BSP and the other glycoproteins in bone; the classic "local factor" in nucleation is one possibility, and a protective action as a cell "coat" is another. However, from the properties as they are so far known, it is evident that they are capable, at least, of providing a carefully balanced system for the control of mineralization.

REFERENCES

Andrews, A. T. deB., and Herring, G. M. (1965). *Biochim. Biophys. Acta* **101**, 239.
Andrews, A. T. deB., Herring, G. M., and Kent, P. W. (1967). *Biochem. J.* **104**, 705.
Andrews, A. T. deB., Herring, G. M., and Kent, P. W. (1969). *Biochem. J.* **111**, 621.
Chipperfield, A. R. (1970). *Biochem. J.* **118**, 36P.
Chipperfield, A. R., and Taylor, D. M. (1968). *Nature (London)* **219**, 609.
Chipperfield, A. R., and Taylor, D. M. (1970). Unpublished results.

II. Role of Calcium in Membrane Structure and Integrity

THE BIIONIC ACTION POTENTIAL AND INDISPENSABILITY OF DIVALENT CATIONS IN THE EXTERNAL MEDIUM FOR NERVE EXCITATION

Akira Watanabe and Ichiji Tasaki

Introduction

In classic theories of nervous excitation, the importance of calcium ions has clearly been recognized (see, e.g., Heilbrunn, 1952; Frankenhaeuser and Hodgkin, 1957). In recent years, however, the emphasis has been placed on the roles played by univalent cations, and divalent cations are regarded as agents which modify permeability changes of the membrane toward sodium and potassium ions. In the course of experiments designed to elucidate the physicochemical mechanisms of excitation phenomena, we have arrived at the conclusion that the role of divalent cations in the external medium of an excitable cell is even more significant than that played by univalent cations.

We now believe that the process of nerve excitation is associated with a physicochemical change of the membrane macromolecules, and this change is triggered by an ion exchange reaction involving univalent and divalent cations in the membrane. Experimentally, the existence of divalent cations in the outside medium appears to be essential for maintaining excitability in almost all the excitable tissues examined, whereas univalent cations in the external medium are, in many excitable tissues, dispensable. (Univalent cations may and often do influence the shape and size of the action potential.) In this article, the experimental evidence which has led us to the above conclusions will be reviewed. A brief description will also be made of a series of fluorescence experiments which have been done more recently and which will serve to specify what kind of physicochemical changes are taking place in the plasma membrane during excitation.

Intracellular Perfusion of the Squid Giant Axon

In 1961, the intracellular perfusion technique was invented by Baker, Hodgkin, and Shaw in England, and by Oikawa, Spyropoulos, Tasaki, and

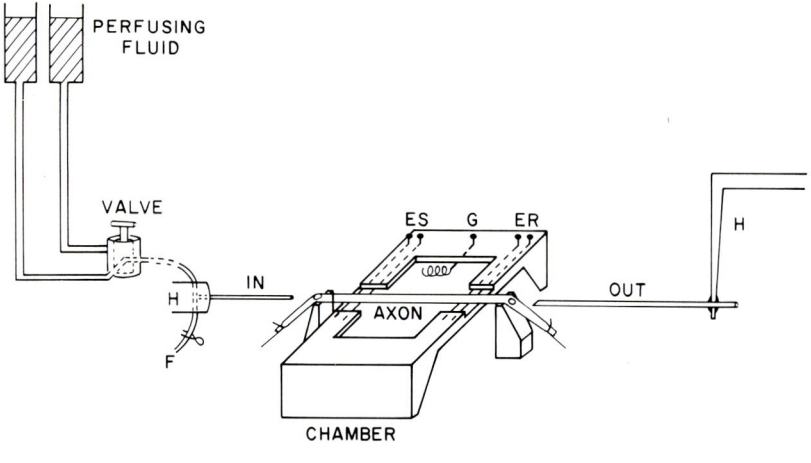

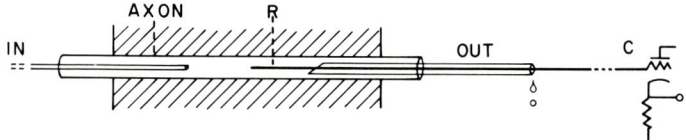

FIG. 1. The experimental setup used for intracellular perfusion of squid giant axons. *Top:* Entire experimental arrangement: (H) holders for inlet (in) and outlet (out) pipettes—these pipettes are moved by the use of micromanipulators; (ES) a pair of platinum wire electrodes used for external stimulation; (G) a wire electrode for grounding the external fluid medium; (ER) a platinum wire electrode used for external recording of conducted nerve impulses. *Bottom:* Pipettes and electrodes inside the squid giant axon: (R) an intracellular recording electrode; (C) an amplifier with a high impedance input stage. Further explanation is in the text. (From Tasaki, 1968.)

Teorell in America. One might say that introduction of this technique marked the beginning of a new era in the field of research on nerve excitation. The biionic action potential and many other important excitation phenomena could be explored only with the help of this technique.

Figure 1 shows the experimental setup used in our perfusion experiments. In a nerve chamber made of Lucite, a squid giant axon with a diameter of 400–700 μ is mounted horizontally. The axon is immersed in either artificial or natural seawater in the chamber. Two glass pipettes are inserted longitudinally through openings made at each end of the axon. Two side pieces are used for the purpose of raising the axon so that the axon does not make direct contact with the bottom surface of the experimental chamber. One of the glass pipettes (in) serves as the inlet for the perfusion fluid and has a diameter of about 150 μ; it is connected to reservoirs of the intracellular perfusing fluid by polyethylene tubing and a switching valve. Another glass pipette (out), which serves as the outlet, has a diameter of about 300 μ. The intracellular perfusion fluid is introduced into the axon through the inlet pipette. The fluid flows through the interior of the axon and is drained through the outlet pipette. A continuous flow of the perfusion fluid is maintained by raising the reservoir above the level of the axon by about 30–100 cm. The flow rate is maintained usually at a level between 10 and 30 mm^3 per minute. Switching of the perfusion fluid is carried out by using the valve. When stopper F shown in the figure is removed, the fluid in the inlet system can be replaced with another new solution very quickly; when the stopper is replaced, the new perfusing fluid starts flowing inside the axon.

Effects of Calcium Ions inside the Axon

The divalent cations are extremely poisonous when they are applied intracellularly (Tasaki *et al.*, 1962, 1967). Figure 2 shows the result of one experiment in which the effect of intracellular perfusion fluid containing 3 mM of calcium ions was examined. Perfusion with this calcium-containing solution brought about a decrease in the membrane resistance of about 20%. There was a corresponding decrease in the time constant of development of an electrotonic potential in response to an anodal current pulse. The amplitude of the action potential was also decreased during intracellular perfusion with a calcium-containing solution, and there was a progressive, irreversible decrease in the resting potential. When the calcium concentration inside the axon exceeded 5 mM, an irreversible loss of excitability was observed.

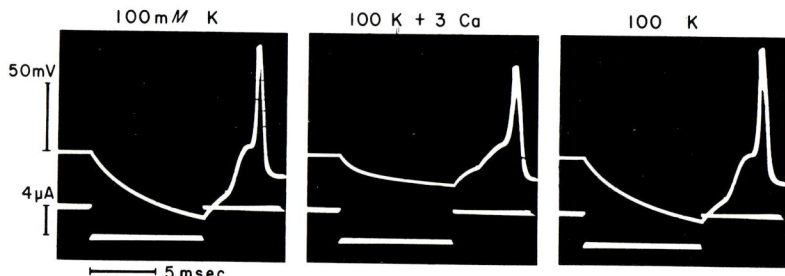

Fig. 2. Effects of calcium ions introduced into the interior of a squid giant axon. External medium contained 450 mM NaCl and 100 mM CaCl$_2$. The composition of the internal fluid is indicated on the top of each figure. The tonicity of the internal solution was maintained with glycerol. The upper oscillograph trace shows the membrane potential; the lower trace, the polarizing current. Following termination of a hyperpolarizing current pulse, a brief depolarizing current pulse was applied to the axon to evoke an action potential. (From Tasaki et al., 1967.)

Such a strong adverse effect of calcium ions was not observed when they were applied externally. Usually an increase in the outside calcium concentration stabilizes the membrane potential, and an adverse effect would never be observed at least up to 100 mM. The membrane reacts very differently to calcium ions, depending on whether they are applied internally or externally. This indicates that the axon membrane is not homogeneous in the radial direction. The axonal membrane must have at least two distinct layers. All theoretical treatments of membrane phenomena which assume that the membrane is uniform in the direction normal to the surface can thus lead to erroneous conclusions.

The Biionic Action Potential

OBJECTIVE OF THE EXPERIMENTS

Even in the inanimate membrane, a general theoretical treatment of the membrane potential or of fluxes is not a simple problem. In a membrane system involving more than two mobile ion species, a simple solution of the flux equation is possible only when the co-ion flux can be neglected and all counter ions have the same valence (Helfferich, 1962). The natural ionic environment of the squid giant axon is far more complicated than such an inanimate system. In the series of experiments to be described in this section, our objective has been to clarify excitability phenomena in the squid axon membrane by investigating the process of action protential production under the simplest possible ionic environments.

To maintain excitability in squid giant axons, the presence of divalent cations in the external medium is essential. Under the conditions of intracellular perfusion, the presence of free Ca^{2+} in the axon interior is detrimental to the axon. Because of these restrictions, we decided to analyze excitation processes under biionic conditions, i.e., under the condition in which only two cations are involved in action potential production. If we introduce a calcium solution outside the axon, for example, and a cesium phosphate solution inside the cell, there are only two cations (i.e., counterions) in the system. We found that excitability of the axon can be maintained under these conditions. The action potential elicited under these conditions is called the biionic action potential.

Experimental Procedure

It is known that the survival time of intracellularly perfused axons is critically influenced by the anions in the intracellular perfusing fluid (Tasaki et al., 1965a). Fluoride and phosphate are the most favorable anions in the axon interior. To demonstrate biionic action potential, we have used these two anions almost exclusively. It is also necessary that the ionic strength of the perfusing fluid be kept at a low level. We have usually used the concentration of less than 50 mM. The tonicity of the media inside and outside the axon is maintained by adding glycerol. When solutions with higher ionic strengths are used, we found it more difficult to demonstrate and to maintain biionic action potentials. This situation created another technical problem. The axoplasm inside the cell forms a rather rigid gel. When a perfusing fluid with a low ionic strength flows through the interior of an axon, the axoplasm swells; consequently, it is difficult to maintain flow of intracellular perfusing fluid under these conditions. To overcome this difficulty, it is imperative that the axoplasm be removed almost completely beforehand. This has been achieved by the use of a proteolytic enzyme, pronase. At the initial stage of perfusion, we perfused the axon with a solution containing pronase (0.05 mg/ml) for about 1.5 minutes. Then the perfusing fluid was switched to an enzyme-free solution. This procedure removes the axoplasm very efficiently, as will be seen in Fig. 3. For further detail of the morphology of axons treated with proteases, see Takenaka et al. (1969).

Two intracellular electrodes were inserted through the outlet pipette. For stimulation, a 50 μ platinum wire electrode was used. This electrode also served to equalize the electric potential throughout the perfusion zone. For

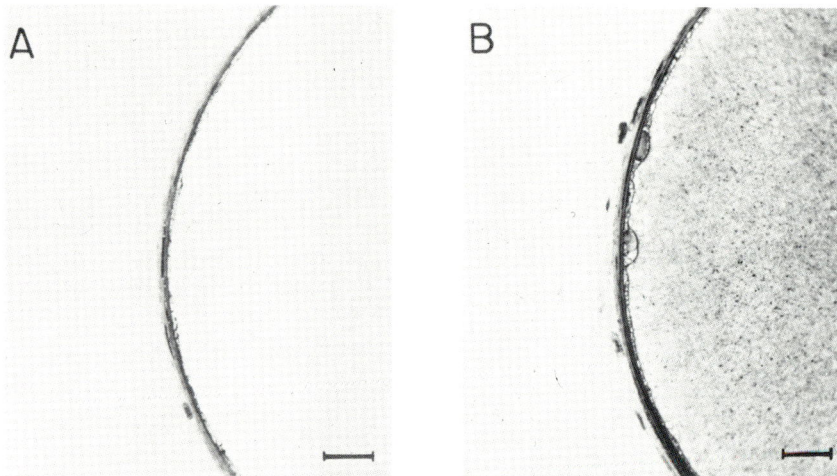

Fig. 3. Photomicrographs of a part of cross-section of a squid giant axon. (A) The axoplasm was removed by perfusion with potassium fluoride solution containing a small amount of pronase; the shape and amplitude of the action potential recorded immediately before fixation of this axon with glutaraldehyde were perfectly normal. (B) An axon fixed without intracellular perfusion. The bars indicate 25 μ. (From Tasaki, 1968.)

recording the membrane potential, a glass pipette electrode filled with 0.6 M KCl–agar gel was inserted. The tip of the recording electrode was placed at the center of the perfusion zone. The length of the perfusion zone was usually between 12 and 20 mm. The external recording electrode was a calomel half cell.

In the following experiments, we maintained a continuous flow of the external medium. The technique employed was simple. Reservoirs of the external fluid media were connected to the nerve chamber by means of polyethylene tubings. The supply of the fluid to the chamber was maintained by raising one of the reservoirs above the chamber. Removal of the fluid was accomplished by using a suction tubing connected to an aspirator.

GENERAL DESCRIPTION OF THE PROPERTIES OF BIIONIC ACTION POTENTIALS

Under continuous internal perfusion with a solution containing phosphate or fluoride salts of various univalent cations and external perfusion with a solution of chloride salt of alkaline earth cations, a squid giant axon produces all-or-none action potentials. The ability of such an axon to produce biionic action potentials can be maintained for more than 2 hours under proper experimental conditions. Therefore, production of biionic action potentials can not be regarded as a transient phenomenon which takes place during the course of deterioration of a normal axon.

The amplitude of the action potential depends on the concentration and ionic species of perfusates inside and outside the axon. It is usually between 50 and 130 mV. The duration of the action potential is generally long. The action potential observed under these biionic conditions has a sharp initial peak, followed by a long-lasting plateau. Termination of the action potential is fairly abrupt. The time course of these action potentials resemble that of cardiac muscle fibers of vertebrates or of crustacean muscle fibers treated by tetraalkylammonium ion. When a biionic action potential is initiated, there is a decrease in the membrane resistance. The decrease is more profound at the initial phase of the action potential. There is a gradual recovery of the membrane resistance during the plateau of the action potential.

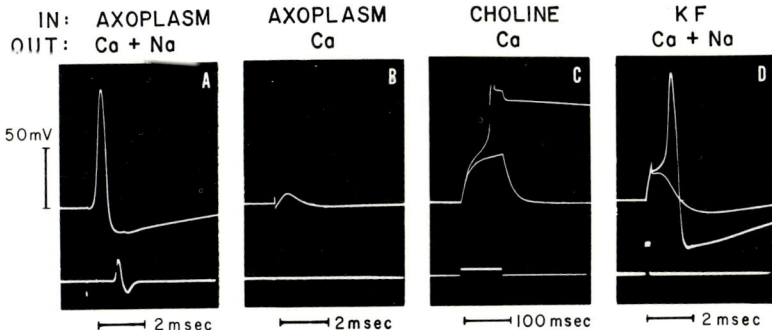

FIG. 4. Demonstration of reversibility of the state of the squid axon membrane following production of a biionic action potential. Records A and B were taken before intracellular perfusion. In A, the external medium contained 300 mM NaCl and 100 mM CaCl$_2$. The upper oscillograph trace shows an action potential recorded internally. The lower oscillograph trace shows a conducted response recorded externally at one end of the axon. Stimuli were applied at the other end of the axon externally. In B, the external medium contained 100 mM CaCl$_2$ and glycerol, but no univalent cations; no action potential was observed. Records C and D were obtained under intracellular perfusion. The upper oscillograph trace indicates the membrane potential recorded internally. The lower trace shows the time course of stimulating current pulses. Two records with sub- and suprathreshold current pulses are superimposed to show the all-or-none behavior of the action potential. In C, the external medium was the same as in B, but the internal medium was a solution containing 25 mM choline phosphate and glycerol. A biionic action potential is seen. Record D was obtained with a mixture of 300 mM NaCl and 100 mM CaCl$_2$ externally and a 400 mM KF solution internally. An action potential with a "normal" size and shape is seen. (From Tasaki et al., 1969c.)

After demonstration of biionic action potentials, it is possible to obtain a typical "normal" action potential by switching the internal and external perfusion solutions to those which are similar in ionic composition to axoplasm and seawater, respectively. Therefore, it is safe to conclude that the alteration of the axon membrane brought about by the biionic environment is reversible (Fig. 4).

Effects of Varying the Composition of the External Perfusion Fluid

For the external solution, we usually used the chloride salt of alkaline earth cations. Bromide was almost as favorable as chloride in producing biionic action potentials. Ethyl sulfate is considered an impermeant anion; this anion gave rise to equally good biionic action potentials. Thus, variation of the external anion species does not have any clear effect on the process of production of the biionic action potential.

Calcium appeared to be the most favorable external cation; most experiments described here were made with calcium. When Ca^{2+} in the external medium was completely replaced with magnesium, excitability of the axon was suppressed reversibly. By adding calcium to the magnesium solution, excitability was promptly restored. Strontium and barium could substitute for calcium to some extent. With cesium internally, strontium was almost as favorable as calcium; but with choline internally, strontium gave rise to smaller action potentials than calcium. Barium did not substitute for calcium effectively; in a medium containing barium as the sole cation species, the amplitude of the action potential was always smaller than those obtained with either calcium or strontium externally.

The external Ca^{2+} concentration could be varied between 400 mM and 50 mM without losing excitability when the internal cation was cesium. A higher calcium concentration gave a larger, shorter action potential with a higher threshold. With other internal cations, the external Ca^{2+} concentration could not be varied in a wide range without complication. For example, when sodium was used as the sole internal cation, sizable biionic action potentials were observed with 100 mM calcium externally. With 200 mM calcium, however, an irreversible deterioration of excitability of the axon was found to set in within a relatively short period of time. With 50 mM calcium externally and 30 mM sodium internally, spontaneous firing of action potentials was frequently observed.

Indispensability of Divalent Cations in the External Medium

To produce biionic action potentials, univalent cations could not be used externally. Figure 5 illustrates this point. An axon was internally perfused

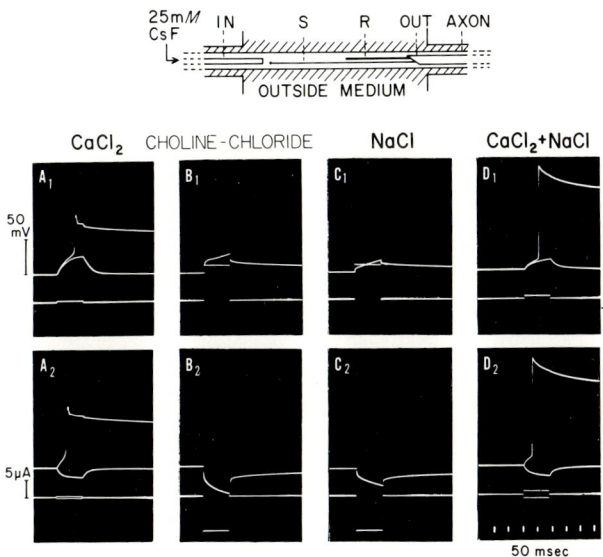

Fig. 5. Demonstration of indispensability of the divalent cation in the external medium for maintaining excitability. The top diagram shows the experimental setup employed: (in) inlet pipette; (out) outlet pipette; (S) stimulating platinum wire electrode inserted into the perfused zone of the axon; (R) recording electrode made of 100 μ glass pipette filled with 600 mM KCl–agar. The bottom records show membrane potential changes (upper trace) produced by stimulating currents (lower trace) through the internal wire electrode. In A_1 and A_2, the external medium contained 200 mM CaCl$_2$ but no univalent cations. An all-or-none biionic action potential was produced in response to stimulating current pulses. In B_1 and B_2, the external medium contained 600 mM choline chloride; the axon showed no sign of excitability. In C_1 and C_2, the external medium contained 600 mM NaCl and 2 mM sodium EDTA; the axon remained inexcitable. In D_1 and D_2, the external medium contained 300 mM NaCl and 200 mM CaCl$_2$; a large action potential is seen. The internal perfusing fluid was a 25 mM CsF solution (with glycerol) throughout. (From Tasaki, 1968.)

with a 25 mM CsF solution (with 10% phosphate as a buffer to maintain the pH at about 7.3). With a 200 mM CaCl$_2$ solution externally, biionic action potentials were observed (Fig. 5A). Then, the external medium was replaced with a 600 mM choline chloride solution. If the external medium was replaced directly with a sodium chloride solution, spontaneous firing of action potentials was almost always observed; a choline solution was used to avoid this complication. After removing the Ca^{2+} in the external medium by this method, a sodium chloride solution was applied to the axon externally. As seen in Fig. 5, no sign of excitability could be observed under these conditions. On addition of calcium in the external medium, excitability could be recovered promptly.

Effects of Varying Cation Species Internally

We have found twelve univalent cations which can be used as internal cations to maintain excitability under biionic conditions (see Fig. 6). If one carried out further experiments along this line, there seems no doubt that many favorable internal cations would be discovered.

Cesium is known to be the most favorable internal cation to maintain excitability (Tasaki et al., 1965a). Attempts to demonstrate biionic potentials were therefore initiated with the use of cesium internally. Solutions of cesium fluoride or cesium phosphate at the concentration level between 3 and 200 mM were used for this purpose, the optimum range being between 10 and 50 mM. With a 200 mM calcium solution externally, the amplitude of the action potential was 80–100 mV, with 120 mV as the largest on the record.

Tetramethylammonium (TMA), tetraethylammonium (TEA), and choline were used as phosphate salts. With these amines internally and with the external calcium concentration of about 100 mM, the excitability was maintained for a long period of time. With choline or TMA internally, axons sometimes gave rise to action potentials up to 120 mV in amplitude. The absolute magnitude of the resting potential was small under these conditions. With choline internally, the membrane potential at rest was often positive inside. The concentrations of these internal cations can be varied between 10 and 100 mM without losing excitability; a 25 mM solution was used most frequently. A detailed description of the results

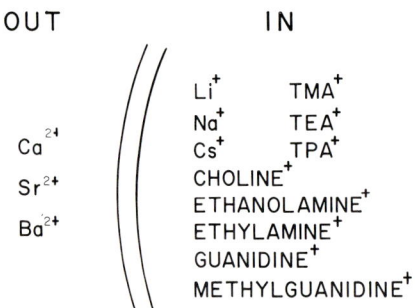

Fig. 6. A list of the ion species which have been used successfully to demonstrate biionic action potentials.

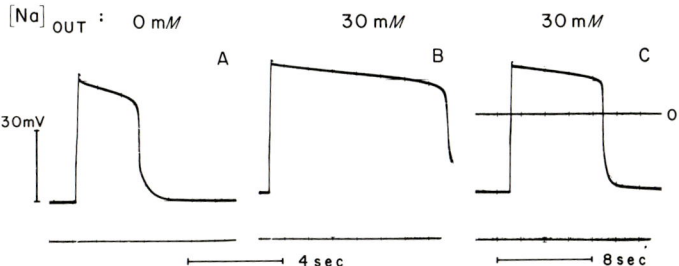

Fig. 7. A record of a biionic action potential observed with sodium as the sole internal cation, and the effect of adding sodium to the external medium. The external calcium concentration was 100 mM. The internal perfusion fluid was 30 mM sodium phosphate solution (the tonicity being maintained with glycerol). Record A shows a biionic potential obtained with calcium as the sole extracellular cation. Records B and C show the effect of 30 mM NaCl added to the external medium. The line 0 indicates the potential level observed with the tip of the recording electrode immersed in the external medium. (From Watanabe et al., 1967.)

obtained with other amines may be found elsewhere (see Tasaki et al., 1969c).

Sodium and lithium were usable as internal cations when the external calcium concentration was about 100 mM (Watanabe et al., 1967). Under these conditions, the ability of axons to develop prolonged all-or-none action potentials could be maintained for a long time with no sign of gradual deterioration in almost all the axons examined. Most experiments with Na^+ internally were carried out in the range of concentration between 10 and 30 mM. As a rule, sodium was used as a phosphate salt at pH 7.3. The amplitude of the biionic action potential was usually 50–60 mV, the largest amplitude observed being 80 mV.

Figure 7A shows an example of biionic action potentials obtained with sodium as the internal cation. Figures 7B and C show the effect of adding 30 mM sodium to the external medium. At this low concentration, the effect of the extracellular sodium on the membrane potential was not very strong. There was a slight decrease in the resting potential, a slight increase in the amplitude of the action potential, and a considerable increase in the duration of the action potential. At the end of these observations, the internal recording electrode was moved out of the axon and was introduced into the external solution. As is seen in the Fig. 7C, the resting membrane potential was found to be about 30 mV and the action potential showed an overshoot of about 20 mV. This experiment simply shows that the amplitude of the action potential cannot be determined by the so-called sodium equilibrium potential, which is zero under the condition of Fig. 7B and C and negative infinity in the case of Fig. 7A.

It was not possible to produce distinct biionic action potentials with the salt of potassium or rubidium internally. With these cations internally, the difference in membrane potential between the resting and excited states of the axon appeared to be too small to create an effective regenerative change in the membrane potential. A detailed discussion of this point will be found in our original paper (Tasaki *et al.*, 1969c). Some axons perfused with rubidium phosphate showed all-or-none activity during direct current hyperpolarization, namely, when a brief stimulating current pulse was superimposed on a steady hyperpolarizing current.

Ionic Mechanism of Nerve Excitation

The biionic action potential represents an excitation phenomenon realized under the simplest possible ionic environments. In inanimate membranes, the biionic potential has been most extensively studied. When the membrane is uniform in the direction normal to the surface, the flux across the membrane, the concentration profile of the counterions, and the membrane potentials can all be theoretically calculated, even in cases where the two counterions have different valences (Helfferich and Ocker, 1957). It is, however, still not quite safe to apply these results directly to the axon membrane, because the axon membrane can not be regarded as uniform in the radial direction. Furthermore, the parameters necessary to characterize the membrane properties (fixed charge density, mobilities, and selectivities of counterions in the membrane) and the effect of the stagnant layers in the membrane are difficult to specify. In spite of these uncertainties, analyses of biionic action potentials lead us to a better understanding of what is happening in the membrane during the process of excitation.

Under biionic conditions, an action potential is produced when an outwardly directed current traverses the membrane. With an inwardly directed current, no excitation phenomenon is observed, provided that the membrane is in the resting state. The effect of passing current across the membrane is to change the ionic concentration profile in the membrane. With an outwardly directed current, the univalent cations tend to go into the membrane and to occupy the negatively charged sites in the membrane, replacing the counterions occupying the sites in the resting state of the membrane. If we assume that in the resting state the sites in the membrane are occupied predominantly by divalent cations, the outward current is expected to decrease the divalent cation concentration and increase the univalent cation concentration within the membrane matrix. The macromolecules of which the membrane is composed are expected to respond to this change in the intramembrane ionic composition with a change in their conformation. Consequently, the mobilities of ions, selectivities, and the fixed charge density could be drastically altered by the applied current. Such ion-exchange processes can proceed cooperatively by virtue of long-range forces acting between different parts of the membrane.

With an inward current applied during the plateau of a biionic action potential, it is possible to terminate the excited state of the membrane prematurely. This is a reverse process of excitation. As the result of the electrophoretic injection of the divalent cations into the membrane matrix, the membrane macromolecules are expected to undergo a conformational change in the reverse direction. Consequently, various electric parameters of the membrane return to their values in the resting state.

The qualitative interpretation of the excitation process described above can probably be applied to excitation phenomena in natural multiionic conditions with little modification. In natural ionic environments, the external medium contains univalent cations as well as divalent cations. It is known that multivalent counterions are absorbed by the charged membrane much more strongly than univalent counterions (see Helfferich, 1962). In fact, some model membranes accumulate calcium much more than the value calculated from a simple Donnan equation (Webb and Danielli, 1940). The hypothesis that the resting membrane is rich in calcium is supported by electrophysiological experiments in which the abrupt transition to the excited state takes place when the external univalent cation concentration is gradually increased (Tasaki *et al.*, 1968a). It is thus concluded that the essential feature of the process of evoking an action potential by electrical stimulation is that a stimulating current injects intracellular univalent cations into the membrane causing an abrupt alteration of the conformation of membrane macromolecules. The membrane potential and impedance in the excited state of the membrane are determined by the membrane parameters (such as fixed charge density, selectivity, and mobilities of ions) in this state.

Change in the Hydrophobicity of the Membrane Macromolecules during Nerve Excitation

Optical Studies of Excitable Axons

In recent years, it was found possible to detect signs of physicochemical changes of the membrane during nerve excitation by various optical techniques. Changes in light scattering and in birefringence were examined

(Cohen et al., 1968; Tasaki et al., 1968b), yielding significant results. One of the most powerful optical techniques of studying macromolecular conformation is to follow changes in fluorescence properties of macromolecules. Ungar and Romano (1962) examined intrinsic fluorescence of nerve; but attempts to detect changes in intrinsic fluorescence during excitation did not yield unequivocal results. Detection of fluorescence changes in nerves stained with different fluorescent dyes, on the other hand, yielded reproducible and significant results which allowed us to draw several important conclusions about the physicochemical nature of the excitable membrane (Tasaki et al., 1968b, 1969a, b).

A group of dyes, called hydrophobic probes, yielded most significant insight into the mechanism of membrane excitation (Tasaki et al., 1968b, 1969b; Kasai et al., 1970). These dyes are almost nonfluorescent when dissolved in water, but are brightly fluorescent when dissolved in less polar solvents or when mixed in protein solutions (Weber and Lawrence, 1954; Stryer, 1968).

Two hydrophobic probes, 8-anilino-1-naphthalenesulfonic acid (ANS) and 2-p-toluidinylnaphthalene-6-sulfonic acid (TNS) were used to stain crab nerves and squid giant axons. When such stained nerves are stimulated electrically, a small change in the intensity of fluorescence could be detected. Recently, fluorescence changes in TNS-stained squid giant axons were studied extensively. Below the results of those extensive studies are presented.

Experimental Setup Used for Detection of Fluorescence Changes in Stained Axons

Figure 8A shows the experimental setup used to detect fluorescence changes in TNS-stained axons. The primary (excitation) light is supplied by a 200 W xenon–mercury lamp (S). With the help of a collimator (L_1) and two cylindrical lenses (L_2 and L_3), a rectangular image of the light source is formed on a stained giant axon, which is mounted horizontally in the nerve chamber. A quasimonochromatic light of 365 mμ wavelength is obtained by inserting an interference filter (F_1) between the lenses and the axon. When necessary, a polarizer (P) is inserted in front of the nerve preparation (see subsequent section). A small portion of the primary light is deflected by a quartz cover slip (R) and sent to a reference photomultiplier (M_2). The output of the reference photomultiplier is used to cancel the fluctuations in the light arising from the xenon–mercury source.

The secondary (fluorescent) light from the axon is collected with the main photomultiplier (M_1), which is placed at a right angle to the direction

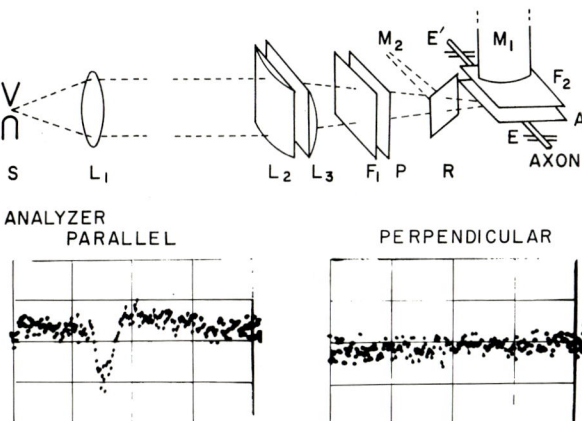

Fig. 8. *Top:* Experimental setup for detecting fluorescence change during excitation (explanation in the text). *Bottom:* Records showing changes in the intensity of the fluorescence light from a TNS-stained axon observed with the analyzer (A) in positions as indicated in the diagram. The direction of the electric vector of the light wave passing through the polarizer was parallel to the longitudinal axis of the axon. The direction of the analyzer (**E** vector) was parallel (left) or perpendicular (right) to the axon. These records were taken after averaging the effect of stimulation over 5000 runs. One vertical division represents a change of 4.3×10^{-5} of the background fluorescence intensity. One horizontal division represents 7.8 mseconds. The experiments were carried out at 7°C. (From Tasaki *et al.*, 1971.)

of propagation of the primary light. An ultraviolet cut-off filter (F_2) is inserted between the axon and the photomultiplier to prevent the primary light scattered by the nerve from reaching the detecter (M_1). In experiments dealing with polarization of fluorescent light (see below), an analyzer (A) is inserted between the nerve and the ultraviolet cut-off filter.

TNS is mixed with a 400 mM potassium phosphate solution at a concentration of 0.5 gm/ml. Because the solubility of TNS in water is low, there are some undissolved particles in the mixture. Approximately 1 mm^3 of the mixture is injected into a single axon.

For stimulating the axon and for recording action potentials, either external electrodes (E and E') or internal twisted platinum wire electrodes are used.

Because the optical signal (i.e., the changing part of the fluorescence) produced in response to stimulation of the axon is small in comparison with the noise level at the output of the photomultiplier, a CAT computer (Mnematron) is used to accumulate optical signals elicited by repetitive stimulation and to improve the signal-to-noise ratio.

Optical Signals Produced by Stimulation of the TNS-Stained Axon

TNS-stained axons give rise to a bluish fluorescent light when illuminated with near-visible ultraviolet light. This fluorescence may be called the resting fluorescence of the axon. Obviously, the major part of the resting fluorescence of the axon derives from the TNS molecules in the axoplasm and in the injected fluid, and only a very small fraction comes from the probes absorbed by the membrane. Note that the ratio of the volume of the membrane to that of the axon interior is of the order of 10^{-4} or 10^{-5}. On excitation of the axon, a rapid and transient decrease in fluorescence intensity is observed (see Fig. 8b, lower left). The magnitude of the decrease is usually between 10^{-4} and 10^{-5}.

As reported earlier (Tasaki *et al.*, 1969b), squid giant axons internally stained with ANS also showed a similar decrease in fluorescence intensity. The results of these experiments and those reported below seem to indicate that during excitation there is a change in hydrophobicity in the membrane.

Spectral Distribution of the Fluorescent Light

With the use of a series of interference filters placed between a TNS-stained axon and the photomultiplier, the spectral distribution of the fluorescent light from the axon was examined. The solid curve in Fig. 9 shows the spectral distribution of the resting fluorescence. As discussed before, a major part of the resting fluorescence of the axon comes from the axoplasm and from the injection fluid. The wavelength at the emission maximum was about 450 mμ.

Because of the interference filter inserted between the axon and the detector, the intensity of the light reaching the detector was very low. For this reason, determination of the spectral distribution of the optical signal was very difficult. In spite of this technical difficulty, the results obtained were clear enough to indicate that the peak of emission lies in the range between 430 and 440 mμ. When an interference filter for 440 mμ wavelength was inserted between the axon and the detector, large optical signals were observed. Only small signals were obtained with an interference filter for 480 mμ, and practically no signals were obtained in the range above 500 mμ.

These experiments show that the spectrum of the portion of the fluorescent light contributing to these optical signals is quite different from that of the resting fluorescence from the axon. From this it follows immediately that the decrease in fluorescent light intensity during nerve excitation is not attributable to the turbidity change observed by Cohen *et al.* (1968) and Tasaki *et al.* (1968b).

The wavelength at which maximum optical signals are observed is shorter than the wavelength of the emission maximum in the resting state of a TNS-stained axon. The best interpretation of this fact suggests that the axonal membrane macromolecules in the resting state are strongly hydrophobic in nature. When such an axon is stimulated electrically, there is a transient decrease in the hydrophobicity of the membrane macromolecules.

Degree of Polarization of the Fluorescent Light

An important piece of information was obtained with the use of polarized light to illuminate a TNS-stained axon and by examining the degree of polarization of the fluorescent light emitted from the axon. When the primary light was polarized with its **E** vector parallel to the axon, it was found that the changing part of the fluorescence light (i.e., the optical signal) was also completely polarized (within the accuracy of the experiment). Thus, when the analyzer (the direction of the **E** vector of the transmitted light wave) was parallel to the axon, the optical signal was large. But when the analyzer was turned away from the parallel position, the size of the signal became smaller. When the analyzer was rotated by 90° from the original position, the signal disappeared completely (see Fig. 8 bottom).

The degree of polarization, P, is defined as $P = (I' - I''/I' + I'')$, where I' and I'' are light intensities observed with the analyzer parallel and perpendicular to the polarizer, respectively. We found that the degree of polarization of the resting fluorescence of the axon was about 0.2. This fact indicates that the dye molecules inside the axon are highly mobile and are fairly randomly oriented. If the dye molecules are bound to large randomly oriented macromolecules in a viscous solvent, the theory of Perrin (1926) and Weber (1953) predicts that the degree of polarization of fluorescence, on excitation at the long wavelength end of the absorption spectrum, is close to 0.5. For optical signals produced in TNS-stained axons, the value of P is close to unity, which exceeds the largest value expected from the theory of randomly oriented macromolecules. Completely polarized fluorescence can be expected when the fluorescent molecules are incorporated in an organized structure so that their transition moments are oriented in one direction (Ziegenpeck, 1944; Feofilov, 1961).

The experimental evidence thus indicates that the molecules in the excitable membrane are highly organized and form a crystalline-like structure, so that the transition moments of TNS molecules are arranged along the direction of the longitudinal axis of the axon.

When the **E** vector of the light passing through the polarizer is perpendicular to the long axis of the axon, no signal is obtained with the analyzer in parallel to the axon. This is reasonable, since the component of the **E** vector of the incident light in the direction parallel to the axon is zero. However, when the analyzer was rotated by 90° from this position, a small increase in fluorescence intensity was observed in response to nerve stimulation. The signal was smaller than the optical signal obtained with both the polarizer and the analyzer parallel to the axon. The interpretation of this fact is unclear at the present time. Probably there is a layer in the membrane where the transition moments of the dye molecules are arranged radially or annularly.

ROLE OF THE HYDROPHOBIC BONDING IN THE EXCITABLE MEMBRANE

Fluorescence changes observed in living axons, using hydrophobic probes, seem to be consistent with the results of recent fluorescence experiments made with membrane fragments. It was found by Chance *et al.* (1969) that fluorescence intensity of the ANS-stained mitochondrial membrane increases on addition of butacaine or calcium. A similar finding was also reported by Feinstein *et al.* (1970) on ANS-stained erythrocyte membrane and several phospholipids. Rubalcava *et al.* (1969) reported that the effect of calcium on intensifying the fluorescence of the ANS-stained erythrocyte membrane is one hundred times stronger than that of sodium. Vanderkooi and Martonosi (1969) observed a similar effect of calcium on the membrane of sarcoplasmic reticulum. It should be recalled that the resting membrane of the squid giant axon is in a calcium-rich state. Transition to the excited state is accompanied by a decrease in the calcium concentration in the membrane. A decrease in fluorescence intensity on excitation of the stained membrane is therefore the result expected from the data on the membrane fragments, and our results are in agreement with the expectation.

Several conclusions can be drawn from the fluorescence study using TNS-stained living axons. The critical layer of the excitable membrane in the resting state has sites which are hydrophobic in nature. The best evidence for this comes from the spectral distribution of the optical response. The fact that the wavelength of the maximum-sized optical response falls between 430 and 440 mμ indicates strongly that the dye molecules are bound to some hydrophobic sites (McClure and Edelman, 1966). This finding further suggests that this hydrophobic bonding is

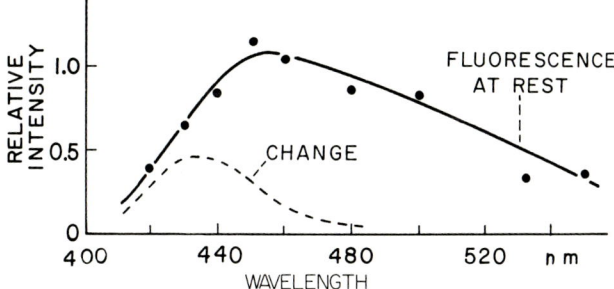

FIG. 9. Spectra of the fluorescence of TNS-stained axons. The solid line indicates the spectrum of the resting fluorescence of the axon. The solid circles indicate the average values from four axons. The broken curve shows an approximate spectral distribution of the changing part of the fluorescence in response to stimulation. (From Tasaki et al., 1971.)

weakened when the stained axon membrane undergoes a transition from the resting to the excited state.

Although fluorescence of TNS molecules can be quenched in many ways, the most important factor is the hydrophobic interactions between the dye molecules and their microenvironment. It is known that TNS fluorescence is not sensitive to pH changes nor to viscosity changes. A decrease in the hydrophobicity of the excitable membrane sites during nerve excitation appears to be the most reasonable interpretation of the results shown in Fig. 9.

Changes in hydrophobicity of the membrane during excitation have been proposed by Tasaki (1968) and Tasaki et al. (1969c). The proposition is based on several independent pieces of evidence:

    1. With a given ionic environment of the membrane, the membrane resistance is a function of its water content; the higher the water content, the lower is the membrane resistance (see Neihof, 1954; Despic and Hills, 1955; Kitchener, 1959; Sollner, 1969). The decrease in membrane resistance in the excited state might be a result of higher water content of the membrane in the excited state.

    2. According to an experiment by Spyropoulos (1961), the excited state can be terminated prematurely by increasing the temperature of the system. It follows from this finding that the transition from the excited to the resting state is an endothermic reaction, and also that there is an increase in entropy associated with the transition. The entropy increase is probably originating from formation of hydrophobic bonding among membrane macromolecules and from reduction of the "iceberg" of water

molecules around the hydrophobic groups in the membrane macromolecules (Kauzmann, 1959). It is known that the water molecules bound to polyanions are released when the salts of calcium or barium are added to the medium; the effect of adding sodium or magnesium salts on bound water is far weaker than that of calcium or barium (Imai and Ikegami, 1962). This effect is also considered to contribute to a decrease in intramembrane water content on termination of an action potential.

3. It is known that some univalent cations in the external medium of the squid giant axon have the ability to increase the amplitude of the action potential (see Tasaki et al. 1965b). These univalent cations are in general more polar and hydrated than those univalent cations which do not show the amplitude-increasing effect. Thus, sodium, lithium, hydrazine, guanidium, hydroxylamine, ammonium, and aminoguanidium show a strong effect, whereas TMA, TEA, choline, and methylguanidium show a very weak or no effect on the action potential amplitude. If one assumes that during excitation the membrane becomes more hydrophilic and, consequently, these polar, hydrated ions are accepted more readily into the membrane, the observed sequence of effectiveness of the ions can be understood.

Conclusions

Based on recent experimental results, excitation phenomena in the squid axon membrane can be interpreted as follows: In the resting state, the negatively charged sites in the membrane are occupied mostly by divalent cations derived from the external medium. The membrane macromolecules assume hydrophobic properties. The water content in the membrane is small and the membrane resistance is accordingly high. In the excited state, the sites in the membrane are occupied mostly by univalent cations. The membrane macromolecules assume hydrophilic properties, and heavily hydrated univalent cations are preferred by the membrane in this state. The water content in the membrane in the excited state is higher than that in the resting state. The membrane resistance is accordingly lower.

Transition from resting to excited state is a result of a cooperative ion-exchange reaction. With stimulating current, the univalent cation in the interior of the axon is electrophoretically injected into the membrane. At a critical ratio between univalent cation concentration and divalent cation concentration, a cooperative conformational change in the macromolecules of the membrane takes place and this change is the fundamental process in the abrupt alteration of the membrane to the excited state.

References

Baker, P. F., Hodgkin, A. L., and Shaw, T. I. (1961). *Nature (London)* **190,** 885.
Chance, B., Azzi, A., Mela, L., Radda, G., and Vainio, H. (1969). *FEBS Lett.* **3,** 10.
Cohen, L. B., Keynes, R. D., and Hille, B. (1968). *Nature (London)* **218,** 438.
Despic, A., and Hills, G. J. (1955). *Trans. Faraday Soc.* **51,** 1260.
Feinstein, M. B., Spero, L., and Felsenfield, H. (1970). *FEBS Lett.* **6,** 245.
Feofilov, P. P. (1961). "The Physical Basis of Polarized Emission." Consultants Bureau, New York.
Frankenhaeuser, B., and Hodgkin, A. L. (1957). *J. Physiol. (London)* **137,** 218.
Heilbrunn, L. B. (1952). "An Outline of General Physiology." Saunders, Philadelphia, Pennsylvania.
Helfferich, F. (1962). "Ion Exchange." McGraw-Hill, New York.
Helfferich, F., and Ocker, H. D. (1957). *Z. Phys. Chem. (Frankfurt am Main)* [N. S.] **10,** 213.
Imai, I., and Ikegami, A. (1962). *J. Polym. Sci.* **56,** 133.
Kasai, M., Podleski, T. R., and Changeux, J. P. (1970). *FEBS Lett.* **7,** 13.
Kauzmann, W. (1959). *Advan. Protein Chem.* **14,** 1.
Kitchener, J. A. (1959). *In* "Modern Aspects of Electrochemistry" (J. O'M. Bockris, ed.), Vol. 2., pp. 87–159. Butterworth, London and Washington, D.C.
McClure, W. O., and Edelman, G. M. (1966). *Biochemistry* **5,** 1908.
Neihof, R. (1954). *J. Phys. Chem.* **58,** 916.
Oikawa, T., Spyropoulos, C. S., Tasaki, I., and Teorell, T. (1961). *Acta Physiol. Scand.* **52,** 105.
Perrin, M. F. (1926). *J. Phys. Radium* [6] **7,** 390.
Rubalcava, B., de Munoz, D. M., and Gitler, C. (1969). *Biochemistry* **8,** 2742.
Sollner, K. (1969). *J. Macromol. Sci., Chem.* **3,** 1.
Spyropoulos, C. S. (1961). *Amer. J. Physiol.* **200,** 203.
Stryer, L. (1968). *Science* **162,** 526.
Takenaka, T., Hirakow, R., and Yamagishi, S. (1969). *J. Ultrastruct. Res.* **25,** 408.
Tasaki, I. (1968). "Nerve Excitation: A Macromolecular Approach." Thomas, Springfield, Illinois.
Tasaki, I., Watanabe, A., and Takenaka, T. (1962). *Proc. Nat. Acad. Sci. U.S.* **48,** 1177.
Tasaki, I., Singer, I., and Takenaka, T. (1965a). *J. Gen. Physiol.* **48,** 1095.
Tasaki, I., Singer, I., and Watanabe, A. (1965b). *Proc. Nat. Acad. Sci. U.S.* **54,** 763.
Tasaki, I., Watanabe, A., and Lerman, L. (1967). *Amer. J. Physiol.* **213,** 1465.
Tasaki, I., Takenaka, T., and Yamagishi, S. (1968a). *Amer. J. Physiol.* **215,** 152.
Tasaki, I., Watanabe, A., Sandlin, R., and Carnay, L. (1968b). *Proc. Nat. Acad. Sci. U.S.* **61,** 883.
Tasaki, I., Carnay, L., Sandlin, R., and Watanabe, A. (1969a). *Science* **163,** 683.
Tasaki, I., Carnay, L., and Watanabe, A. (1969b). *Proc. Nat. Acad. Sci. U.S.* **64,** 1362.
Tasaki, I., Lerman, L., and Watanabe, A. (1969c). *Amer. J. Physiol.* **216,** 130.
Tasaki, I., Watanabe, A., and Hallett, M. (1971). *Proc. Nat. Acad. Sci. U. S.* (in press).
Ungar, G., and Romano, D. V. (1962). *J. Gen. Physiol.* **46,** 267.
Vanderkooi, J., and Martonosi, A. (1969). *Arch. Biochem. Biophys.* **133,** 153.
Watanabe, A., Tasaki, I., and Lerman, L. (1967). *Proc. Nat. Acad. Sci. U.S.* **58,** 2246.
Webb, J., and Danielli, J. F. (1940). *Nature (London)* **146,** 197.
Weber, G. (1953). *Advan. Protein Chem.* **8,** 415.
Weber, G., and Lawrence, D. J. R. (1954). *Biochem. J.* **56,** xxxi.
Ziegenpeck, von H. (1944). *Kolloid-Z.* **106,** 62.

Discussion

Dr. Armstrong: I, as chairman, would first like to invite any extemporaneous and brief contributions having to do strictly with calcium in relation to cell membrane structure and integrity from those individuals who do not have an assigned position on the program.

Dr. Schraer: Dr. Armstrong, do you think that membranes have the same structure throughout the cells and subcellular structures?

Dr. Armstrong: According to the unit membrane hypothesis, all membranes, whether plasma membranes, cytoplasmic membranes, or organelle membranes, are constituted of a bilayer of lipids with a protein layer on each side. Undoubtedly, basically all membranes must have a composition and constitution which are very much alike, but I think there must be variations, or else the peculiarities of permeability or lack of permeability would not be exhibited.

Dr. Martonosi: In this context, it may be interesting to draw attention to a major review by Stoeckenius and Engelman [*J. Cell Biol.* **42,** 613 (1969)], dealing with the problem of reconciliation between the unit membrane structure, as earlier proposed by Danielli and Davson, and the criticism of that structure by Korn [Science **153,** 1491 (1966)]. Stoeckenius and Engelman propose that most biological membranes may be viewed as a mosaic-type structure in which lipoprotein globules are immersed into extended phases of lipid bilayers. The lipoprotein globules may represent functional centers, and they are expected to be more frequent in specialized membranes which have an extensive range of transport functions. Lipid bilayer phases would dominate in membranes where the transport function is less pronounced, and the lipid bilayer portions of all membranes would serve primarily as permeability barriers. We may have a whole spectrum of membranes based essentially on the same structural elements. I believe all the evidence collected so far is in agreement with this unified proposal.

Dr. Matthews: Dr. Lucy of London, a proponent of the mosaic substructure model of membranes, showed that the globular dimensions of certain isolated membranes differ from those of the erythrocyte membrane. On another matter, we demonstrated, using microincineration techniques, that desmosomes of epithelial tissue and nerve synapses have at least ten times as much mineral as adjacent membranes. This applies to both the presynaptic and postsynaptic membranes of nerve.

Dr. Copp: Dr. Watanabe, I wondered if you could discuss the mechanism for the increase of nervous excitability associated with low ionic calcium levels which we commonly call tetany.

Dr. Watanabe: It is known that with low calcium concentrations in the external medium, the axon tends to fire spontaneously. With higher calcium concentrations, the membrane stays in the resting state. This is called the stabilizing action of calcium. With higher calcium concentration in the outside medium, the ratio of calcium ions to the univalent cations in the membrane increases, and this is the condition which keeps the membrane in the resting state.

Dr. Armstrong: Dr. Watanabe, you mentioned that, when you perfused the nerves with fluoride solution, it allowed maintenance of excitability, quite in contrast to the circumstances that occurred when chloride was used in the perfusions. Is that a correct statement of your findings?

Dr. Watanabe: Yes. If we use, for instance, potassium chloride instead of potassium fluoride or potassium phosphate, we cannot maintain excitability for any length of time.

Dr. Armstrong: What was the concentration of fluoride?

Dr. Watanabe: The concentration of fluoride that was used depended on the ion species in the medium. If we use for the outside medium a sodium–calcium mixture, and for the inside potassium, we can use a high concentration (up to 600 mM) of potassium fluoride. If we go to the biionic situation, we have to lower the ionic strength of the outside and inside solutions. For the outside medium, we use about 100 or 200 mM calcium chloride, and for the inside medium we use, for example, 50 mM cesium fluoride or cesium phosphate. If the ionic strength of the inside medium is over 100 mM, we cannot get a biionic action potential.

Dr. Armstrong: Do you think there is a possibility that fluoride ion did not actually perfuse through the nerve, but that it was bound by calcium and by protein and was effectively not an ion?

Dr. Watanabe: We do not think that the effect of fluoride is its ability to form a complex with calcium. Axoplasm might bind calcium, but the binding sites would be rapidly saturated. Also, if we later perfuse with EDTA, we do not see any improvement in the state of the axon membrane. Further, Dr. Tasaki and his collaborators, Dr. Takenaka and Dr. Singer, showed that the survival time of the axon depends on the order in the lyotropic series of the anions which were used to perfuse inside the axon, and the lyotropic series is not always correlated with calcium-binding activity.

Dr. H. E. Harrison: What was the concentration of the hydrogen ion in the outside solution when you used 100 mM calcium? Couldn't hydrogen ion be the monovalent cation which was substituting for sodium ions in these experiments?

Dr. Watanabe: It is at pH 8.

Dr. Harrison: How do you get pH 8?

Dr. Watanabe: We use about 1 mM of tris–HCl buffer. The existence of tris buffer is not essential, however, to get the biionic action potential. Several times we used an unbuffered outside solution and we could get the biionic action potential, although the pH must have been changing rapidly. The axon is not too sensitive to the pH of the outside medium. The excitability is maintained if the outside medium has a pH between 6.5 and 8.5.

We believe that hydrogen ion plays a role in excitation. We tried many experiments on the effect of pH, but the results have never been clear. We see some deterioration of excitability when we go to the extreme end of the allowed range of pH. The effect is mostly irreversible.

Dr. Nichols: Dr. Watanabe, I was very interested in your model, the changes in fluorescence which you see, and particularly with the shift in the polarization of light. You said that these indicated to you that there was one structure in the membrane which was not changed during stimulation, while another one probably was, because of the decrease in fluorescence. I wonder if you could tell us how you see the model in the membrane which has a structure which in one orientation is not changed and in another is changed.

Dr. Watanabe: This is a very interesting problem for us. What we found was that if we put the **E** axis of the analyzer in the vertical position with respect to the nerve, we see no optical response at all. In fact, what we wanted to see was the change in degree of polarization of the fluorescent light during excitation, because we expected that the viscosity of the membrane might change during excitation.

If we have some protein solution or any other solution of macromolecules and determine the degree of polarization, it should be between 0.5 and 0. If the viscosity of the solution is very high, so that the direction of the dipole moment of the dye molecules doesn't change during the period of molecular excitation, the degree of polarization would become 0.5. Experimentally, we found that the degree of polarization of the optical response was very close to unity. This fact means that the theory of Perrin, which is applicable to protein solutions, can't be applied to the axon membrane. What we are treating here is a fibrous structure or crystalline structure rather than an isotropic protein solution.

We think that the dipole moment of the dye molecule is arranged parallel with the axon membrane. It can be argued, then, that rotation of the dipole moment of the dye molecule is not enough to explain the intensity of change in fluorescence. Then the only possibility is to assume that quenching is going on during nerve excitation. There are many quenching mechanisms. TNS is supposed to change by a change in the hydrophobicity of the medium. McClure and Edelman state that TNS is not sensitive to pH change. It changes by changing the viscosity of the medium, but only very little. The most dramatic change comes from the change in polarity of the solvent. A simple solution of TNS in water doesn't fluoresce much. But if protein is added to the solution, it becomes more fluorescent. We see a decrease in fluorescence intensity on nerve excitation. This is a sign that the hydrophobicity of the nerve membrane has decreased during excitation.

Dr. Martonosi: The conventional interpretation given to changes in the fluorescence intensity of various hydrophobic probes in membrane systems is that they indicate changes in the hydrophobicity of the environment. However, there are many observations in the literature which suggest that microsome–ANS or phospholipid–ANS systems yield marked changes in intensity of fluorescence when there are changes in the ion concentration of the environment. For example, by raising the concentration of sodium or potassium from 0 to 10 mM, the fluorescence intensity increases by approximately 200%, and 10^{-4} M lanthanum produces about a 800% increase in fluorescent intensity. Because of this, I would find it hard to exclude the possibility that a 0.01% change in fluorescent intensity was not due to changes in the internal ion concentration of the giant axon during the action potential, instead of the postulated changes in protein.

Dr. Watanabe: It is certainly possible that the fluorescence change comes from the ion concentration change, not from the conformational change. In fact, we believe that the latter phase of the fluorescence change is mainly due to changes in ionic concentration rather than the drastic conformational change of membrane macromolecules themselves. However, we cannot really separate these two causes in a rigorous way. On excitation, we believe that calcium ions are chased out of the membrane, and there is a conformational change of the membrane macromolecules because of the ion exchange reaction in the membrane. In mitochondria or red blood cell membranes, too, I believe they use membrane fragments, and they add some ANS or TNS and change the calcium concentration. Small ions would not change fluorescence by themselves. At least for the initial phase of the fluorescence change, if we say this is due to the conformational change of the membrane macromolecules, triggered by the ion concentration change in the membrane, I think we can put it in a better way.

THE CALCIUM HOMEOSTATIC SYSTEM AS A PHYSIOLOGICAL REGULATOR OF CELL PROLIFERATION IN MAMMALIAN TISSUES*

A. D. Perris

Introduction

The concentration of calcium in the external environment of isolated cells has been known for many years to be a crucial component in the sequence of events which leads up to mitosis. Thus, the absence of calcium in the medium prevents or severely delays the entry of many different mammalian and invertebrate cell types into mitosis, whereas elevated calcium levels hasten this process (1–11). However, it was not until 1967, when it was observed that calcium chloride injections stimulated mitotic activity in the thymus gland of the rat (12) that these *in vitro* findings acquired a relevance to the control of cell division in the whole animal.

Since then, a large amount of material has appeared, principally from our laboratory under the direction of Dr. J. F. Whitfield, which has expanded these observations and suggested a mechanism by which calcium and other agents might effect these changes in mitotic activity (13–23). The principal purpose of this review is limited to a summary of those

* Issued as NRCC No. 11988.

results which have physiological meaning for the whole animal. In at least three areas—(a) the growth of the animal, (b) thymic lymphopoiesis and structure, and (c) erythropoiesis—the calcium homeostatic hormones will be shown to play a vital role in the physiological control of cell division.

Basic Phenomena

By stopping the progression of cells through the various stages of mitosis at metaphase with colchicine (or colcemid), the rate of flow of nucleated

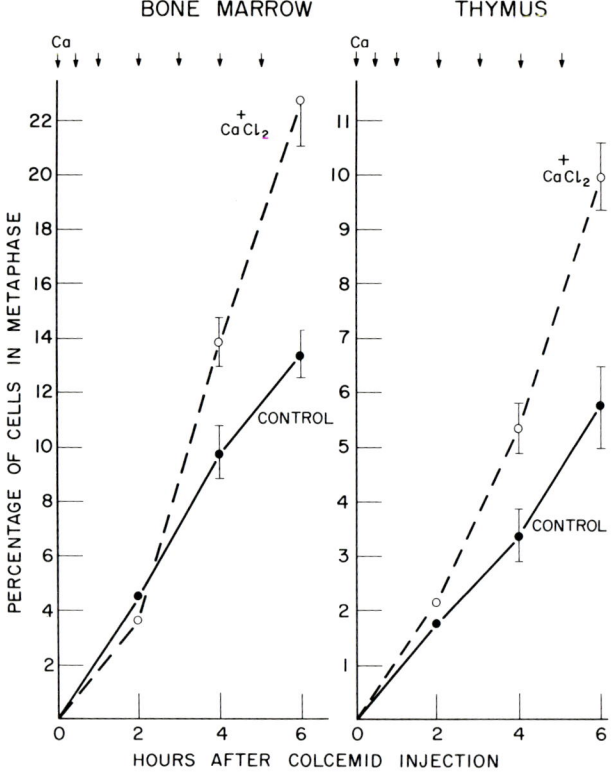

FIG. 1. Effect of calcium on mitotic activity in bone marrow and thymus. Colchicine was given i.p. (0.2 mg per 100 gm of rat) at 0 and 3 hours, and the percentage of nucleated bone marrow or thymus cells in the total population arrested in the colchicine metaphase configuration scored at 2, 4, and 6 hours after the first injection. Experimental animals also received a series of i.p. calcium chloride injections at times indicated by the arrows. Each injection was 1 ml of a 62.5 mM solution. Each point is a mean value ± S.E.M. derived from at least six rats in each case.

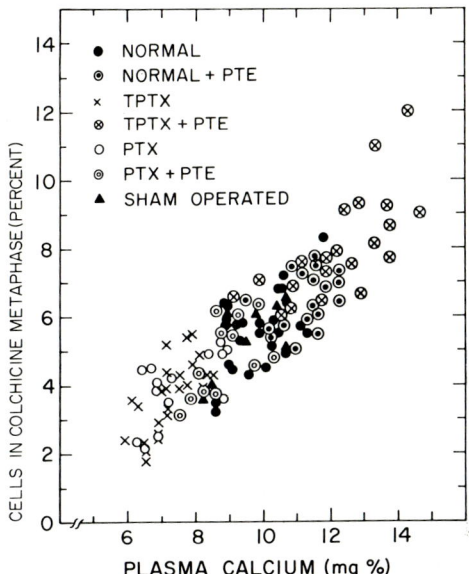

Fig. 2. Effect of plasma calcium concentration on mitotic activity in rat bone marrow. The percentage of bone marrow cells arrested at metaphase over a 6 hour period in the colcemid-treated rat was measured after different treatments. PTE = parathyroid extract. [From Rixon (16).]

bone marrow or thymus cells into mitosis can be simply and very accurately assessed by plotting the progressive accumulation of colchicine–metaphase figures (14, 24). Thus in the male Sprague–Dawley rat (200 gm), there is a regular and linear progression of cells into division over a 6 hour period following the injection of colcemid, implying that there is neither any significant cell death nor escape from the metaphase block under these conditions (Fig. 1).

When rats received a series of intraperitoneal calcium chloride injections, there was a highly significant increase in mitotic activity in these tissues (Fig. 1). Dr. R. H. Rixon then showed that parathyroid extract also stimulated mitotic activity in rat bone marrow (14, 16) and that the proliferation of marrow cells was reduced in the aparathyroid condition. In addition, a direct proportionality was found between the concentration of calcium in the plasma and mitotic activity in this tissue (16) (Fig. 2).

Mechanism

Using suspension cultures of rat thymic lymphocytes maintained *in vitro*, Drs. J. P. MacManus and J. F. Whitfield have developed a cogent

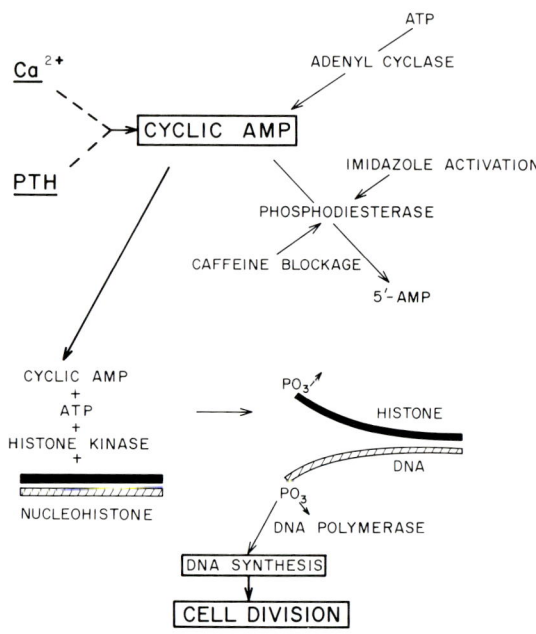

Fig. 3. Proposed reaction scheme for calcium-, PTH-, and cyclic AMP-induced mitogenesis.

hypothesis to explain the mitogenic effect of calcium. The response, in fact, emanates from the ability of calcium to cause a rapid initiation of DNA synthesis in those cells which are poised at the G_1–S boundary of the cell cycle. This early triggering of DNA synthesis is ultimately followed a few hours later by the entry of the stimulated cells into mitosis (19). In addition to calcium, a wide variety of other agents and hormones (such as agmatine, detergents, bradykinin, parathyroid hormone, growth hormone, prolactin, and the neurohormones) can all stimulate cell division of isolated thymic lymphocytes, provided calcium is also present in the culture medium (18, 25). These compounds seem to function by sensitizing the cell to the ambient calcium ion which is the actual mitogenic agent. Acting in some way upon the cell membrane, and ultimately upon the systems which organize the formation and destruction of cyclic adenosine 3'5'-monophosphate (cyclic AMP), calcium with or without a sensitizing agent such as parathyroid hormone (PTH) increases the intracellular concentration of this nucleotide (26, 26a). Cyclic AMP might then stimulate the phosphorylation of histone, which would disrupt the nucleohistone complexes (20, 27, 28) and thereby permit replication of DNA to commence as a preface to cell division. This hypothesis is supported by the observations that cyclic AMP itself stimulates DNA synthesis and mitotic activity, both in the presence and absence of calcium (22). Furthermore, a phosphodiesterase stimulant imidazole, which promotes the breakdown of cyclic AMP, inhibits cyclic AMP-, PTH-, and calcium-induced mitotic stimulation (20, and unpublished observations). It is of interest here to mention that the natural antagonist of PTH, thyrocalcitonin, which may be the physiological equivalent of imidazole, will inhibit PTH- and cyclic AMP-induced mitogenesis (23). On the other hand, caffeine, a phosphodiesterase inhibitor, which retards the breakdown of cyclic AMP, potentiates the mitogenic effect of calcium, PTH, and the cyclic nucleotide (20, and unpublished observations). A diagrammatic summary of these proposed and actual events is shown in Fig. 3.

Physiological Significance

Growth of the Animal

When considering various physiological situations in which fluctuations in cell division might occur, it was immediately obvious that compensatory

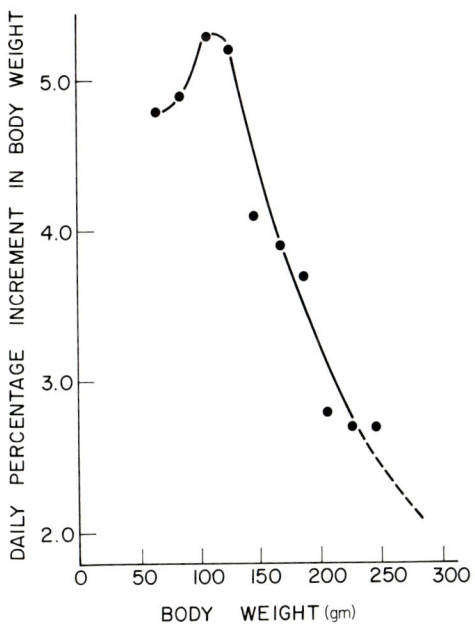

Fig 4. Growth curve of male Sprague–Dawley rats. [From Perris et al. (15).]

or parallel changes in the level of cell division in various tissues must accompany the growth of an animal. As the rat increased in body weight from 70 to 120 gm, the growth rate of the animal increased to a maximum, and then, although the rat continued to increase in size, the growth rate subsequently declined (Fig. 4). As the growth rate of the rat rose to its maximum value there was a marked and progressive increase in mitotic activity in both bone marrow and thymus (Figs. 5 and 6). As the growth rate subsequently declined, so also did mitotic activity (Figs. 5 and 6). However, at any stage throughout this growth period it was possible to enhance the level of mitotic activity in the bone marrow and thymus by artificially elevating plasma calcium concentrations by means of a series of intraperitoneal calcium chloride injections (Figs. 5 and 6).

Since artificially increasing the calcium concentrations stimulated mitosis in thymus and bone marrow (Figs. 5 and 6), it was important to

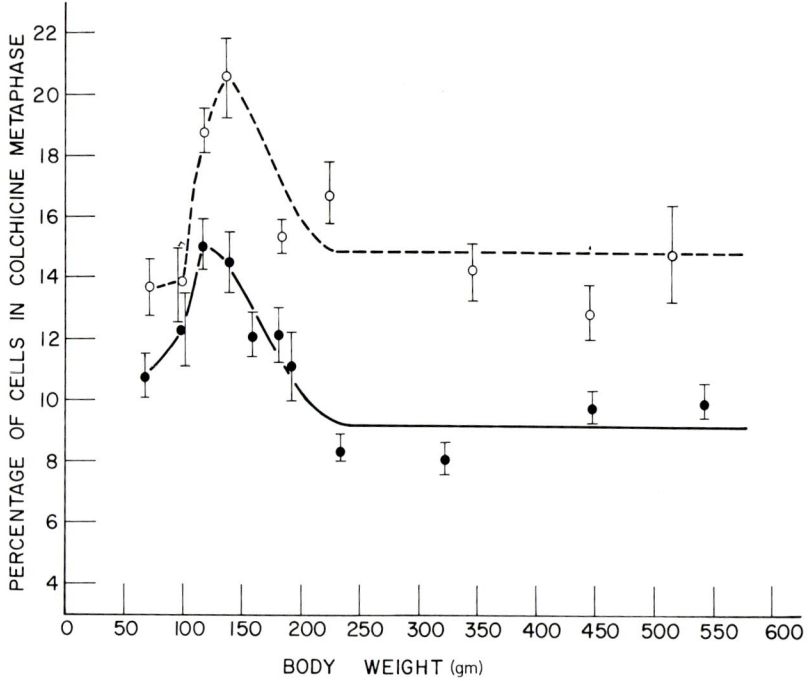

FIG. 5. Variations in bone marrow mitotic activity in rats of different weight. Accumulation of colchicine metaphase figures over a 6 hour period was assessed in norma- (solid line) and calcium chloride-injected (broken line) rats. Calcium chloride was administered as in Fig. 1. Each point is the mean value ± S.E.M. derived from between five and twelve rats in each case. [From Perris et al. (15).]

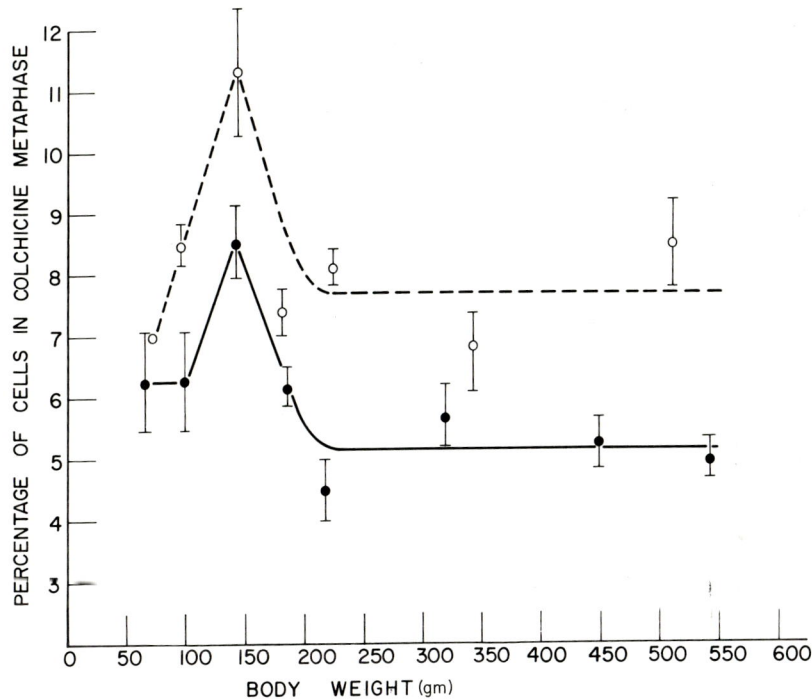

FIG. 6. Variations in thymus mitotic activity in rats of different weight. Details as in Fig. 5.

know whether there were any natural changes in plasma calcium levels associated with the normal physiological alterations in mitotic activity during growth. Both total and ionized plasma calcium concentrations were therefore measured in rats of different body weight (Fig. 7). When the physiologically pertinent ionized calcium fraction was studied, it was apparent that the changing levels of mitotic activity were indeed paralleled by remarkably large shifts in plasma calcium concentration (compare Figs. 5, 6, and 7). Thus, the calcium homeostatic system must be intimately involved in these age-dependent alterations in mitotic activity (15).

Thymic Structure and Lymphopoiesis

Lymphopoietic activity in the thymus is rapid, the total population of small lymphocytes in the thymus cortex being replaced every 3–4 days

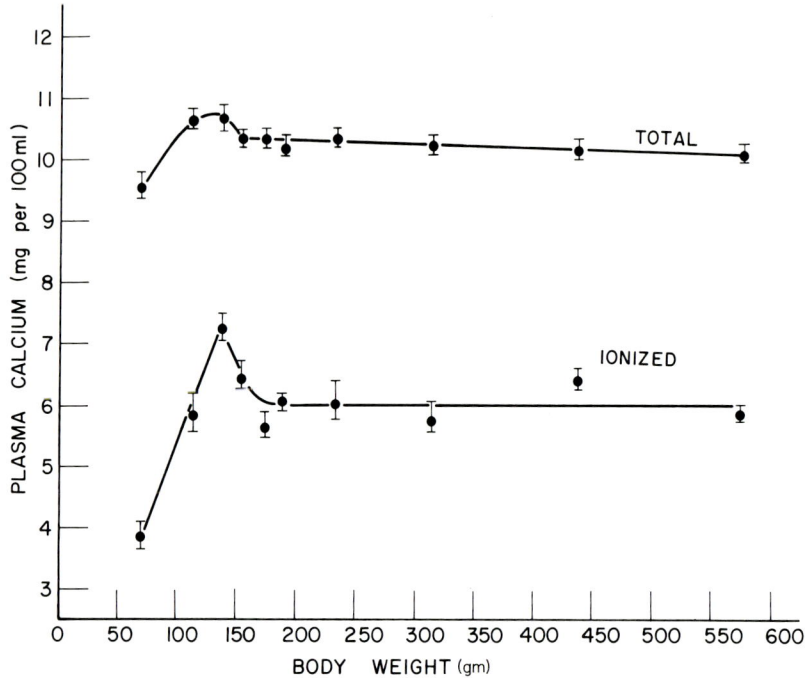

FIG. 7. Variations in total and ionized plasma calcium concentrations in rats of different weight. [From Perris et al. (15).]

(29, 30), yet the size of the thymus gland remains relatively constant over long periods of time in the adult animal. Cell production must therefore be balanced by cell loss due to death or emigration (31). Although experiments on the growth behavior of thymic grafts have implied that the stimulus for the proliferation of thymic lymphocytes is largely intrinsic and depends upon the epithelial cytoreticulum of the donor tissue (32–37), the *in vivo* studies described above (Figs. 1 and 6) and the profound effect of calcium and PTH on thymocyte mitosis *in vitro* (6, 12–14, 18) almost demanded that these agents must also influence thymocyte proliferation *in vivo*. This was proven by the fact that thyroparathyroidectomy (TPTX) caused a very large reduction in mitotic activity in the thymus (38) (Fig. 8). Since TPTX so strongly reduced cell production, we reasoned that this should be followed by thymic atrophy. This was confirmed by the observation that thymic dry weights in TPTX rats dramatically declined from the normal value of 121 ± 8 mg to only 10 ± 5 mg over a 9 day period (Fig. 9). This profound involution of the thymus after TPTX was not a result of the loss of thyroid tissue, since it also occurred in the parathyroidectomized (PTX) rat (Fig. 10). Either the loss of endogenous PTH itself or the associated hypocalcemia was the principal cause of this atrophy, for it could be retarded by either PTH injections or the provision of calcium gluconate in the drinking water (Fig. 10). It should be remembered that the PTH injections were only given every other day and the animal's drinking is only spasmodic. Thus, these treatments would not be expected to maintain the normal plasma calcium concentration, nor would they be expected to completely prevent the ensuing thymic atrophy in the TPTX rat.

When adrenalectomized and orchidectomized rats were also parathyroidectomized, thymic involution still occurred (Fig. 11). This atrophic response cannot therefore be due to a secondary release of the cytolytic adrenal or gonadal sterioids (39–42) and must be ascribed to the inhibition of thymic lymphopoiesis rather than the increased destruction of lymphocytes.

The effects of parathyroidectomy on those cell-mediated immunological reactions which are controlled by the thymus gland have not been tested (31). Tissue function, however, must depend in part upon the cellularity of that tissue. The dramatic effect of the removal of the parathyroid glands on the mitotic activity of thymic lymphocytes and thymic weight suggests

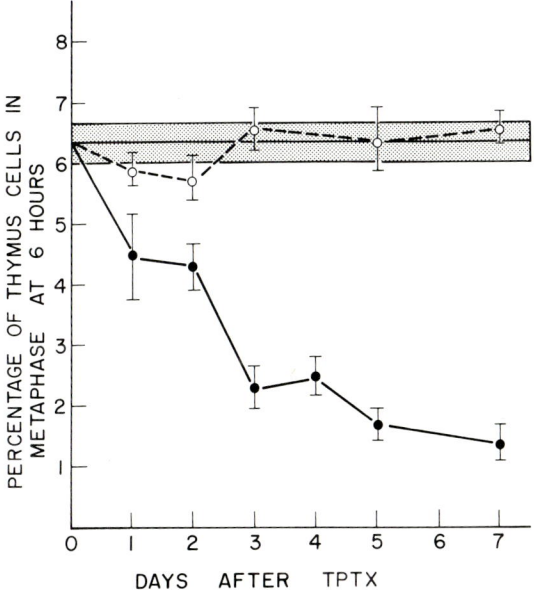

FIG. 8. Mitotic activity in the thymus after thyroparathyroidectomy. Values shown for TPTX (solid line) or sham operated (broken line) animals are means ± S.E.M. derived from at least five rats in each case. Mean value and standard error for normal control rats is indicated by the horizontal line and shaded area. [From Perris et al. (38).]

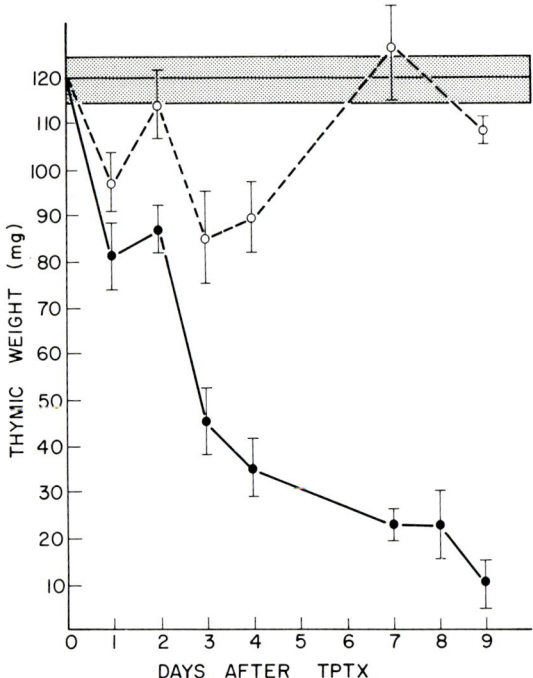

FIG. 9. Thymic weight after TPTX. Values shown for TPTX (solid line) or sham operated (broken line) animals are means ± S.E.M. derived from between three and twenty-five rats in each case. Mean value and standard error for normal control rats is indicated by the horizontal line and shaded area. [From Perris et al. (38).]

the role of the parathyroid gland on such immunological processes may well be important.

Erythropoiesis

Since experimentally created increases and decreases in the level of environmental calcium caused significant parallel changes in bone marrow mitotic activity (13–16), it seemed likely that erythropoiesis would also be affected. The surge of cell division induced by a series of calcium chloride injections was in fact followed 1 day later by a surge of reticulocytes in the bone marrow and peripheral blood (Fig. 12). A single injection of PTH had a similar effect. In contrast, parathyroidectomy which reduces bone marrow cell division (Fig. 2) also produced a reticulocytopenia (Fig. 13). One week after the parathyroids were removed, reticulocyte levels in both the bone marrow and peripheral blood were reduced dramatically (Fig. 13), but PTH injections on three successive days completely reversed this effect and restored levels to normal again (Fig. 13). It might be mentioned parenthetically that Dr. Helen J. Morton of our laboratory has shown increased environmental calcium also increases cell division and reticulocyte production in cultures of isolated bone marrow (11).

In addition to using reticulocyte production as an indicator of erythropoiesis, we have also utilized the radioactive iron incorporation technique (43). As expected, calcium and PTH significantly stimulated ^{59}Fe incorporation into peripheral red blood cells of the normal rat, but parathyroidectomy profoundly depressed the incorporation of isotope (44) (Table I). Furthermore, in the aparathyroid rat, injections of PTH and calcium significantly raised ^{59}Fe uptake.

This ability of calcium and PTH to increase cell division in rat bone marrow and to thereby stimulate erythropoiesis (as judged by both reticulocyte production and ^{59}Fe incorporation) was not due to a secondary release or activation of erythropoietin. In both nephrectomized and polycythemic rats [where the major source of erythropoietin is removed

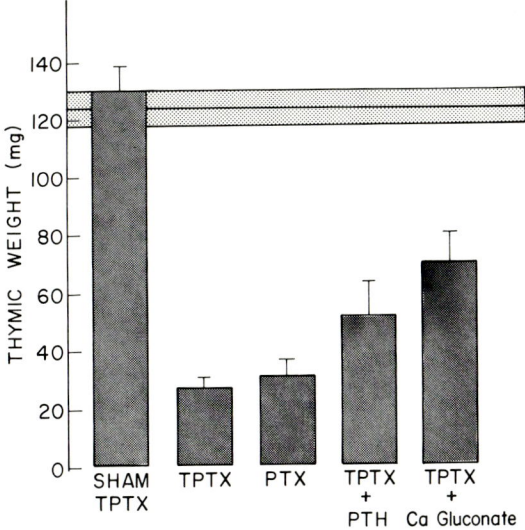

FIG. 10. Thymic weight 7 days after various operations and treatments. Values are means ± S.E.M. derived from between six and twenty-five rats in each case. Mean value and standard error for normal control rats is indicated by the horizontal line and shaded area. [From Perris et al. (38).]

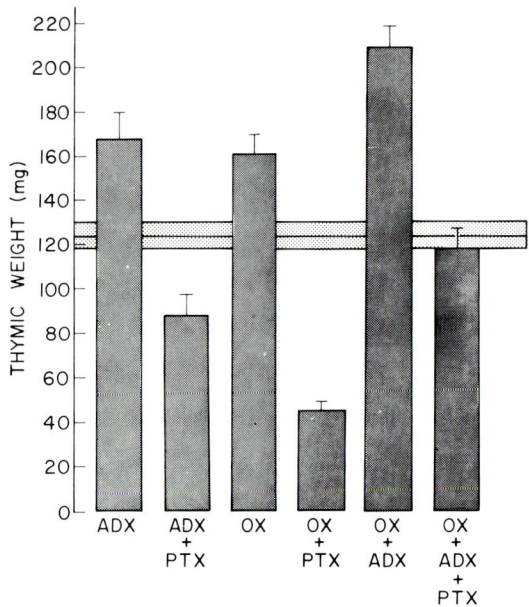

FIG. 11. Thymic weight 7 days after various operations and treatments. ADX = adrenalectomy, OX = orchidectomy. Values are means ± S.E.M. derived from between four and twelve rats in each case. Mean value and standard error for normal control rats is indicated by the horizontal line and shaded area. [From Perris et al. (38).]

and the circulating level reduced to very low levels, respectively (45–48)], calcium and PTH still stimulated bone marrow mitosis (44).

Since we had already seen there were age-dependent variations in bone marrow mitotic activity (Fig. 5) associated with physiological shifts in calcium concentration (Fig. 7), it followed that there might be accompanying calcium-dependent alterations in erythropoietic activity with age. Reticulocyte levels in bone marrow and peripheral blood did indeed parallel the age-dependent changes in ionized calcium concentration (Fig. 14), thus confirming our belief that the calcium homeostatic hormones were involved in the physiological regulation of erythropoiesis. The need for an adaptive increase in red cell production to transport oxygen to the increasing tissue mass in the rapidly growing rat is obvious. It may be effected via the increase in bone marrow cell division which accompanies the increase in ionized calcium concentration, which itself is presumably a reflection of an altered balance between PTH and thyrocalcitonin.

In addition to participating in the prolonged maintenance of an adequate red cell population during growth, the calcium homeostatic system also provides for the rapid production of erythrocytes following hemorrhage. One day after an acute blood loss, mitotic activity in the bone marrow was increased, and associated with this increase in cell division was a significant hypercalcemia (Fig. 15). This hypercalcemia was the result of the loss of blood cells rather than the hypovolemia or hypotension associated with the blood loss. When the blood sample removed was reinfused within 1 minute, no hypercalcemia developed 1 day later, whereas if an equal volume of homologous rat plasma was reinfused equally rapidly, it did (Fig. 16). The conclusion that it was the loss of blood cells that was responsible for the hypercalcemia was reinforced by the observation that the elevated calcium concentration and the heightened mitotic activity in the bone marrow persisted until the hematocrit returned to normal (Fig. 17).

Both the post-hemorrhagic hypercalcemia and stimulation of bone marrow mitosis were mediated by the parathyroid gland, since neither response occurred in the bled TPTX rat (Table II). The importance of a

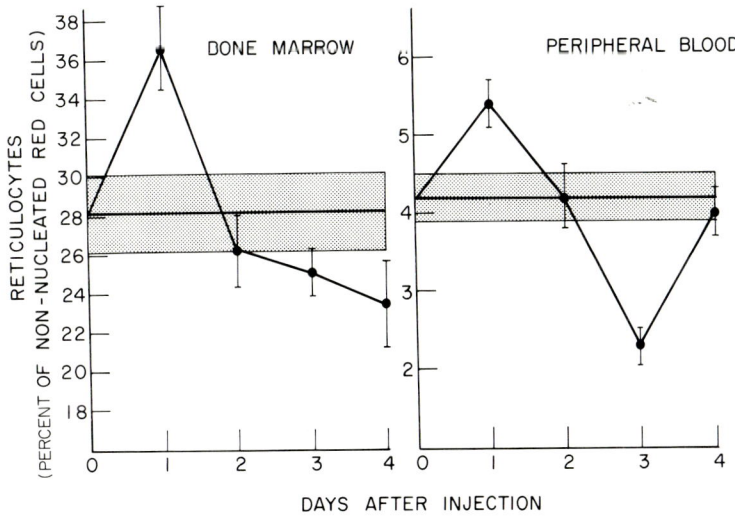

FIG. 12. Effect of calcium chloride injections on reticulocyte production in bone marrow and peripheral blood. Animals received seven 1-ml injections of 62.5 mM CaCl$_2$ on day 0 as described in Fig. 1. Reticulocytes were scored as the percentage of the total non-nucleated red cell population. Values are means ± S.E.M. derived from between eleven and twenty-four animals for each point. Mean value and standard error for control animals is indicated by the horizontal line and shaded area. [From Perris and Whitfield (48).]

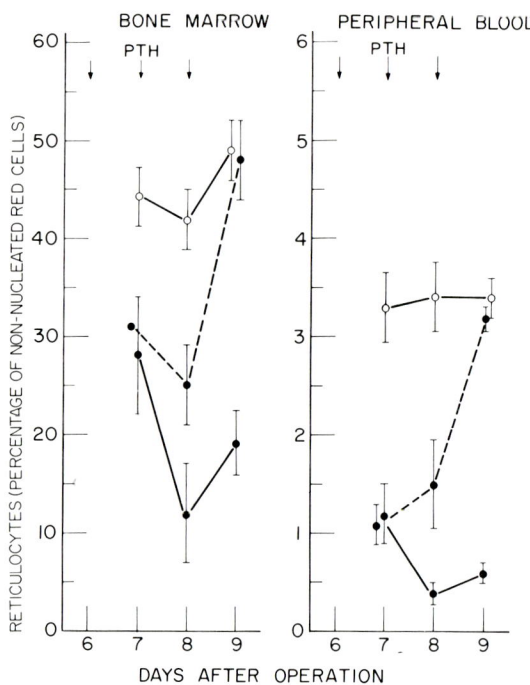

Fig. 13. Effect of highly purified PTH on reticulocytes in TPTX rats. ●——● TPTX; ●---● TPTX + PTH; ○——○ sham operated controls. Values are means ± S.E.M. derived from three or four animals in each case. Fifty units of PTH per 100 gm of rat were given subcutaneously each day for 3 days commencing 6 days after the TPTX operation. [From Perris and Whitfield (48).]

functional parathyroid gland for increasing cell division in the bone marrow after blood loss is shown by the very much slower rate of recovery of the hematocrit in bled TPTX rats compared to sham-operated bled controls (Fig. 18). The loss of thyroid tissue is of consequence here, since the same effect has been demonstrated in the PTX rat (48). Furthermore, administration of purified PTH to the bled aparathyroid rat raised the rate of erythrocyte replenishment to its normal value (Fig. 18).

Since the normal stimulus for a release of parathyroid hormone is a lowering of plasma calcium concentration (49–51), it was not at first clear how the loss of red cells per se could affect this release. However when we examined calcium concentrations immediately after hemorrhage it was evident that there was initially a hypocalcemia of sufficient magnitude to stimulate PTH secretion (50) (Fig. 19). The release of PTH restored normal calcium levels within 20 hours of the blood loss and then, presumably because of an excessive and protracted secretion, caused the post-hemorrhagic hypercalcemia already described (Figs. 15, 16, 17, and 19 and Table II). Although the cause of this early hypocalcemia is not known, it has been suggested that it may be related to the hypoxia which accompanies the blood loss (52). Whatever the cause, the hypocalcemia sets in motion a train of events leading ultimately to a parathyroid-mediated normal rate of restoration of red cell proportions.

Finally, to emphasize the crucial role of the calcium homeostatic system in the control of erythropoiesis, we examined the changes in bone marrow mitotic activity and plasma calcium concentrations which occur under other conditions which are known to affect erythropoiesis. Erythropoiesis is stimulated after injection of the hormone erythropoietin or the salt co-

TABLE I

Effect of Calcium Chloride and PTH Injections on the Incorporation of ^{59}Fe into Peripheral Red Blood Cells in Normal, TPTX, and PTX Rats[a]

Condition	No. of rats	Average percentage ^{59}Fe uptake in RBC ± S.E.M.
Normal control	12	50.7 ± 1.1
Normal + CaCl$_2$	6	65.6 ± 2.4
Normal + PTH	6	65.4 ± 1.6
Sham operated	6	47.7 ± 3.7
TPTX control	23	7.8 ± 0.6
PTPX + CaCl$_2$	8	15.2 ± 1.2
TPTX + PTH	4	13.6 ± 1.8
PTX control	11	6.4 ± 0.7
PTX + CaCl$_2$	5	11.4 ± 2.1
PTX + PTH	3	9.8 ± 0.3

[a] Treated animals received either seven 1 ml intraperitoneal injections of 62.5 mM CaCl$_2$ as described in Fig. 1 or a single subcutaneous injection of highly purified PTH (50 units per 100 gm of rat). Iron-59 was given 6 hours after the first calcium chloride or the PTH injection, and the percentage of the injected dose incorporated into red blood cells (RBC) were assessed 18 hours later. TPTX and PTX rats were used 6 days after the respective operations. Iron-59 incorporation in calcium chloride- or PTH-treated normal rats was significantly higher than in control rats ($p < 0.001$). Calcium chloride and PTH also significantly increased ^{59}Fe incorporation in aparathyroid rats ($p < 0.02$ and $p < 0.05$, respectively). Iron-59 incorporation in aparathyroid rats was significantly lower than in normal and sham operated controls ($p < 0.001$). [From Perris and Whitfield (44).]

baltous chloride and during pregnancy (53–55). One day after injection of erythropoietin or cobaltous chloride, and during the second and third weeks of pregnancy, both plasma calcium concentrations and bone marrow mitotic activity were increased (Fig. 20). In contrast, when erythropoiesis was depressed in polycythemic rats, plasma calcium concentrations and cell proliferation in the bone marrow decreased. In fact, there was a direct proportionality between plasma calcium concentrations and the level of bone marrow mitosis under all these conditions (Fig. 20).

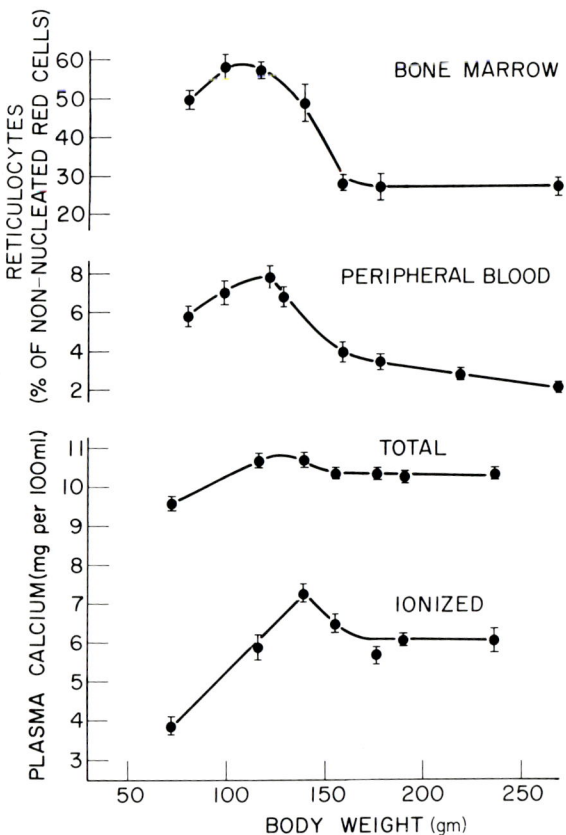

FIG. 14. Comparison of plasma calcium concentrations and reticulocyte patterns in rats of different body weight. Animals were divided into several groups according to weight (the weight range being 20 gm in each case). Each point is a mean value ± S.E.M. derived from between five and seventeen animals.

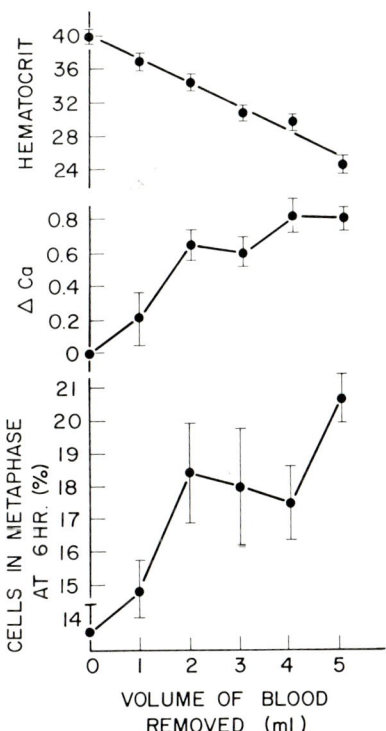

FIG. 15. Effect of hemorrhage on hematocrit, plasma calcium, and bone marrow mitotic activity. One day after different volumes of blood were removed from the rat, the following parameters were examined: *Hematocrit:* For all blood volumes taken, hematocrits are significantly different from controls ($p < 0.001$). Between six and fifty-two rats were used to establish each point. *Change in total plasma calcium concentration:* Plasma calcium concentration was measured in individual rats on the day of bleeding and repeated 1 day later, each rat serving as its own control. The average increment in plasma calcium, Δ Ca, in milligrams per 100 ml of plasma, for each sample volume is shown. For blood samples of between 2 and 5 ml, the increments were significantly different from zero ($p < 0.001$). Between six and forty-two rats were used to establish each point. *Mitotic activity in bone marrow:* One day after bleeding, animals were treated with colcemid as described in the text. Six hours later, the percentage of nucleated femoral bone marrow cells in metaphase was determined. Between four and six rats were used to establish each point. For blood samples, between 2 and 5 ml mitotic activity is significantly different from controls ($p < 0.001$). All points shown are mean values ± S.E.M. [From Perris et al. (52).]

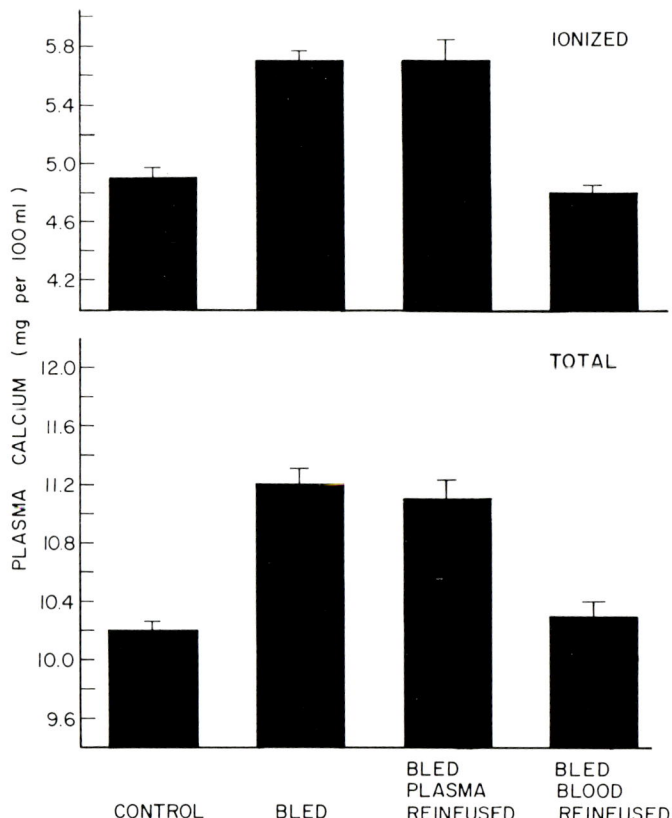

FIG. 16. Effect of bleeding and reinfusion of homologous plasma or blood on total and ionized plasma calcium concentration one day after 5 ml blood loss. Five milliliters of blood or plasma was reinfused within 1 minute of taking the original blood sample. Each value is a mean ± S.E.M. derived from between six and seventeen rats in each case. [From Perris et al. (52).]

Summary

The present considerations must lead to the conclusion that in at least three areas, those of growth, the control of thymic structure and lymphopoiesis, the calcium homeostatic system plays a vital role. Not only do experimentally created alterations in calcium balance affect mitotic activity in hemopoietic and lymphoid tissue, but also, and perhaps more importantly, when there is a physiological requirement for changes in the rate of cell division in these tissues, the rat utilizes its calcium homeostatic machinery to effect this process.

Although we have concentrated upon only two tissues, there may well be more general significance to these results. During growth, many tissues are obviously increasing in size, and this must partly be due to increased cellularity as well as perhaps an increase in size of individual cells. Aparathyroid animals in our experience do not grow, and this could be attributed in part to reduced calcium mobilization which inhibits bone growth and remodelling, and in part to the stress of hypocalcemia. However, the fact that there is a direct correlation between ionized plasma calcium concentrations and the growth rate of the rat (Fig. 5 and 8) and the fact

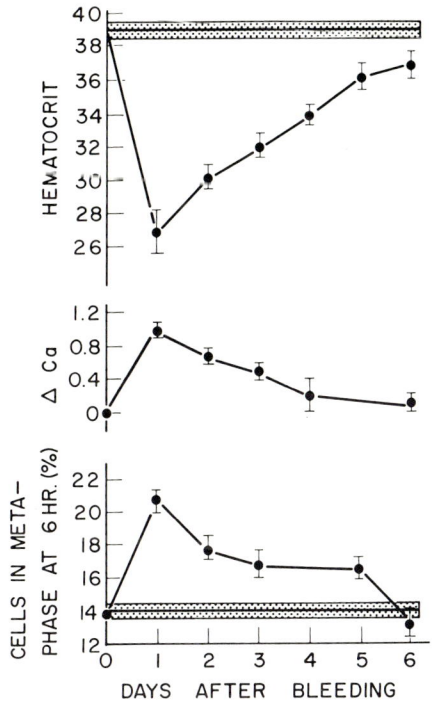

FIG. 17. Variation in hematocrit, plasma calcium, and bone marrow mitotic activity with time after hemorrhage. Five milliliters of blood were removed from rats on day 0, and at daily intervals thereafter the different parameters were examined as in FIG. 15. All values shown are mean values ± S.E.M. derived from between six and forty rats in each case. The horizontal line and shaded area represents the mean values and S.E.M. for normal rats. [From Perris et al. (52).]

TABLE II

Bone Marrow Mitotic Activity and Plasma Calcium Concentrations 24 Hours after 5 ml Blood Loss in Normal and TPTX Rats[a]

Condition of rat	Total plasma calcium (mg per 100 ml)	P	Percentage of cells in metaphase at 6 hours	P
Normal control	10.2 ± 0.06 (17)	<0.01	16.7 ± 1.3 (6)	<0.05
Normal bled	11.2 ± 0.1 (15)		20.7 ± 1.1 (6)	
TPTX	5.6 ± 0.17 (15)	>0.05	12.6 ± 1.4 (7)	>0.8
TPTX bled	5.2 + 0.11 (16)		12.2 ± 0.8 (7)	

[a] From Perris et al. (52).

that calcium and PTH influence cell division in a wide variety of different cell types *in vitro* (1–11, 18, 20, 26, 56, 57) suggest that mitotic activity in many tissues of the body like the lymphoid and hemopoietic tissues may be influenced by the endogenous secretion of PTH and thyrocalcitonin.

In the case of erythropoiesis, the interplay of these two polypeptide hormones definitely provides an important regulatory device for the control of this function (Figs. 12–14, 18, and 20 and Table I). In a wide variety of heightened and depressed erythropoietic circumstances, there are invariably parallel changes in the concentration of calcium in the plasma and the mitotic activity in the bone marrow (Figs. 14–17, 20). In many of these cases, it is impossible at the present time to state whether the calcium changes are due to altered rates of secretion of PTH or calcitonin, or whether the classic target tissues for these hormones, bone, kidney, or gut, have an altered sensitivity to the hormones. However, there is no doubt that after hemorrhage the hypocalcemia which develops over the first few hours (Fig. 19) act as a provocative stimulus for PTH release. Furthermore, the presence of the parathyroid gland and this release of PTH are essential for the increase in bone marrow mitosis and the normal rapid rate of erythrocyte restoration after bleeding (Table II and Fig. 18). This suggests that the important regulatory function of PTH is to stimulate proliferation in the bone marrow, thus providing a larger base of cells upon which erythropoietin may subsequently act as a differentiating agent and thus channel more cells along the erythroid developmental pathway (58).

Similarly where the calcium homeostatic system exercises a regulatory role on thymic lymphopoiesis (Figs. 1, 6, and 8), it may be important to have an adequate population of cells of thymic origin, with which antigens or other differentiating agents can subsequently react. The dramtic loss of thymic weight and the ultimate elimination of a supply of lymphocytes of thymic origin which accompanies parathyroidectomy (Figs. 8–11) must

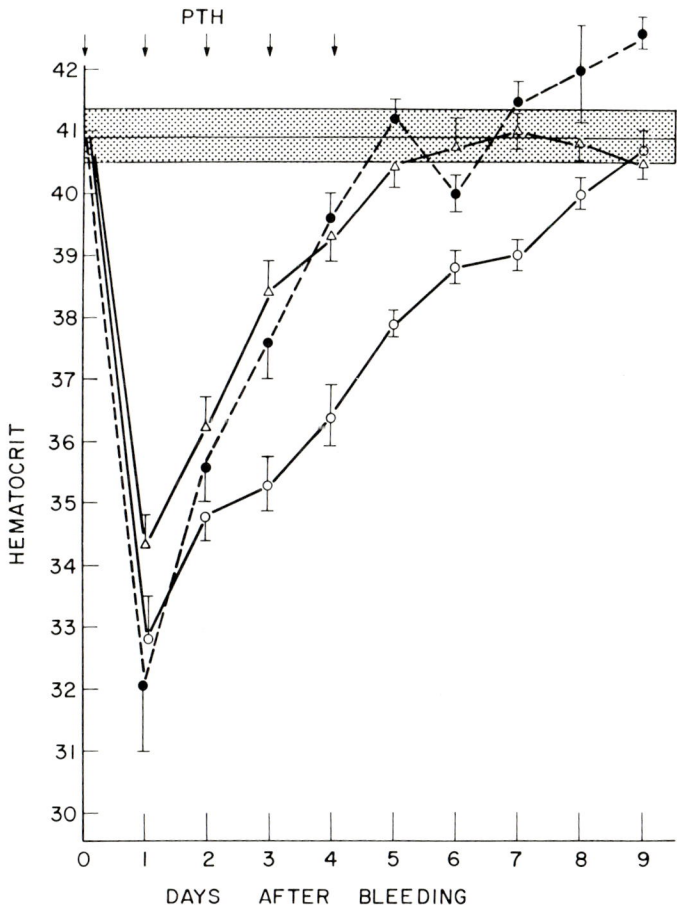

FIG. 18. Variation in hematocrit with time after hemorrhage in control and TPTX rats. Two days after the real or sham operation, 3 ml of blood were removed from each rat and the hematocrit was then measured at daily intervals. Each value is a mean ± S.E.M. derived from between six and ten rats in each case. The horizontal line and shaded area represent the mean and S.E.M. for normal untreated rats. ●---● Sham-operated pair-fed control rats; O——O TPTX rats; △——△ TPTX rats treated daily with PTH (50 units per 100 gm of rat) as shown by the arrows. [From Perris et al. (52).]

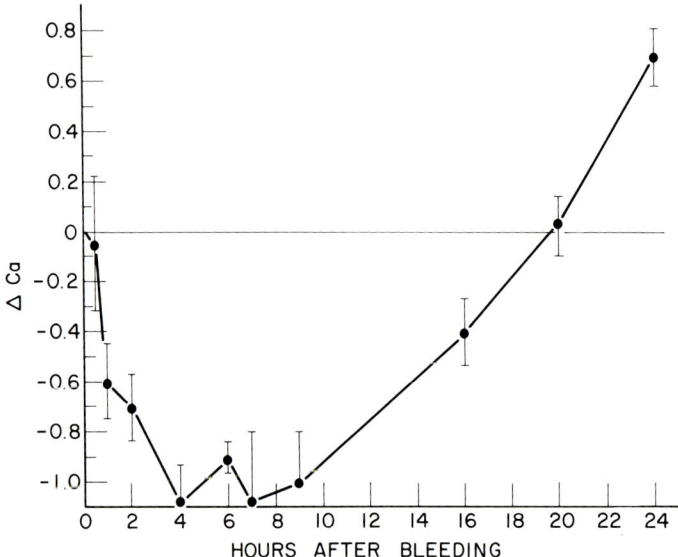

FIG. 19. Changes in plasma calcium concentrations in the rat immediately after 5 ml-blood loss. At intervals after the initial bleeding a second sample was taken. Final plasma calcium concentrations were compared with the initial concentration, each animal thus serving as its own control. Δ Ca is the difference between the final and initial plasma calcium concentrations (mg per 100 ml). Values are means ± S.E.M. derived from between four and nineteen animals. [From Perris et al. (52).]

surely affect whatever immunological function the thymus normally exercises in the adult animal (31).

We have stressed the role of calcium and PTH as mitogenic agents. This capacity, in fact, depends ultimately upon a cyclic AMP-mediated initiation of DNA synthesis (20–23), and thus the problem is really only a particular case of genetic expression. In the very rapidly proliferating thymic lymphocyte, exogenous or endogenous cyclic AMP induces the initiation of DNA synthesis within 1 hour (20–22). In cells and other tissues, such as peripheral blood lymphocytes and parotid glands, phytohaemagglutinin- or isoproterenol-induced cyclic AMP formation first stimulates nuclear RNA synthesis, and it is only many hours later that DNA synthesis and cell division occur (59–62). Perhaps because of its known ability to participate in the phosphorylation of histones (27, 28), the cyclic AMP causes derepression of the nucleohistone complex permitting in some cases transcription and in others replication of DNA. Certainly histone phosphorylation does precede the initiation of DNA synthesis and mitosis, and

The Homeostatic System and Cell Proliferation 123

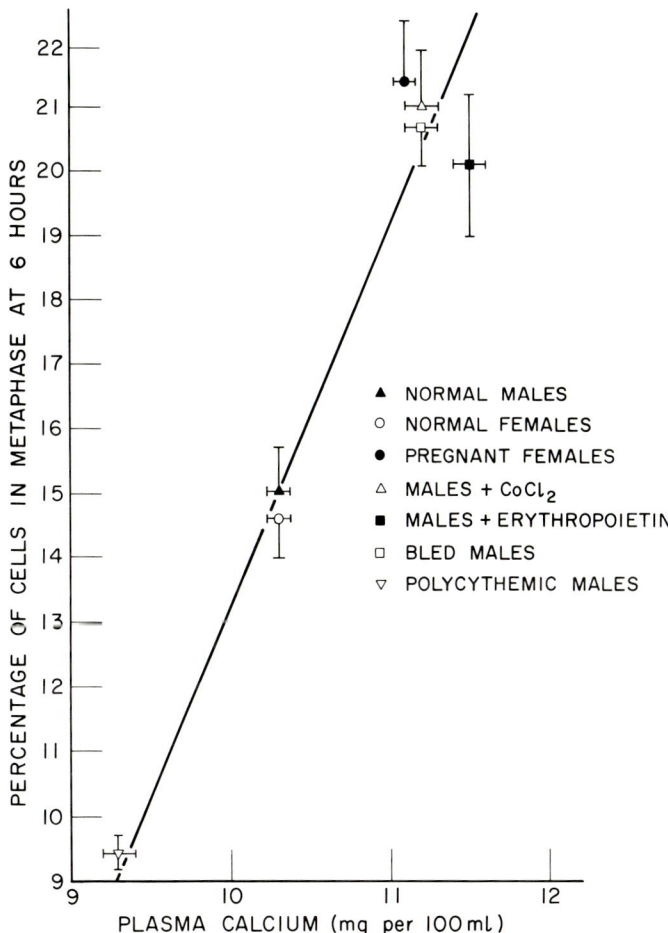

FIG. 20. Correlation between plasma calcium and bone marrow mitosis under different erythropoietic conditions. Pregnant rats were used at any time during the second and third weeks of pregnancy. Cobaltous chloride was given subcutaneously, dissolved in 0.5 ml saline at a dose of 5 μmoles per 100 gm of rat. Erythropoietin (Step I, Connaught Labs., Toronto, Canada) was dissolved in saline and a 0.5 ml subcutaneous injection was given containing 10 units per 100 gm rat. In the bled male rats, 5 ml of blood was removed by cardiac puncture. Plasma calcium and bone marrow mitotic activity was assessed 24 hours after cobaltous chloride, administration, erythropoietin, or bleeding. Polycythemia was induced by intraperitoneal injections of 2 ml of saline-washed packed red cells each day for 4 days and the rats were used 1 day after the last injection. Each point is a mean value ± S.E.M. derived from at least six rats in each case.

in the derepressed dispersed euchromatin, as opposed to repressed compact heterochromatin granules in the mammalian cell, there is a greater degree of histone phosphorylation (63-67). Cyclic AMP may thus be intimately in the regulation of genetic expression for both differentiation and proliferation. It should be pointed out here that in some autonomously growing tumors, the adenyl cyclase system responsible for cyclic AMP formation no longer responds to hormonal treatment, and such cells have excessively high levels of adenyl cyclase activity (68, 69).

Via their effect on the formation and degradation of cyclic AMP, the polypeptide hormones of the thyroparathyroid complex thus assume, in addition to their classic function of calcium homeostatic control, the equally important role of regulators of cell proliferation in mammalian tissues. The vast array of effects of calcium and these hormones on immunological, hemopoietic, and perhaps many other tissue functions awaits investigation.

ACKNOWLEDGMENTS

I would like to pay tribute to the extensive help and advice of Dr. J. F. Whitfield, with whom many of the experiments described here were conducted; to my other colleagues Drs. Helen J. Morton, R. H. Rixon, and J. P. MacManus, who allowed me to use their results; and to Messrs. L. A. Weiss, P. K. Tölg, C. Ibey, and Mlle V. Bibor, who provided me with excellent technical assistance at all times. Mrs. G. O. Barker has been a constant help with the literature associated with this work, as have Miss E. Monson and Mrs. C. Gobey with their secretarial assistance.

REFERENCES

1. Carlson, J. G., and Gaulden, M. E. (1961). In "The Initial Effects of Ionizing Radiations on Cells" (R. J. C. Harris, ed.), pp. 201-209. Academic Press, New York.
2. St. Amand, G. A., Anderson, N. G., and Gaulden, M. E. (1966). *Exp. Cell Res.* **20**, 71-76.
3. Whitfield, J. F., and Rixon, R. H. (1962). *Exp. Cell Res.* **27**, 154-157.
4. Whitfield, J. F., Brohée, H., and Youdale, T. (1966). *Exp. Cell Res.* **41**, 49-54.
5. Whitfield, J. F., and Youdale, T. (1966). *Exp. Cell Res.* **43**, 602-610.
6. Tyler, A. (1941). *Biol. Rev.* **16**, 291-335.
7. Heilbrun, L. V. (1952). "An Outline of General Physiology," pp. 728-743. Saunders, Philadelphia, Pennsylvania.
8. Hollingsworth, J. (1941). *Biol. Bull.* **81**, 261-276.
9. Fautrez-Firlefyn, N., and Fautrez, J. (1967). *Int. Rev. Cytol.* **22**, 171-204.
10. Morton, H. J. (1968). *Proc. Soc. Exp. Biol. Med.* **128**, 112-116.
11. Yang, D-P., and Morton, H. J. (1971). *J. Nat. Cancer Inst.* **46**, 505-516.
12. Perris, A. D., and Whitfield, J. F. (1967). *Nature (London)* **214**, 302-303.
13. Perris, A. D., and Whitfield, J. F. (1967). *Nature (London)* **216**, 1350-1351.
14. Perris, A. D., Whitfield, J. F., and Rixon, R. H. (1967). *Radiat. Res.* **32**, 550-563.

15. Perris, A. D., Whitfield, J. F., and Tölg, P. K. (1968). *Nature (London)* **219**, 527–529.
16. Rixon, R. H. (1968). *Curr. Mod. Biol.* **2**, 68–74.
17. Whitfield, J. F., Perris, A. D., and Youdale, T. (1968). *Exp. Cell Res.* **53**, 155–165.
18. Whitfield, J. F., Perris, A. D., and Youdale, T. (1969). *J. Cell. Physiol.* **73**, 203–212.
19. Whitfield, J. F., Rixon, R. H., Perris, A. D., and Youdale, T. (1969). *Exp. Cell Res.* **57**, 8–12.
20. Whitfield, J. F., MacManus, J. P., and Rixon, R. H. (1970). *J. Cell. Physiol.* **75**, 213–224.
21. MacManus, J. P., and Whitfield, J. F. (1969). *Proc. Soc. Exp. Biol. Med.* **132**, 409–412.
22. MacManus, J. P., and Whitfield, J. F. (1969). *Exp. Cell Res.* **58**, 183–191.
23. MacManus, J. P., and Whitfield, J. F. (1970). *Endocrinology* **86**, 934–939.
24. Bertalanffy, F., and Lau, C. (1962). *Int. Rev. Cytol.* **13**, 357–366.
25. Perris, A. D., and Whitfield, J. F. (1969). *Proc. Soc. Exp. Biol. Med.* **130**, 1198–1201.
26. MacManus, J. P., Perris, A. D., Whitfield, J. F., and Rixon, R. H. (1970). *In* "Proceedings of the Fifth Leukocyte Culture Conference." (J. Harris, ed.) Academic Press, New York, pp. 125–142.
26a. MacManus, J. P., Youdale, T., Whitfield, J. F., and Franks, D. J. (1971). Proceedings of the Fourth Parathyroid Hormone Conference (R. V. Talmago, ed.) Excerpta Medica, Amsterdam (in press).
27. Langan, T. A. (1968) *Science* **162**, 579–580.
28. Langan, T. A. (1969). *J. Biol. Chem.* **244**, 5763–5765.
29. Borum, K. (1964). *Abstr. Congr. Int. Soc. Haematol.*, *10th 1964* Sect. H., p. 20.
30. Metcalf, D. (1966). *Thymus: Exp. Clin. Stud., Ciba Found. Symp.*, 1965 pp. 242–287.
31. Miller, J. F. A. P., and Osoba, D. (1967). *Physiol. Rev.* **47**, 437–520.
32. Metcalf, D., Sparrow, N., Nakamura, K., and Ishidate, M., Jr. (1961). *Aust. J. Exp. Biol. Med. Sci.* **39**, 441–453.
33. Pepper, F. J. (1961). *J. Endocrinol.* **22**, 349–359.
34. Metcalf, D. (1964). Thymus, *Symp.*, 1964 No. 2, pp. 53–73.
35. Metcalf, D. (1964). *In* "The Thymus in Immunobiology" (R. A. Good and A. E. Gabrielson, eds.), pp. 150–182. Harper (Hoeber), New York.
36. Dukor, P., Miller, J. F. A. P., House, W., and Allman, V. (1965). *Transplantation* **3**, 639–668.
37. Matsuyama, M., Wiadrowski, M. N., and Metcalf, D. (1966). *J. Exp. Med.* **123**, 559–576.
38. Perris, A. D., Weiss, L. A., and Whitfield, J. F. (1970). *J. Cell. Physiol.* **76**, 141–150.
39. Dougherty, T. F. (1952). *Physiol. Rev.* **32**, 379–401.
40. Kaplan, H. S., Nagareda, C. S., and Brown, M. (1954). *Recent Progr. Horm. Res.* **10**, 293–338.
41. Shewell, J. (1957). *Brit. J. Pharmacol.* **12**, 133–139.
42. Ishidate, M., Jr., and Metcalf, D. (1963). *Aust. J. Exp. Biol. Med. Sci.* **41**, 637–649.
43. Fried, W., Plzak, L., Jacobson, L. O., and Goldwasser, E. (1956). *Proc. Soc. Exp. Biol. Med.* **92**, 203–207.
44. Perris, A. D., and Whitfield, J. F. (1971). *Can. J. Physiol. Pharmacol.* **49**, 22–35.
45. Zanjani, E. D., Contrera, J. F., Cooper, G. W., Gordon, A. S., and Wong, K. K. (1967). *Science* **156**, 1367–1368.
46. Zanjani, E. D., Cooper, G. W., Gordon, A. S., Wong, K. K., and Scribner, V. A. (1967). *Proc. Soc. Exp. Biol. Med.* **126**, 540–542.

47. Wong, K. K., Zanjani, E. D., Cooper, G. W., and Gordon, A. S. (1968). *Proc. Soc. Exp. Biol. Med.* **128,** 67–70.
48. Adamson, J. W., and Finch, C. A. (1968). *Ann. N.Y. Acad. Sci.* **149,** 560–563.
49. Copp, D. H., and Davidson, A. G. F. (1961). *Proc. Soc. Exp. Biol. Med.* **107,** 342–344.
50. Sherwood, L. M., Mayer, G. P., Ramberg, C. F., Kronfeld, D. S., Aurbach, G. D., and Potts, J. T. (1968). *Endocrinology* **83,** 1043–1051.
51. Talmage, R. V., and Toft, R. (1961). *In* "The Parathyroids" (R. O. Greep and R. V. Talmage, eds.), pp. 224–242. Thomas, Springfield, Illinois.
52. Perris, A. D., MacManus, J. P., Whitfield, J. F., and Weiss, L. A. (1971). *Amer. J. Physiol.* **220,** 773.
53. Jacobson, L. O., and Goldwasser, E. (1958). *Brookhaven Symp. Biol.* **10,** 110–131.
54. Jepson, J., and Lowenstein, L. (1968). *Brit. J. Haematol.* **14,** 555–562.
55. Contopoulos, A. N., Van Dyke, D. C., and Simpson, M. E. (1956). *Proc. Soc. Exp. Biol. Med.* **93,** 424–428.
56. Borle, A. B. (1968). *J. Cell Biol.* **36,** 567–582.
57. Borle, A. B., and Neumann, W. F. (1965). *J. Cell Biol.* **24,** 316–323.
58. Goldwasser, E. (1966). *Curr. Top. Develop. Biol.* **1,** 173–209.
59. Smith, J. W., Steiner, A. L., and Parker, C. W. (1970). *Fed. Proc. Fed. Amer. Soc. Exp. Biol.* **29,** 369 (abstr.).
60. Hirschhorn, R., Grossman, J., and Weissmann, G. (1970). *Proc. Soc. Exp. Biol. Med.* **133,** 1361–1365.
61. Baserga, R., Sasaki, T., and Whitlock, J. P. (1969). *In* "Biochemistry of Cell Division" (R. Baserga, ed.), pp. 77–90. Thomas, Springfield, Illinois.
62. Malamud, D. (1969). *Biochem. Biophys. Res. Commun.* **35,** 754–758.
63. Stevely, W. S., and Stocken, L. A. (1968). *Biochem. J.* **109,** 24P.
64. Stevely, W. S., and Stocken, L. A. (1968). *Biochem. J.* **110,** 187–191.
65. Ord, M. G., and Stocken, L. A. (1969). *Biochem. J.* **112,** 81–89.
66. Littau, V. C., Burdick, C. J., Allfrey, V. G., and Mirsky, A. E. (1965). *Proc. Nat. Acad. Sci. U.S.* **54,** 1204–1212.
67. Allfrey, V. G., Pogo, B. G. T., Pogo, A. O., Kleinsmith, L. V., and Mirsky, A. E. (1966). *In* "Histones" (A. V. S. de Reuck and J. Knight, eds.), pp. 42–62. Churchill, London.
68. Brown, H. D., Chattopadhyay, S. K., Spjut, H. J., Spratt, J. S., and Pennington, S. N. (1969). *Biochim. Biophys. Acta* **192,** 372–375.
69. Brown, H. D., Chattopadhyay, S. K., Morris, H. P., and Pennington, S. N. (1970). *Cancer Res.* **30,** 123–126.

Discussion

Dr. Simmons: Dr. Perris, when one wants to consider colchicine metaphases, one worries about the variation owing to diurnal changes in the numbers of cells in a tissue undergoing replication [D. J. Simmons, *Nature (London)* **202,** 906 (1964); D. J. Simmons and G. Nichols, Jr., *Amer. J. Physiol.* **210,** 411 (1966)].

Dr. Perris: There certainly are diurnal variations in bone marrow mitotic activity. We always assess mitosis at the same time each day in both control and treated rats, thus avoiding the problem. I do hope to look at calcium levels at different times of the day to see whether there are changes associated with diurnal alterations in mitosis.

Dr. Frame: It has been suggested that a relative excess of PTH may play a role in the endosteal bone loss which occurs in osteoporosis. There is also the possibility that the endosteal bone loss in osteoporosis is secondary to primary changes in the bone marrow. Since you found evidence of increased cellular mitoses and proliferation in the bone marrow after the administration of PTH, I wonder if you observed any evidence of enhanced endosteal bone resorption?

Dr. Perris: I really have no idea. We don't work with human material, of course. The only comment I have is that both exogenous and endogenous PTH increase DNA synthesis in bone cells [H. Rohr, *Klin. Wachenschr.* **42**, 1209 (1964); H. Z. Park and R. V. Talmage, *Endocrinology* **80**, 552 (1967)].

Dr. Bergstrom: Dr. Fernando Canas found adrenal hypertrophy in rats 48 hours after bilateral nephrectomy [F. M. Canas, W. H. Bergstrom, and S. J. Churgin, *Metab. Clin. Exp.* **16**, 670 (1967)]. This did not occur in rats thyroparathyroidectomized at the time of nephrectomy; these animals had an average serum calcium concentration of 7.2 mg%. The calcium concentration did not rise after nephrectomy alone. Has the effect of calcium on cell multiplication been demonstrated in other than hematopoietic tissues?

Dr. Perris: With the exception of lymphoid tissue, as you have seen, I don't think it has been shown *in vivo*. Certainly, *in vitro* things as diverse as grasshopper neuroblasts, L-cells, Hela cells, and thymic cells all respond to calcium, and in some cases to PTH as well. After nephrectomy, I certainly think there would be an increase in secretion of PTH. Dr. Talmage's studies showed this. It could very well have an effect on hypertrophy of the adrenal, as you mentioned.

Dr. MacIntyre: I think you inferred that the changes in total plasma calcium after hemorrhage were in fact due to changes in ionic plasma calcium. Did you make any measurements of this?

Dr. Perris: We have measured both total and ionized calcium, and they both change in parallel with each other. During the initial hypocalcemia immediately after hemorrhage, we can detect a lowering of both total and ionized calcium. The subsequent hypercalcemia is also in terms of both ionized and total calcium.

Dr. MacIntyre: Do you have any explanation on the mechanism of the changes?

Dr. Perris: We presume it is a release of PTH which is causing the subsequent hypercalcemia.

Dr. MacIntyre: I meant the initial hypocalcemia.

Dr. Perris: We think in some way this is probably related to hypoxia. In support of this, we can assume, I think, that after removal of 33% of the rat's blood volume, they are at least temporarily hypoxic. As you have seen, the plasma calcium goes down. If we treat the rat with cobaltous chloride, which causes histotoxic hypoxia, again plasma levels of calcium fall. Further, if we keep the rats in a hypoxic chamber and expose them either briefly to 10% oxygen or, in a more protracted sense, to 15% oxygen (in contrast to the normal 20%), again we get a lowering of plasma calcium.

We think that hypoxia may inhibit the pump which normally excludes calcium from the cell interior. If this pump is inhibited, it may lead to an influx of calcium into the cells from the extracellular fluid and perhaps from the plasma, which may be of sufficient magnitude to cause the initial posthemorrhagic hypocalcemia.

Dr. Heaney: Dr. Perris, you have proposed a plausible explanation for the transiently increased parathyroid activity after hemorrhage, but this does not seem a suitable explanation for continued hypercalcemia, so long as the hematocrit remains low, nor does it explain the hypercalcemia of pregnancy and that occurring during the most rapid phase of growth.

Dr. Perris: No, it doesn't.

Dr. Heaney: You have shown or presented evidence for a rather dramatic change in the ionized calcium, from about 4 to about 7 mg%, as I recall. Do you have any thoughts on this rather dramatic readjustment of the reference level to which the homeostatic system is attempting to adjust the plasma calcium?

Dr. Perris: The protracted hypercalcemia which exists as long as the hematocrit remains subnormal is something of a puzzle. It may be that in some way the release of erythropoietin which accompanies hemorrhage and pregnancy, for example, could sensitize the appropriate end organs to the ambient PTH, and thus lead to increased plasma calcium concentration. However, there may not be any protracted increase in PTH concentration in the circulation. It is rather difficult to measure in the rat, of course.

Dr. Radde: We have some confirmatory evidence. Very premature babies, during the most rapid phase of growth at 1-3 months of age, have significant hypercalcemia, with ionized calcium levels going up to about almost 3 meq/liter. Their total calcium was not elevated quite as markedly. Can you explain the proliferative effect of hypomagnesemia on lymphocytes reported by Dr. Jasmin of Montreal in magnesium-deficient rats?

Dr. Perris: Hypomagnesemia is well known to provoke a release of PTH which could, independently of its calcium elevating capacity, stimulate cell division in the thymocyte.

Dr. Spencer: You mean that the low magnesium was acting as a provocative stimulus for PTH release as well? That could be true. I should mention here, prehaps, that magnesium on its own is also mitogenic. The mechanism is a little less certain than the one I described to you for calcium. However, I hadn't measured magnesium concentrations.

Dr. Massry: Do you think that this phenomenon will play any role in carcinogenesis? This question is posed because we have just reviewed some 160 cases of parathyroid adenoma and were surprised to find that the incidence of other malignancies, such as those of gastrointestinal tract, thyroid, and breast, were significantly higher than the incidence in a similar group of similar age and sex.

Dr. Perris: That is very exciting. As an additional comment to this, I think that I implied that the effect of calcium and PTH on mitosis in fact emanates from an ability of calcium or PTH to increase the intracellular concentration of cyclic AMP. In certain tumors the activity of adenyl cyclase (which is responsible for the formation of cyclic AMP) is markedly elevated [H. D. Brown, S. K. Chattopadhyay, H. J. Spjut, J. S. Spratt, and S. N. Pennington, *Biochim. Biophys. Acta* **192**, 372 (1969); *Cancer Res.* **30**, 123 (1970)].

Dr. Kuettner: I think your observation on the thymus may be extremely interesting for the immunologist. Do you see any implication of coinjection of antigen and calcium, or even combination of the treatment of PTH with the antigen or any influence of calcitonin in antibody formation?

Dr. Perris: We don't have the answers. I hope to indulge in some of these things in the near future.

Dr. Bordier: It is well known that, in the presence of PTH, bone progenitor cells differentiate mainly into osteoclasts. Is it possible that increased calcium concentration inside the progenitor cells (as an effect of PTH upon the entry of calcium into the cell) is a stimulus for the differentiation or division of the cells?

Dr. Perris: I suppose it could. Certainly a differentiation process or model of such a differentiation process has been derived for the peripheral blood lymphocytes after treatment with phytohemagglutinin. Phytohemagglutinin induces an increase in the intracellular concentration of cyclic AMP in these cells [J. W. Smith, A. L. Steiner, W. N. Newberry, Jr., and C. W. Parker, *J. Clin. Invest.* **50,** 432 (1971).] In such repressed cells, it takes several days before DNA synthesis is initiated. After the initial event (increased cyclic AMP concentration), first of all, RNA synthesis is stimulated, then protein synthesis, and ultimately DNA synthesis. A few days after exposure to PHA these peripheral blood lymphocytes ultimately enter division. I think there is a good case for involving cyclic AMP and perhaps PTH in differentiation processes.

Dr. Rich: Dr. Perris, your beautiful work invites speculation about possible extension of your concepts to other systems in which tissue function is dependent upon rapid proliferation of cells. In hypoparathyroid patients, one occasionally sees, not only the failure to absorb calcium, but failure to absorb fat as well. I wonder whether this failure could be the consequence of reduced mitogenesis leading to a hypoplastic intestinal mucosa. I don't know of any work that relates to this possibility and wonder if you do.

Dr. Perris: No.

Dr. Copp: This elegant demonstration of the effect of calcium on cell reproduction and growth by Dr. Perris may help to explain the effects on growth which we have observed in young rats and chicks given daily injections of salmon calcitonin. The rats, which received the hormone from birth to 23 days of age, grew consistently slower than the control group injected with vehicle. In view of the hypocalcemia associated with calcitonin administration, this would fit in with Dr. Perris' hypothesis. In the case of chicks injected daily with 1 MRC unit salmon calcitonin from hatching to 3 months of age, growth of the hormone-treated birds was approximately 25% faster than in the controls. These birds do not get hypocalcemic, and there is the possibility of secondary hyperparathyroidism which might, according to Dr. Perris' work, explain the enhanced growth rate. It is also possible that calcitonin may have had a direct effect on intracellular calcium. In any case, I feel that the linking of growth and calcium may be of great significance.

Dr. Matthews: We have been looking at calcium in the cells in cooperation with Dr. Lynn of our Department of Pathology, and we have now looked at over three hundred mammary gland tumors. The electron micrographs of the nuclei of the cells are of particular interest. One sees fine dots associated with the chromatin material called perichromatin granules. We analyzed these granules and showed that they were calcium by EGTA resorption and other methods. When we count these granules, their number correlates with the state of malignancy as determined morphologically.

Dr. Perris: We are not entirely sure whether the effect of calcium is via surface events on the plasma membrane or are cytoplasmic events or via some direct effect on nuclear metabolism. Some Australian investigators recently have studied isolated nuclei from both liver and the thymus, and found that calcium elevation does increase DNA synthesis in these isolated nuclei [L. A. Burgoyne, M. A. Waqar, and M. R. Atkinson, *Biochem. Biophys. Res. Commun.* **39,** 918 (1970)].

Dr. Mills: I was fascinated by your work, partly because we see a similar thing in rabbits at the costochondral junction, where the entire cell population seems to change markedly when you inject calcium or conversely, when you inject EDTA to remove calcium. You are probably familiar with the work of Lippman [M. Lippman, *in* "Epithelial-Mesenchymal Interactions," pp. 208–229. Williams & Wilkins, Baltimore, Maryland, 1968] which shows that in the cell cycle, calcium initiates mitosis until nucleic acids are reduced and mitosis is stopped, and that this is followed by a cycle of protein synthesis. Have you done any work on protein synthesis at various times in the cycle?

Dr. Perris: No, we haven't. If I recall Lippman's work correctly, she interpreted the effect of calcium on mitotic activity as being a prophase event and in some way related to the coiling of chromosomes as a preface to cell division. Our work shows the effect emanates from somewhere much further back in the cell cycle; in fact, from the initiation of DNA synthesis.

Dr. Sabet: Did you investigate lymph node cells, particularly in the light of the significant number of cells in the lymph nodes being thymus derived?

Dr. Perris: No, we haven't looked at lymph nodes yet.

Dr. W. P. L. Myers: I wonder whether others observed, as we have, the occurrence of anemia in spontaneous hyperparathyroidism. Albright and Reifenstein [F. Albright and E. C. Reifenstein, Jr., *in* "The Parathyroid Glands and Metabolic Bone Disease," pp. 62 and 67. Williams & Wilkins, Baltimore, Maryland, 1948] have described this in their book, and we have observed one patient with profound anemia which was reversed by parathyroidectomy, the patient having had primary hyperparathyroidism. Also, have you studied the effect of vitamin D in this system?

Dr. Perris: We haven't studied the effects of vitamin D. In response to your first question, I can't explain the effect, but I should point out that we are not claiming that the requirement for PTH following hemorrhage, for example, is absolute. In the TPTX rat, the hematocrit does eventually come back to normal after bleeding, despite the fact that there are no parathyroids. So other things must certainly be operating. Erythropoietin is an obvious possibility. Antidiuretic hormone, which is released after hemorrhage, might also have some effect on the rate of hematocrit restoration since it, too, is mitogenic. There is no absolute requirement for PTH, but it is essential for the normal rapid rate of erythrocyte restoration. In these experiments, one must be very careful to distinguish between what may be hemodilution or hemoconcentration and anemia or polycythemia.

Dr. Howell: Is there any information on intracellular calcium requirements for effective muscle spindle formation of the contractile proteins which are involved with mitosis?

Dr. Perris: Do you mean is there any requirement for calcium in the formation of the mitotic apparatus? Yes, there is, but that is not what we are looking at. Our effects of calcium on mitosis emanate from the S-phase of the cell cycle, long before the spindle has, in fact, become apparent. But there may be a requirement for calcium for the contraction and separation of the chromosomes at anaphase and in the actual formation of the mitotic apparatus.

Dr. Eisenberg: Were the TPTX rats given thyroid supplements? Also, I was wondering if you had observed the initial hypocalcemia in the bled animals when they are reinfused with plasma.

Dr. Perris: Yes, bled rats reinfused with plasma do develop hypocalcemia. In regard to thyroid supplementation, I believe we gave 3 μg per day in some cases, which is adequate to replace the lost thyroid function. We get no effect of thyroxin on mitotic activity in the bone marrow under these circumstances. The administration of L-thyroxine to a TPTX bled rat also has no effect on the rate of hematocrit restoration.

Dr. Eisenberg: Parenthetically, I would like to say we have made the observation that parathyroidectomy relieves anemia in the absence of any change in renal function in hyperparathyroid patients.

Dr. King: I would like to comment that, in animals which we treat with the diphosphonate [ethane-1-hydroxy-1,1-diphosphonate (EHDP)], we see a rise in blood calcium levels. Simultaneous with this, we also have good histological evidence of increased osteoblastic activity in the bone.

Dr. Harrison: On the relation of ionized calcium and total calcium to the age or the

The Homeostatic System and Cell Proliferation

size and growth of the animal, I noticed that the ionized calcium rose from about 40% to about 60%. Was there less serum protein in the older animal? Or do we have to assume that the binding capacity of the protein is altered so that a higher proportion of the calcium is ionized at the same concentration of albumin in the plasma?

Dr. Perris: I don't know. It could be that pH and/or phosphate changes are also involved. These haven't been measured.

Dr. Goldhaber: If I understood the point brought up before about those cases having parathyroid tumors also having other tumors correctly, I am not so sure that this situation would be limited only to the parathyroids. I believe it is well known that there is a greater incidence of multiple tumors in patients who have other tumors. I suggest that one should look at other types of tumors besides parathyroid tumors. Another point: heparin does drastically affect mitosis and reduces it.

Dr. Perris: Yes, if you raise the heparin concentration high enough, the ionized plasma calcium is decreased as a consequence. This could be one reason why it does so.

Dr. Frame: I would like to comment on your evidence that increased calcium levels increase cell mitoses in certain tissues and also on Dr. Massry's comment regarding an increased incidence of malignancies in primary hyperparathyroidism. I have been interested in the syndrome of multiple endocrine adenomatosis where hypercalcemia due to hyperparathyroidism is often present for many years before there is evidence of other endocrine hyperplasia and hyperfunction. I would like to ask whether you think the longstanding hypercalcemia might play a role in the hyperplastic and adenomatous changes that occur in several of the endocrines in this syndrome.

Dr. Perris: I am pleased to hear about it. The cart does really come before the horse in this case. Many people have said to me that the hypercalcemia will develop after the advent of the tumor, but in your case the hypercalcemia comes prior to the development of the malignancy.

Dr. Hastings: Did you determine the effect of calcium on liver regeneration?

Dr. Perris: Not yet.

III. Calcium Transfer across Cell and Subcellular Membranes

A CALCIUM PUMP IN RED CELL MEMBRANES

Frank F. Vincenzi

The late J. B. Kahn, in his review of glycoside actions (1962), noted the superficial absurdity of scientists who, wishing to know about the actions of digitalis on the heart, spent their time studying the red blood cell (RBC), or even broken-up pieces of RBC membrane. I hasten to point out that our work on the movement of calcium across RBC membranes is also based on the kind of reasoning to which Dr. Kahn alluded. However, I must add that the use of the RBC as a model of the myocardial cell may not be quite as absurd as might first appear. Certainly, the RBC has been an extremely useful model in working out the now widely accepted notions about sodium–potassium transport and the actions of digitalis thereon. The model is obviously far from complete, for in spite of a mountain of circumstantial evidence, the relationship (if any) between the inhibition of sodium–potassium transport in heart cells and the positive inotropic (and other) cardiac actions of glycosides is not entirely clear (Glynn, 1964). Some very attractive evidence has recently appeared linking inhibition of sodium–potassium–magnesium-activated ATPase (also called sodium–potassium-activated ATPase or transport ATPase) with positive inotropism (Schwartz *et al.*, 1969; Akera *et al.*, 1970). Nevertheless, the relationship is still circumstantial.

With the general acceptance of the central role of calcium as the link in excitation–contraction coupling, the attention of many workers turned to possible glycoside actions on active calcium as well as active sodium–potassium transport. We reasoned that, in spite of intriguing studies with isolated sarcoplasmic reticular fragments (Lee and Choi, 1966), a simpler model would be useful. Because the RBC had been so useful in working out sodium-potassium transport mechanisms, we reasoned that it might also be useful in studying calcium transport. Of course, in thinking of the RBC as a model of calcium transport, the first question was whether RBC's in fact transport calcium. A second major question was whether such calcium transport be influenced by cardiac glycosides. As a working hypothesis, we proposed that active membrane calcium transport did exist and that such transport would be associated with membrane ATPase activity.

Early experiments (Schatzmann, 1966) were encouraging and suggested that active calcium transport did occur, and that it was not inhibited by ouabain. It was decided to pursue these findings and to apply more rigorous criteria for establishing active transport. Most of our findings, outlined below, have been published (Schatzmann and Vincenzi, 1969).

From earlier workers (Passow, 1961, 1963; Rummel et al., 1962) there was reason to believe that RBC membranes were relatively impermeable to calcium, and that normal calcium content of the RBC is extremely low. Our findings were in agreement with these expectations. We found extremely slow passive influx of ^{45}Ca in cold-stored RBC's. Porzig (1970) has concluded that such passive calcium movements fit saturation kinetics and also that there is a calcium–calcium exchange diffusion mechanism. Calcium content of RBC's in our experiments was approximately 6×10^{-5} moles per liter of cell water. The concentration of free Ca^{2+} in the cell ($[Ca]_i$) is certainly less than this when one considers that a sizeable, but admittedly unknown, fraction of the calcium is bound to various cell constituents such as ATP and ADP. In any event, considering the plasma calcium concentration ($[Ca]_o$) it is clear that a large inward gradient for calcium exists across the RBC membrane. Whether this is maintained only by low permeability to calcium or also by an active outward transport of calcium needed investigation.

Several important advancements in the field of membrane transport lay the foundation for our approach. For example, in 1953 Schatzmann described the specific action of cardiac glycosides on the active transport of sodium and potassium across the RBC membrane. This action has now been amply confirmed in nearly all tissues (Glynn, 1964). Second, Skou (1957) described an ATPase in isolated crab nerve membrane which was activated (in the presence of magnesium and ATP) by the simultaneous presence of sodium and potassium and which was likewise specifically inhibited by cardiac glycosides. These phenomena have also been amply confirmed in many tissues. The work of hundreds of investigators since these observations has formed the basis of overwhelming circumstantial evidence linking membrane-bound sodium–potassium–magnesium–activated

ATPase activity with the active transport of sodium and potassium. By analogy, we therefore predicted that the active transport of calcium would be associated with a calcium-activated ATPase. Of course, a calcium-activated-magnesium-dependent-ATPase (or calcium–magnesium-activated ATPase) had been known in RBC membranes for some time (Dunham and Glynn, 1961; Wins and Schoffeniels, 1966a). Since we were searching for a model of active calcium transport in muscle, we noted that the isolated actomyosin systems of skeletal and cardiac muscle are activated when the [Ca] is about 10^{-7} M or above, with half maximal activation occurring at about $10^{-6.2}$ M (Katz and Repke, 1966). To learn if the calcium–magnesium-activated ATPase of RBC membranes would be stimulated by similarly low [Ca]'s we carefully quantified activation of RBC membrane ATPase as a function of [Ca]. The results (Vincenzi and Schatzmann, 1967) indicated that the threshold for activation was about 10^{-7} M, with peak activation at about 10^{-4} M. This therefore seemed to be a reasonably sensitive system. Interestingly, the calcium–magnesium-activated ATPase was not inhibited by 10^{-4} M ouabain. We shall return to this point. It was also of interest that the magnitude of the calcium–magnesium-activated ATP splitting was about five times that of the ouabain-inhibitable ATPase. Since the ouabain-inhibitable activity has become synonymous with the sodium–potassium–magnesium activated ATPase activity, and in turn with sodium–potassium transport, this was an extremely exciting finding. Here was an ATPase which, under proper conditions would split five times as much substrate as the sodium–potassium transport ATPase. We concluded (see below) that active calcium transport is related to a calcium–magnesium-activated ATPase. However, recent findings suggest the existence of a number of calcium-activated ATPases in the RBC (Marchesi and Steers, 1968; Rosenthal et al., 1970; Schatzmann, 1970a). The relationships of the variously determined calcium-activated ATPases to each other and to various cellular functions is uncertain. Until the pattern is more clearly defined, stoichiometric comparisons between ATPase activity and other functions must remain circumspect.

The next question was obviously whether the calcium–magnesium-activated ATPase was, in fact, associated with active calcium transport, whether it had other functions (Wins and Schoffeniels, 1966b), or even no apparent biological function. In experiments to test whether calcium is transported by RBC membranes (Schatzmann, 1966), we loaded RBC's with calcium using the reversible hemolysis technique (Whittam, 1962). Much of the usefulness of the RBC, in addition to its relative simplicity, is based on this phenomenon of reversible hemolysis. Exactly how reversible hemolysis works is unknown. In simplified terms, it might be said that during hypotonic shock, RBC membranes become "leaky." Thus, substances such as calcium or hemoglobin, which normally do not pass the membrane well, do so readily. The critical part of the phenomenon is that the "leakiness" is not irreversible, and that if cells are soon returned to normal tonicity (usually by addition of hypertonic potassium chloride), they somehow "reseal" and regain low permeability. Thus, one may load cells with particular substances and then reseal the cells. Such cells are usually referred to as resealed ghosts.

For transport experiments, then, red cell ghosts prepared from starved (see below) RBC's were loaded with calcium and ATP–magnesium, or

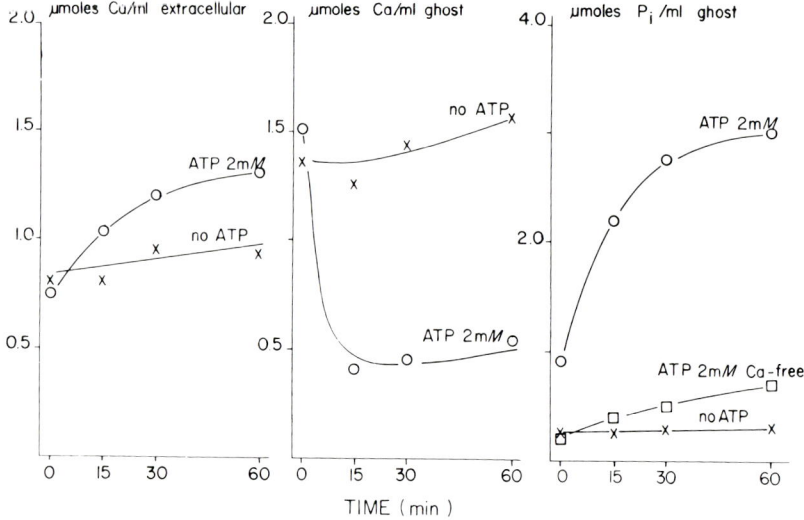

FIG. 1. Active extrusion of calcium from red cell ghosts prepared from starved RBC's and correlation with inorganic phosphate (P_i) release. Cells were starved by preincubation at 37°C for 17 hours in the absence of glucose. Cells were then reversibly hemolyzed at room temperature and washed once at 0°C. Hemolyzing solution contained 1 mM $CaCl_2$; 2 mM $MgCl_2$; with (○) or without (×) 2 mM $ATPNa_2$. An additional group of cells was treated similarly and loaded with $MgCl_2$ and $ATPNa_2$ in the absence of $CaCl_2$, and without $CaCl_2$ in the extracellular medium (□). Ghosts were then incubated at 37°C in medium containing 130 mM NaCl, 5 mM KCl, 1 mM $CaCl_2$, 20 mM tris buffer (pH 7.4), and ouabain 10^{-4} gm/ml, with a hematocrit of approximately 0.3. Note that in the ATP-loaded cells there is a rapid disappearance of calcium from the ghost and appearance of calcium in the extracellular medium, with the final cell content being less than medium content. This transport of calcium was associated with the liberation of P_i in the ghost above levels for ATP-loaded–calcium-free ghosts, or calcium-loaded–ATP-free ghosts.

with calcium and magnesium, but without ATP. The ghosts were washed once at 0°C in medium containing 130 mM NaCl, 5mM KCl, 2 mM MgCl$_2$, and 20 mM tris buffer (pH 7.4). When subsequently incubated in the same medium at 37°C, calcium and ATP–magnesium loaded cells exhibited a rapid disappearence of calcium from the ghosts and a simultaneous appearance of calcium in the external medium. There was likewise appearance of inorganic phosphate (P$_i$) in the ghosts. These results were not seen in cells loaded with calcium and magnesium without ATP. In a typical experiment, as shown in Fig. 1, the final content of calcium in the extracellular fluid always exceeded that in the ghosts with ATP (in spite of overestimation of cell calcium content, because ghosts were not washed in calcium-free medium prior to analysis). Thus, the movement of calcium was against a chemical gradient, and in view of the membrane potential of the ghost, which is similar to the normal RBC [8 mV, negative inside (Jay and Burton, 1969)], was thermodynamically uphill. A number of possible artifactual explanations for these observations were considered and were dismissed (Schatzmann and Vincenzi, 1969). In short, we concluded that there exists in the RBC membrane an outwardly-directed active calcium transport mechanism associated with the extrusion of calcium from the cell. Other workers have come to the same conclusion (Olson and Cazort, 1969; Lee and Shin, 1969; Porzig, 1970).

We also concluded that active calcium transport was associated with the hydrolysis of ATP. During the initial phase of calcium transport, 1.3 moles of P$_i$ appeared per mole of calcium transported. On the other hand, the ATP requirement for active transport was unclear in our earliest transport experiments, in which only calcium was measured. In such early experiments, fresh (rather than starved, see above) RBC's were divided into two groups, one of which was loaded with calcium and ATP–magnesium, the other with only calcium and magnesium. A typical result is shown in Fig. 2. Although apparent calcium transport was less for control cells (without ATP), these cells, nevertheless, seemed to extrude calcium against a chemical gradient. Since this is a basic criterion for active transport, this was disturbing to say the least. The results seemed to imply either a systematic error in calcium analysis, or a lack of ATP-dependence of the presumably active extrusion mechanism, or both. However, when we correlated the appearance of P$_i$ with the transport of calcium (as in Fig. 3), it became clear that ghosts prepared from fresh RBC's contained enough endogenous ATP to support calcium transport, even when ATP was not added during reversible hemolysis. Cells which were starved so as to deplete endogenous ATP (by incubation at 37°C for 17 hours in the absence of glucose) before reversible hemolysis did not transport calcium when ATP was not added, but did when the energy source was provided, as in Fig. 1.

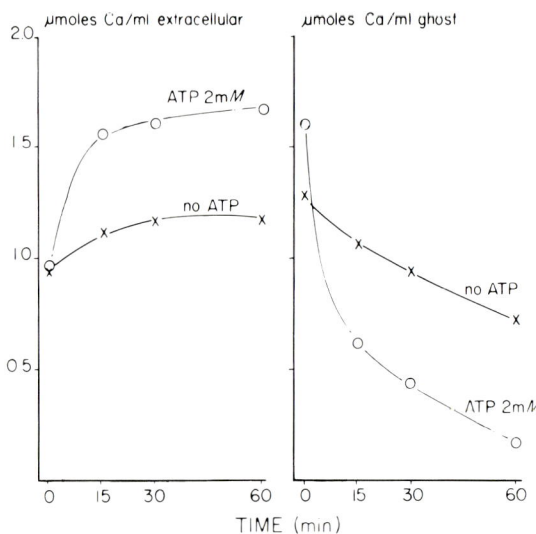

Fig. 2. Active extrusion of calcium from red cell ghosts prepared from fresh RBC's. Experimental design and symbols as in Fig. 1, except that ghosts were prepared from fresh RBC's. Transport of calcium was less in the ghosts to which no ATP was added during hemolysis. Nevertheless, ghosts appeared to extrude calcium against a chemical gradient.

Clearly, reversible hemolysis had not caused complete loss of endogenous ATP from fresh RBC's. Other endogenous compounds are also not completely lost during the procedure. For example, our subsequent attempts to clearly demonstrate a dependence of calcium transport on $[Mg]_i$ (see below) were thwarted somewhat by the fact that endogenous magnesium is not removed by reversible hemolysis.

Once the initial demonstration of uphill, energy-dependent transport of calcium was complete other factors were investigated and were found to reinforce the view that we were, in fact, dealing with an active transport system for calcium. The dependence on internal ATP, temperature (Q_{10} = 3.5), and apparent dependence on $[Mg]_i$ are all consistent with this notion. Transport of calcium appears to be unaffected by $[Mg]_o$, or by the P_i gradient. The Ca+Mg-activated ATPase of resealed ghosts is stimulated only by internal, and not external calcium. This assymetric activation of a membrane-bound ATPase implicated in calcium transport is exactly analogous to the situation for sodium–potassium–magnesium-activated ATPase. That is, the ion activates the ATPase (and the transport) on the side of the membrane from which the ion is actively transported (Whittam, 1962).

A Calcium Pump in Red Cell Membranes

The Na/K ratio does not appear to affect either the activity of isolated RBC membrane calcium–magnesium-activated ATPase, or active extrusion of calcium from the RBC ghost. Recent findings (Schatzmann, 1970a), however, may modify our early view that these ions do not influence the calcium–magnesium-activated ATPase.

The search for specific inhibitors of the active calcium transport system has met with only limited success. The active extrusion of calcium is not inhibited by ouabain (10^{-4} gm/ml). This is in contrast to sodium–potassium which is inhibited by low concentrations of ouabain. On the other hand, like sodium–potassium transport, calcium transport appears to depend on ATP. Olson and Cazort (1969) concluded that ITP, GTP, and UTP could also support calcium transport. This observation needs confirmation and proof that endogenous ATP is not synthesized by nucleoside phosphotransferase. If the calcium pump can utilize ITP (and/or GTP, etc.), it will be of interest since the sodium–potassium transport system is

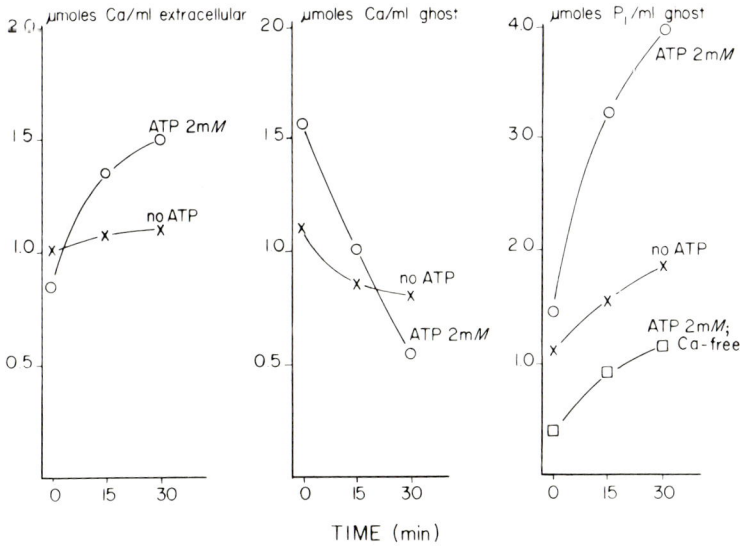

FIG. 3. Active extrusion of calcium from red cell ghosts prepared from fresh RBC's and correlation with inorganic phosphate release. Experimental design and symbols as in Fig. 1, except that ghosts were prepared from fresh RBC's. Note that there was transport of calcium against a chemical gradient even from ghosts with no added ATP. Compare the appearance of P_i in "no ATP" ghosts with the same measurement in Fig. 1. This appearance of P_i, and active transport of calcium in the "no ATP" ghosts appears to be due to endogenous ATP.

quite specific for ATP (Hoffman, 1962). Testing for possible calcium–magnesium-activated ITPase (or GTPase or UTPase) activity of isolated membranes might provide a clue here.

Strontium was considered as a possible competitive antagonist of calcium transport, but calcium transport was not reduced in the presence of an equal amount of strontium. In fact, strontium is itself transported apparently by the system which transports calcium (Schatzmann and Vincenzi, 1969; Olson and Cazort, 1969), and strontium transport rate is reduced in proportion to $[Ca]_i$. Conversely then, internal calcium is an antagonist of strontium transport under conditions in which calcium is itself transported. Interestingly, strontium transport, like calcium transport, depends on $[Mg]_i$. Furthermore, while strontium can replace calcium in the activation of both the ATPase and the transport system, it can not substitute for magnesium. Thus, one may describe a strontium–magnesium-activated ATPase, but calcium does not activate ATPase when strontium and ATP are present in the absence of magnesium. For consideration of divalent cation dependence of sodium–potassium–magnesium-activated ATPase, see Skou (1960).

Mela and Chance (1969) observed that the trivalent lanthanides, holmium and praseodymium could decrease the initial rate of calcium uptake in mitochondria. Recent experiments show that these ions are also capable of inhibiting calcium extrusion from the RBC (Schatzmann, 1971). Results with the lanthanides are compatible with, but do not prove, the suggestion that these ions compete at the calcium-specific site, rather than the magnesium-(or ATP–magnesium-) specific site.

Figure 4 illustrates the effect of ethacrynic acid (ETHA) on active calcium transport. Following prolonged exposure, ETHA does appear to inhibit the calcium transport system. Results in Fig. 4 were obtained using starved RBC's which were treated with 10^{-3} M ETHA during the final 8.5 hours of a 17 hour preincubation to exhaust endogenous ATP. ETHA was also added to the hemolyzing fluid during reversible hemolysis and to the final extracellular incubation medium. Similar experiments with fresh RBC's in which ETHA was added, either to the hemolyzing fluid or to the extracellular medium, or both, did not yield a clear inhibition of calcium transport by ETHA. This may be related to the protective effect of ATP and ADP on sulfhydryl group inhibitors such as ETHA (Hasselbach, 1966). The transport inhibition illustrated in Fig. 4 is probably not specific. ETHA inhibition of the isolated membrane calcium–magnesium-activated ATPase was indistinguishable from inhibition of sodium–potassium–magnesium-activated ATPase. ETHA is probably a rather nonspecific sulfhydryl group inhibitor and is capable of inhibiting both ATPases, and presumably, both transport systems. It is interesting to note that Makinose

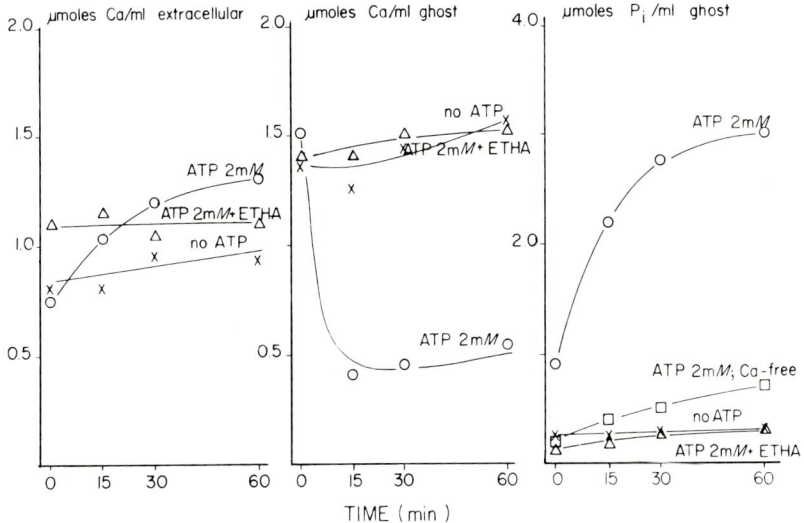

FIG. 4. Ethacrynic acid (ETHA) inhibition of active extrusion of calcium from red cell ghosts. Experimental design and symbols as in Fig. 1. Cells were starved by preincubation at 37°C for 17 hours in the absence of glucose. Cells were treated with ETHA (10^{-3} M) during the final 8.5 hours of preincubation. In addition, 10^{-3} M ETHA was present in both the hemolyzing and extracellular fluid. ETHA inhibited both active extrusion of calcium and the appearance of P_i associated with such extrusion.

(1969) concluded that free sulfhydryl groups were important to calcium transport in sarcoplasmic reticulum.

Mersalyl appeared to block calcium transport in rather high concentrations, but it also appeared to affect membrane permeability, and it is uncertain if block of active transport was achieved. Chlorpromazine causes incomplete inhibition of calcium transport at 10^{-4} M (Schatzmann, 1970b). The significance of inhibition at such concentrations is unclear. Chlorpromazine induces structural changes in RBC membrane proteins (Holmes and Piette, 1970) at such concentrations, but how this might affect active transport is not known at this time.

Discussion of inhibitors would be incomplete without mentioning substances which do not inhibit active calcium transport across the RBC membrane. Caffeine was ineffective at 1 mg/ml. Oligomycin, which inhibits the RBC sodium–potassium–magnesium-activated ATPase, sodium–potassium transport, and the calcium pump of mitochondria (Brierly et al., 1964), was likewise ineffective. The lack of glycoside action on both Ca+Mg-activated ATPase activity and on active calcium transport bears repeating. Since Na+K+Mg-activated ATPase and sodium–potassium transport are specifically inhibited by low concentrations of glycosides and by oligomycin, the calcium pump of the RBC membrane is quite independent of sodium–potassium transport. However, the converse may not be true (see below). In addition, calcium transport does not depend on the sodium (or potassium) gradient. All in all, these findings support the suggestion that, in the RBC, active transport of calcium is somewhat different than in mitochondria, in which active uptake of calcium is highly dependent on the Na/K ratio of the medium (Dransfeld et al., 1967), and in nerve, where uphill movement of calcium is apparently driven by downhill movement of sodium along its electro-chemical gradient (Tower, 1968; Blaustein and Hodgkin, 1969; Baker et al., 1969; Stahl and Swanson, 1971), but may be similar to that in sarcoplasmic reticulum, in which glycosides probably do not affect transport (Lee and Choi, 1966; Dransfeld et al., 1969; Klaus and Lee, 1969; Lee et al., 1970).

Comparison of RBC membranes with nerve or other membranes raises some other interesting points. Since RBC's do not, so far as we know, undergo the periodic influx (or internal release) of calcium which occurs in excitable cells, one may ask why a calcium pump is necessary for the RBC. It is too early to give a definitive answer, but two obvious possibilities are already fairly clear. First, under conditions in which calcium accumulates in the RBC (e.g., in the presence of certain metabolic inhibitors, such as as iodoacetamide) a number of authors have found results which suggest an increased permeability to potassium or to potassium and sodium (Hoffman, 1966; Whittam, 1968; Lew, 1970). Lew concluded that this phenomenon is manifest at $[Ca]_i$ as low as 10^{-6} M. Thus, in terms of efficiency of sodium–potassium transport, it would be to the cell's advantage to maintain a very low $[Ca]_i$. This has been pointed out by Hoffman (1962).

A second "reason" for maintenance of low $[Ca]_i$ is, and has been inferred (Hoffman, 1962) from data on membrane ATPases. As indicated, the notion is purely inferential, since meaningful experiments on transport are not yet available. However, if one accepts that the specific ion-activated, membrane-bound ATPases are a biochemical expression of specific active transport systems, then one is led to an interesting prediction concerning the relationship between active sodium–potassium transport and active calcium transport. It has been known for some years that rather low [Ca] would inhibit sodium–potassium–magnesium-activated ATPase of isolated RBC membrane fragments (Dunham and Glynn, 1961; Hoffman, 1962). Similar inhibition by calcium has been noted for Na+K+Mg-activated ATPase of nerve (Skou, 1960), brain (Jarnefelt, 1962), heart (Lee and Yu, 1963), and kidney (Epstein and Whittam, 1966). It should be clear that the site of this action is on the inner membrane surface. One may therefore sug-

A Calcium Pump in Red Cell Membranes

gest that active calcium transport, or more specifically, the resultant low $[Ca]_i$, is a necessary (although obviously not sufficient) condition for active sodium–potassium transport (Vincenzi, 1968). Since sodium and calcium are thought to be competitive at a number of membrane sites, it seems likely that calcium competes with sodium at the sodium-specific site on the inner surface of the membrane. Regardless of the detailed mechanism of inhibition, one obvious prediction results from this observation. If Ca_i inactivates the sodium–potassium pump, then the active calcium transport system (or whatever system is normally responsible for maintenance of low $[Ca]_i$) should be activated by $[Ca]_i$'s not greater than those which would inactivate the sodium–potassium pump. Otherwise, calcium would accumulate in the cell and inactivate the sodium–potassium pump. Considering the nearly ubiquitous nature of the sodium–potassium pump, an equal

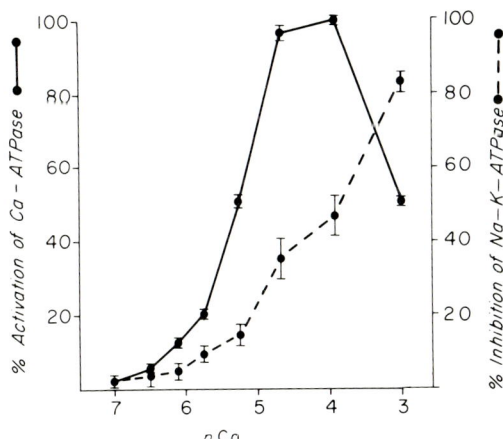

Fig. 5. Activation of calcium–magnesium-activated ATPase and inhibition of sodium–potassium–magnesium-activated ATPase as a function of calcium concentration, using isolated RBC membranes. ATPase activity was assayed by the P_i release in 60 minutes at 37°C with 3 mM tris ATP, 3 mM MgCl$_2$, 80 mM NaCl, 15 mM KCl, 30 mM tris HCl (pH 7.1), and 4 mM EGTA. Calcium–magnesium-activated ATPase was measured as the difference in P_i release between zero calcium and a given [Ca] in the presence of ouabain 10^{-4} M. Sodium–potassium–magnesium-activated ATPase (NaK–ATPase) was taken as the ouabain-inhibitable activity at each pCa. Respective 100% activities were 3.6 ± 0.2 and 0.8 ± 0.1 μmoles P_i mg protein^{-1} hour^{-1}. Each point represents the mean from five independent experiments on different days with RBC membranes from different blood samples and independently prepared calcium buffers. Vertical bars represent 2 SE. Over the range of pCa 6.1–3.9, the activation of Ca–ATPase was significantly greater ($P < .05$) than was inhibition of NaK–ATPase.

ubiquity of low [Ca]$_i$ is suggested. This, of course, agrees with our present knowledge of calcium in a number of tissues (Bianchi, 1968).

One way of investigating the above suggestion in a preliminary way might be to quantify the actions of calcium on ATPase activity of isolated RBC membrane fragments. Results of such a preliminary study are presented in Fig. 5 (Davis and Vincenzi, 1971). The data in Fig. 5 illustrate activation of calcium–magnesium-activated ATPase and inhibition of sodium–potassium–magnesium-activated ATPase of isolated RBC membranes as a function of pCa ($-\log[\text{Ca}]$). The data confirm both the activation of calcium–magnesium-activated ATPase by low [Ca]'s (Vincenzi and Schatzmann, 1967) and the inhibition of sodium–potassium–magnesium-activated ATPase by calcium. Germane to the present discussion is the demonstration that over the range of pCa 6.1 to pCa 3.9, the activation of calcium–magnesium-activated ATPase was significantly greater ($P < .05$) than was inhibition of sodium–potassium–magnesium-activated ATPase. Of course, the relationship to transport is not defined by these data, so this discussion must remain speculative. The fact that activation of calcium–magnesium-activated ATPase occurs at [Ca]'s not more than those which inhibit sodium–potassium–magnesium-activated ATPase is consistent with the suggested indirect dependence of sodium–potassium transport on calcium transport in the RBC. The notion that sodium–potassium transport and that monovalent ion permeability may depend on active membrane transport of calcium is reminiscent of the intriguing suggestion by Duncan (1967) concerning the general control of cell membrane permeability by ouabain-insensitive membrane ATPase. Whether the active calcium transport of RBC membrane will remain a model only unto itself or will be more widely useful must remain a problem for the future.

ACKNOWLEDGMENTS

This work was supported in part by a National Science Foundation Postdoctoral Fellowship. I thank Drs. W. L. Stahl and P. D. Swanson for providing a prepublication copy of their interesting paper. Professor H. J. Schatzmann provided inspiration and information for all phases of this work.

REFERENCES

Akera, T., Larsen, F. S., and Brody, T. M. (1970). *J. Pharmacol. Exp. Ther.* **173,** 145.
Baker, P. F., Blaustein, M. P., Hodgkin, A. L., and Steinhardt, R. A. (1969). *J. Physiol. (London)* **200,** 431.
Bianchi, C. P. (1968). "Cell Calcium." Butterworth, London and Washington, D.C.
Blaustein, M. P., and Hodgkin, A. L. (1969). *J. Physiol. (London)* **200,** 497.
Brierly, G. P., Murer, E., and Bachmann, E. (1964). *Arch. Biochem. Biophys.* **105,** 89.
Davis, P. W., and Vincenzi, F. F. (1971). *Life Sci.* **10,** 401.

Dransfeld, H., Greeff, K., Hess, D., and Schorn, A. (1967). *Experientia* **23,** 375.
Dransfeld, H., Greeff, K., Schorn, A., and Ting, B. T. (1969). *Biochem. Pharmacol.* **18,** 1335.
Duncan, C. J. (1967). "The Molecular Properties and Evolution of Excitable Cells." Pergamon Press, Oxford.
Dunham, E. T., and Glynn, I. M. (1961). *J. Physiol. (London)* **156,** 274.
Entman, M. L., Cook, J. W., and Bressler, R. (1969). *Circ. Res.* **24,** 793.
Epstein, F. H., and Whittam, R. (1966). *Biochem. J.* **99,** 232.
Glynn, I. M. (1964). *Pharmacol. Rev.* **16,** 381.
Hasselbach, W. (1966). *Ann. N.Y. Acad. Sci.* **137,** 1041.
Hoffman, J. F. (1962). *Circulation* **26,** 1201.
Hoffman, J. F. (1966). *Amer. J. Med.* **41,** 666.
Holmes, D. E., and Piette, L. H. (1970). *J. Pharmacol. Exp. Ther.* **173,** 78.
Jarnefelt, J. (1962). *Biochim. Biophys. Acta* **59,** 643.
Jay, A. W., and Burton, A. C. (1969). *Biophys. J.* **9,** 115.
Kahn, J. B. (1962). *Proc. Int. Pharmacol. Meet. 1st, 1961* Vol. 3, pp. 111–135.
Katz, A. M., and Repke, D. I. (1966). *Science* **152,** 1242.
Klaus, W., and Lee, K. S. (1969). *J. Pharmacol. Exp. Ther.* **166,** 68.
Lee, K. S., and Choi, S. J. (1966). *J. Pharmacol. Exp. Ther.* **153,** 114.
Lee, K. S., and Shin, B. C. (1969). *J. Gen. Physiol.* **54,** 713.
Lee, K. S., and Yu, D. H. (1963). *Biochem. Pharmacol.* **12,** 1253.
Lee, K. S., Hong, S. A., and Kang, D. H. (1970). *J. Pharmacol. Exp. Ther.* **172,** 180.
Lew, V. L. (1970). *J. Physiol. (London)* **206,** 35P.
Makinose, M. (1969). *Eur. J. Biochem.* **10,** 74.
Marchesi, V. T., and Steers, E. (1968). *Science* **159,** 203.
Mela, L., and Chance, B. (1969). *Biochim. Biophys. Res. Commun.* **35,** 556.
Olson, E. J., and Cazort, R. J. (1969). *J. Gen. Physiol.* **53,** 311.
Passow, H. (1961). *Colloq. Ges. Physiol. Chem.* **12,** 54.
Passow, H. (1963). *In* "Cell Interphase Reactions" (H. D. Brown, ed.), pp. 57–107. Scholar's Library, New York.
Porzig, H. (1970). *J. Membrane Biol.* **2,** 324.
Rosenthal, A. S., Kregenow, F. M., and Moses, H. L. (1970). *Biochim. Biophys. Acta* **196,** 254.
Rummel, W., Seifen, E., and Baldauf, J. (1962). *Arch. Exp. Pathol. Pharmacol.* **244,** 172.
Schatzmann, H. J. (1953). *Helv. Physiol. Pharmacol. Acta* **11,** 346.
Schatzmann, H. J. (1966). *Experientia* **22,** 364.
Schatzmann, H. J. (1970a). *Experientia* **26,** 687.
Schatzmann, H. J. (1970b). *In* "Symposium on Calcium and Cellular Function" (A. W. Cuthbert, ed.), pp. 85–95. Macmillan, New York.
Schatzmann, H. J. (1971). *Experientia* **27,** 59.
Schatzmann, H. J., and Vincenzi, F. F. (1969). *J. Physiol. (London)* **201,** 369.
Schwartz, A., Allen, J. C., and Harigaya, S. (1969). *J. Pharmacol. Exp. Ther.* **168,** 31.
Skou, J. C. (1957). *Biochim. Biophys. Acta* **23,** 394.
Skou, J. C. (1960). *Biochim. Biophys. Acta* **42,** 6.
Stahl, W. L., and Swanson, P. D. (1971). *J. Neurochem.* **18,** 415.
Tower, D. B. (1968). *Exp. Brain Res. (Berlin)* **6,** 273.
Vincenzi, F. F. (1968). *Proc. West. Pharmacol. Soc.* **11,** 58.
Vincenzi, F. F., and Schatzmann, H. J. (1967). *Helv. Physiol. Pharmacol. Acta* **25,** CR233.
Whittam, R. (1962). *Biochem. J.* **84,** 110.

Whittam, R. (1968). *Nature (London)* **219,** 610.
Wins, P., and Schoffeniels, E. (1966a). *Biochim. Biophys. Acta* **120,** 341.
Wins, P., and Schoffeniels, E. (1966b). *Arch. Int. Physiol.* **74,** 812.

Discussion

Dr. Assali: What do you feel is the influence of intracellular pH on calcium transport?

Dr. Vincenzi: There was little difference between pH 6.6 and 7.1 in terms of the absolute calcium-activated ATPase activity. But we have no information on calcium transport.

Dr. Martonosi: You mentioned that sodium is not a counterion for calcium transport. Is there any indication that perhaps there is a counter proton transfer?

Dr. Vincenzi: With respect to hydrogen, I don't know. Magnesium, phosphate, sodium, and potassium gradients were obvious possibilities, and we did look at those, but there is no counterion as far as we know yet. During the initial phases of transport there were 1.3 moles of inorganic phosphate appearing per mole of calcium transported. Some people get very upset when you come up with a number that is not an integer and it bothered us at first. On the other hand, maybe it isn't supposed to be 1:1 or perhaps there is a significant back-leak of calcium. One can imagine all kinds of possibilities.

It is too early to say anything here about what it means, but very recent data have indicated that the calcium-activated ATPase is certainly not a homogeneous enzyme. At least some of the calcium-activated ATPase is dependent on the presence of either sodium or potassium. We spent some time testing a hypothesis for digitalis action in which we predicted that slight changes in intracellular sodium and potassium would lead to large changes in calcium transport. We did not find anything like this. About this time, Dransfeld and Greeff showed that the uptake of calcium in mitochondria was highly dependent on the Na/K ratio. Perhaps we put our money on the wrong membrane.

Dr. Mulrow: Certain species of sheep and other animals have high intracellular sodium and low sodium–potassium-activated ATPase in their red cells. I wondered if you had looked at the calcium levels in those cells?

Dr. Vincenzi: No, but I have wondered if maybe there is a little more calcium in low-potassium cells that inhibits the sodium–potassium transport. That might explain part of the difference. I don't want to put too much emphasis on that, because, as you know if one isolates the sodium–potassium ATPase, there is less sodium–potassium ATPase activity per milligram of membrane. I agree with you that it is a very interesting observation that really should be followed up.

Dr. Armstrong: I am sure you have tried metabolic inhibitors with the intact cells.

Dr. Vincenzi: If one preincubates the cells with ethacrynic acid and then puts it inside and outside the cells, one can totally inhibit the ATPase activity and calcium transport. This is not specific, I am sure, because inhibition of the sodium–potassium-activated ATPase and inhibition of the calcium ATPase were essentially superimposable over the whole dose–response curve. I think this probably does imply that phosphorylation is important and that sulfhydryl groups are important since ethacrynic acid is thought to be a sulfydryl inhibitor, but it is nonspecific. As a pharmacologist I would like to have a very specific inhibitor, such as the sodium–potassium people have. These people have glycosides. We need that kind of tool.

Question: You mentioned that the ATPase has a high affinity for calcium on the inside and was asymmetric with regard to calcium. It is also sensitive to magnesium. Where does the magnesium enter the picture?

Dr. Vincenzi: This is really a messy proposition. The conclusion that I have come to, at least tentatively, is that magnesium–ATP complex at one site somehow sets up the system so that it is ready to transport calcium. When calcium arrives at another site, the calcium-specific site, the ATP is split, maybe through the intermediary of the phosphorylating system, and then subsequently, the phosphate comes off. Thus, there are probably magnesium or magnesium–ATP-specific sites and calcium-specific sites. If magnesium is too high, you inhibit by competing at calcium sites. If calcium is too high, it competes with magnesium at the magnesium site. This gets messy when you try to make a very clear picture quantitatively, but qualitatively it fits.

CALCIUM TRANSPORT IN KIDNEY CELLS AND ITS REGULATION*

André B. Borle

Calcium metabolism is presumably regulated at the cellular level. The hormones and the vitamins involved in calcium homeostasis probably act through some mechanism located in the cells of their respective target organs. Cellular calcium metabolism is not only important for calcium homeostasis, which involves shifts of calcium from one body compartment to another, but also for the regulation of physiological and metabolic processes of the cell itself. It comprises the influx and efflux of calcium in and out of the cell, its distribution between subcellular pools, the shifts of calcium from one cell compartment to another, and the rise and fall of the concentration of ionized calcium in the cytoplasm.

By kinetic analyses of calcium movements in isolated cells, it is possible to detect several calcium compartments and to measure their rate of exchange (Borle, 1969a, b, 1970a, b). I have studied several types of cells (Table I) and observed that the fluxes and compartment sizes are not very different from one cell strain to another. The fast compartment, which represents extracellular binding, shows the greatest variation. This could reflect quantitative or qualitative differences between the various extracellular cell coats or the different techniques used in isolating the cells. The

---

* This work was supported by USPHS Grant AM 07867 from The National Institutes of Health.

TABLE I

CALCIUM FLUXES AND CALCIUM POOL SIZE OF DIFFERENT CELL STRAINS

Cell strain	Fast compartment		Slow compartment	
	Flux (pmoles/ mg protein · minute)	Pool size (nmoles/mg protein)	Flux (pmoles/ mg protein · minute)	Pool size (nmoles/mg protein)
Human HeLa cells[a]	948	1.06	120[b]	2.69
Monkey kidney[c]	1160	1.90	96	3.21
Dog kidney[b]	3124	3.87	118	2.62
Human intestine[d]	1115	1.82	82	2.92
Rat thymocytes[e]	1003	1.87	40	1.31

[a] From Borle, 1969a.

[b] The studies with HeLa cells were performed with monolayers in which half of the cell surface is unavailable for exchange. The flux actually measured has been multiplied by 2 in this table to be comparable to the other values obtained in cell suspensions. See discussion in Borle (1970a).

[c] From Borle, 1970a.

[d] From Borle, 1968.

[e] From Shematek and Borle, 1971.

parameters of the slow compartment are very similar in all cells, except in thymocytes. In this case, the smaller flux and pool size of the slow compartment can be attributed to a significant difference in cell size*, to their low cytoplasmic to nuclear mass ratio or to their comparatively small number of mitochondria. Since the fluxes and compartment sizes of these various cells are of the same order of magnitude, we can assume that the resting level of calcium exchange is not very different from cell to cell. In this presentation, I shall limit my observations to the monkey kidney cells.

Although it is commonly assumed that the intracellular concentration of ionized calcium is very low and relatively constant, the total cell calcium varies considerably. Increasing the medium calcium to 5 mM causes the total cell calcium to rise from 13 to 222 nmoles per milligram of cell protein (Fig. 1). Extracellular phosphate also influences the total cell calcium (Fig. 2). Obviously, calcium must be sequestered in several cellular compartments. Let us consider then the size of the different calcium pools and their calcium fluxes obtained by kinetic analyses.

---

* Thymocytes have a cell diameter of 9 μ, as compared to 17–19 μ for the other epithelial cells (Shematek and Borle, 1971).

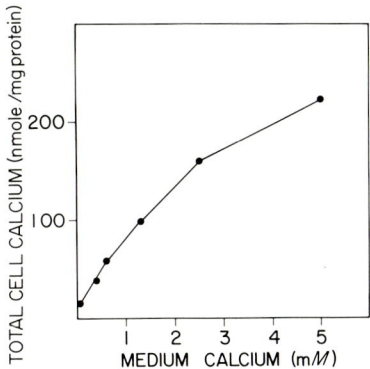

FIG. 1. Influence of the medium calcium concentration on the total cell calcium. The cells were incubated for 5 hours in a Krebs–Ringer solution, tris buffer at pH 7.45. The medium phosphate was 1.0 mM.

Calcium Pools

The curves of calcium-45 uptake in isolated cells reveal at least two kinetic phases (Borle, 1970a, b): a fast component with a half-time of about 1 minute, and a slow component with a half-time of 26 minutes. The exchange of calcium of the first phase is so fast that it can only represent extracellular binding. The slow phase, on the other hand, represents one or more intracellular compartments. The arguments in favor of these identifi-

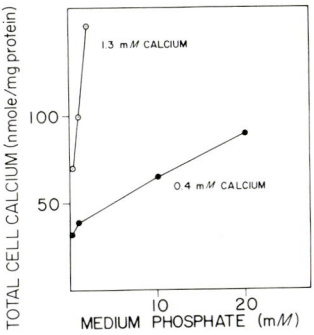

FIG. 2. Influence of the medium phosphate concentration on the total cell calcium. The cells were incubated for 5 hours in a Krebs–Ringer solution, tris buffer at pH 7.45. The medium calcium concentration was 0.4 mM (lower line) or 1.3 mM (upper line).

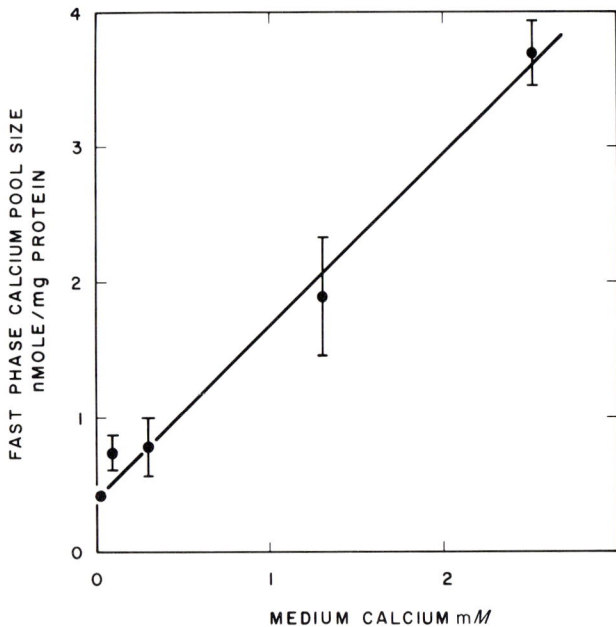

FIG. 3. Influence of the medium calcium concentration on the pool size of the fast component of calcium uptake. The cells were incubated for 3 hours in a Krebs–Ringer solution, bicarbonate buffer at pH 7.45. The medium phosphate concentration was 1.0 mM. (From Borle, 1970a.)

cations have already been published (Borle, 1970a). The compartment size of the fast and slow compartments are, respectively, 1.9 and 3.3 nmoles of calcium per milligram of cell protein. Both increase with increasing medium calcium. Raising the medium calcium from 0 to 2.5 mM increases the fast phase from 0.4 to 3.7 and the slow phase from 0.9 to 5.7 nmoles per milligram of protein (Figs. 3 and 4). Extracellular phosphate also increases the slow calcium compartment (Borle, 1970b) from 3.0 to 8.2 nmoles per milligram of protein between 0 and 10 mM phosphate (Fig. 5) (Borle, 1970a, b). But the most dramatic expansion of the intracellular compartment is obtained with pyrophosphate (Borle and Herold, 1971). With physiological concentrations of calcium and phosphate (1.3 and 1.0 mM, respectively) the pool size increases from 3.5 to 30 nmoles per milligram of protein between 0 and 0.5 mM pyrophosphate in the medium (Fig. 6).

Several conclusions can be drawn from these few examples. (1) Cellular calcium can be divided at least in two compartments, one extracellular and one intracellular. (2) Both compartments are markedly affected by the extracellular concentrations of calcium, phosphate, and pyrophosphate. (3) The intracellular calcium can rise to such high concentrations that it must be sequestered in some subcellular compartment. (4) The intracellular free calcium concentration cannot be identified with any of these pools.

Recently, I have been able to identify another intracellular calcium compartment by calcium efflux experiments. Figure 7 reveals that the amount of radioactive calcium left in the cell after a period of repeated washout is dependent on the length of time of the labeling period. With a labeling period of 10 minutes, only 2% of the total radioactivity taken up remains in the cell after 2 hours of desaturation. With a labeling of 1 hour, 8% is left in the cell, and with a 3 hour uptake 14% remains, suggesting the progressive sequestration of calcium-45 into a very slowly exchangeable compartment. This very slow compartment can be detected only when

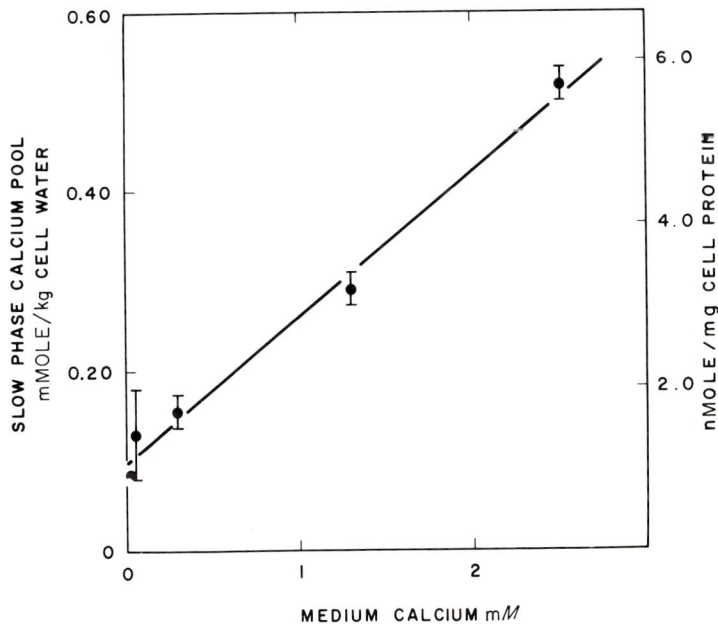

Fig. 4. Influence of the medium calcium concentration on the pool size of the slow component of calcium uptake. Experimental conditions as in Fig. 3. Since monkey kidney cells contain 11 mg water per milligram of cell protein, the data can be expressed in millimoles per kilogram of cell water (left ordinate) or in nanomoles per milligram of protein (right ordinate); 0.1 mmole of calcium per kilogram of cell water = 1.1 nmole per milligram of cell protein. (From Borle, 1970a).

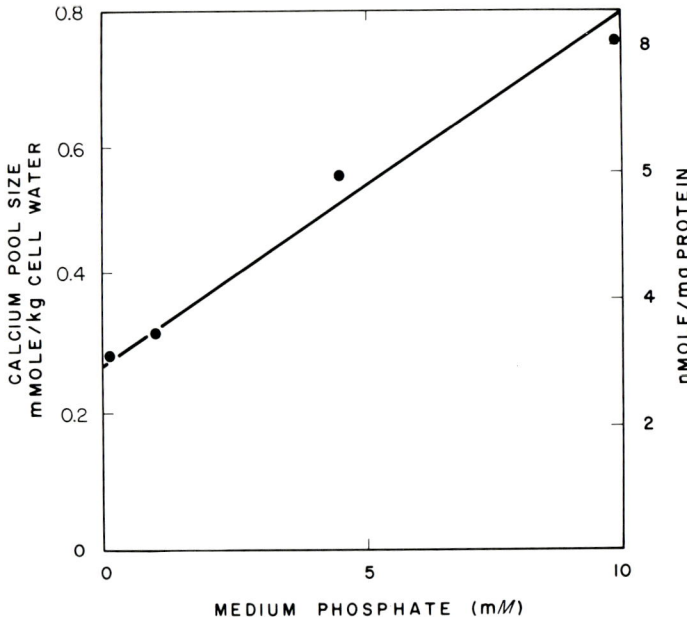

FIG. 5. Influence of the medium phosphate concentration on the pool size of the slow component of calcium uptake. The medium calcium was 1.3 mM, otherwise the experimental conditions were identical to those of Fig. 3. For the unit conversion from right to left ordinate, see legend of Fig. 4. (From Borle, 1970b).

phosphate is present in the medium. Figure 8 shows one experiment performed with 1 mM phosphate and another in phosphate-free medium. In the first case, 20% of the calcium-45 is left in the cell after 2 hours of efflux, while in the second, only 2% remains. There is a direct relationship between the slow compartment size and the medium phosphate concentration. The isotope left in the cells after 2 hours of efflux varies from 2.9 to 27% between 0 and 20 mM phosphate (Fig. 9). The medium calcium concentration has also a marked influence on the third compartment and this effect is best seen at high phosphate concentrations. Figure 10 shows a progressive sequestration of calcium from 10% of the total uptake at 0.4 mM calcium to 30% at 0.6 mM and 53% at 1.3 mM.

It is well known that mitochondria can accumulate significant amounts of calcium and that this uptake is markedly increased by phosphate and completely inhibited by antimycin A and warfarin* (see reviews by Borle,

* 3-(α-Acetonylbenzyl)-4-hydroxycoumarin.

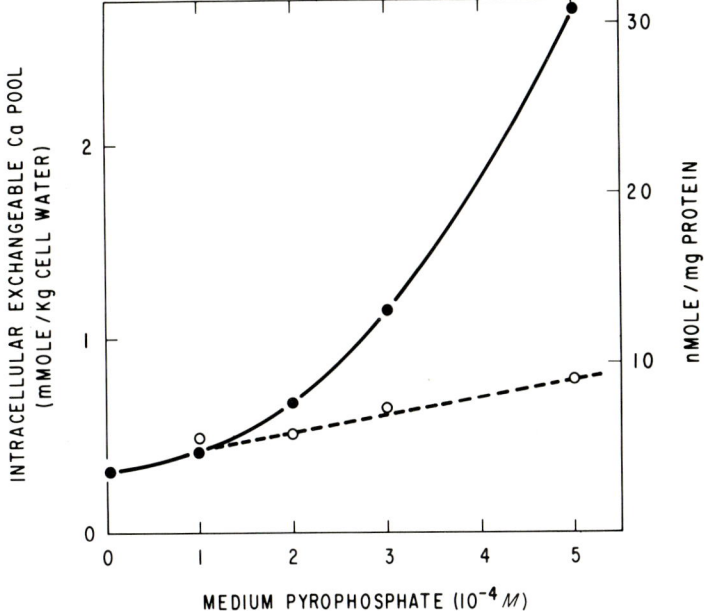

Fig. 6. Influence of medium pyrophosphate concentration on the pool size of the slow component of calcium uptake. The cells were incubated for 3 hours in a Krebs–Ringer solution, tris buffer at pH 7.45. The medium calcium was 1.3 mM. The medium phosphate was 0 (broken line) or 1 mM (solid line). For the unit conversion from right to left ordinate, see legend of Fig. 4. (From Borle and Herold, 1971).

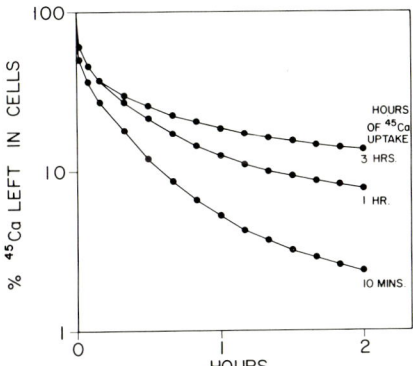

Fig. 7. Influence of the labeling period on the calcium-45 left in the cells during 2 hours of desaturation. The medium was a Krebs–Ringer solution, tris buffer at pH 7.45, containing 1.3 mM calcium and 1.0 mM phosphate.

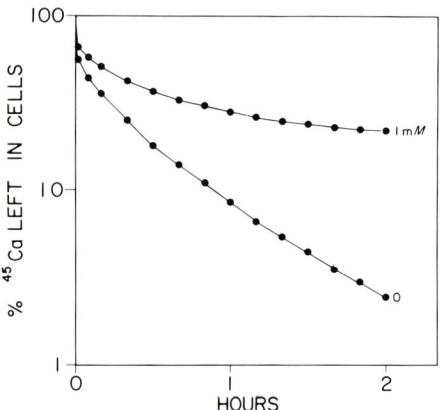

FIG. 8. Influence of phosphate on calcium efflux. The cells were labeled with calcium-45 for 1 hour. The medium was a Krebs–Ringer solution, tris buffer, containing 1.3 mM calcium. The medium phosphate was 1 mM in the upper curve. The lower curve was obtained in phosphate-free medium.

1967; Lehninger *et al.*, 1967). In an attempt to identify the third compartment, I studied the effects of these mitochondrial inhibitors. Antimycin A completely suppresses the intracellular sequestration of calcium observed with 5 mM phosphate and 1.3 mM calcium (Fig. 11). The control cells

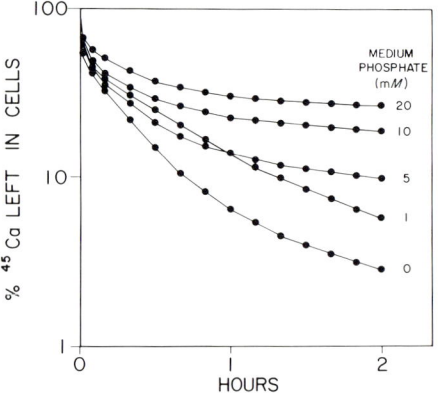

FIG. 9. Influence of the medium phosphate concentration on calcium efflux. The cells were labeled with calcium-45 for 1 hour. The medium was a Krebs–Ringer solution, tris buffer, containing 0.4 mM calcium.

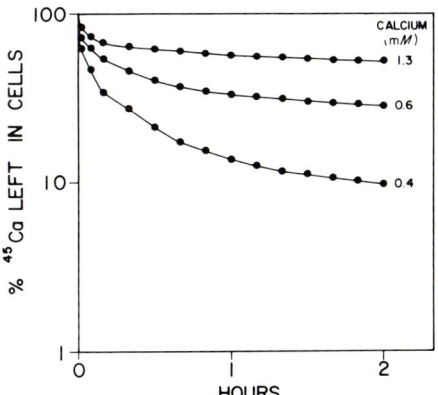

Fig. 10. Influence of the medium calcium concentration on calcium efflux. The cells were labeled with calcium-45 for 1 hour. The medium was a Krebs–Ringer solution, tris buffer, containing 5 mM phosphate.

retain 53% of the isotope originally incorporated, whereas the cells treated with 10^{-5} M antimycin A lose all but 4% of their calcium-45. If one accepts antimycin A to be a specific mitochondrial inhibitor, this experiment indicates that the third slow component of calcium efflux represents calcium

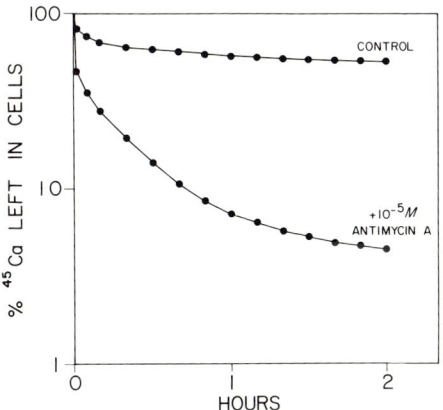

Fig. 11. Effect of antimycin A on calcium efflux. The cells were labeled with calcium-45 for 1 hour. The medium was a Krebs–Ringer solution, tris buffer, containing 1.3 mM calcium and 5 mM phosphate. The upper curve was obtained with control cells. The lower curve was obtained with cells incubated in a medium containing 10^{-5} M antimycin A during the labeling and the efflux period.

TABLE II

Influence of Phosphate on the Intracellular Distribution of Calcium

Medium		Calcium distribution (nm/mg protein)[a]		
Calcium (mM)	Phosphate (mM)	Toal cell calcium	Pool 2	Pool 3
1.3	0	70.1	1.27	0.91
1.3	1	98.2	1.60	2.53
1.3	2	152	3.09	10.3
1.3	3	149	2.39	12.2
1.3	5	748	6.00	457

[a] Values are the mean of two experiments.

trapped in mitochondria. Table II compares the influence of various medium concentrations of calcium and phosphate on the total cell calcium with the actual pool size of the two intracellular compartments. Raising the medium phosphate from 0 to 5 mM increases the total cell calcium tenfold. Most of the calcium taken up by the cell appears in pool 3 which increases five hundredfold; pool 2 increases only fivefold, a ratio of 100 to 1. Figure 12 shows the differences in pool 2 and 3 obtained with a medium calcium of 0.4 mM and a medium phosphate increasing from 0 to 20 mM.

The effects of antimycin A and warfarin have been studied at 2 different

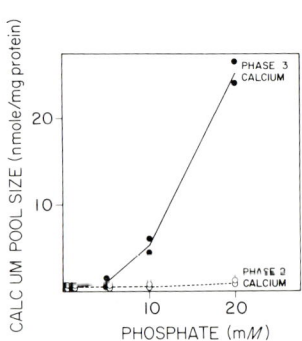

Fig. 12. Influence of the medium phosphate concentration on the pool size of two slowest phases of calcium efflux. The medium was a Krebs–Ringer solution, tris buffer. The medium calcium was 0.4 mM so that the medium phosphate could be increased to 20 mM.

TABLE III

Effects of Mitochondrial Inhibitors on the Calcium Distribution

Medium		Inhibitor (10^{-5} M)	Calcium distribution (nmoles/mg protein)[a]		
Calcium (mM)	Phosphate (mM)		Total cell calcium	Pool 2	Pool 3
1.3	5	—	748	6.00	457
1.3	5	Antimycin A	117	1.02	1.68
1.3	5	Warfarin	85	1.42	1.00
0.6	5	—	107	1.72	32.2
0.6	5	Antimycin A	18	0.94	0.35
0.6	5	Warfarin	86	1.32	0.97

[a] Values are the mean of two experiments.

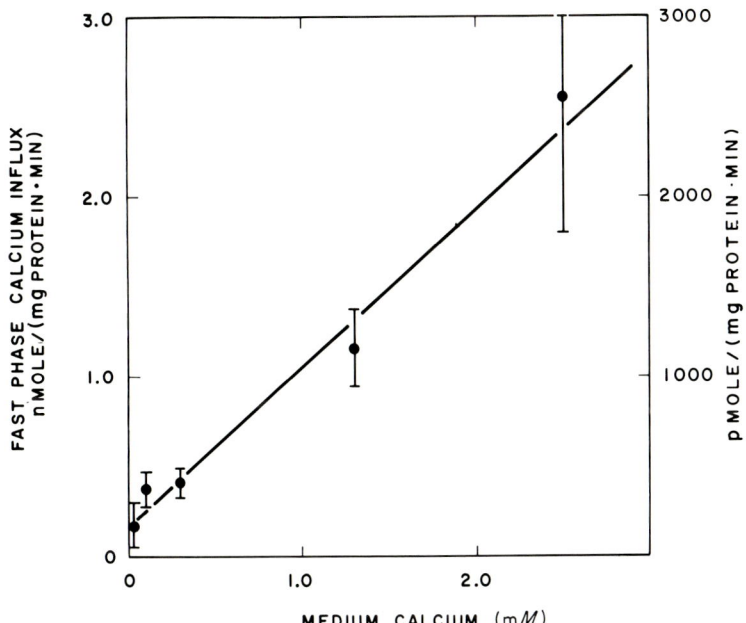

Fig. 13. Influence of the medium calcium concentration on the calcium influx of the fast component of uptake. The medium was a Krebs-Ringer solution, bicarbonate buffer, with a phosphate concentration of 1 mM. (From Borle, 1970a).

calcium concentrations. Table III shows that they reduce the mitochondrial pool to the low levels obtained in phosphate-free medium. The second pool is also reduced, reflecting, perhaps, an influence of the mitochondria pool on the cytoplasmic calcium. The difference between the sum of pool 2 and 3 and the total cell calcium represents binding of calcium to the faster extracellular pools. It varies linearly with the medium calcium and phosphate.

Calcium Fluxes

Uptake studies reveal that calcium exchange with the first extracellular phase is ten to twenty times faster than calcium influx into the second phase (Figs. 13 and 14) (Borle, 1970a). With a medium calcium of 1.3 mM, the

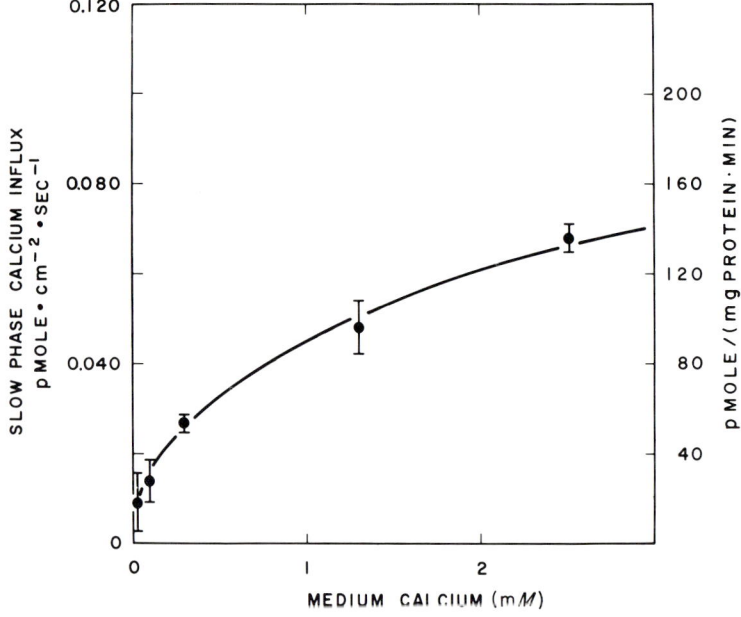

FIG. 14. Influence of the medium calcium concentration on the calcium influx of the slow component. The experimental conditions are the same as in Fig. 13. The data are expressed in picomoles per square centimeter per second (left ordinate) and in picomoles per milligram of protein per minutes (right ordinate). Since the cell surface is 33.5 cm² per milligram of protein, the conversion factor is 2000: 0.050 pmoles cm^{-2} sec^{-1} = 100 pm/(mg protein·minute). (From Borle, 1970a).

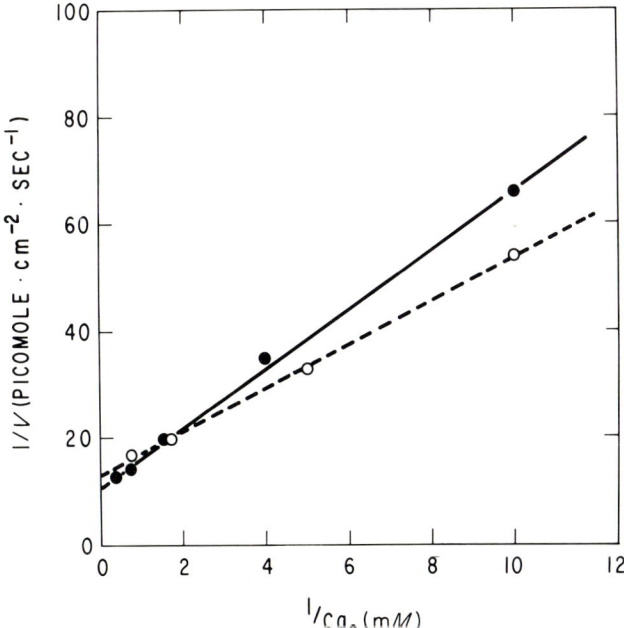

Fig. 15. Lineweaver Burk plot of calcium influx of the slow component of uptake. The medium was a Krebs–Ringer solution, bicarbonate buffer, containing 1.3 mM calcium and 1.0 mM phosphate. Influx was measured in magnesium-free medium (solid line) or with 2 mM MgCl$_2$ (broken line).

fast influx is 1160 compared to an influx into the second phase of 96 pmoles/(mg protein·minute), a twelvefold difference. It is obvious that only kinetic analyses can detect changes in the slow phase, since a 50% rise in slow influx represents only 2–4% of the total uptake.

There is another important difference between the fast and slow influx. The fast influx varies linearly with increasing medium calcium (Fig. 13), whereas calcium influx into the slow compartment follows the pattern of saturation kinetics (Fig. 14). This suggests a carrier-mediated transport and supports our assumption that calcium influx into the cell is a facilitated diffusion process. The transport mechanism seems to be specific for calcium because magnesium is not a competitive inhibitor. Far from being inhibited by magnesium, calcium influx is slightly greater in presence of 2 mM MgCl$_2$ than in magnesium-free medium (Fig. 15).

Phosphate and pyrophosphate stimulate calcium influx into the second compartment. Raising the phosphate concentration to 10 mM doubles

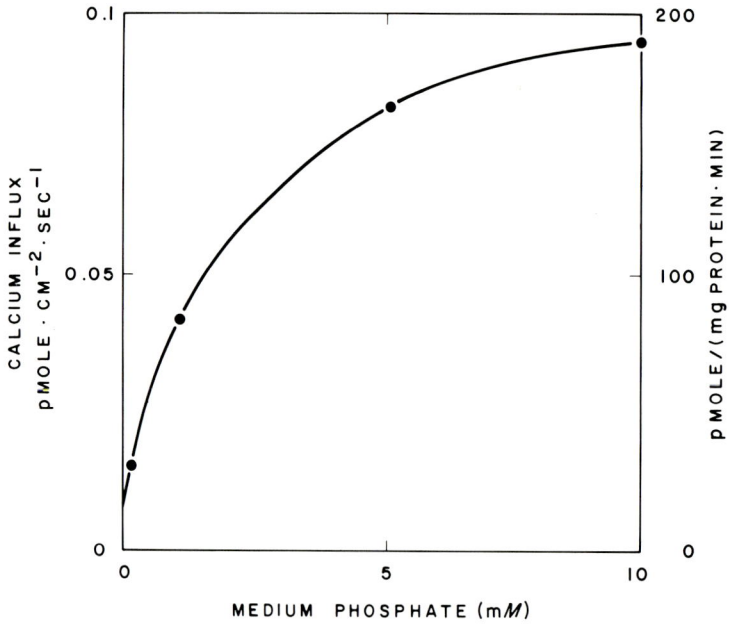

Fig. 16. Influence of the medium phosphate concentration on the calcium influx of the slow component of uptake. The medium calcium was 1.3 mM. For the unit conversion from right to left ordinate, see legend of Fig. 14. (From Borle, 1970b).

calcium influx (Fig. 16). The effects of pyrophosphate are still more impressive; 0.5 mM pyrophosphate stimulates calcium influx tenfold in physiological conditions (Fig. 17).

There is a good agreement between the calcium fluxes measured by uptake experiments and those obtained by calcium efflux. Table IV shows that calcium efflux from pool 2 varies from 25.5 to 96.5 fmoles·cm^{-2}·second^{-1} between 0 and 5 mM extracellular phosphate. This compares well with the range of 15.5–82.0 fmoles·cm^{-2}·second^{-1} observed in influx experiments (Fig. 17). The effects of the medium calcium concentration on the calcium fluxes to and from pool 2 agree equally well regardless of the methods.

Calcium efflux from the third pool varies more widely; it can increase fiftyfold from 2.95 to 165 fmoles·cm^{-2}·second^{-1} (Table IV), but it is totally suppressed by the mitochondrial inhibitors antimycin A and warfarin (Table V). This suggests again that pool 3 represents mitochondria which may act as an intracellular calcium buffer system.

Calcium Transport in Kidney Cells

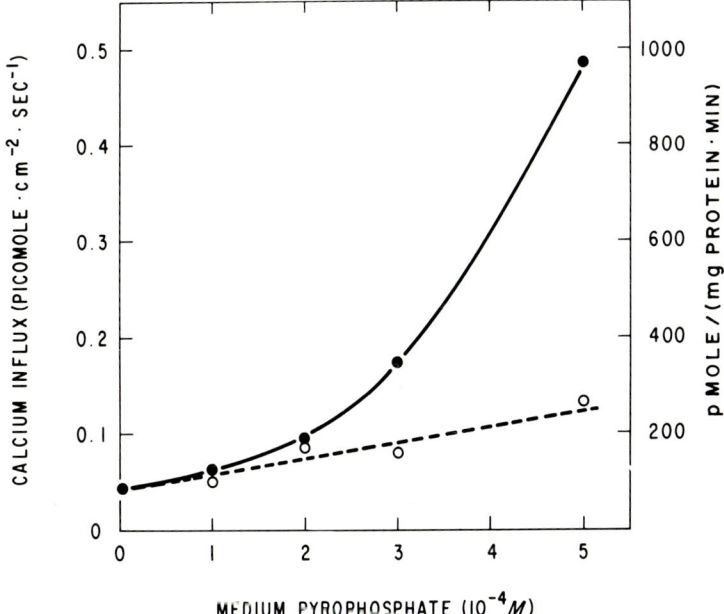

Fig. 17. Influence of the medium pyrophosphate concentration on calcium influx of the slow component of uptake. The medium calcium was 1.3 mM and the medium phosphate was either 0 mM (broken line) or 1 mM (solid line). For the unit conversion from right to left ordinate, see legend of Fig. 14. (From Borle and Herold, 1971).

Finally, I have attempted to measure how fast calcium can shift from one compartment to another. By running simultaneously two desaturation experiments from cells uniformly labeled, one can perturb the calcium efflux of one group and compare it with the control group. Figure 18

TABLE IV
Calcium Fluxes Measured by Calcium-45 Efflux

Medium		Efflux[a] (fmoles·cm^{-2} seconds^{-1})[b]	
Calcium (mM)	Phosphate (mM)	Pool 2	Pool 3
1.3	0	25.5	2.95
1.3	1	32.3	4.55
1.3	2	50.8	11.2
1.3	3	37.0	10.1
1.3	5	96.5	165.0

[a] Values are the mean of two experiments.
[b] 1 fmole (femtomole) = 10^{-15} moles or 10^{-3} pmoles.

TABLE V
Effects of Mitochondrial Inhibitors on Calcium Efflux

Medium		Inhibitor (10^{-5} M)	Efflux[a] (fmoles·cm^{-2} seconds^{-1})[b]	
Calcium (mM)	Phosphate (mM)		Pool 2	Pool 3
1.3	5	—	96.5	165
1.3	5	Antimycin A	23.5	1.65
1.3	5	Warfarin	24.7	1.50
0.6	5	—	30.3	17.1
0.6	5	Antimycin A	14.0	0.68
0.6	5	Warfarin	22.8	1.74

[a] Values are the mean of two experiments.
[b] 1 fmole (femtomole) = 10^{-15} moles or 10^{-3} pmoles.

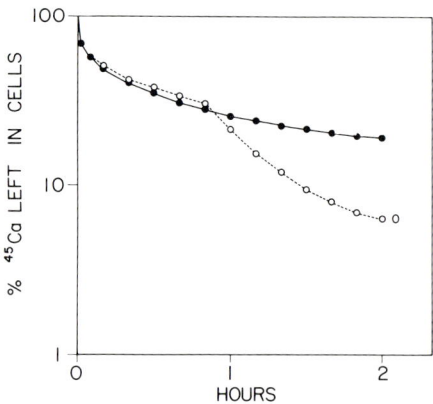

FIG. 18. Effect of the sudden removal of phosphate from the medium during a desaturation experiment. Two groups of cells were labeled with calcium-45 for 1 hour. The medium contained 1.3 mM calcium and 1.0 mM phosphate. Until 50 minutes, efflux was performed in both groups in a medium of the former composition. From that time one group was desaturated in phosphate-free medium (broken line), while the other group was still exposed to 1 mM phosphate (solid line).

* 1 fmole (femtomole) = 10^{-15} moles or 10^{-3} pmoles.

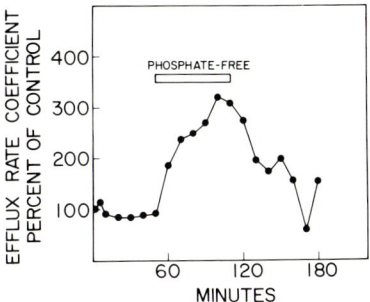

FIG. 19. Effect of the temporary removal of phosphate from the medium on the efflux rate coefficient of calcium (see methods in Borle, 1969b). The cells were labeled and desaturated in 1.3 mM calcium and 1.0 mM phosphate. From 50 to 110 minutes, phosphate was removed from the medium of the experimental group.

demonstrates such an experiment. From 0 to 50 minutes both groups are desaturated in 1 mM phosphate and 1.3 mM calcium. When the cells of one group are placed in a phosphate-free medium, calcium efflux increases immediately. Figure 19 shows the efflux rate coefficient of the experimental group compared to its control. Efflux increases threefold and returns to control levels when the cells are replaced in 1 mM phosphate. Figure 20 illustrates the reverse experiment; efflux begins in a phosphate-free medium, and 1 mM phosphate is added from 50 to 110 minutes. Calcium efflux drops immediately to 25% of the control values. When phosphate is later removed from the medium, efflux returns to control levels. These experiments

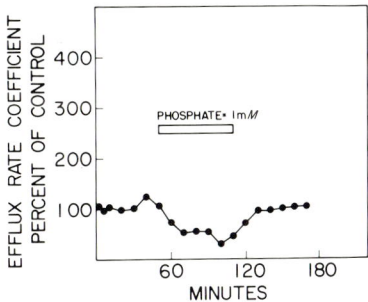

FIG. 20. Effect of the temporary addition of 1 mM phosphate on the efflux rate coefficient of calcium. The cells were labeled and desaturated in a phosphate-free medium containing 1.3 mM calcium. From 50 to 110 minutes, 1 mM phosphate was added to the medium of the experimental group.

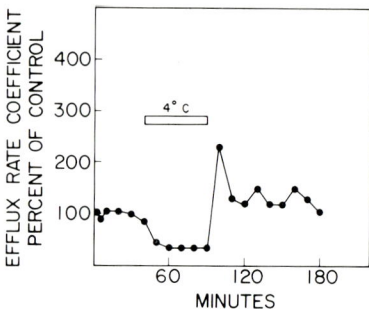

Fig. 21. Effect of a temporary decrease in temperature to 4°C on the efflux rate coefficient of calcium. The cells were labeled and desaturated in 1.3 mM calcium and 1.0 mM phosphate at 37.5°C. From 40 to 90 minutes, the temperature of the incubating medium of the experimental group was lowered to 4°C. At 90 minutes, the cells were replaced at 37.5°C.

demonstrate that the shifts of calcium from one compartment to another are rapid and reversible. The effects of phosphate could be explained as follows: (1) phosphate may inhibit the calcium pump located in the cell membrane; (2) increasing the medium phosphate could lower the intracellular calcium activity by raising the intracellular phosphate; (3) since phosphate stimulates the accumulation of calcium by mitochondria, a sudden increase in phosphate could cause a shift of calcium from cytoplasm to mitochondria and a transient fall in the cytoplasmic calcium activity. Conversely, removal of phosphate could release calcium from the mitochondria, raise transiently the calcium activity in the cytoplasm, and secondarily stimulate calcium efflux.

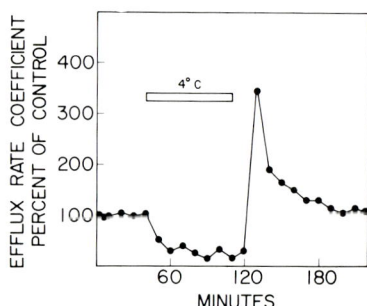

Fig. 22. Effect of a temporary decrease in temperature to 4°C on the efflux rate coefficient of calcium. The conditions are identical to those described in Fig. 21 except for the length of the cold period. In this case, the period of cold exposure lasted 70 minutes.

Calcium Transport in Kidney Cells

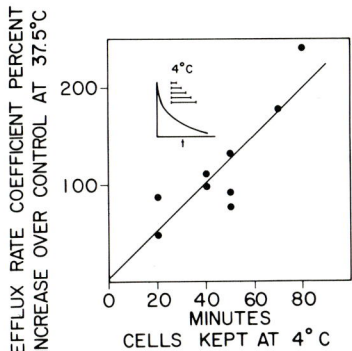

FIG. 23. Relationship between the period of cold exposure at 4°C and the rebound in calcium efflux when the cells are replaced at 37.5°C. In this series of experiments, the cells were all placed at 4°C at the same time of desaturation, i.e., 40 minutes. They were replaced at 37.5°C at various times: 60, 80, 70, 110, and 120 minutes. The linear regression equation, $y(x) = 4.5 + 2.4x$, and the coefficient of correlation, $R = 0.86$, were obtained by computer.

If the intracellular calcium activity influences calcium efflux, inhibiting the calcium pump should in turn increase the calcium activity of the cytoplasm. The rise in cellular calcium should be proportional to the period of inhibition. I tested this hypothesis by placing the cells at 4°C for various lengths of time during efflux and then replacing them at 37°C. After an inhibition of 50 minutes, calcium efflux jumps to twice the control rate

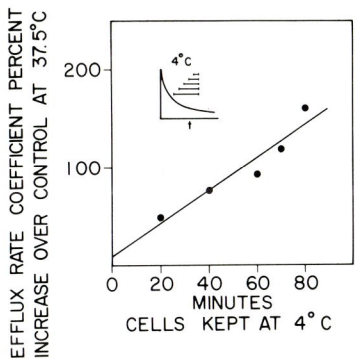

FIG. 24. Relationship between the period of cold exposure and the rebound in calcium efflux when the cells are replaced at 37.5°C. In these experiments, the cells were placed at 4°C at various times: 40, 50, 60, 80, and 100 minutes. They were all replaced at 37.5°C at the same time of desaturation, i.e. 120 minutes. The linear regression equation, $y(x) = 8.5 + 1.66x$, and the coefficient of correlation, $R = 0.95$, were obtained by computer.

(Fig. 21), and after 70 minutes, it rebounds to 350% before returning to control values (Fig. 22). The magnitude of the rebound is proportional to the period of cold exposure, regardless of the initial or final time of the inhibition (Figs. 23 and 24). Apparently, inhibiting the calcium pump increases the intracellular calcium activity, which in turn stimulates calcium efflux as soon as the inhibition is released.

A Model for Cellular Calcium Metabolism

The data I have just presented can be summarized in the model shown in Fig. 25. The cell calcium is divided into several extracellular and intracellular compartments. On the outer surface of the cell, calcium is bound to the plasma membrane and to the mucoproteins of the glycocalyx. This accounts for about 90% of the total cell calcium. The intracellular calcium concentration is about 0.3 mM. However, since the ratio of calcium uptake between mitochondria and cytoplasm can be as high as 100 to 1, the cytoplasmic calcium may actually be of the order of 10^{-6} M. In addition, cytoplasmic calcium is bound to cell proteins and other subcellular components (represented as X in the model) that would further reduce its activity.

Calcium influx into the cell is only 5–10% of the total calcium uptake. The rest represents calcium exchange with the extracellular pools. It is a carrier-mediated process, specific for calcium. This transport is going down an electrochemical gradient and can be described as a facilitated diffusion process. Calcium efflux is an active transport which is proportional to the calcium activity of the cytoplasm. A rise in free calcium stimulates the calcium pump, and conversely, inhibition of the pump causes the cell calcium to rise at least temporarily.

Mitochondria act as a buffer mechanism and as a calcium trap. Phosphate has a marked influence on this exchange. It stimulates calcium uptake and

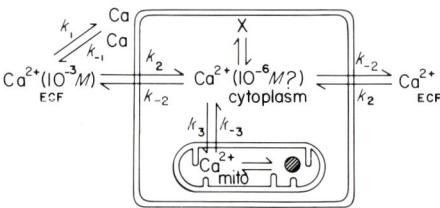

FIG. 25. Model representing the different extra- and intracellular compartments of calcium, and the tentative identification of the three rates of calcium exchange obtained by kinetic analyses of calcium-45 movements in isolated cells.

its sequestration by mitochondria. The very slowly exchangeable fraction of calcium probably represents precipitation of calcium phosphate inside the mitochondria. Shifts of calcium from one intracellular compartment to the other are fast and reversible. Consequently, the levels of free calcium ion in the cytoplasm may be regulated mainly by the exchange of calcium between mitochondria and cytoplasm and to a lesser extent by the influx and efflux of calcium in and out of the cell.

This is, of course, a tentative model, but the experimental tools which I have described might ultimately be useful for locating the cellular site of action of the hormones and vitamins involved in the regulation of calcium metabolism.

REFERENCES

Borle, A. B. (1968). Unpublished data.
Borle, A. B. (1967). *Clin. Orthop. Related Res.* **52**, 287.
Borle, A. B. (1969a). *J. Gen. Physiol.* **53**, 43.
Borle, A. B. (1969b). *Endocrinology* **85**, 194.
Borle, A. B. (1970a). *J. Gen. Physiol.* **55**, 163.
Borle, A B. (1970b). *Endocrinology* **86**, 1389.
Borle, A. B., and Herold, E. (1971). Submitted for publication.
Lehninger, A. L., Carafoli, E., and Rossi, C. S. (1967). *Advan. Enzymol. Relat Areas Mol. Biol.* **29**, 259.
Shematek, J., and Borle, A. B. (1971). Submitted for publication.

Discussion

Dr. Raisz: I gather that pyrophosphate causes a larger entry of calcium than phosphate. In this case, one wonders whether the calcium could get into pool 3. Have you measured pool 3 calcium in the high pyrophosphate circumstance?

Dr. Borle: I did not study the influence of pyrophosphate on the third pool. But I would suspect that most of the calcium which entered the cell would ultimately be found in the third pool.

Dr. Lloyd: I would like to ask about your kinetic analysis procedure. Am I right in thinking that you determined ^{45}Ca uptake by isolated cells, plotted these data as a function of time, split the curve into three exponentials, and from this, calculated pool sizes? I have had some experience in trying to strip exponential curves in order to estimate pool sizes in respect to other body functions. I found this particularly difficult to do. I wonder how sure one can be of the results and whether you could show an example of the curves so we can get some idea of how you arrived at these numbers.

Dr. Borle: Influx experiments in a closed system are, of course, more difficult to analyse than in an open system. Since I have described the method in detail in a recent paper [A. B. Borle, *J. Gen. Physiol.* **55**, 163 (1970)], I didn't go into the details of the technique. In the appendix, I made some remarks about the limitations of the method for measuring pools and fluxes in such a system. The precision and the accuracy of the measurements of the second pool—that is, the intracellular pool are quite good—of the order of a few percent. The first pool, however, can be subject to large errors, something like 25%. I am quite aware of this uncertainty. That is why I did not investigate the effect of phosphate on the first pool. But I am quite confident of the accuracy in the second pool. I was very glad to see that the values obtained for the second pool by efflux studies in an open system matched the values obtained by influx experiments in a closed system. It is not easy to obtain nice smooth curves. We usually use twenty-four points to establish one single curve, and with a good and careful technique, the reliability is quite good. But one needs some skill and some experience.

Dr. Wallach: Dr. Borle, I wonder if you can say a few words about the characteristics of the active efflux process. Specifically, do you think that decreased intracellular binding of calcium at the area you refer to as X might create a favorable gradient for efflux on one side of the cell?

Dr. Borle: I have no evidence on which to base an answer. However, I will say, no. Perhaps Dr. Vincenzi and Dr. Martonosi can give you more information on the intracellular concentration of ionized calcium. I believe that the intracellular calcium ion concentration is below 10^{-5} or even below 10^{-6} M. I would doubt that a decrease in calcium binding to X, whatever X represents, would increase the ionized calcium in the cell from below 10^{-6} M to 10^{-3} M, which is the calcium concentration in the extracellular fluids. Furthermore, I have shown that metabolic inhibitors inhibit calcium efflux. There is also a less specific inhibition of calcium efflux by lowering the temperature. In this case there is a rebound in the efflux after the period of inhibition which also suggests that calcium efflux is by active transport.

Dr. Nichols: I was interested particularly in the experiments in which you showed the effect of low phosphate media on the efflux from the third compartment. I wondered whether you had studied phosphate shifts directly, because it seemed to me that there are many parts of this whole model which are enormously dependent on the shifts of phosphate into and out of the mitochondria, and while they have been shown in isolated systems, do we know for sure that external phosphate influences the phosphate concentration in those very critical areas?

Dr. Borle: Yes, I agree with you. I think there are several possible explanations for these shifts. Since phosphate increases the uptake of calcium in mitochondria *in vitro*, it is possible that increasing phosphate outside the cell might secondarily increase the phosphate inside the cell. This could cause a shift of calcium and phosphate in the mitochondria. It is a possibility, but it is not a complete explanation, because I think that in mitochondria at least, phosphate follows calcium uptake. It is fairly well established now that the active transport in mitochondria is a cation transport, and that phosphate follows calcium passively.

Of course, phosphate will increase the calcium uptake by mitochondria, not because it stimulates the influx but because it creates a calcium trap inside the mitochondria. Thus, the mitochondria may accumulate a greater amount of calcium without the influx being significantly affected by phosphate.

Dr. MacIntyre: Dr. Borle, in your earlier experiments, I think you postulated an effect of calcitonin on calcium extrusion from a different sort of experiment. When you studied it with your new system, could you confirm such an effect?

Dr. Borle: The effects of calcitonin on calcium efflux were obtained in such a system, studying efflux directly. I perturbed the steady state by adding calcitonin and observed a drop in the efflux rate coefficient. In these experiments I did not measure all the kinetic parameters, but I plan to do so in the future.

Dr. Cohn: I was struck with the similarity in the uptake of calcium by your intact cells with the way in which mitochondria behave when they are studied *in vitro* with calcium and phosphate. Specifically, one adds calcium to solutions containing mitochondria with phosphate present, and the mitochondria continue to take up calcium phosphate. For a while, the mitochondria are metabolically active and retain respiratory control. At a certain point, however, they become what Lehninger's group called "heavily loaded." Then, if they are warmed up or allowed to stand, they rapidly discharge their content of calcium and phosphate. During the final stages of calcium loading and during the unloading process, the mitochondria lose most of their physiological properties, though they still take up oxygen. The question I have, therefore, is, if you have measured some metabolical or physiological parameters of your kidney cells during the final stages of uptake and efflux to find out if you are studying physiological sequestration and release, or whether you have perhaps turned your cells into a damaged mitochondrial preparation.

Dr. Borle: My answer is an unequivocal, no. I am sure that my cells are in a physiological state. When you isolate mitochondria and expose them to 1.3 mM calcium and 5 mM phosphate, of course you are going to damage them. You may have mitochondrial swelling, lysis, etc. But don't forget that these mitochondria are not exposed to 5 mM phosphate, the cells are. In fact, you can grow kidney cells and HeLa cells in suspension in commercial media containing 20 mM phosphate, and these cells grow normally. I doubt that anything goes wrong with my cells in 5 mM phosphate, when I can grow them very successfully in 20 mM phosphate. As far as the calcium is concerned, the highest concentration I used with high phosphate concentrations was 1.3 mM. Therefore, I think that the changes I observed by kinetic analysis were not pathological but physiological events.

Dr. Massry: Dr. Borle, I would like to try to transfer your elegant data to the intact kidney and intact animal where we know that calcium and sodium transport by the renal tubules is closely and intimately interrelated. Do you have any data about the role of sodium in the media in your studies? Secondly, it was surprising to find that changes in magnesium concentration in the media did not affect the influx of calcium, since we know that elevation in serum magnesium or magnesium in the renal tubular fluid causes a decrease in the tubular reabsorption of calcium by the nephron.

Dr. Borle: We were very interested by the observations of Blaustein and Hodgkin suggesting that part of the calcium efflux in the squid axon may be coupled to sodium entry [H. P. Blaustein and A. L. Hodgkin, *J. Physiol.* (*London*) **200**, 497 (1960)]. We were fortunate to have Dr. Blaustein stay for a few days in our laboratory in Pittsburgh and we did a few experiments on calcium efflux from kidney cells. We tried to test in kidney cells his theory of exchange of calcium for sodium ions. The two experiments we did were not convincing to me because we could not see a drop in calcium efflux when we replaced sodium by lithium or choline chloride in the media. However, lithium and choline chloride themselves have an effect on calcium efflux, so that these experiments were not that clear cut. But as far as I can interpret two single experiments, I would say that I have not found any convincing evidence for an exchange of sodium for calcium in kidney cells.

Concerning the lack of inhibition of calcium influx by magnesium, I should emphasize that what I measured was the influx of calcium from the extracellular phase to the second phase, that is, the intracellular compartment. One should be careful not to identify this influx, which is only one step of the calcium transport process, with the transcellular calcium transport across an epithelium. Of course, calcium has to enter the cell to go through, but it still has to get out of the cell. What magnesium does at the exit side of the cell I don't know. Perhaps magnesium does inhibit calcium efflux. The clinical or experimental evidence of magnesium inhibiting calcium reabsorption in the nephron is not necessarily in conflict with the fact that magnesium does not inhibit that single step that I measure: the influx of calcium from the extracellular fluids to the intracellular compartment.

Dr. Urist: This has been an awesome demonstration of measurements of calcium in micromoles, nanomoles, and picomoles per milliliter of cell water or per milligram of cell protein. As a hard-tissue physiologist, who measures calcium in relatively gross quantities, millimoles per kilogram, I would like to ask Dr. Borle about influx of cell calcium. This afternoon I made a demonstration of the capacity of cells of the intact rabbit's ear to tolerate microperfusion of concentrations of at least 20 mmoles per liter of calcium ion without any evidence of tissue damage. Is this high level of tolerance evidence of a unique capacity of the living cell to resist influx, or to employ active transport mechanisms for efflux? Can you measure the true proportion of influx and efflux of calcium ions?

Dr. Borle: I am not sure that I know what you mean by "true proportion," but I will try to answer your question this way. If we assume that the calcium influx that I have measured in kidney cells is a necessary step in the overall directional transport, this passive influx, although limiting, should be sufficient to account for the total calcium resorption in the nephron [A. B. Borle, *J. Gen. Physiol.* **55**, 163 (1970)]. With an average glomerular filtration rate of 120 ml/minute and a normal filterable calcium of 1.6 mmoles/liter, the total calcium filtered per day in man is 276 mmoles, or 11.0 gm. The proximal tubule is reported to have a diameter of 60 μm and a length of 14 mm. In addition, the microvilli increase the cellular surface area some forty times. Since up to 4.5 million nephrons per kidney have been reported in man, the total surface area available in the proximal tubule alone is 9.5×10^6 cm^2. With calcium influx rates ranging from 50 to 300 femtomoles·cm^{-2}·sec^{-1}, calcium reabsorption can fluctuate between 2 and 10 gm/day. If one takes into account the physiological effects of the parathyroid hormone normally present, it is evident that our measurements of calcium influx can explain the total calcium reabsorption in the proximal tubule alone. I made the same calculations for the intestine and I got the same agreement between the flux measurements and absorption. I hope that this answers your question.

Dr. Armstrong: I have two very short questions which Dr. Borle can quickly answer. The first is what is the counterion involved in the efflux of calcium? The second is is there any need now to postulate a pumping of magnesium into the cell, in view of the fact that the intracellular magnesium concentration in liver and muscle is maintained without change over long periods of magnesium deficiency?

Dr. Borle: To answer the first question, I don't know, really, what is the counterion. I would guess that it is phosphate that follows calcium passively. Another possibility would be an exchange with the hydrogen ion. Or it could be an exchange for sodium ions as shown by Blaustein and Hodgkin in nerve. In answer to your second question, is there a magnesium pump to maintain a constant concentration of magnesium in magnesium deficiency? I do not know. I did not study magnesium transport in any of these cellular systems, so I have no idea what the mechanism is.

RECENT OBSERVATIONS ON THE MECHANISM OF CA^{2+} TRANSPORT BY FRAGMENTED SARCOPLASMIC RETICULUM MEMBRANES*

A. Martonosi, A. G. Pucell, and R. A. Halpin

Introduction

Fragmented sarcoplasmic reticulum vesicles, isolated from white skeletal muscles of rabbit, actively accumulate Ca^{2+} at the expense of energy derived from ATP hydrolysis (Ebashi and Lipmann, 1962). The hydrolysis of ATP occurs through an ATPase enzyme which is tightly linked to the microsomal membrane and requires Mg^{2+} and small concentrations of Ca^{2+} for activity (Hasselbach and Makinose, 1961). The hydrolysis of ATP and the active Ca^{2+} transport are inhibited by treatment of microsomes with phospholipase C, parallel with the hydrolysis of membrane lecithin into diglycerides and phosphorylcholine (Martonosi, 1963, 1964; Martonosi et al., 1968). The inhibited ATPase and Ca^{2+} transport of lipid depleted microsomes are reactivated by micellar suspensions of synthetic or natural lecithin or lysolecithin preparations, indicating a requirement for phospholipids in these functions (Martonosi, 1963; Martonosi et al., 1968).

* The work was supported by research grants GB 7136 from the National Science Foundation and NS 07749 from the National Institute of Neurological Diseases and Stroke.

During ATP hydrolysis, phosphorylation of membrane proteins occurs, and the phosphoprotein (E $\sim$ P) is presumed to be an intermediate in the ATP–ADP exchange and calcium transport processes (Yamamoto and Tonomura, 1967; Martonosi, 1967, 1969a; Makinose, 1969). The principal evidence relating the phosphorylated intermediate to Ca^{2+} transport is the marked and similar dependence of phosphoprotein formation, ATPase activity, and calcium transport on the free Ca^{2+} concentration of the incubation medium (Yamamoto and Tonomura, 1967; Makinose, 1969).

The subject of this chapter is (a) the analysis of the mode of involvement of phospholipids in the ATPase activity and calcium transport, (b) the isolation and characterization of the transport protein, (c) fragmentation of the transport protein by proteolytic enzymes and the isolation of the active center phosphopeptide.

Role of Phospholipids in ATPase Activity and Calcium Transport

The hydrolysis of ATP by fragmented sarcoplasmic reticulum membranes may be represented schematically as follows:

$$AT^{32}P + \text{enzyme} \underset{}{\overset{(1)}{\rightleftarrows}} E \sim {^{32}P} \overset{(2)}{\rightarrow} E + {^{32}P_i}$$
$$+$$
$$ADP$$

Step 1, in the direction of upper arrow, represents the formation of phosphoprotein intermediate (E $\sim$ P), with the liberation of ADP. Reversal of this step leads to ATP–ADP exchange. Step 2 is the hydrolytic decomposition of E $\sim$ P with the liberation of inorganic orthophosphate.

It is expected that selective inhibition of step 1 leads to a decrease, while that of step 2 to an increase in the steady state concentration of phosphoprotein intermediate, and therefore, by measuring the concentration of E $\sim$ P, conclusions may be drawn regarding the point of action of various inhibitors. The concentration of E $\sim$ ^{32}P complex can be readily estimated after stopping the reaction with trichloroacetic acid by measurement of protein bound radioactivity.

The marked inhibition of ATPase activity and calcium transport which results from hydrolysis of microsomal membrane phospholipids with phospholipase C (*Clostridium welchii*) is accompanied by accumulation of phosphoprotein intermediate in the presence of 5 mM $MgCl_2$ and 0.5 mM EGTA, as compared with untreated control microsomes (Table I).

From these observations, it may be concluded that hydrolysis of membrane phospholipids interferes primarily with the second phase

TABLE I

Effect of Phospholipase C Treatment[a] on the ATPase Activity,[b] Calcium Transport,[c] and Phosphorylated Intermediate[d]

Treatment	ATPase activity (μmole P_i/mg protein/ minute)	Ca uptake (μmole Ca^{2+}/mg protein)	Phosphorylated intermediate with 5 mM mg and 0.5 mM EGTA (moles/ 10^6 gm protein)	Phosphorylated intermediate with 5 mM $CaCl_2$ (moles/10^6 gm protein)
Phospholipase C treatment 20 minutes				
Treated microsomes	0.11	0	2.03	2.02
Control microsomes	1.20	8.10	0.11	2.74
Phospholipase C treatment 60 minutes				
Treated microsomes	0.18	0.15	2.16	2.15
Control microsomes	1.17	8.90	0.13	2.69
Phospholipase C treatment 180 minutes				
Treated microsomes	0.20	0	2.38	2.35
Control microsomes	0.95	9.10	0.11	2.84

[a] Phospholipase C treatment was carried out in a medium of 0.1 M KCl, 10 mM imidazole, 2 mM $CaCl_2$, 10 mg/ml microsomal protein, and 1 mg/ml phospholipase C (*Cl. welchii*), at 21°C temperature for times indicated in the table. After incubation, the suspension was diluted threefold with cold water and centrifuged in Spinco preparative centrifuge at 26,000 rpm for 1 hour. The washing was repeated once more. The final sediment was suspended in water to a protein concentration of 10 mg/ml and stored in ice. Control samples were subjected to the same treatment without phospholipase C.

[b] ATPase assay system contained 0.05 M KCl, 5 mM imidazole, 5 mM $MgCl_2$, 5 mM ATP, 0.05 mM $CaCl_2$, and 0.03 mg microsomal protein per milliliter. Incubation was for 10 minutes at 25°C.

[c] Ca^{2+} transport assay system contained 0.1 M KCl, 10 mM imidazole, 5 mM oxalate, 5 mM $MgCl_2$, 5 mM ATP, 9.4×10^{-5} M $^{45}CaCl_2$, and 0.01 mg microsomal protein per milliliter. After 5 minutes of incubation at 25°C, reaction was stopped by Millipore filtration, and the radioactivity of the microsome-free filtrate was determined (Martonosi and Feretos, 1964).

[d] Phosphorylated intermediate assay system contained 0.05 M KCl, 5 mM imidazole, 0.5 mM $AT^{32}P$, 1 mg microsomal protein per milliliter, and either 5 mM $CaCl_2$ or 5 mM $MgCl_2$ and 0.5 mM EGTA as activators. Incubation was carried out in ice for 20 seconds. Reaction was stopped, and the samples were processed as described earlier (Martonosi, 1969a).

(step 2) of the overall ATP hydrolysis, i.e., the decomposition of phosphorylated intermediate, leaving the first step, the formation of enzyme $\sim$ P complex relatively unaffected (Martonosi, 1967, 1969a).

The Ca^{2+} sensitivity of the enzyme system is markedly changed as a result of phospholipase C treatment. While formation of maximum levels of E $\sim$ P complex in untreated microsomes requires the presence of 5 mM Mg^{2+} and higher than 10^{-6} M Ca^{2+}, the phosphoprotein concentration of phospholipase C-treated microsomes is only slightly influenced by medium Ca^{2+} concentration in the range of 10^{-8} to 10^{-3} M (Fig. 1).

These observations do not support the widely held view that the formation of phosphoprotein intermediate is absolutely dependent on Ca^{2+} as E $\sim$ P accumulates to maximum concentrations in phospholipase C-treated microsomes at medium free Ca^{2+} concentrations as low as 10^{-8} M. It is likely, however, that Ca^{2+} accelerates the rate of E $\sim$ P formation in

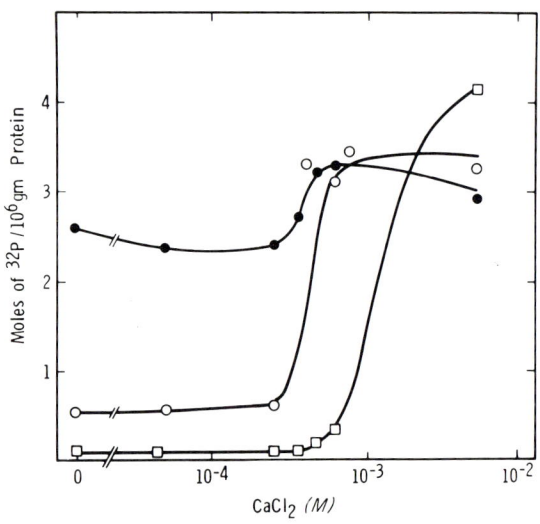

FIG. 1. Effect of Ca^{2+} concentration on the phosphorylated intermediate in control and phospholipase C-treated microsomes. Phosphorylated intermediate was assayed in a medium of 0.05 M KCl, 5 mM imidazole, 0.5 mM AT^{32}P, 5 mM MgCl$_2$, 0.5 mM EGTA, and 1 mg microsomal protein per milliliter. Incubation was for 20 seconds at 0°C. Calcium was added to final concentrations indicated on the abscissa. □ and ○ indicate control microsomes; the two experiments are included to illustrate the range of variation which was encountered among different preparations. ● indicates phospholipase C-treated microsomes; treatment was carried out for 60 minutes under conditions described in Table I.

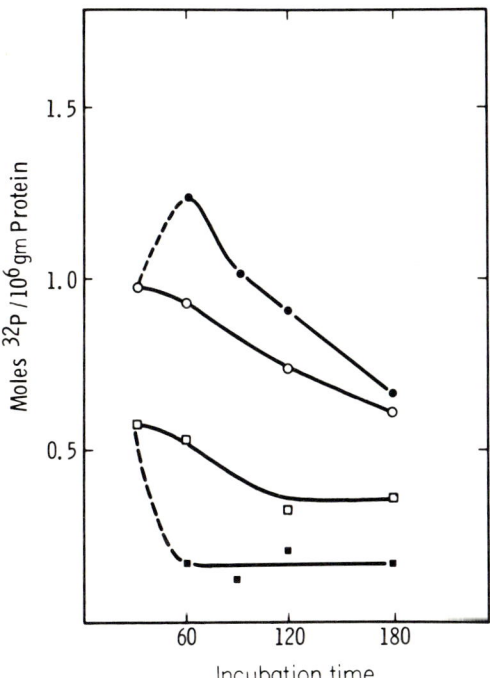

FIG. 2. The rate of decay of phosphorylated intermediate upon magnesium and EDTA addition. Samples containing control (□) or phospholipase C-treated microsomes (○) were incubated in a medium which contained 0.05 M KCl, 5 mM imidazole, 1 mM CaCl$_2$, 0.5 mM AT^{32}P, and 1 mg microsomal protein per milliliter. Portions were taken after 30, 60, 120, and 180 seconds of incubation for the determination of phosphorylated intermediate. To a second set of samples containing control (■) or phospholipase C-treated microsomes (●), 5 mM EGTA and 5 mM MgCl$_2$ were added after 30 seconds of incubation in ice, and portions were taken for assay of phosphorylated intermediate after 60, 90, 120, and 180 seconds of incubation.

control microsomes resulting in high E ∼ P levels in spite of rapid ATP hydrolysis. The effect of Ca^{2+} on the rate of formation of E ∼ P could not be investigated due to the high velocity of this reaction.

The apparently selective requirement for phospholipids in the decomposition of E ∼ P is further emphasized by the slower rate of decomposition of previously formed E ∼ P in phospholipase C-treated, as compared with control microsomes, in the presence of magnesium and EGTA (Fig. 2). With 5 mM calcium as activator, the phosphoprotein accumulates to

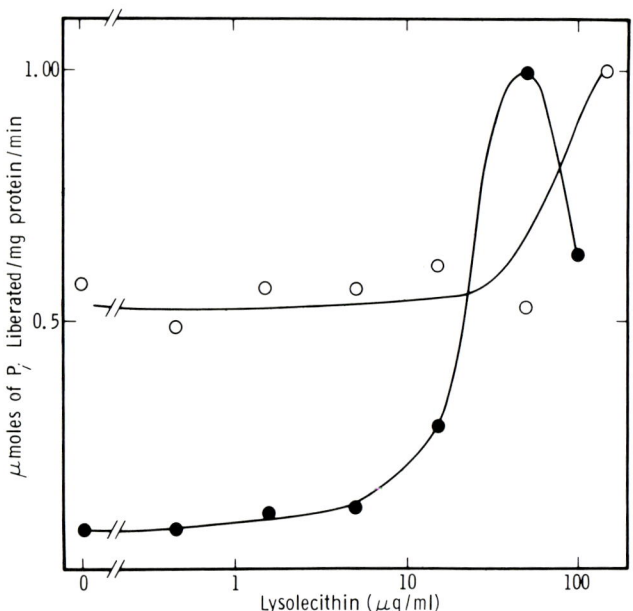

FIG. 3. Effect of lysolecithin on the ATPase activity. Microsomes (0.15 mg protein per milliliter) were incubated for 5 minutes at 21°C with lysolecithin at concentration stated in the abscissa (microgram per milliliter), in a medium of 0.05 M KCl, 5 mM imidazole, 5 mM MgCl$_2$, and 0.05 mM CaCl$_2$, pH 7.3. Reaction was started with addition of ATP to a final concentration of 5 mM. Incubation time 10 minutes; ○——○, control microsomes; ●——●, phospholipase C-treated microsomes.

similar levels in control and phospholipase C-treated systems, even in the absence of magnesium (Table I). The inhibition of ATP hydrolysis and accumulation of E $\sim$ P in the presence of 5 mM Ca^{2+} suggests a specific role for magnesium in the hydrolysis of E $\sim$ P complex. Lysolecithin, at concentrations which produce optimal activation of the hydrolysis of ATP by phospholipase C-treated microsomes (Fig. 3), reduces the E $\sim$ P concentration nearly to control level with 5 mM MgCl$_2$ and 0.5 mM EGTA as activators (Fig. 4). This effect is readily explained by assuming phospholipid involvement in the decomposition of E $\sim$ P complex (Martonosi, 1967, 1969a). Lysolecithin is much less effective in altering the level of E $\sim$ P in the presence of 5 mM calcium, i.e., under conditions when the hydrolysis of E $\sim$ P is severely inhibited even in control microsomes (Fig. 5).

Variation of ATP concentration between 10^{-5} and 10^{-3} M does not influence qualitatively the above conclusions (Fig. 6). The abrupt rise in the level of E $\sim$P at ATP concentrations exceeding 1 mM is of uncertain significance, as these values are based on small differences in protein-bound radioactivity, and calcium introduced as contaminant with ATP may elevate the free calcium concentration of the system to levels where its influence on the concentration of E $\sim$ P becomes marked, especially in control microsomes.

Inhibition of ATPase activity and Ca^{2+} transport by extraction of microsomes with 90% acetone was accompanied by marked inhibition of the formation of E $\sim$ P complex, both with magnesium or calcium as activators. Neither functions could be restored by readdition of extracted phospholipids or other synthetic or natural phospholipid preparations. These experiments may indicate the requirement for phospholipids other than lecithin for the formation of E $\sim$ P, although irreversible denaturation of transport ATPase caused by acetone extraction is a likely alternative.

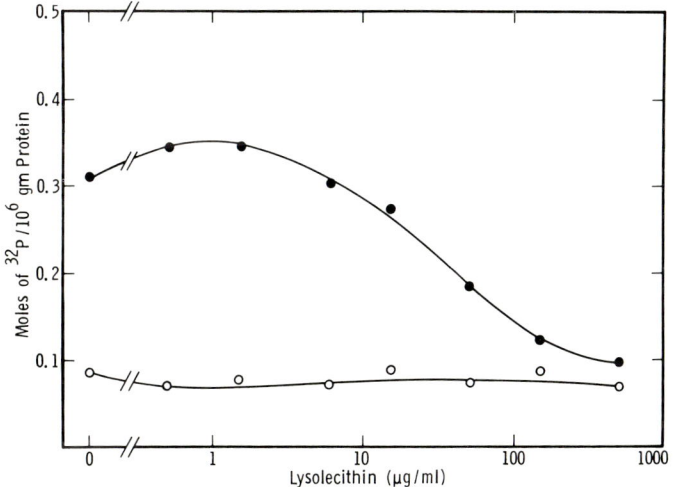

FIG. 4. Effect of lysolecithin on the phosphorylated intermediate with magnesium–EGTA. Microsomes (1 mg protein per milliliter) were exposed to lysolecithin at stated concentration for 5 minutes, at 2°C, in a medium which contained 0.05 M KCl, 5 mM imidazole, 5 mM MgCl$_2$, and 0.5 mM EGTA at pH 7.3. Reaction was started with addition of AT^{32}P to a final concentration of 0.5 mM. After 20 seconds of incubation at 2°C, the reaction was stopped and protein-bound phosphate was assayed as described in legend to Table I. ○, Control microsomes; ●, phospholipase C-treated microsomes.

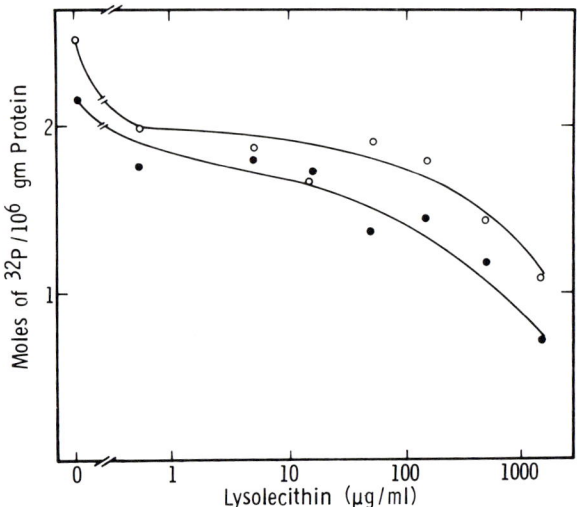

Fig. 5. Effect of lysolecithin on the phosphoprotein intermediate with 5 mM CaCl$_2$ as activator. Experiments were carried out as described in legend to Fig. 4, except that instead of magnesium–EGTA, the assay system contained 5 mM CaCl$_2$. ○, Control microsomes; ●, phospholipase C-treated microsomes.

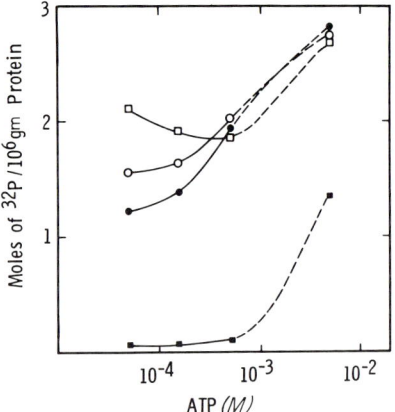

Fig. 6. Effect of ATP concentration on the level of phosphorylated intermediate. Microsomes (1 mg protein per milliliter) were incubated in a medium of 0.05 M KCl, 5 mM imidazole, and either 5 mM MgCl$_2$–0.5 mM EGTA or 5 mM CaCl$_2$, at ATP concentrations stated on the abscissa for 20 seconds at 2°C. Protein-bound phosphate was measured as described in legend to Table I. ○, 5 mM CaCl$_2$, phospholipase C-treated microsomes; ●, 5 mM CaCl$_2$, control microsomes; □, 5 mM MgCl$_2$–0.5 mM EGTA, phospholipase C-treated microsomes; ■, 5 mM MgCl$_2$–0.5 mM EGTA, control microsomes.

The mechanism of Ca^{2+} transport may be represented in the following hypothetical scheme:

Outside surface

$$E + AT^{32}P \rightleftarrows E \sim {}^{32}P + ADP \qquad (1)$$

$$E \sim P + Ca^{2+} \rightleftarrows E \sim P - Ca \qquad (2)$$

Inside surface

$$E^* \sim P - Ca + H_2O \rightarrow E^* + P_i + Ca^{2+} \qquad (3)$$

$$E^* \rightarrow E \qquad (4)$$

It is an essential feature of this scheme that the formation of $E \sim {}^{32}P$ complex is not absolutely dependent upon Ca^{2+}. The interaction of Ca^{2+} with the energized carrier leads to Ca^{2+} translocation from the external to the internal membrane surface followed by hydrolysis of the $E \sim P$ bond with release of Ca^{2+}. The phospholipid requirement is probably connected with the translocation step or the subsequent hydrolysis of $E \sim P$ complex

The accumulation of phosphorylated intermediate to maximum levels in phospholipase C-treated microsomes with 5 mM $MgCl_2$–0.5 mM EGTA or with 5 mM $CaCl_2$ as activators contrasts the recent findings of Fiehn and Hasselbach (1970) that phospholipase A treatment of microsomes inhibits the formation of intermediate. As inhibition is never observed with phospholipase C even after extensive treatment, the inhibiting effect of phospholipase A may result from the liberation of fatty acids or from the hydrolysis of phospholipids other than lecithin.

Recent studies in our laboratory (Martonosi et al., 1971) indicate, however, that phospholipase C of B. cereus (similarly to that of Cl. welchii) does not inhibit the formation of phosphoprotein, even under conditions when phosphatidylserine, phosphatidylethanolamine, and phosphatidylcholine were largely degraded, with massive inhibition of ATPase activity and Ca^{2+} transport.

Protein Composition of Sarcoplasmic Reticulum Membranes

Separation of proteins from solubilized membranes of fragmented sarcoplasmic reticulum may be easily accomplished by electrophoresis in 0.1 M sodium phosphate buffer containing 0.1% SDS on polyacrylamide gels (Fig. 7a). In addition to proteins, a fast moving band which contains most of the lipid content of microsomes appears after periodate–Schiff reaction (Fig. 7b). The lipid band disappears on extraction of microsomes

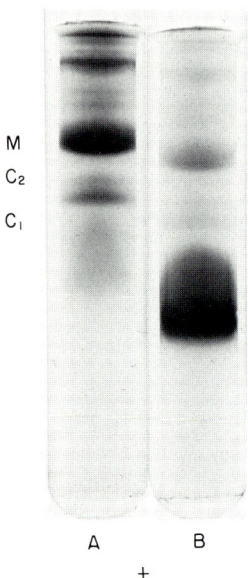

Fig. 7. Separation of microsomal phospholipids from proteins on polyacrylamide gels. Electrophoresis was carried out using 0.1 M sodium phosphate, 0.1% sodium dodecylsulfate, pH 6.0 buffer at 5 mA per tube for 10 hours on polyacrylamide gel. The gel contained 10 gm Cyanogum 41, 0.34 ml dimethylaminopropionitril, and 0.5 gm ammonium persulfate in a total volume of 200 ml. Samples of 0.1–0.2 ml containing 1–3 mg protein per milliliter, 0.4% sodium dodecylsulfate, 6.5% sucrose, and 0.05 M sodium phosphate, pH 6.0, were layered on the surface of the gel under the buffer (Martonosi, 1969b). Sample A was stained with amido black and sample B with periodate–Schiff reaction. For periodate–Schiff staining, the gels were extruded and exposed to the following solutions, in succession: (1) 0.5% periodic acid in 90% acetic acid for 5 minutes; (2) 15% sodium metabisulfite in 1.5 N HCl for 5 minutes; (3) 0.2% pararosaniline in 0.5% sodium metabisulfite for 10 hours. The gels were stored in 10% acetic acid.

with 90% acetone (Fig. 8b) or chloroform methanol (Fig. 8c) and may be recovered from the corresponding extracts (Figs. 8d and e) with virtually unchanged mobility.

Electrophoresis of microsomes previously labeled with $AT^{32}P$ or acetyl-^{32}P permitted the identification of a major protein band (M) with the ATPase enzyme involved in calcium transport as the only region of the gel which retained significant radioactivity during prolonged electrophoresis (Martonosi, 1969b).

Various methods were developed for the isolation of ATPase enzyme from microsomes:

1. Pure but inactive enzyme protein may be obtained (Martonosi, 1970) from microsomes solubilized with sodium dodecylsulfate by preparative electrophoresis on polyacrylamide gel (Fig. 9). The pure M protein emerged in pooled fractions 7 and 8 as evidenced by analytical polyacrylamide electrophoresis of the dialyzed and concentrated material.

2. A simple method for the isolation of enzymically active, nearly homogeneous M protein is the ammonium sulfate fractionation of microsomes solubilized with cholate and deoxycholate (Martonosi, 1968). The floating layer of protein and phospholipids obtained at 50–55% saturation consists of nearly pure enzyme protein with specific ATPase activity 1.6 times that of the starting material (Fig. 10). The clear supernate contains in virtually pure form the two fast moving proteins (C_1 and C_2) which are enzymically inactive. C_1 and C_2 proteins are also released selectively from the membrane by treatment of microsomes with EDTA at pH 8–9, indicating that divalent cations are involved in their interaction with the microsomes (Duggan and Martonosi, 1970).

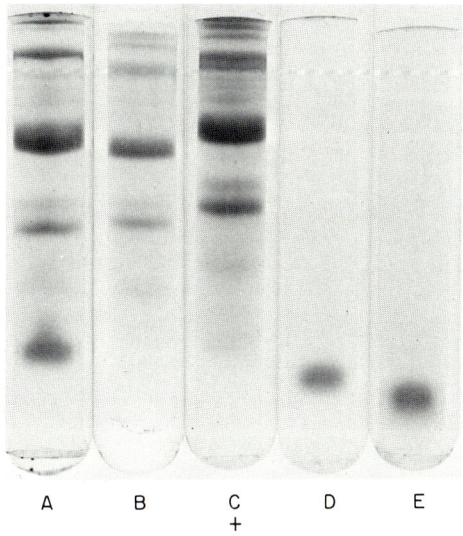

FIG. 8. Staining of microsomal lipids with periodate–Schiff reagent. Electrophoresis was performed as described under legend to Fig. 7. Key: (A) control microsomes; (B) microsomes extracted with 90% acetone; (C) microsomes extracted with chloroform–methanol (2:1) mixture; (D) lipids extracted from microsomes with acetone; (E) lipids extracted from microsomes with chloroform-methanol. All samples were stained first with amido black and subsequently with periodate–Schiff reaction as described under legend to Fig. 7.

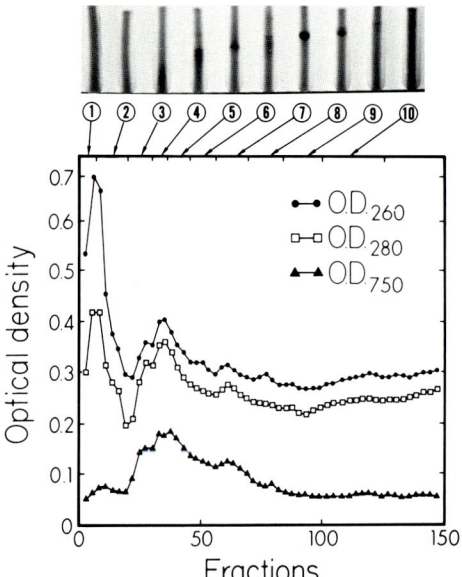

Fig. 9. Separation of microsomal proteins by preparative electrophoresis on polyacrylamide gel. Electrophoresis was carried out on Shandon preparative apparatus using 40 ml gel of the following composition: 10 gm Cyanogum 41, 0.34 ml dimethylaminopropionitrile, 0.5 gm ammonium persulfate in 200 ml of 0.1 M sodium phosphate, 0.1% SDS solution, pH 6.0. Sample containing 37.5 mg protein in 1.75 ml solution of 0.5% sodium dodecylsulfate, 4.6% sucrose, and 6.7 mM phosphate buffer at pH 7.0 was layered on the surface of the gel. Electrophoresis was carried out at room temperature using tap water for cooling.

The contents of the upper and lower buffer reservoirs were continually mixed by pumping the lower buffer with a peristaltic pump into the upper reservoir and draining by gravity the overflow from the upper reservoir into the lower one. In this manner, the pH was maintained within ±0.1 pH units during electrophoresis lasting for several days. A solution of 0.1 M sodium phosphate and 0.1% sodium dodecylsulfate was used for elution with Buchler polystaltic pump at a flow rate of 2.8 ml in 1 hour. Fractions were collected at 20 minute intervals. Electrophoresis was started at 30 mA current, which was raised after 2 hours to 80 mA and maintained at that level throughout.

The collected fractions were analyzed for ultraviolet absorption at 280 and 260 mμ. Lowry protein determinations were carried out with assay at 750 mμ. The fractions were pooled as indicated, dialyzed exhaustively against water, and lyophilized. The lyophilized fractions were subjected to analytical polyacrylamide electrophoresis as described in legend to Fig. 7. The resulting patterns are represented in the upper portion of the figure.

The molecular weight of the M protein was close to 100,000 (Fig. 11), while those of C_1 and C_2 proteins were 61,000 and 67,000, respectively. The amino acid composition of the transport protein is similar to that of intact microsomes (Table II).

The molecular weight of 100,000 is considerably larger than the 6000–17,000 value reported by Yu and Masoro (1970) for a rat sarcoplasmic reticulum fraction. It seems likely that if the ATPase protein consists of subunits, the rabbit enzyme used in our work is considerably more resistant to dissociating conditions than its rat counterpart. The value of 100,000 is

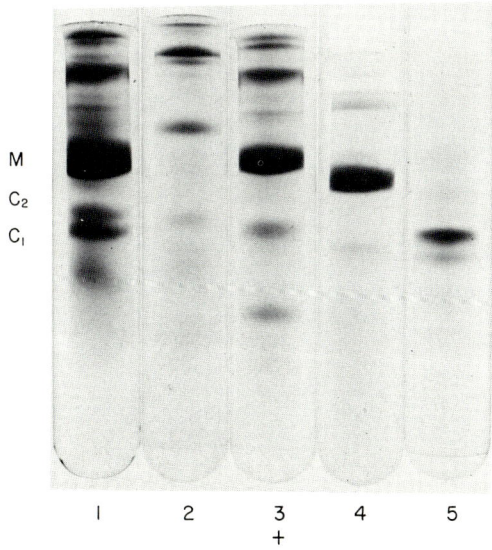

FIG. 10. Fractionation of microsomal proteins with ammonium sulfate (Martonosi, 1968). Microsomes (5 mg protein per milliliter) were suspended in a solution which contained in final concentration 0.1 M KCl, 10 mM Tris (pH 7.65), 6.5% sucrose, 2.5 mg per milliliter sodium cholate and 2.5 mg per milliliter sodium deoxycholate. Following sonication (four times for 5 seconds with 2 minute intervals in ice), the solution was centrifuged at 30,000 rpm for 30 minutes. Sediment was suspended in water and dialyzed (sample 2). To the supernate, saturated ammonium sulfate solution was added to 33% saturation. Fifteen minutes later, the precipitate was collected by centrifugation at 10,000 rpm for 30 minutes, suspended in water, and dialyzed (sample 3). To the supernate, ammonium sulfate was added to 50% saturation. On centrifugation at 10,000 rpm for 30 minutes, a floating layer formed on the surface. The floating layer was dissolved in water and dialyzed (sample 4). The clear supernate was dialyzed, lyophilized, and dissolved in water (sample 5). Sample 1 represents untreated control microsomes. Electrophoresis was carried out as described in legend to Fig. 7.

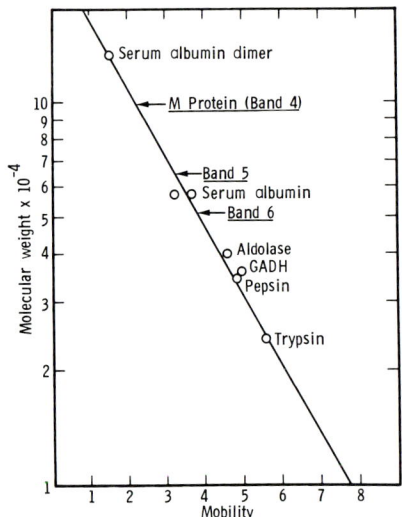

FIG. 11. Molecular weight of microsomal proteins. Electrophoresis was carried out as described in the legend to Fig. 7.

compatible with early estimates on the number of ATPase sites in microsomes (Martonosi, 1964) and close to the combining weight derived from the maximum level of protein-bound phosphate generated from $AT^{32}P$ or acetyl-^{32}P during enzymic reaction. These similarities may imply that the M protein fraction isolated by ammonium sulfate fractionation or polyacrylamide gel electrophoresis represents the undissociated ATPase protein.

Isolation of a Phosphopeptide from Microsomal Membranes Labeled with $AT^{32}P$ or Acetyl-^{32}P

Following incubation of microsomes with $AT^{32}P$ or acetyl-^{32}P, the reaction was stopped with 5% trichloroacetic acid, and after extraction of lipids with 90% acetone, the proteins were hydrolyzed in 0.01 N HCl with pepsin for 2 hours at room temperature (microsomal protein:pepsin weight ratio; 20:1) (Martonosi, 1969a). The mixture of peptides was fractionated either by a combination of paper chromatography and paper electrophoresis, or by Dowex 50 column chromatography according to Schroeder et al. (1962).

High voltage electrophoresis in pyridine acetate at pH 3.5 separates the peptic peptides into a large number of bands. The radioactivity is largely confined to a slow-moving band which does not correspond to any of the main ninhydrin staining fractions. Additional weak radioactive bands are frequently present. These may be due to incomplete digestion or secondary aggregation, although the existence of more than one distinct phosphopeptide cannot be excluded.

A fingerprint made by chromatography in butanol:acetic acid:water (4:1:5), followed by high voltage electrophoresis in pyridine-acetate at pH 3.5, is shown in Fig. 12. The peptide-bound radioactivity is confined largely to a single compact spot of relatively low mobility; three additional regions of much weaker radioactivity are present.

TABLE II

AMINO ACID COMPOSITION OF SKELETAL MUSCLE MICROSOMES AND THE PURIFIED M PROTEIN[a]

Amino acid	Content	
	Microsomes (mole percent)	M Protein (Gel Electrophoresis) (mole percent)
Lysine	6.04	5.84
Histidine	2.36	1.52
Arginine	4.00	4.76
Aspartic	10.45	9.70
Threonine	5.65	5.53
Serine	5.65	5.49
Glutamic acid	13.19	12.20
Proline	4.48	5.05
Glycine	7.22	8.45
Alanine	8.88	9.80
½ Cystine	1.31	1.26
Valine	7.65	7.55
Methionine	1.37	1.36
Isoleucine	5.64	5.60
Leucine	10.80	9.81
Tyrosine	2.08	2.15
Phenylalanine	4.08	3.94

[a] M protein was isolated by preparative polyacrylamide gel electrophoresis as described in legend to Fig. 9. Amino acid analysis was carried out on Beckman 120C amino acid analyzer using Spackman's procedure (1967).

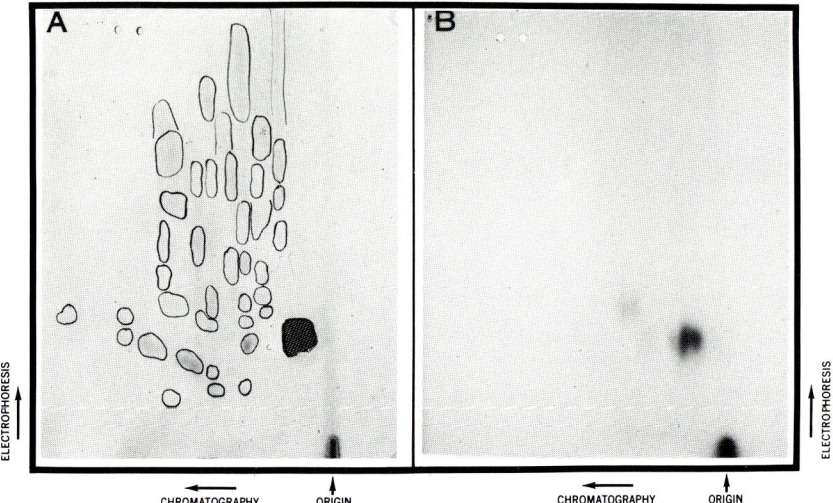

FIG. 12. Fingerprint of peptic digest of ^{32}P-labeled microsomal membrane proteins. Radioactive labeling and peptic hydrolysis were performed as described earlier (Martonosi, 1969a). Following chromatography in the upper phase of butanol:acetic acid: water (4:1:5) mixture, electrophoresis was carried out in pyridine:acetate pH 3.5 buffer at 3000 V for 90 minutes at 15 C. The chromatogram was exposed on x-ray. (A) Position of ninhydrin staining peptides; the shaded area indicates the principal radioactive spot. (B) corresponding autoradiogram.

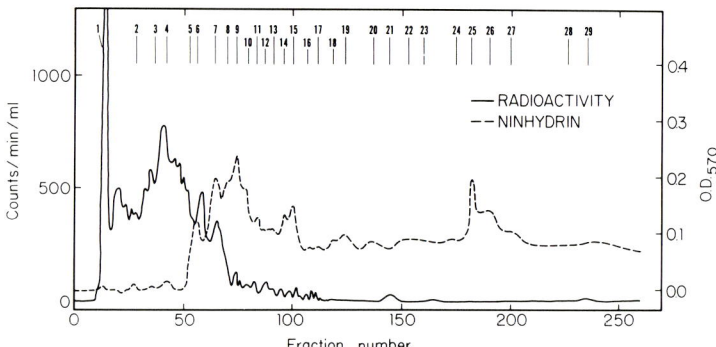

FIG. 13. Chromatography of microsomal peptides on Dowex-50 column with pyridine acetate. The procedure was essentially that of Schroeder *et al.* (1962) adapted for Beckman 120 C autoanalyzer equipped with a stream divider. Radioactivity measurements were carried out on the collected fractions. Solid line indicates radioactivity; broken line indicates ninhydrin reaction.

On chromatography using a Dowex 50 column, the radioactive peptides emerge shortly after inorganic phosphate (Fig. 13) and considerably ahead of the major ninhydrin staining fractions. The main radioactive peak eluted from a Dowex-50 column contained three distinct peptides with amino acid compositions characterized by high concentration of acidic amino acids. Further studies are required to clarify the relationship of the three peptides to each other and to the active center phosphopeptide.

It is tempting to speculate that carboxyl functions of acidic amino acids at the active site of the transport enzyme may constitute a chelating structure of sufficient affinity, specificity, and flexibility to create the Ca^{2+} binding site of the hypothetical carrier. The phosphorylation of the membrane may influence calcium affinity through conformational changes in the protein which alter the relative arrangement of the carboxyl groups.

REFERENCES

Duggan, P. F., and Martonosi, A. (1970). *J. Gen. Physiol.* **56,** 147.
Ebashi, S., and Lipmann, F. (1962). *J. Cell Biol.* **14,** 389.
Fiehn, W., and Hasselbach, W. (1970). *Eur. J. Biochem.* **13,** 510.
Hasselbach, W., and Makinose, M. (1961). *Biochem. Z.* **333,** 518.
Makinose, M. (1960). *Eur. J. Biochem.* **10,** 74.
Martonosi, A. (1963). *Biochem. Biophys. Res. Commun.* **13,** 273.
Martonosi, A. (1964). *Fed. Proc., Fed. Amer. Soc. Exp. Biol.* **23,** Suppl., 913.
Martonosi, A. (1967). *Biochem. Biophys. Res. Commun.* **29,** 753.
Martonosi, A. (1968). *J. Biol. Chem.* **243,** 71.
Martonosi, A. (1969a). *J. Biol. Chem.* **244,** 613.
Martonosi, A. (1969b). *Biochem. Biophys. Res. Commun.* **36,** 1039.
Martonosi, A. (1970). *Abstr. Biophys. Soc.* 10, 8A.
Martonosi, A., and Feretos, R. (1964). *J. Biol. Chem.* **239,** 648.
Martonosi, A., Donley, J., and Halpin, R. A. (1968). *J. Biol. Chem.* **243,** 61.
Martonosi, A., Donley, J., Pucell, A. G., and Halpin, R. A. (1971). *Arch. Biochem. Biophys.* **144,** 529.
Schroeder, W. A., Jones, R. T., Cormick, J., and McCalla, K. (1962). *Anal. Chem.* **200,** 803.
Spackman, D. H. (1967). *Methods Enzymol.* **11,** 3–15.
Yamamoto, T., and Tonomura, Y. (1967). *J. Biochem. (Tokyo)* **62,** 558.
Yu, B. P., and Masoro, E. J. (1970). *Biochemistry* **9,** 2909.

Discussion

Dr. Mechanic: Apparently your fingerprint of the active center just showed one major spot, and your elution diagram showed many peaks. How would you reconcile this?

Dr. Martonosi: In approximately one-third of our experiments we get, for some reason, incomplete digestion or secondary aggregation. In that particular experiment which I used for illustrating the elution diagram, we had picked one in which the triple band arrangement is pronounced. If that system had been digested longer, the additional bands would have disappeared. The three radioactive bands are probably peptides containing the same basic sequence, with some amino acids attached in unidentified places.

Dr. Mechanic: Have you hydrolyzed the active center and looked for the possibility of the phosphate being attached to serine, so you would have serine phosphate?

Dr. Martonosi: Serine phosphate can be probably excluded. The compound is reasonably stable at acid pH down to pH 2. It is very alkaline labile and is readily decomposed by hydroxylamine. So most of the characteristics are that of an acyl phosphate rather than phosphoserine. It may be glutamyl phosphate, aspartyl phosphate, or phosphate linked to terminal carboxyl.

Dr. Mechanic: But hydroxylphosphoserine, after all, is just an ester, and I would imagine hydroxylamine, being such a powerful neutrophilic agent, would hydrolyze the serine phosphate.

Dr. Martonosi: The pH dependence of decomposition is different. Phosphoserine is stable over a wide pH range. With our phosphopeptide, the decomposition begins at pH 5, and at pH 9 it proceeds so fast that it is hard to measure. Phosphoserine was, of course, proposed [K. Ahmed and J. D. Judah, *Biochim. Biophys. Acta* **71**, 295 (1963)] to form in mitochondria under certain conditions. The phosphoserine, which they observed is not an intermediate in the oxidative phosphorylation.

Dr. Mechanic: The point is, if it is a phosphate bond broken by hydroxylamine, you should have a hydroxylamide. Have you corrected for this?

Dr. Martonosi: The situation is the following: The concentration of phosphoprotein intermediate is only about 2 moles per 10^6 gm protein. The conventional assay for hydroxamate detection is approximately one thousand times less sensitive than what we need, so instead of the hydroxamate formation we measure the liberation of ^{32}P from protein-bound phosphate.

Dr. Anderson: Which membrane phosphate groups are being split out by phospholipase C and how is this affecting calcium bound in the membrane? Does the removal of these phosphate groups influence the transfer of calcium across muscle membrane, for it is known that red cell membrane structure remains largely intact after phospholipase C treatment [J. Lenard and S. C. Singer, *Science* **159**, 738 (1968)]? Have you measured calcium influx into the cells after phospholipase treatment?

Dr. Martonosi: We have never measured calcium fluxes in intact cells. These are all isolated membrane preparations. Phospholipase C hydrolyzes lecithin into diglycerides and phosphorylcholine. The phosphorylcholine moiety is water soluble and is removed during the subsequent washing procedure. Diglycerides are released from the membrane. They are shown to accumulate by electron microscopy as osmiophilic droplets still attached to the microsomes, but nearly all the diglycerides can be shown to be separated from the membrane. Calcium fluxes in this system are affected by phospholipase C treatment in various ways: (a) The Ca^{2+} transport system is inhibited, as indicated by inhibition of ATP hydrolysis to something like 10% of its original value, (b) the hydrolysis of lecithin seems to increase the calcium permeability of the membrane. This can be demonstrated by accumulating calcium into the microsomes and then exposing them to phospholipase C. Native membranes are able to retain calcium for a fairly long time. After phospholipase C is added to the preparation, the Ca^{2+} begins to pour out within 30 seconds.

Dr. Dirksen: Correct me if I am mistaken, but does not phospholipase C hydrolyze other glycerol phospholipids other than the one you mentioned? Have you tried adding phospholipids other than lysolecithin?

Dr. Martonosi: Different types of phospholipases hydrolyse different phospholipids. The kind we used here is obtained from *Cl. welchii*. This phospholipase is reasonably specific for phosphatidylcholine and for sphingomyelin. There is a phospholipase C in culture filtrates of *Bacillus cereus* which is able to hydrolyze, in addition to phosphatidylcholine, phosphatidylethanolamine and phosphatidylserine. The results obtained with *B. cereus* phospholipase C, under conditions when phosphatidylethanolamine and phosphatidylserine were extensively degraded, did not differ from that obtained with *Cl. welchii* enzyme.

As we can obtain full reactivation of ATPase activity with lysolecithin, even in those cases when phosphatidylethanolamine and phosphatidylserine were hydrolyzed, it appears that these two phospholipids are not necessary for the ATPase activity.

Phospholipase A has also been used. The problem with phospholipase A is that it releases fatty acids and lysophosphatides as products, and fatty acids are powerful inhibitors of the system. For this reason the consequences of phospholipase A treatment are suspect, even if carried out in the presence of serum albumin, because the observed effects may be due to the liberated fatty acids.

IV. Cell Mechanisms in Mineralized Tissues

THE CONCEPT OF A BONE MEMBRANE: SOME IMPLICATIONS*

William F. Neuman and Warren K. Ramp

Since the days of the Macy Conferences on Bone (Reifenstein, 1950), a number of basic questions have plagued the chemists and physiologists interested in skeletal physiology and metabolism. Is serum saturated with respect to calcium and phosphate? Are the $Ca \times P_i$ ion products of serum low during periods of negative calcium balance? Are these ion products high during periods of positive balance? Clinically, disease states present a confounding array of serum compositions. Every conceivable combination of high, normal, or low calcium values in serum may be associated with high, normal, or low phosphate values in serum. This is an impossible situation chemically. In the presence of literally pounds of finely divided extracellular bone salt, the blood may exhibit a composition (with respect to Ca/P ratios and Ca × P products) that varies all over the chemical map.

In retrospect, the whole issue now appears irrelevant. It should have been as obvious then as it is now. The mineral salts deposited in the skeleton are not in chemical equilibrium with the blood. It really doesn't matter what the nature of the mineral phase actually is, nor does it matter

---

* This work was supported in part by Public Health Service Training Grant No. 1 Tl DE-175 and in part by the United States Atomic Energy Commission Contract No. At-30-1-49 and has been assigned Report No. UR-49-1339.

what its solubility properties might be. The clinical data are clearly describing a case of disequilibrium. It is no accident that the first person to state unequivocally that bone possesses a membrane or its functional equivalent that separates it from the circulation was a clinician. It was John E. Howard (1956) and he didn't invoke physicochemical principles, rather he drew entirely from clinical experience.

However, without the benefit of hindsight, I returned from the Macy Conferences determined to settle these primal issues. Eight years later, a number of aspects were indeed experimentally clarified (Neuman and Neuman, 1958). We had established, as others before, that the aqueous calcium phosphate system at neutral pH is a miserable system in chemical terms. Nonetheless serum and serum ultrafiltrates were clearly undersaturated with respect to the spontaneous formation of new mineral and highly supersaturated with respect to the dissolution of pre-existing crystals (Neuman and Neuman, 1958). These findings gradually gained general acceptance and provided the basis for the views that nucleation phenomena are involved in the calcification (Strates et al., 1957; Glimcher et al., 1957) process and that cellular mechanisms [acid production (Neuman et al., 1956) and lysozomal release (Vaes, 1966)] are needed for resorption.

All this was gratifying and internally consistent as far as it went. However, in the adult, there is precious little new mineral formed or old mineral resorbed in comparison to the fluxes of ions entering and leaving mature established bone. Moment to moment regulation of serum calcium is a problem almost unrelated to processes of nucleation and bone formation or lysozomal resorption. We plan to belabor this point because, in recent years, the literature dealing with calcitonin and parathyroid hormone has commonly accepted what we believe to be a fallacious presumption: that serum calcium levels are raised or lowered by the hormonal control of resorption.

Let us examine some very approximate calculations to put the matter in perspective, i.e., resorption rates versus moment-to-moment fluxes. While estimates of skeletal turnover vary a great deal, most center around a figure of about 3% per year for the human adult (Frost, 1964).

Given: 3% turnover per year; 1000 gm Ca in skeleton; 300 days per year; 25 hours per day; 400 seconds per hour.

resorption and replacement would normally remove from and add to the skeleton:

$$(.03 \times 1000) \div (300 \times 25 \times 400) = 10 \gamma \text{ Ca/second or 100 mg per day}$$

All will agree that this amount is miniscule compared to the rates of calcium movement required for the replacement of calcium which has been removed from the blood (Hastings, 1951), or for the removal of an injected calcium load (Chen and Neuman, 1955), or for the fluxes suggested by ^{45}Ca exchange (Bauer *et al.*, 1956). For example, if ^{45}Ca entered the skeleton only via the resorption–replacement mechanism, an injected dose would require 24 hours to decline 1%. This is ridiculously out of step with observation. Clearly, the fluxes of ionic calcium into and out of the skeleton are more than four orders of magnitude greater than the fluxes related to resorption and remodeling. What is it we are trying to describe? There are pounds and pounds of bone present. This solid phase simply has to be in an equilibrium with the fluids in bone. But the fluids in bone are not in equilibrium with the E. C. F. In terms of a crude model, the situation may be pictured:

$$\text{Bone mineral surface} \longleftrightarrow \text{Bone fluid} \longleftrightarrow \text{E.C.F.}$$

Large translations of ions are occurring across the two interfaces without invoking mechanisms of resorption or bone formation. Some very approximate calculations of the quantitative relationships can be made.

Given: 1000 gm skeletal calcium; 30% of apatite crystals are in surfaces; 20% of ions in surface crystals are available for surface interactions; 1 liter of bone water; 0.5 mM Ca^{2+} in bone water; 1.5 gm of Ca^{2+} in the E.C.F.

Then, in terms of our model, we have:

$$\text{Surface Ca}^{2+} \text{ in bone} = 60 \text{ gm} \qquad \text{Ca}^{2+} \text{ in bone fluid} = 20 \text{ mg}$$
$$\text{Ca}^{2+} \text{ in E.C.F.} = 1.5 \text{ gm}$$

Even if one challenges the accuracy of the assumptions we've made, the calculated results are certain to remain valid in order of magnitude. Thus, a 10% increase in serum Ca^{2+} could be transferred to bone mineral altering the overall composition (.15 gm/1000 gm) or the surface composition (.15 gm/60 gm) from 0.01 to 0.3%. Such compositional changes are inconsequential in terms of the total skeletal mass. The only point of control available is at the interface between bone fluid and the E. C. F. Therefore, the control of the composition of the E. C. F. must reside at that interface.

Changes involving 10% of the E. C. F. (150 mg) can take place very quickly by interfacial transfers, whereas by a complete shutoff of either formation or resorption, 36 hours would be required to accomplish the same result. I will not deny that resorption and remodelling rates play a dominant role in long-term balances. I will not deny that, integrated over time, resorption-remodeling rates determine the net skeletal substance in any one individual. I am trying to emphasize the point that ion movements resulting from bone formation and resorption have very little, if any, effect on circulating levels of calcium on a moment to moment basis.

Let us be even more explicit. Calcitonin causes serum calcium to decrease. Calcitonin is said to inhibit resorption. It seems commonly accepted that the two phenomena are causally related. This is nonsense. If resorption were completely blocked by calcitonin, the resultant fall in serum calcium would be a percent or two and would require days to develop. In an analogous fashion, the rise in serum calcium from parathyroid administration and its fall after parathyroidectomy cannot be explained in terms of the hormone's action on resorption rates.

Important as they may be in the overall economy of the skeleton, bone resorption and bone formation rates have next to nothing to do with the moment to moment regulation of calcium homeostasis. Moreover, the mineral phase of bone is not in equilibrium with the circulating fluids. What is it that accounts for this compartmentalization and makes possible the regulation of circulating calcium? Today, at least, we must consider that the evidence favors the existence of a membrane or membrane function—a membrane which normally controls the fluxes of ions to and from the bone substance. I'd like now to summarize very briefly some of our recent evidence for the existence of such a membrane. This summary represents the collaborative efforts of a number of colleagues, F. Cañas, J. Geisler, J. Triffitt, B. J. Mulryan, and A. R. Terepka.

We've had, for some time, bits and pieces of evidence of the existence of the bone membrane. For example, bone contains too much strontium (Neuman, 1964) to be a passively accumulated substituent. Very recently, we've found that there is too little magnesium to be in equilibrium with serum (Neuman and Mulryan, 1971). We also found too much carbonate in the bones of teleosts (Neuman and Mulryan, 1968). These and many other odd facts suggested but did not prove unambiguously that the fluids surrounding bone mineral are different in composition from the composition of an ultrafiltrate of serum.

Almost by accident, we discovered that potassium is the one ionic constituent of bone that uniquely proves the compartmentalization of the bone fluid. Although some potassium, usually 20% or less, has to be ascribed to intracellular fluid, 80% or more of the potassium of cortical bone has to be assigned to the extracellular fluid (Geisler and Neuman, 1969). Moreover, *in vitro* it is not significantly incorporated into the mineral phase (Neuman *et al.*, 1962), it is not concentrated by mucopolysaccharides (Boyd and Neuman, 1951), it is not bound to collagen, it is completely and readily exchangeable (Triffitt *et al.*, 1968), and finally, it passively leaches out of nonvital bone (Geisler and Neuman, 1969). Potassium resides, then, in the extracellular fluid, compartment of bone.

By physiological experiments, we were able to show that this extracellular potassium of bone is quite independent of the levels of potassium in the general circulation. For example, in young bone, its concentration in bone water may be as high as twenty-five times that of the general extracellular fluids (Neuman, 1969). Similar calculations show its concentration in long bone declines with decreasing growth rate in the two species tested, chick and rat (Canas et al., 1969). Its concentration falls after hypophysectomy (Canas et al., 1969). In both instances, serum levels of K^+ are constant. The high concentration in bone is maintained in severe potassium deficiency when serum levels fall by 50% (Canas et al., 1969). Finally, its concentration in bone falls markedly in vitamin D deficiency and rebounds dramatically when the vitamin is returned to the diet (Canas et al., 1969). Incidentally, reciprocal changes were seen in the sodium content of these same bones. During these changes in bone, serum levels of sodium and potassium remain normal.

The only reasonable explanation for such a disassociation of bone potassium from that in the circulation rests in some mechanism for a highly selective compartmentalization of the bone fluids. These data minimally prove that large ion gradients are maintained in bone and that these gradients are influenced by a vitamin and a hormone. By all odds, the most likely mechanism is a functional membrane. However, the acceptance of a concept involving a bone membrane(s) raises many unanswered questions of a very fundamental character:

1. In anatomical terms, what is or are the membrane(s) of bone?
2. On physicochemical grounds our laboratory would predict that the fluids in mature bone are, relative to serum, rich in potassium and strontium, low in sodium and magnesium, even lower in calcium. Are these predictions in fact even close to the mark?
3. Obviously such a membrane must be responsible for the regulation of serum calcium, but is the serum level an integrative average of a wide variety of gradients or do all osteones regulate simultaneously to the same target (serum) value? Is the fluid in bone everywhere the same, or does it differ from unit to histological unit? If such variations exist, are they related to localized bone resorption and bone formation?
4. What is the role of potassium? Why is potassium level high in growing bone and low in nongrowing bone?

We could go on and on, posing such questions. For example, we've not raised any of the issues related to the acute and chronic response of the bone regulatory membrane(s) to hormones.

Let's deal with these questions in turn as best we can, considering first the problem of anatomy. Such a membrane might reasonably be hypothesized for trabecular bone. If properly fixed, sections of trabecular

TABLE I

Comparison of Bovine Plasma with Bovine Bone "Fluid"

Material	Electrolyte content (mM)					
	Ca	Mg	K	Na	P_i	Cl
Plasma	1.5	0.7	4	140	1.8	100
Bone "fluid"	0.48	0.4	25	125	1.8	130

bone never show bare, trabecular substance. There is always a layer of cellular material, a full cellular layer covering the surface of each trabecula. In fact, the histological case for a cellular covering of trabeculae was summarized as early as 1956 by Howard. On the other hand, these cellular coverings are merely that—cell bodies enclosing each trabecula. They are bone cells and do not, at least to my knowledge, appear to evince structural evidence of any specialized membrane function.

When we turn to Haversian systems in cortical bone, the anatomical picture is even more cloudy to say the least. Yet, we would remind you that the potassium data just cited was based on analyses of cortical bone (Neuman, 1969). The evidence of compartmentalization, therefore, is strongest for cortical bone.

Neither the electron microscopists nor the electron micrographs I have seen give me any clear picture of a cellular or membrane compartmentalization in Haversian systems. Frankly, I am very puzzled and can only put my view in the form of a question. Is it possible that the Haversian blood vessels have a specialized membrane function? High resolution electron micrographs from Robinson's laboratory show Haversian vessels to have thick cellular walls, and between the cells are tight junctions (Cooper *et al.*, 1966). Moreover, the cell walls show intense pinocytic activity. Surely, this doesn't give the impression of a simple passive filtration process. But, even if the blood vessels do possess special pumping functions, we have to assign to the periosteum and the endosteum the role of providing a semipermeable and selective barrier to ion diffusion as an envelope to the organ system as a whole. How could such a system of envelope and vascular tree be integrated? We really are in a terrible state of ignorance with respect to the anatomical nature of bone compartmentalization.

This ignorance prevents us from obtaining answers to all the other fundamental questions. For example, are the fluids of bone consistent with our physicochemical expectations? Since we cannot sample bone fluids, we cannot answer the question. However, we tried an indirect approach. We powdered fresh cortical veal bone. By repeated (over fifty) equilibrations with buffers, each time adjusting the buffer's composition, Frank Eisenmont in our laboratory finally arrived at a buffer which did not significantly change in composition when exposed to a fresh charge of new bone powder. The composition of that buffer is given in Table I.

If this is a valid procedure and if the buffer approximates the average composition of bone fluid, then our physicochemical expectations are more or less met; i.e., the [Ca] is less than in serum, the Ca:P_i product is much less than serum, the [K] is high and the [Na] and [Mg] are low. The principal point to emphasize is that the bone envelope, in this instance and on the average, is pumping calcium toward the circulation. It is maintaining an electrochemical gradient by an outward directed pump.

Immediately the question arises as to the validity and meaning of such an averaged result. From the physicochemical standpoint, it would make good sense for the pumps to shut off or reverse in areas of new mineralization, i.e., to permit the Ca $\times$ P_i to rise and therefore permit nucleation and growth of crystals. Conversely, it would also make good sense in an area of resorption to pump even more actively and thereby lower the Ca $\times$ P_i and ease the cells' task in dissolving preformed mineral. We have no information bearing on these issues, and to my knowledge there is none.

It is appropriate at this point to wonder why there are so may questions and so few answers. After all, our laboratory has been searching for the membrane for over 10 years. The potassium data are now several years old, and we at Rochester are by no means the only ones thinking in terms of the membrane concept (Talmage, 1969; Howard, 1956). The answer, of course, is that there exists no generally acceptable experimental model by which the function of the bone membrane can be studied. On the face of things, the outlook for the development of such an experimental model appears rather gloomy. However, we are hopeful and would share with you what is now no more than a hopeful hunch. It is my hunch that the membrane compartmentalization in long bones is managed by the periosteum and

TABLE II

Effect of P_i on Culture

Medium P_i (mM)	C/U Ratio				Lactate Production (μg/mg N/hour)
	Ca	P_i	N	K	
1	0.83	0.87	1.28	1.23	166
3	1.83	1.55	1.27	1.19	165

endosteum plus the walls of the blood vessels. At least, our limited experience with the incubation and culture of embryonic chick tibia suggests that such specimens maintain some of the major properties of the bone with a membrane. For illustration, I'd like to present some results which show the profound effects of disruption of the bone membranes by splitting embryonic tibia lengthwise. These are experiments performed by Dr. Warren Ramp (Ramp and Neuman, 1971).

In Table II are assembled the results of a 4-day incubation of 10-day embryonic chick tibiae in MEM (minimum essential medium), a chemically defined modified Eagle's medium. The results are expressed as paired ratios ($n \simeq 4$), cultured to noncultured, and show the importance of P_i levels in the culture medium, a phenomenon stressed by Raisz and Niemann (1969). At 1 mM P_i, the bones lost both calcium and P_i. They grew as shown by the increases in nitrogen and potassium. At 3 mM P_i, growth was unaffected, but the bones showed partial mineralization.

Table III shows the comparison of such cultured controls, which are growing and mineralizing, with paired contralateral tibiae which were either poisoned with iodoacetate, 10^{-3} M, or were simply split longitudinally. Poisoning the cells with iodoacetate stopped lactate production and caused a loss of potassium and nitrogen, but permitted a massive mineralization over and above that which was occurring in the control cultures. Merely splitting the bones did not affect cellular proliferation and the potassium loss was very small, but again, the treatment permitted massive mineralization to occur. Lactate production, though considerable, was markedly reduced.

These results provide strong presumptive evidence, it seems to us, that the endosteal and periosteal membranes in the intact embryonic limb buds normally prevent a large influx of calcium and phosphate from the culture medium. That they also influence the ionic environment of many cells is suggested by the lactate data. Figure 1 shows the time sequence of

TABLE III

Effects of IAA and Splitting

Treatment	T/C ratio				
	Ca	P_i	N	K	Lactate
IAA	2.27	2.22	0.44	0.16	0.07
Split	2.18	2.22	0.94[a]	0.88[a]	0.68

[a] Not significant.

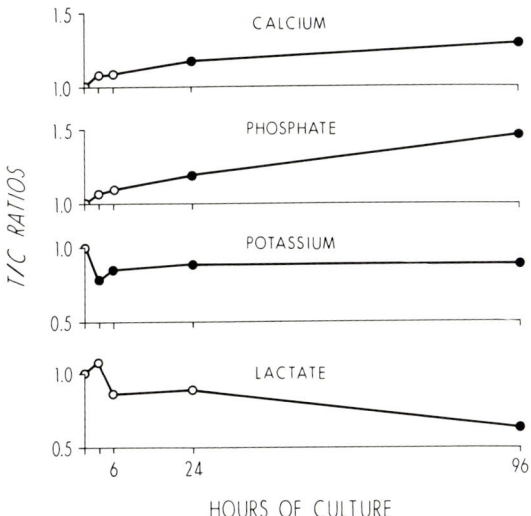

FIG. 1. Data showing the time sequence of changes induced by splitting embryonic tibia. The T/C ratio is the comparison of treated tibia (split) with contralateral controls unmanipulated but cultured under comparable conditions. Values differing from unity significantly ($p < .05$) are represented by filled circles.

the effects of splitting. This time, the P_i was reduced to 2 mM, at which concentration, the control cultures mineralize only slightly. In this case, the first significant change (at 3 hours) was a loss of tissue potassium (presumably extracellular). By 24 hours a significant increase in mineralization was observed. Though lactate production fell early, significant changes were not seen until 4 days of culture. We are puzzled about the importance and function of extracellular potassium. At the moment, there is no clue as to its role. The correlation between potassium concentration and bone growth and mineralization is, however phenomenal (Canas *et al.*, 1969: Neuman and Mulryan, 1972).

It is clear, after 20 years, that serum is normally supersaturated with respect to existing bone mineral and that this disequilibrium is maintained and regulated by a functional membrane compartmentalization of the bones' extracellular components. Beyond this, we are pretty ignorant, and further study is obviously imperative. Until we have a much clearer understanding of the bone membrane(s), its anatomical nature, its normal function and the hormonal and dietary factors which affect its function, we will necessarily possess only a rudimentary understanding of the regulation of serum calcium and the effects of hormones on calcium homeostasis.

References

Bauer, G., Carlsson, A., and Lindquist, B. (1956). *Metab., Clin. Exp.* **5,** 573.
Boyd, E. S., and Neuman, W. F. (1951). *J. Biol. Chem.* **193,** 243.
Canas, F., Terepka, A. R., and Neuman, W. F. (1969). *Amer. J. Physiol.* **217,** 117.
Chen, P. S., Jr., and Neuman, W. F. (1955). *Amer. J. Physiol.* **180,** 623.
Cooper, R. R., Milgram, J. W., and Robinson, R. A. (1966). *J. Bone Joint Surg., Amer. Vol.* **48,** 1239.
Frost, H. M. (1964). *In* "Bone Biodynamics," Chapter 18, p. 315. Little, Brown, Boston, Massachusetts.
Geisler, J. Z., and Neuman, W. F. (1969). *Proc. Soc. Exp. Biol. Med.* **130,** 608.
Glimcher, M. J., Hodge, A. J., and Schmitt, F. O. (1957). *Proc. Nat. Acad. Sci. U.S.* **43,** 860.
Hastings, A. B. (1951). *Conf. Metab. Interrelations, Trans.* **3,** 38.
Howard, J. E. (1956). *Bone Struct. Metab., Ciba Found. Symp., 1955* p. 206.
Neuman, W. F. (1964). *In* "Bone Biodynamics," Chapter 21, p. 393. Little, Brown, Boston, Massachusetts.
Neuman, W. F. (1969). *Fed. Proc., Fed. Amer. Soc. Exp. Biol.* **28,** 1846.
Neuman, W. F., and Mulryan, B. J. (1968). *Calcif. Tissue Res.* **2,** 237.
Neuman, W. F., and Mulryan, B. J. (1971). *Calcif. Tissue Res.* **7,** 1.
Neuman, W. F. and Mulryan, B. J. (1972). Unpublished observations.
Neuman, W. F., and Neuman, M. W. (1958). "Chemical Dynamics of Bone Mineral." Univ. of Chicago Press, Chicago, Illinois.
Neuman, W. F., Firschein, H., Chen, P. S., Jr., Mulryan, B. J., and DiStefano, V. (1956). *J. Amer. Chem. Soc.* **78,** 3863.
Neuman, W. F., Toribara, T. Y., and Mulryan, B. J. (1962). *Arch. Biochem. Biophys.* **98,** 384.
Raisz, L. G., and Niemann, I. (1969). *Endocrinology* **85,** 446.
Ramp, W. K., and Neuman, W. F. (1971). *Amer. J. Physiol.* **220,** 270.
Reifenstein, E. C. (1950). *Conf. Metab. Interrelations, Trans.* **2,** 279.
Strates, B., Neuman, W. F., and Levinskas, G. L. (1957). *J. Phys. Chem.* **61,** 279.
Talmage, R. V. (1969). *Clin. Orthop. Related Res.* **67,** 210.
Triffitt, J. T., Terepka, A. R., and Neuman, W. F. (1968). *Calcif. Tissue Res.* **2,** 165.
Vaes, G. (1966). Thesis de grade d'Aqréqé, Université Catholique de Louvain, E. Warny, Louvain.

Discussion

Dr. Talmage: I enjoyed the delightful talk given by Bill Neuman and would only take issue with one point, namely, that I really feel that the anatomical picture of bone surface is much clearer than Bill suggests. I hope that when Les Matthews finishes his talk this morning, Bill will be convinced of this. Blood vessels as they pass through blood channels in bones are lined with the usual endothelial cells, but in addition, the surface of the bone is covered with cells called lining cells. The existence of these is well documented and have been demonstrated by many electron microscopists.

The second point I would like to make is to review very briefly some of our recent studies which support Neuman's concept of the existence of a membrane covering bone, a membrane which I believe is made up of a layer of cells. Femurs of young adult rats were incubated for 4 hours. The left femur was incubated intact, while the opposite femur was broken into five or six pieces. This simple procedure produces marked different effects in the two bones on the rate of calcium movement in and out of the medium, and the rate of collagen synthesis. To me these studies demonstrated not only the existence of a membrane, but that those cells synthesizing collagen are part of this membrane.

Dr. Neuman: May I rebut just a little. You will recall that I prefaced my remarks about our ignorance of the anatomical nature of the membrane by the two words "to me." I remain unconvinced, but I don't think that should bother you at all, Dr. Talmage, because there were many years in which I didn't even believe in morphology at all.

Dr. Urist: Observations on the capillary wall as a functional membrane regulating influx of calcium is well established. The capillary walls, as observed in our experiments using microperfusion, can be exposed without injury to concentrations of calcium ions of 2–25 mM, except perhaps over periods of time in excess of a few hours. However, short term experiments suffice to demonstrate that capillary endothelium is a functional membrane regulating with great efficiency the influx of calcium ions.

I would question the data on calcium fluxes derived from an experiment on the split tibia *in vitro*. Embryonic cartilaginous bones will heal *in vitro* as a fracture heals *in vivo*. If a split bone behaves like a fractured bone, the question is is the measured influx of calcium due to regeneration of bone? Active accumulation of apatite from calcification in new tissue, not the pre-existing tissue under culture, occurs with regeneration of bone. New tissue formed in response to injury would produce new local conditions, circumstances not previously in existence. Accordingly, a boundary membrane enclosing the system, such as periosteum, would not account for the ion fluxes as much as new tissue accumulating calcium by increased numbers of new osteoblasts through the process of regeneration.

Dr. Neuman: I think the answer is, "most unlikely," because of the iodoacetate controls. Here, development and growth are completely blocked by iodoacetate. Yet, they show essentially the same kind of mineralization we observed in the split bone. Also, the mineral is seen to deposit in the bone area rather than in the cartilage area in both iodoacetate and the split cultured bone.

Dr. Urist: The hypertrophic cartilage of the epiphysial plate of the growing bone does not regenerate. This cartilage is replaced by bone.

Dr. Posner: May I ask you to define what you mean by bone fluid? Does it include the hydration layer on the crystal and the intracellular fluid?

Dr. Neuman: I think that you knew I am in trouble before you even asked that question. This is one of the lovely problems that arose when we discovered that bone crystals hydrate. If you put bone crystals in a free aqueous suspension, they take a weight of water equal to the mineral phase. Therefore, on this basis, the bone water in mature bone should never drop below something like 30 or 40%. It is shocking, then, to find when you correct for cells and cell volume and canaliculae and so on, that there is only something of the order of 7 or 8% water in really mature bone. This isn't enough water to hydrate the crystals and it isn't enough to hydrate the collagen. There just isn't enough water there. So, how much of that which is there is in which compartment, at this moment, is impossible to say. That is why I used the quotes around "fluid." It includes fluid between cells and it includes hydration water of those crystals which are available for ion transfer.

Dr. Posner: Couldn't the hydration layer be the membrane you speak of?

Dr. Neuman: That is quite true. If you assume that bone water was just hydration water related to the crystals, it would have a composition quite different from that of the extracellular fluid. On the other hand, if you equilibrate crystals with their little hydration jackets with varying concentrations of potassium, the potassium goes up and down with the passage of this fluid into the external medium. We wouldn't expect the inverse relationships observed in the physiological experiments.

Dr. Harrison: I was struck particularly by the concentration of potassium in the hypothetical bone fluid because it does bring up the possibility of a role of potassium in the exchange of calcium between the mineral phase of bone and the extracellular fluid. This might fit in with a rather mysterious clinical situation which occurs and has never been explained.

I refer to the occasional occurrence of hypocalcemia in acute and chronic hypokalemic states. There are certain patients with severe potassium deficiency who develop an intractible hypocalcemia associated with very marked hypophosphatemia. They have both a deficiency of calcium and of phosphate in extracellular fluid. No one has ever offered a suitable explanation of this. Your suggestion that potassium is enriched in bone fluid offers the possibility that this ion plays a role in the transfer of calcium across a barrier. Have you studied the effect of potassium deficiency on the rate of solubilization of calcium or the movement of calcium from the solid phase into the bathing fluid?

Dr. Neuman: No, we haven't. I don't think we have an explanation for the syndrome you described, but it does open some possibilities. Since you brought up potassium, I would like to mention a model we are developing to study membrane function which is with chick embryonic calvaria. The increase of mineralization in chick calvaria begins at about day 15 or 16, and after a few days, the rate falls off with the lowest rate of mineralization occurring just at the time of hatching. After hatching, there is another spurt of mineralization.

When potassium levels in the calvaria are superimposed on this growth curve, it was seen that there was a direct relationship between the rate of mineralization and the level of potassium in the tissue. The potassium level drops at the point of hatching and again bounces up after hatching to correspond to the burst of mineralization which occurs post hatching. This relationship between growth and potassium has never been considered or dealt with before.

Dr. Harrison: You think potassium might work in both directions?

Dr. Neuman: At this moment, yes.

Dr. Hirsch: You originally emphasized that in man, the rate of bone resorption and accretion is very low, and that hormonal changes would take a long time to occur. I think this point is well taken, but, in the rat, calcitonin will cause a marked hypocalcemic response in a relatively short time. Many of us have interpreted this as an inhibition of bone resorption. Are we interpreting this wrong in the rat?

Dr. Neuman: I wouldn't say "wrong," and I don't mean that facetiously. In the young rat, the rate of growth is fantastic, like 15% per day. Bone resorption must also be very fast. But, I still think that even those rates that can be calculated will not account for all the variations seen in serum calcium. In other words, in the young rat, serum calcium control is probably a mixed bag of resorption rates and regulation.

I guess the thing I am really appealing for here is that we clean up our semantics and not use "resorption" as such an all-inclusive term, in one case to mean regulation and in another case to mean actual removal of bone. It is sloppy. I think our present nomenclature and its usage is confused.

Dr. Talmage: I would like to second Bill's suggestion. However, his definition of resorption is different from that given by the "pure" anatomist. To anatomists bone resorption is that process by which bone is broken down by osteoclasts. To others, an inhibition of bone resorption implies inhibiting all calcium removal from bone, not just that resorbed by osteoclasts.

Dr. Barzel: We have demonstrated that continuous feeding of ammonium chloride to normal adult rats caused bone resorption, and that feeding potassium containing bicarbonate stimulated bone formation and prevented osteoporosis from developing in these rats when fed a low calcium diet [U. S. Barzel and J. Jowsey, *Clin. Sci.* **36**, 517 (1969)]. Since hydrogen ion and potassium ion do exchange intracellularly under varying physiological conditions, I would postulate that bone cell potassium or hydrogen ion concentration may have an effect on formation or resorption activity. Do you have information on the hydrogen ion concentration in the models you have studied?

Dr. Neuman: That is a perfectly good possibility, but I can't measure pH values in bone either directly or by interpolation. At one time I thought we could by measuring bicarbonate loss on heating, since there is a relationship between bone pH and the percentage of carbon dioxide loss when you heat it. Obviously, with the low pH, there is more bicarbonate and you get greater loss of carbon dioxide than a high pH, but when the slope of the curve is in the physiological range, the relationship is not sufficiently precise to permit an interpolation of the pH in bone. It is a fine idea, and I think a very reasonable one, but I can't devise an experimental approach to check it.

Dr. Heaney: I would judge that most skeletal physiologists would be very happy with your compartmentalization. I find your results fascinating and your conclusions convincing. It is with the *a priori* assumptions which led to them that I take issue. To begin with, there is a quite good relationship between the magnitude of calcitonin-produced hypocalcemia and the rate of skeletal turnover. In fact, current estimates of adult skeletal turnover (5 mg Ca/kg/day) explain why calcitonin does not lower plasma calcium detectably in normal adults. Only with much higher skeletal turnovers (as in Paget's disease) do we see a clear calcitonin effect. So, far from demonstrating the inadequacy of kinetic estimates, your calculation confirms what they predict. Furthermore, we have made and published these same calculations ourselves [R. V. Talmage and L. Belanger, eds., "Parathyroid Hormone and Thyrocalcitonin (Calcitonin)," p. 85. Excerpta Med. Found., Amsterdam, 1968].

Furthermore, let me add for the record that clinicians who have to work with hypercalcemia have realized for a long time that a simple balance between bone formation and bone resorption (however defined) is inadequate to explain hypercalcemia. This is why your results and conclusions are so satisfying. It is not necessary to set kinetic estimates up as a straw man and then proceed to demolish them. To begin with, your evidence is not in conflict with kinetic estimates, and secondly, the kinetic values are now supported by an increasing body of both morphometric and quantitative microradiographic data.

Dr. Kenny: Is your hypothetical membrane maintained, with respect to the potassium data, by bone in tissue culture?

Dr. Neuman: If you take, for example, calvaria from newly born rat pups, unless you handle them gently, they lose potassium. You can dip them in saline, and if you have been rough, they will lose 30% of the potassium. If you incubate them in a protein-free solution, they will lose 70% of their potassium in 6 hours. On the other hand, if you incubate them in the presence of serum, they will maintain their potassium content. Thus, the envelope and its sensitivity to maintenance and retention of potassium at high concentration in bone, I think, is experimentally established.

BONE CELLS, CALCIFICATION, AND CALCIUM HOMEOSTASIS

George Nichols, Jr., Peter Hirschmann, and Peggy Rogers

As has been pointed out, calcium is critical to the organization and function of a number of vital biological systems, ranging from the stability of membrane structures through the control of muscle contraction, to providing the rigidity of bone. All depend ultimately on the ready availability of a limitless pool of calcium ions at a precisely regulated concentration. This pool is provided, of course, by the extracellular fluid whose calcium concentration is protected from moment to moment by the movement of ions into and out of the large stores of calcium present in bone.

The central importance of the skeleton in the homeostasis of the serum calcium concentration was first clearly pointed out by Hastings and Huggins (1933), and the ways in which the distribution of calcium between bone and the circulating fluids were regulated through the action of hormones on skeletal mechanisms became the ruling passion of Franklin McLean's later scientific life. Yet, despite the efforts of these men and the scores of able investigators whom they inspired, the nature of the mechanisms being controlled by the hormones continued to remain uncertain beyond the obvious deduction that they were located in the cellular elements of the tissue rather than in its calcified extracellular matrix.

The involvement of the bone cells in calcification and serum calcium homeostasis, on the other hand, seemed rather indirect, being limited to the formation of a calcifiable matrix and the production of organic acids—processes which, while they appeared to be influenced by the appropriate hormones, seemed either to be inadequate to account for the precise control of serum calcium concentration which obviously existed or failed to explain why additional factors such as vitamin D were needed for normal mineral deposition in osteoid.

Part of the problem lay in the mechanical difficulties inherent in attempting to measure the ways in which a widely scattered cell population could affect calcium transfer into and out of a tissue, the major portion of which consisted of a dense, heavily calcified organic matrix. Quite recently, however, three difference approaches have been used to solve this problem by three different groups, each of which has provided evidence pointing to the direct, intimate involvement of bone cells in these processes. Kashiwa (1970) has used the calcium-specific stain glyoxal bis (2-hydroxyanil) (GBHA) as well as other histochemical techniques to demonstrate the apparent presence of large numbers of calcium-containing granules in bone and cartilage cells, especially osteocytes, and their increase following injection of parathyroid extract (PTE) into the animal. Matthews and his collaborators (this volume) have, in a series of elegant electron microscopic studies, demonstrated the presence of what are presumed to be calcium (and probably phosphorus) containing granules in mitochondria and other subcellular organelles of bone, cartilage, and gut mucosal cells whose numbers and size are affected by such "calcium-active agents" as parathyroid hormone (PTH) and vitamin D (Martin and Matthews, 1970; Sampson *et al.*, 1970), and my collaborators and I have attempted to study the same phenomena by separating the bone cells from their calcified extracellular material and measuring directly their content of calcium and the way it exchanges with the calcium in incubation media *in vitro* under a variety of conditions (Nichols *et al.*, 1969; Nichols and Rogers, 1971).

Needless to say, we have all faced serious problems both with methodology and interpretations. Kashiwa has had to deal with the problem of proving the specificity of the GBHA stain and the possibility of serious artifacts developing from secondary effects of the extremely alkaline conditions required for staining. Matthews has had to contend with the possibility of artifactual appearance, growth, or loss of granules during fixation for electron microscopy and the proof that the electron-dense particles he sees are indeed calcium. Both have been limited by the problems of precise quantitation inherent in morphological techniques. Our greatest problems have been to be sure that the large amounts of calcium which we find in bone cell preparations are not just residual contamination with fragments of the calcified extracellular material; to be sure that the cells we obtain are still relatively intact and viable so that mineral exchanges can be examined in relationship to metabolic processes, and in terms of movement between an intracellular and an extracellular compartment; and finally, to find ways of proving that the cells we are examining are, in fact, bone cells and of identifying which of the several kinds present in these tissues contain calcium.

Since Dr. Matthews and Dr. Kashiwa describe their work in other chapters of this volume, I will not attempt to review their work, but instead will concentrate on our own observations. In doing so I will discuss our initial observations, the evidence we have regarding the identity of the cells we are examining, the location of the calcium in them, their turnover of calcium and how it is affected by various factors, and how we think these observations relate to calcium metabolism in the skeleton and through it to homeostasis of the serum calcium concentration.

In 1961, Dr. Woods, then seeking a collagenase in bone cells, first noted that when fresh minced bone was ground with isotonic buffer in a mortar the cellular elements of the tissue tended to separate intact from the calcified extracellular matrix and float up into the supernatant solution from which they could be harvested free of calcified collagen by centrifugation (Woods and Nichols, 1963). This observation opened the way to the study of aspects of cell composition and function which because of the abundance and particular composition of the extracellular material of the tissue could not be conveniently examined in slices or minces. The possibilities for studying a variety of features of cell behavior such as amino acid transport, protein synthesis, and the presence and intracellular distribution of such enzymes as collagenase, and phosphatases both acid and alkaline were exploited by us in subsequent years and by Peck and his collaborators (1964) using cells isolated by enzymic rather than mechanical means, but for some obscure reason none of us looked at the inorganic ion content of these cells.

Observations which turned our attention from the organic to the inorganic metabolism of bone cells are illustrated in Fig. 1. At the time (1967), we were collaborating with Dr. Wasserman in a search for his calcium binding protein which we both felt might be present in bone cells as it seemed to be in the other two tissues chiefly involved in calcium transport, gut and kidney. While we failed to identify his protein in our bone cells we found that they contained anywhere from ten to fifty times more calcium than soft tissues taken from the same pigs and analyzed simultaneously. Several questions immediately arose. Was this calcium associated with bone cells or was it merely contamination with extracellular material of either bone or marrow cells?

The method usually used for preparing the cells (shown in Fig. 2) (Nichols and Rogers, 1971), is identical to the one devised by Dr. Woods and me in 1961, except that for these studies the cells were harvested by centrifugation over a layer of 30% w/v dextran which has a density of 1.11.

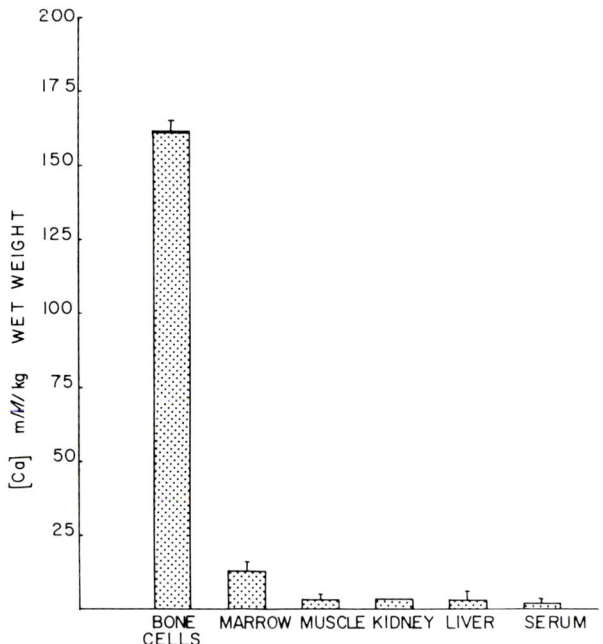

Fig. 1. Mean calcium content expressed as millimoles per kilogram of fresh wet weight of tissue in bone cells and several other tissues from suckling pigs. One standard deviation is indicated above each bar. [From Nichols and Rogers (1971).]

This modification was introduced in the hope that any fragments of calcified collagen contaminating the cells would pass through to the bottom of the tube, while the cells, we already knew, would float on top. Since trials showed that the calcium content of cell samples prepared by our original method were often reduced by 5–40% by a single sedimentation over dextran but remained constant thereafter through several subsequent repetitions of the procedure, two sedimentations were made part of the standard preparative procedure in all subsequent experiments. While significant contamination with loose extracellular material thus seemed to be eliminated in the preparation of the cells, the possibility remained that fragments of calcified collagen or crystals of mineral might be either adhering to the surface of or even have been engulfed by either bone or marrow cells. Our attempts to answer these two questions are summarized in Figs. 3 and 4.

The question of adherent material was attacked in two ways. Cells prepared by grinding washed trabecular bone from young pigs as described in Fig. 1 were incubated for 1 hour at 37°C in Krebs–Ringer solution, bicarbonate buffer pH 7.4, with glucose as substrate and various hydrolytic enzymes, as indicated in Fig. 3. As can be seen, none of these lowered the cell calcium content. Even the addition of low concentrations of EDTA in

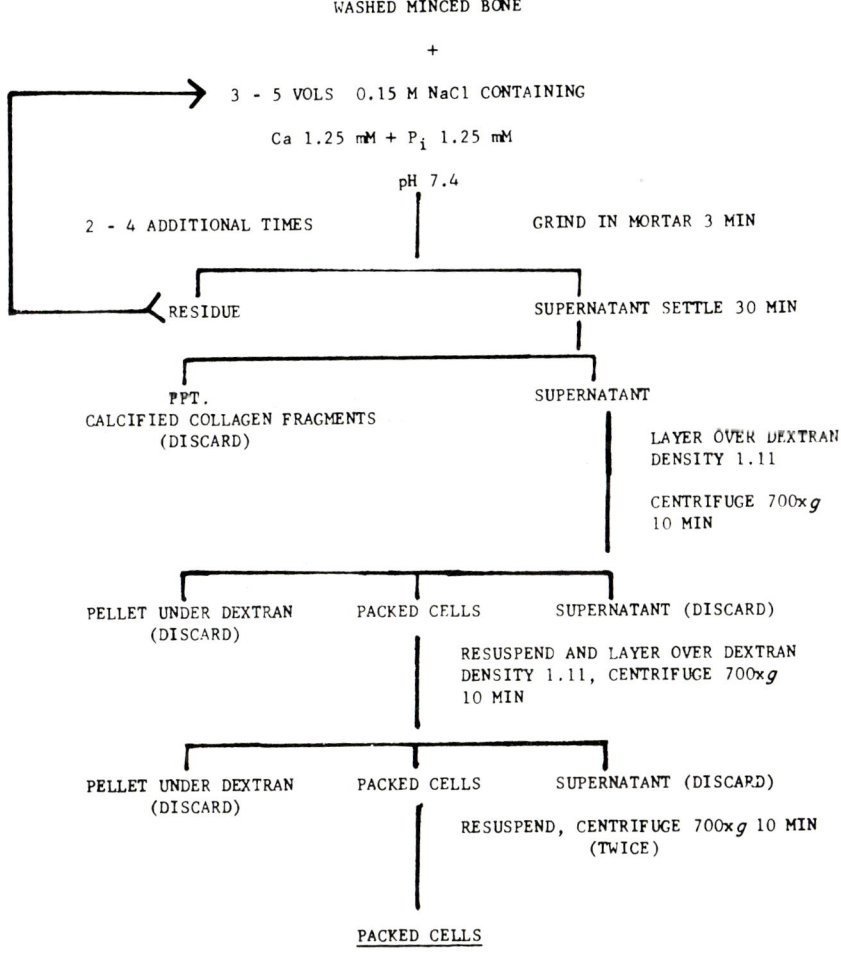

Fig. 2. A schematic representation of the method customarily used to separate bone cells from the calcified extracellular matrix. [From Nichols and Rogers (1971).]

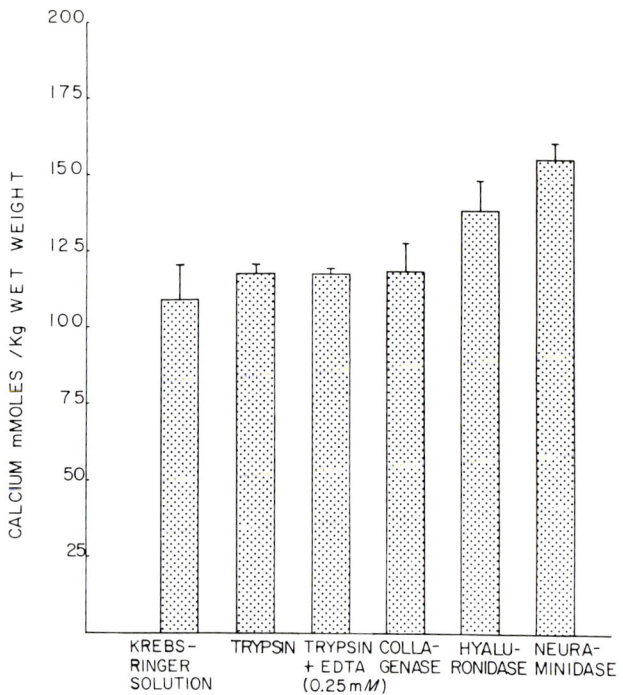

FIG. 3. The mean calcium concentrations found in portions of pig bone cells after incubation for 1 hour at 37°C in Krebs–Ringer solution, bicarbonate buffer, pH 7.3. The various enzymes were added in the following concentrations: crystalline trypsin, Sigma Type I, 2.5 mg/ml; bacterial collagenase, Sigma Type III, 0.1 mg/ml; hyaluronidase, Sigma Type III, 0.1 mg/ml; and neuraminidase from *Vibrio cholera* (Hoechst Pharmaceuticals Co.) 200 units per milliliter. Ethylenediaminetetraacetic acid at a final concentration of 0.25 mM was added to the trypsin in one set of incubations. One standard deviation of the mean is indicated in each case. Three samples were used to determine the means in all cases save the experiments with trypsin, where eighteen are included.

the experiments with trypsin—conditions which Borle (1968) has shown removes 90% of the calcium of HeLa cell preparations—was without effect. While these data served to indicate that the calcium was probably not bound to a surface coating on the cells, the possibility of artifactual phagocytic uptake of fragments of extracellular material released during grinding remained.

This and the question of possible marrow contamination of bone cell samples were tackled in another series of experiments as shown in Fig. 4. Cells were harvested from dense cortical diaphyseal pig bone and calvarium

—both virtually marrow free—by three different methods: (1) by our usual grinding technique, (2) by digestion of the minced tissue with crude bacterial (Sigma Type I) collagenase for 1 hour at 37°C at pH 7.4 followed by vigorous hand shaking of the mixture for 1 minute, and (3) by scraping the surface of the bone with a sharp knife followed by vigorous shaking of the scrapings with cold isotonic buffer. Cells in each case were harvested from the supernatant incubation or washing medium by centrifugation after the large particles had been allowed to sediment to the bottom of the flask. All three methods yielded cells containing the same high concentrations of calcium. Indeed, the values in cells isolated by grinding or with enzyme and no grinding were virtually identical with those shown in Fig. 1, while somewhat lower values were found in cells harvested from bone surfaces by scraping, a finding which may have indicated that this method harvests

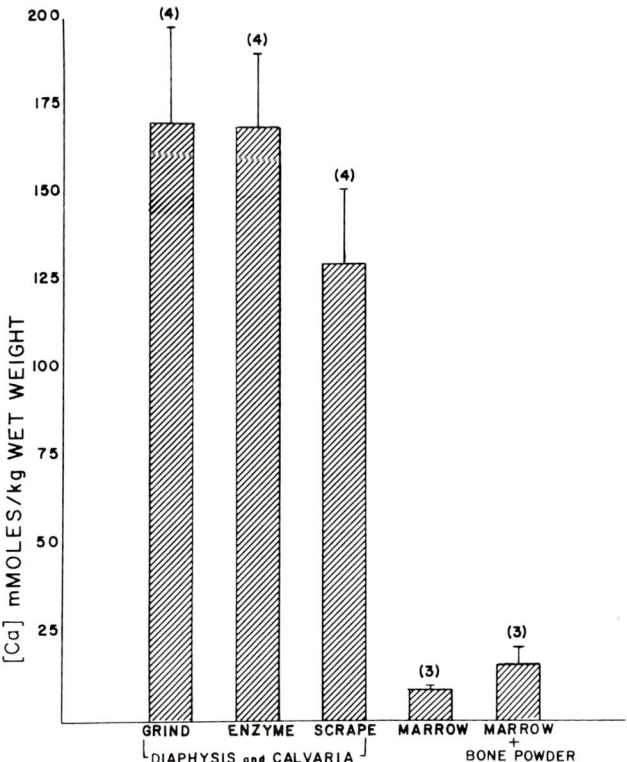

FIG. 4. Mean calcium concentrations in bone cells and marrow prepared in a variety of ways (see text). One standard deviation is indicated for each by the vertical bar. The numbers above each bar indicate the number of samples included.

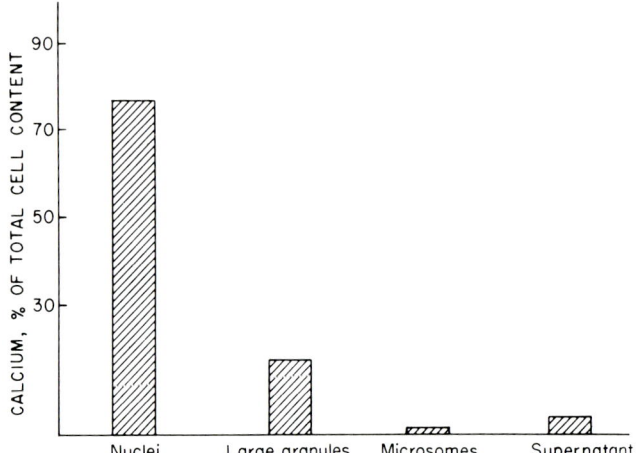

FIG. 5. The distribution of calcium in various fractions of bone cell homogenates prepared in 0.25 M sucrose buffered to pH 7.4 with 0.010 M tris by internal cavitation with nitrogen gas and separated by differential centrifugation. The various fractions have been defined as follows: nuclei—the pellet from centrifugation of the whole homogenate for 10 minutes at 700 g; large granules—the pellet separating after 10 minutes at 15,000 g from the nuclear supernatant; microsomes—the pellet separating after 60 minutes at 105,000 g from the large granule supernatant; supernatant—the supernatant from the microsome separation.

more osteoblasts and fewer osteocytes than the others. The significance of this idea will be more apparent later on.

Possible phagocytosis of bone fragments by marrow elements during grinding was further tested by grinding marrow cells (harvested by washing minced trabecular bone with ice cold buffer) as we would bone to harvest bone cells with dry defatted human bone powder and then separating bone powder from cells by sedimentation on top of a dextran barrier as in Fig. 2. Even though this procedure nearly doubled the calcium content of the cell samples, the total calcium content so accumulated was still far too low to explain the calcium content of the bone cell samples even if all the cells harvested were in fact marrow.

Altogether, these data plus the low levels of hydroxyproline which can be found on analysis, and the rarity with which any fragments of collagen fibers can be found by histochemistry or electron microscopy of bone cell samples combine to make it seem quite unlikely that the high concentrations of calcium found in the bone cells represent accidental contamination during preparation.

Two facts, the data in Fig. 3 and the large amounts of calcium found in bone cell preparations, as well as the work of Kashiwa and later Matthews suggested that the calcium was bound inside the cells, the former by excluding a location in an extracellular "coat" and the latter because considerations of osmotic balance and electroneutrality made the existence of such a concentration of divalent cation free in the cytosol virtually impossible. Biochemical confirmation of this view soon was obtained in a series of experiments in which the distribution of calcium in homogenates of bone cells was examined by differential centrifugation. Figure 5 shows that more than 90% of all the calcium in homogenates prepared in tris-buffered isotonic sucrose sedimented in centrifugal fields of 15,000 g or less, the balance being present probably as free ions in the supernate. Indeed, the major portion of the calcium sedimented at 700 g in the fraction which, in soft tissue homogenates at least, contains largely nuclei and unbroken cells, suggesting that the density of the calcium-containing particles might well be very high.

The nature of the calcium-rich particulate fraction of bone cells has now been studied in more detail by Dr. Hirschmann who has taken advantage of its density to partially purify it by centrifugation through a 70% sucrose barrier after preliminary digestion with DNAse to remove the very variable amounts of DNA found in it (Hirschmann and Nichols, 1971). While the details of his work are beyond the scope of the present discussion, a couple of characteristics of this fraction should be noted. As can be seen from Table I, calcium and phosphorus accounted for 10% of the dry weight of the

TABLE I

CHEMICAL COMPOSITION OF THE CALCIUM-RICH PARTICULATE CELL FRACTION[a]

Component	Composition (% dry weight[b])	
Calcium	6.75 ± 0.39	(10)
Phosphate	3.38 ± 0.18	(9)
Protein	51.90 ± 2.70	(7)
RNA	7.10 ± 0.39	(8)
Total lipid	33.60 ± 3.30	(4)
Phospholipid	10.50 ± 2.10	(3)
Hydroxyproline	0.0056 ± 0.0003	(3)
Hexose	4.50 ± 1.65	(4)
Hexosamine	0.368 ± 0.10	(4)
Sialic acid	0.0013 ± 0.00015	(7)

[a] From Hirschmann and Nichols (1971).
[b] ±S.E.M., the number of samples in parentheses.

fraction which proved to be rich in protein and lipid, including phospholipid, but poor in hexosamine, hydroxyproline, and sialic acid, suggesting that the Ca/P was associated with subcellular membranes and not elements of the extracellular matrix. It also contained considerable RNA, indeed almost 60% of the total present in the total homogenate. A survey of the enzymic activity of the fraction suggested that it contains mitochondria, endoplasmic reticulum, and some plasma membrane fragments but relatively few lysosomes, an impression of heterogeneity which has been confirmed by electron microscopic examinations of the pellet kindly prepared by Drs. Marijke Holtrop and Micheline Federman. These data are consistent with the findings of both Kashiwa and Matthews of an intracellular particulate location for calcium and seem to fit particularly well with the latter's view that it is associated with both mitochondria and endoplasmic reticulum.

Both osteoblasts and osteocytes have been implicated in calcium transport largely on morphological grounds—the former in connection with the formation of new bone (Hancox and Boothroyd, 1965; Kashiwa, this volume; Woods and Nichols, 1963) and the latter in connection with the parathyroid-stimulated osteocytic osteolysis by Belanger et al. (1963) and more recently by Kashiwa (1970). Although osteoclasts have been shown to contain calcium too, at present this seems probably to relate to their phagocytic function in active bone resorption rather than to calcium homeostasis and so does not seem germane to our present consideration (Nichols, 1970). Unfortunately, two facts have made progress toward positive identification of the cells involved difficult. Just as the morphologists are hampered in measuring rates of transfer by the nature of the techniques they use, we have been hampered by the difficulty of identifying and then sorting into pure samples the several kinds of bone cells which are inevitably mixed together in our cell suspensions. We have attempted to approach this problem by taking advantage of special features of bone and bone cells. The results of three such approaches, all of which seem to point toward the osteocyte as the major contributor to skeletal calcium metabolism are summarized in the next few figures.

In the experiments illustrated in Fig. 6, advantage was taken of the fact that when bone is ground, the first cells which would be expected to be released are the surface osteoblasts and any marrow elements which might remain, while osteocytes would not be expected to be freed until later when the tissue was more thoroughly macerated (Nichols and Rogers, 1971). Therefore, by grinding the same lot of minced bone repeatedly and collecting the cells released by each grinding separately, one could expect to have samples which were progressively richer in osteocytes as the grind number increased. When such cell samples are analyzed, as can be seen in

Bone Cells, Calcification, and Homeostasis

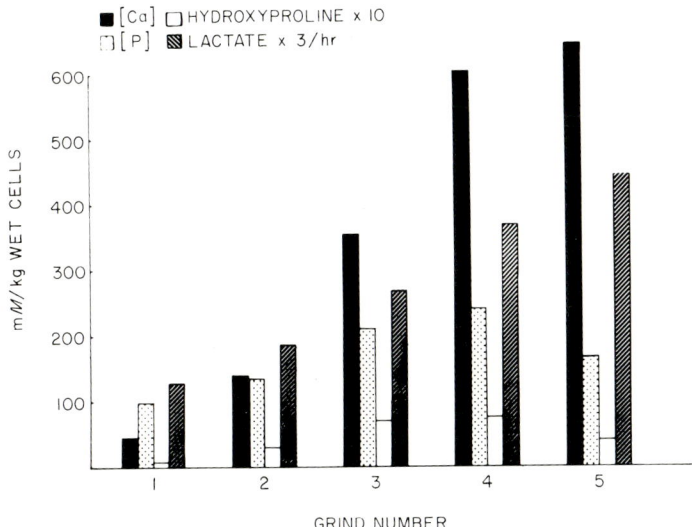

FIG. 0. Calcium, phosphate, and hydroxyproline content and lactate production of five lots of cells derived sequentially by repeatedly grinding the same bone fragments and harvesting each lot of cells so released separately. Note that the values for lactate have been multiplied by three and for hydroxyproline by ten to permit plotting all data on the same coordinates. [From Nichols and Rogers, 1971.]

this figure, the calcium content rises progressively as the osteocyte content of the sample increases. The phosphorus content rises also but not as strikingly, suggesting that some of the calcium in the cells is associated with anions other than phosphate. Although the small amounts of hydroxyproline present (measured to assess possible contamination with extracellular debris) also increase at first, they later decrease in the fractions with the most osteocytes. The low concentration of this material, its pattern of distribution, together with the changing Ca/P ratio in the cell samples made it seem most unlikely for the increasing cell calcium to be due to increasing contamination with extracellular material released by the successive grinding. To our surprise, the rate at which lactate was produced from glucose by the cells on incubation at 37°C increased as dramatically in the osteocyte-rich fractions as did the calcium. This plus an equally striking increase in O_2 uptake shown in other experiments (Nichols, 1967) first suggested to us that the osteocyte may well be the bone's most actively metabolizing cell, rather than its least as used to be thought.

The notion that high cell calcium concentration and high levels of energy

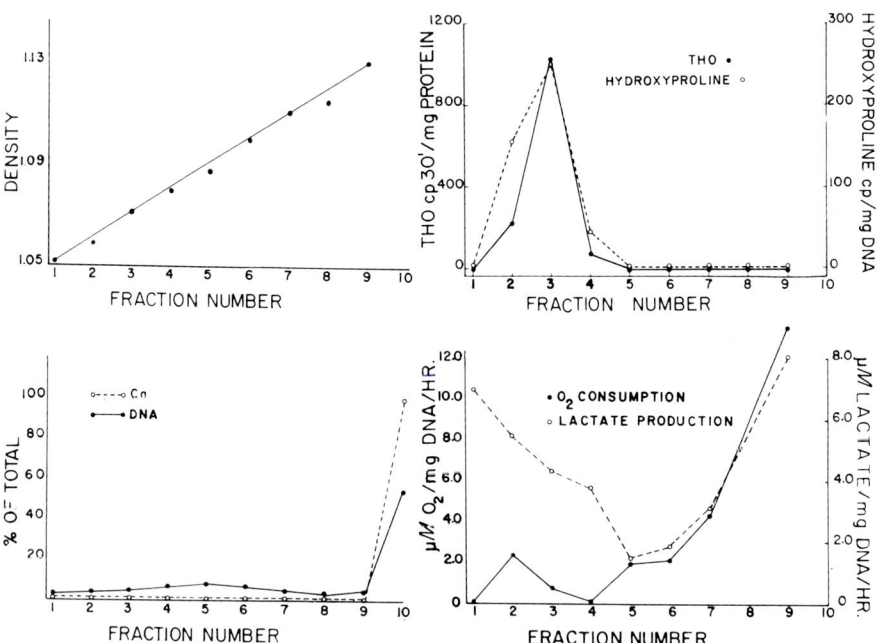

Fig. 7. The distribution of calcium, DNA, and a variety of cell fractions in populations of bone cells separated by their buoyant density in albumin density gradients. Nine fractions and a pellet of cells (designated as fraction 10) were separated. Proline hydroxylase activity (*upper right*) was measured by the release of tritium (^{3}H) counts from a previously labeled hydroxyproline-free protocollagen substrate derived from embryonated eggs. This and the presence in the cells of labeled hydroxyproline were used as markers to locate collagen biosynthesis. Other measurements plotted are self-explanatory. (Combined from unpublished experiments by Flanagan and Nichols, 1966 and 1970).

production are associated in a cell population different from the one concerned with matrix synthesis was also suggested in experiments in which attempts were made to separate the different cell populations present in the cell suspension by their buoyant density in albumin density gradients. These are summarized in Fig. 7. The important features to note here are that the heaviest cells not only have all the calcium in them but also have the highest rates of lactate production and O_2 uptake, while the collagen biosynthetic system located by the ability of the cells to hydroxylate proline seems to exist only in the lighter cells which contain little calcium and float at the other end of the gradient.

Additional evidence implicating the osteocyte in bone mineral metabolism has come from another quarter. Tetracycline was noted several years ago to be deposited in areas of new bone formation which could be identified in microscopic sections by the characteristic fluorescence of the drug under ultraviolet light as long as the sections were not decalcified prior to examination, for procedures which removed the mineral from the bone removed the drug as well. Although opinions differ regarding how tetracycline comes to be localized to such areas and how it is bound there, it occurred to us that it might be deposited by the bone cells with the mineral in new bone formation and therefore might serve as a useful marker to differentiate bone cells in general and "mineralizing" cells in particular in mixed suspensions of marrow and bone cells. The rapid uptake of tetracycline into bone cells was demonstrated, as shown in Fig. 8, by finding, in fresh wet preparations viewed under ultraviolet light, brightly fluorescent granules in most of the bone cells harvested by grinding 15 minutes after injection of 50 mg tetracycline intraperitoneally into a 10 kg suckling pig. Moreover, examination of fresh samples of marrow from the same animals showed that while all cells showed faintly fluorescent nuclear and cell membranes, the occasional contaminating bone cell was easily distinguished by its content of brightly fluorescent granules, which when compared to the fluorescent granules appearing in some granulocytes are much larger and tend to be clustered at one side of the cell.

Confirmation of these findings can be obtained by measuring the tetracycline content of bone and marrow cell homogenates chemically. Ten times more tetracycline (measured by its absorbance of ultraviolet light at 380 mμ wavelength in 0.1 N HCl and ethyl acetate extracts of the tissues) was present in bone than in marrow cells. Furthermore, this difference was entirely due to uptake into the particulate fraction of these cells—the same fraction which has been shown to contain the calcium.

While these data suggest that the bone cells involved in calcium transport can be identified in cell suspension by their content of tetracycline-labeled and calcium-containing granules, the demonstration of these granules in fixed microscopic sections of bone in which the identity of the cells which contain them could be established has yet to be accomplished because of the problems of preparing undecalcified sections of the requisite thickness. In fact, the only evidence we have on this point at present is shown in Fig. 9. This is a photograph of a fresh wet spicule of bone from one of our young tetracycline-labeled pigs viewed under ultraviolet light. It can be seen that the osteocytes and their processes, or perhaps their lacunae and canaliculi, appear to contain most of the label. Some label also appears at the surface of the bone, but whether this is in the osteoblasts cannot be ascertained because of the thickness of the preparation.

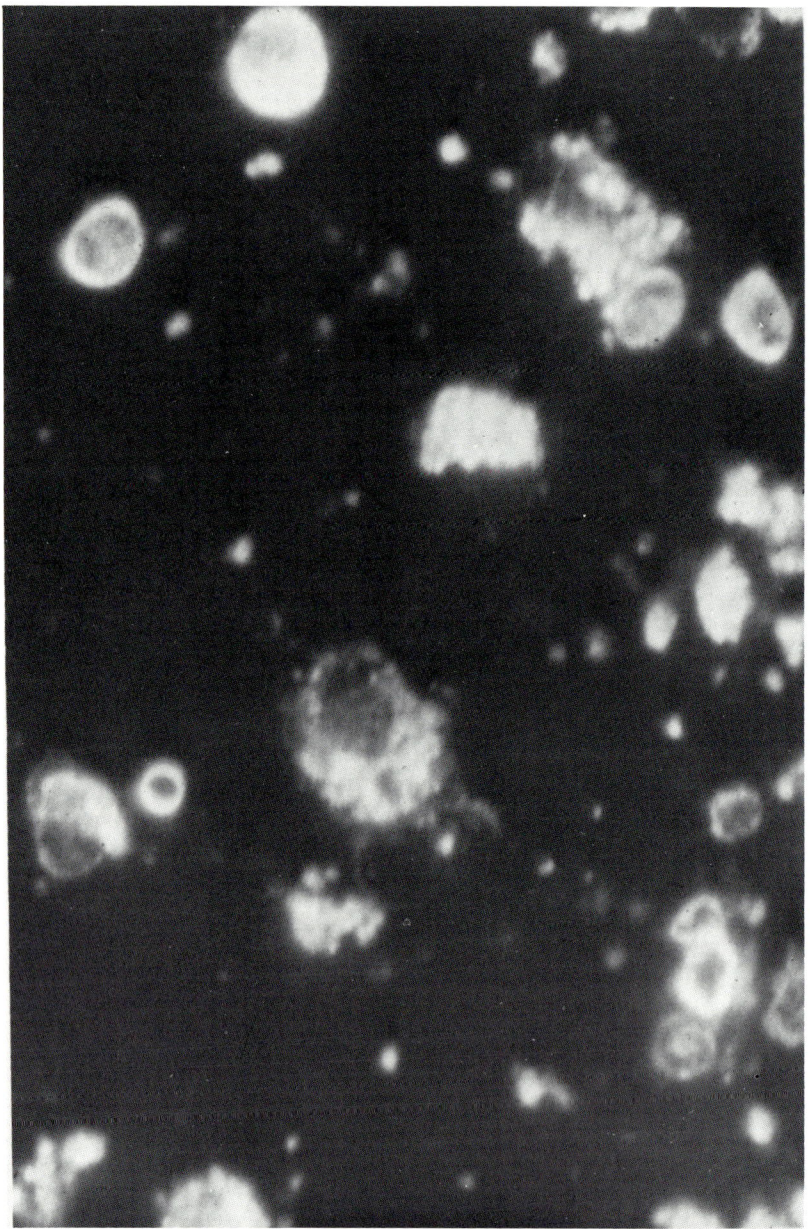

Fig. 8. Unfixed fresh bone cells taken from a young pig previously given tetracycline viewed under ultraviolet light. See text for details. (About 1000 ×.)

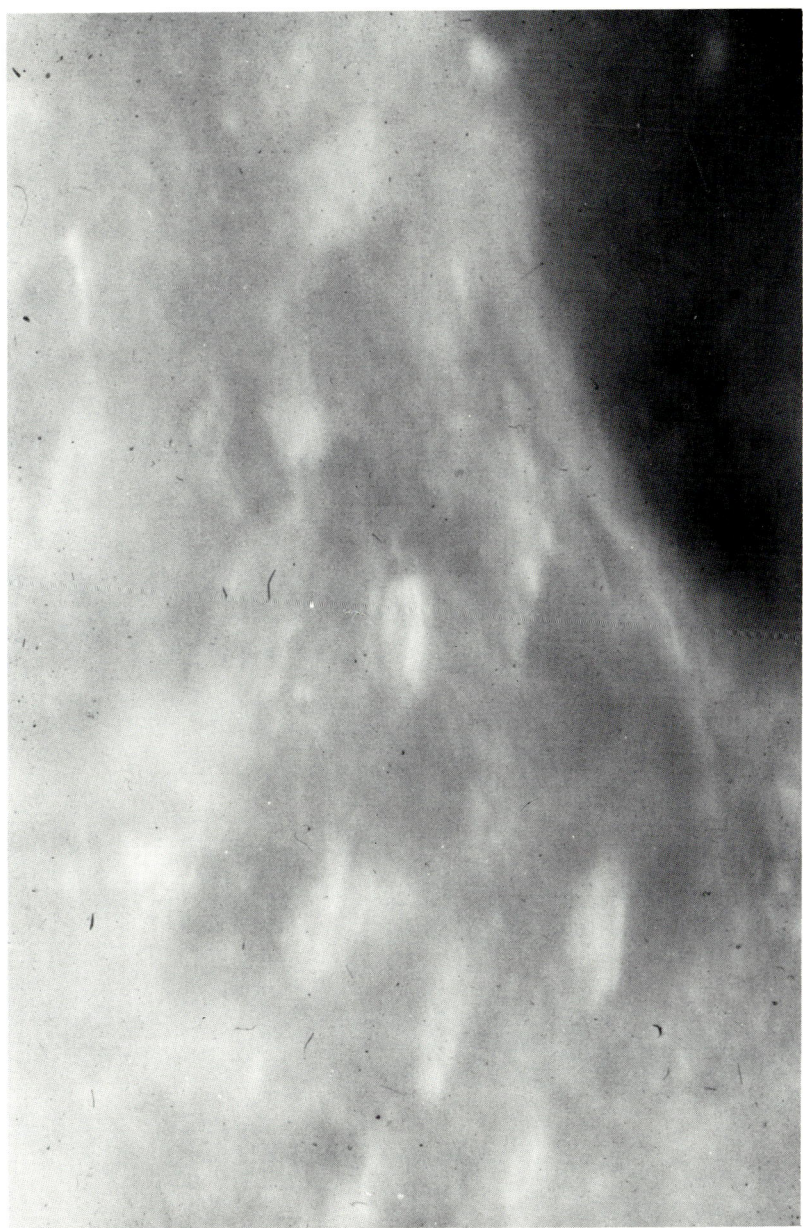

Fig. 9. A fresh spicule of trabecular bone from a young pig injected with tetracycline viewed by transmitted ultraviolet light. See text for details. (About 400 ×.)

While these data and those of Kashiwa (1970) and Martin and Matthews (1970) point strongly to the presence of large amounts of calcium collected into dense cytoplasmic granules in the osteocytes and perhaps osteoblasts, they do not in themselves shed any light on the significance of this fact with respect to skeletal mineral metabolism. Here the isolated cell approach offers unique experimental advantages for it allows one to measure changes in calcium content, and, with isotopes, calcium flux into and out of the cells in response to various stimuli, and through the use of inhibitors etc., to examine how these may relate to metabolic processes in the cells. The results of some studies of bone cell mineral content and exchange under various conditions and the ways in which we see the cells working in relation to mineral metabolism in bone and the circulating fluids are summarized in the remainder of the figures.

Although bone cell and medium calcium concentrations tended to remain stable during *in vitro* incubations in Krebs–Ringer bicarbonate buffer, cell content of both calcium and phosphorus proved to be in part dependent upon their concentration in the medium during incubation, as illustrated in Fig. 10. Increasing the medium calcium concentration from 0 to 10 mM led after 1 hour of incubation at 37°C to a 38% increase in cell calcium content, while a similar increase in medium phosphorus concentration led to a 47% increase in cell phosphorus.

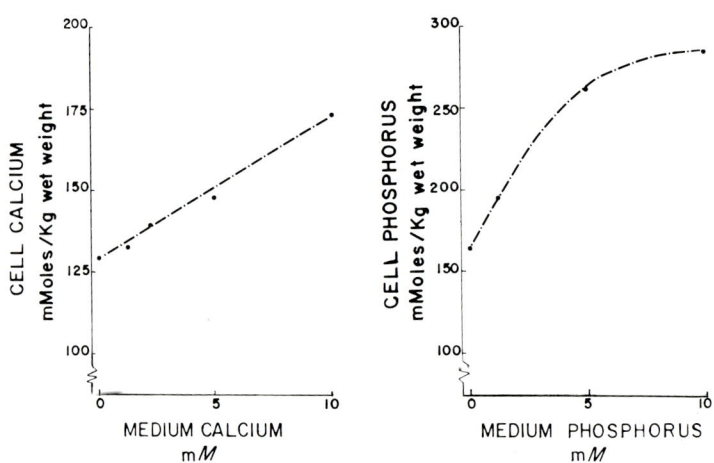

FIG. 10. Bone cell calcium and phosphorus concentrations in relation to their concentrations in incubation medium after 1 hour incubation at 37°C. All media were Krebs–Ringer solution, bicarbonate buffer, with glucose 11.1 mM as substrate.

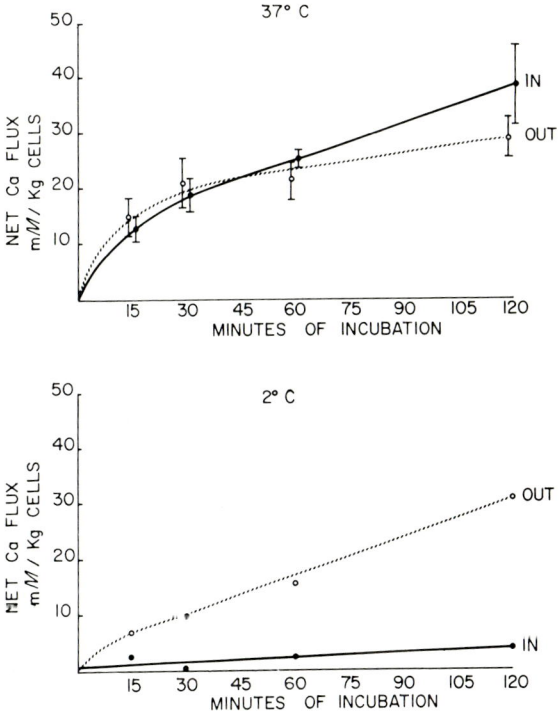

FIG. 11. Net calcium fluxes into and out of bone cells during incubation at 37°C and 2°C in Krebs–Ringer solution, bicarbonate buffer, with 1.25 mM calcium and glucose as substrate. [From Nichols and Rogers (1971).]

These findings suggested that, despite the stability of cell and medium calcium concentration during incubation, calcium could penetrate bone cells under *in vitro* conditions. This was amply confirmed by experiments in which a rapid uptake of ^{45}Ca from incubation media into the supernate and particulate calcium fractions of bone cells during incubation at 37°C was easily demonstrated both by the appearance of counts in the cell fractions and by their disappearance from the incubation medium. Since the calcium concentration changes in cells and medium were far smaller in these experiments than the changes in radioactivity, it was clear that rapid exchange between intra- and extracellular calcium could occur under *in vitro* conditions. Moreover, net movements of ^{45}Ca inward and ^{40}Ca outward could be calculated and the balance between the two examined in relation to any changes in cell calcium content which might occur. The really considerable magnitude of these exchanges and the close correlation between net movement of calcium in with net movement of calcium out of the cells at 37°C is illustrated in Fig. 11. These facts are important, not only because they explain why bone cell calcium stores seem to be stable *in vitro*, but because they point out that these cells can turn over calcium at a rapid rate. Indeed this rate is rapid enough to explain all the exchanges of calcium which go between bone and blood. Also shown is the fact that at 2°C almost no ^{45}Ca is taken up by the cells. However, calcium efflux from the cells seems to proceed under these conditions at a rate similar to that occuring at 37°C, and is reflected by a slow loss of cell calcium which occurs with incubation in the cold. These data appear to indicate that uptake of calcium is metabolically dependent while outflow is not, which is at variance with Dr. Stern's reported observations (Stern and Austin, 1970). Our experience to date with metabolic inhibitors other than cold suggests that only actinomycin D affects calcium exchange and that it may block both influx and efflux.

Having shown that the calcium stores in bone cells were indeed in some sort of dynamic equilibrium with the calcium outside them, we examined the ways in which various agents known to affect calcium metabolism and serum calcium concentration might affect bone cell calcium content and exchange.

Some effects of parathyroidectomy, thyroparathyroidectomy, and parathyroid extract on bone cell calcium content in rats are shown in Fig. 12. As can be seen, parathyroidectomy tended to raise but thyroparathyroidectomy to lower cell calcium. Chronic administration of parathyroid extract tended to lower cell calcium in normal rats but raised it to supernormal levels when given 2 hours before sacrifice to fasted thyroparathyroidectomized animals. It was also found in chicks that vitamin D deficiency markedly lowered cell calcium content, findings which we have had difficulty reproducing more than partially in rats, probably because of the difficulty of inducing complete D deficiency in this species. While these findings indicated that bone cell calcium content was affected when calcium metabolism was perturbed, they shed little light on the mechanisms involved, so we turned to an examination of the effects of these procedures on calcium fluxes as a next step.

Our initial experience with the repair of thyroparathyroidectomized rats with parathyroid extract indicated that while their bone cell calcium content was raised to normal 18 hours after hormone injection, the only effects we could find on bone cell calcium flux rates was an increase in efflux, a paradox which seemed explicable only by the possibility that the rise in cell calcium which characterized such animals had been induced by an increased influx which had faded by the time the animals were sacrificed.

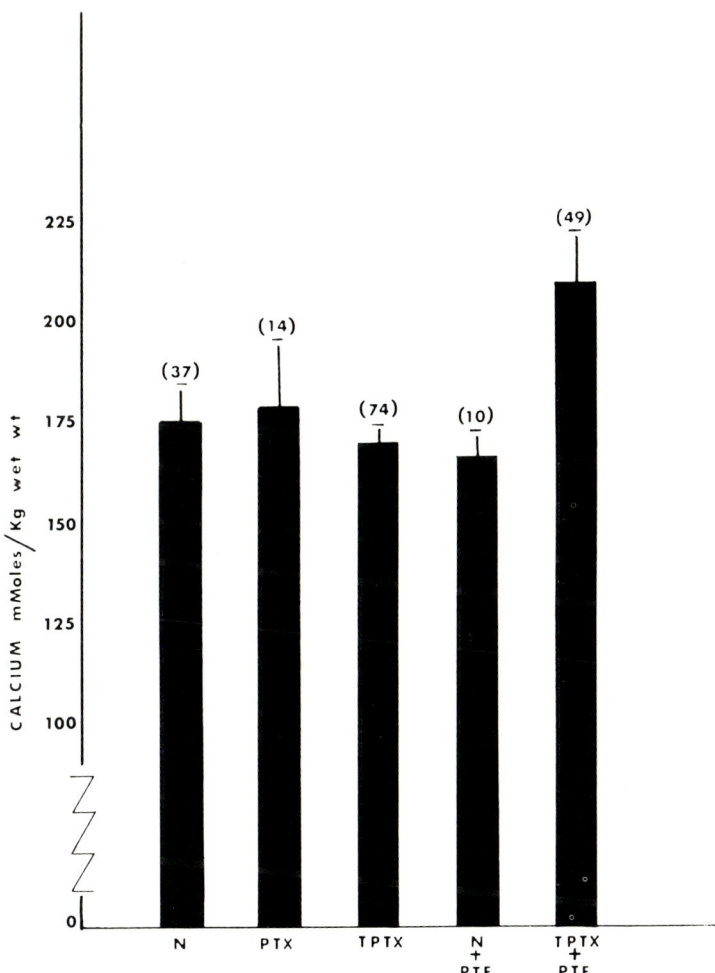

FIG. 12. Mean calcium concentrations found in bone cells from rats following various manipulations of their parathyroid and thyroid status. One standard deviation of the mean and the number of samples included in the mean are indicated above each bar. PTX = parathyroidectomized; TPTX = thyroparathyroidectomized; PTE = Lilly parathyroid extract given subcutaneously at a dose of 1 unit per gram body weight either 2 hours before or in two or three repeated doses over the 36 hours preceeding sacrifice.

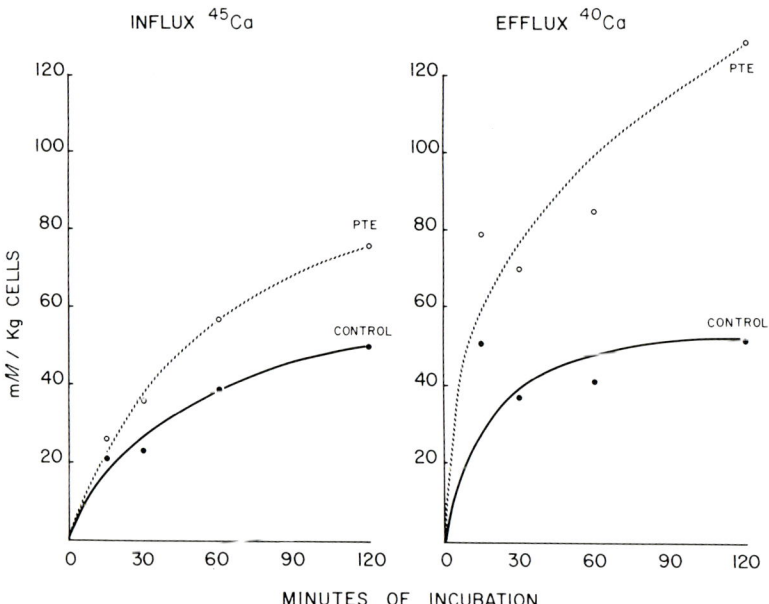

FIG. 13. Net cumulative fluxes of calcium into and out of bone cells from thyroparathyroidectomized rats that had received 1 unit per gram of PTE 2 hours before sacrifice, compared to cells from animals which had not been treated. See text. [From Nichols and Rogers, 1971.]

This idea was confirmed when fluxes were measured in cells from animals which had received their hormone just 2 hours before sacrifice, as can be seen in Fig. 13. Here, a clearcut increase in calcium influx could be demonstrated to account for the concomitant rise in cell calcium content observed. However, an even larger increase in efflux was also found. These data suggested to us that the rate of efflux of calcium from bone cells might be related in some way to the maintenance of the serum calcium concentration and that it might be controlled in part by such factors as calcitonin and phosphorus. Moreover, changes in the latter are induced by nonskeletal actions of parathyroid hormone. Both are known to block parathyroid hormone-stimulated calcium movement out of bone both *in vivo* and in tissue culture.

It was not surprising, therefore, when the ambient phosphorus concentration proved to have effects on bone cell calcium metabolism, although these proved considerably more dramatic than anticipated. As shown in Fig. 14 calcium influx increased progressively as the ambient phosphorus concentration was increased. Even more impressive was the decrease in efflux which occured simultaneously. In fact, at medium phosphorus concentrations of 5 mM or more, calcium movement into the medium was completely blocked. The finding of decreased calcium concentrations in the medium confirmed the validity of these observations.

Unfortunately, because of difficulties experienced in obtaining pure material, the effects of calcitonin on these variables have been examined only indirectly until very recently. However, the data on cell calcium content (Fig. 12) suggested that when calcitonin is available, cell calcium concentrations are higher than when it is not, and therefore, that like phosphorus, it blocks calcium efflux from bone cells, an impression which appeared to be confirmed in a very recent experiment. Whether it has any effect on influx remains to be discovered.

The way in which we currently assemble these and other data available in the literature into a model of how the osteocyte and perhaps the osteoblast functions as the chief mediator of bone mineral metabolism is shown in Fig. 15. The general features of this scheme were postulated by Drs. Flanagan and van der Sluys Veer and me (Nichols et al., 1969) about 2 years ago on the basis of the few data we had available then. Although we have learned a great deal about bone cells and their calcium metabolism

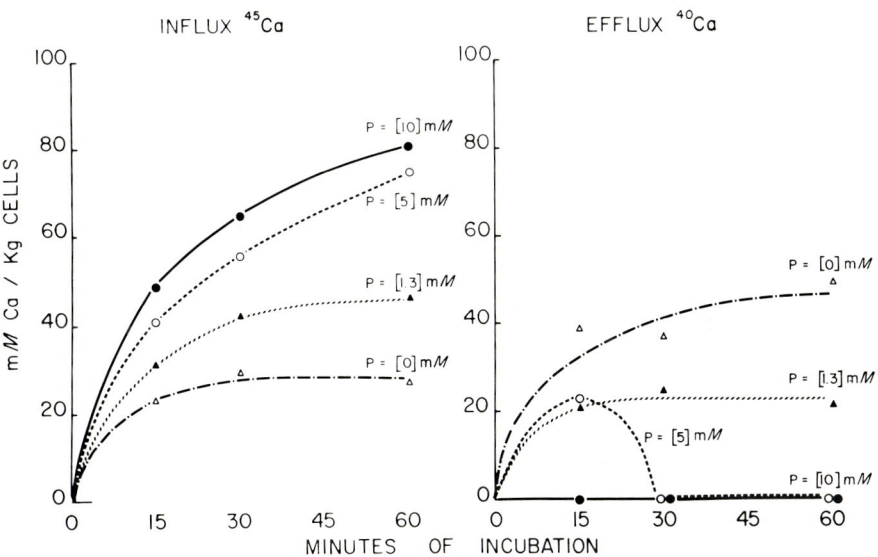

Fig. 14. Net cumulative fluxes of calcium into and out of pig bone cells incubated for various periods at 37°C in Krebs–Ringer solution, bicarbonate buffer, containing 1.25 mM calcium and the different concentrations of phosphorus indicated.

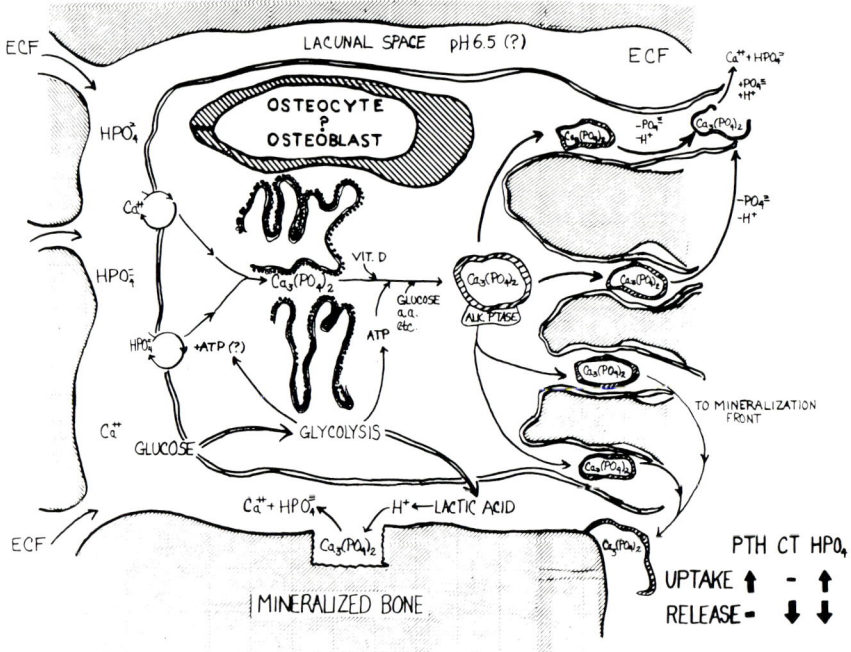

Fig. 15. A model of a bone cell, perhaps an osteocyte or an osteoblast, indicating the authors' present concept regarding the mechanisms such cells contain for the uptake, storage, and release of calcium. See text for details.

since, few things have had to be changed from the model we drew at that time, but there have been some important additions.

An osteocyte is pictured ensconced in its lacuna with its cell processes extending out to either the perivascular space or the mineralization front. Calcium and phosphorus, we believe, are taken up from the large volumes of extracellular fluid flowing through the cannalicular system by the cell, perhaps by an ATP-dependent process, and are combined in the endoplasmic reticulum with organic components into a granule. Whether the organic material forms a coat on the outside of the mineral salt as is pictured or serves as a core around which it aggregates is not clear and is probably unimportant to understanding the function of the system. What is important, however, is that formation of these granules we believe is an *active* process which involves the biosynthesis of at least protein and lipid components and requires vitamin D or one of its active metabolites, substrates such as amino acids and ATP. The energy to drive this process, we feel, is probably largely derived from glycolysis, although some ATP may be generated by an O_2-dependent electron transport pathway. Once formed, we think some granules are stored in the cells while others pass along the cell processes to be extruded intact either at the mineralization front or into the perivascular space. In either case we propose that the alkaline phosphatase in their walls [Doty et al. (1968) have demonstrated that there is one in granules in osteocytes] is activated by the low PO_4^{-3} and H^+ ion concentrations in the local area, and the wall of the package is destroyed. The mineral crystals so released at the mineralization front form the nucleus for new crystal formation there, while the calcium and phosphorus needed to support the circulating concentrations of these ions are provided by the solubilization of these crystals in the fluids adjacent to the capillaries.

The action of the parathyroid hormone on the system, we believe from the data cited above, is to increase the active uptake of calcium by the cells from the lacunal fluid, an action which is enhanced by increasing the calcium and/or phosphorus concentrations there. The action of calcitonin, on the other hand, would seem to be to block the exit of calcium from the cells. Phosphate, we know, has a similar action, and in addition, we know from older work (Borle et al., 1960) that it inhibits glycolysis. Thus, both the availability of ATP for ion transport and granule synthesis and the release of H^+ and lactate ions into the lacunal space would be decreased by local increase in phosphate concentration. Whether an additional control exists which regulates the total number of granules which can accumulate in the cells and thus limits their maximum calcium concentration is not known.

A couple of other features of this model have interesting implications which are worthy of passing comment. For example, it can act as a biological amplifier of the parathyroid response to hypocalcemia in the following way (Nichols, 1970): Parathyroid hormone not only increases cell calcium uptake, but stimulates glycolysis and therefore the release of organic acids from the bone cells as well. The latter will lower the pH of the lacunal fluid and hence tend to increase the dissolution of the surrounding bone mineral. This in turn will raise the [Ca] in the lacuna and hence promote cell calcium uptake. A built-in regulator of the system is provided by the phosphate, which must be released from the mineral stores along with the calcium. As its concentration increases, it will tend to block the activity of the system both by blocking granule exit and reducing available energy for transport and granule synthesis, thus preventing its running out of control.

Moreover, as we pointed out in connection with the earlier version of this scheme, it provides an explanation for the long argued phenomenon of excessive bone resorption in acidotic states. For, a fall in blood pH would produce a similar fall in bone extracellular fluid pH, including that in the lacunae, and so would enhance or mimic the effects of parathyroid hormone.

How much of this model is fancy and how much will ultimately be proved to be fact is, of course, purely a matter of conjecture at present. All that can be said for it so far is that it seems to be consistent with the facts we currently have available and so provides a framework for the design of further experiments. It also has recently provided an intriguing and perhaps correct explanation of some at first rather surprising findings in respect to the calcium concentration found in the bone cells of patients with disturbances of parathyroid function.

The bone cell [Ca] of two ladies with hypoparathyroidism proved high and that of one with hyperparathyroidism low, as can be seen in Figure 16. The model suggests that this state of affairs should hold, since it states that bone cell calcium content depends on the balance between uptake and outgo, and the latter is extremely sensitive to blockade by phosphorus. If the high serum phosphorus concentration characteristic of the hypoparathyroid state were acompanied by a high bone fluid phosphorus concentration as we suspect, the high bone cell calcium in such patients was to be

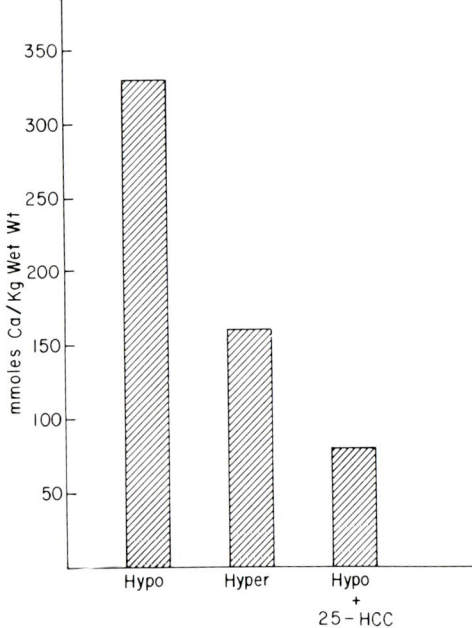

FIG. 16. The calcium content found in the bone cells of four patients—two with untreated hypoparathyroidism (mean value shown), one with hyperparathyroidism, and one of the two hypoparathyroid patients following repair of serum calcium concentration with the active metabolite of vitamin D-25 hydroxycholecalciferol.

expected as was the low cell calcium of the hyperparathyroid patient where low plasma phosphorus concentrations are the rule. Confirmation of this view was provided by a second observation in one of the former just after serum calcium and phosphorus had been returned to normal by vitamin D therapy. As can be seen in the last column, bone cell calcium had at that time fallen to one-third its previous level.

ACKNOWLEDGMENTS

Needless to say, a number of colleagues have contributed importantly to this work and to the development of our ideas about it. We would like to take this opportunity to acknowledge the contributions of Drs. Barry Flanagan, John Woods, Jaap van der Sluys Veer, Elizabeth Lloyd, Marijke Holtrop, James Irving, and more recently, Dr. Micheline Federman, all of whom have collaborated in various aspects of the overall project, only a small part of which is discussed here. Invaluable technical help has been provided by Mrs. S. Ault and Misses M. Overman, R. Wolpert, and B. Stolberg. Without their help little would have been accomplished.

REFERENCES

Belanger, L. F., Robichon, J., Migicovsky, B. B., Copp, D. H., and Vincent, J. (1963). *In* "Mechanisms of Hard Tissue Destruction," Publ. No. 75, p. 531. Am. Assoc. Advance. Sci., Washington, D.C.
Borle, A. B. (1968). *J. Cell Biol.* **36,** 567.
Borle, A. B., Nichols, N., and Nichols, G., Jr. (1960). *J. Biol. Chem.* **235,** 1211.
Doty, S. B., Schofield, B. H., and Robinson, R. A. (1968). *In* "Parathyroid Hormone and Thyrocalcitonin" (R. V. Talmage, L. F. Belanger, and I. Clark, eds.), p. 169. Excerpta Med. Found., New York.
Flanagan, B., and Nichols, G., Jr. (1966 and 1970). Unpublished experiments.
Hancox, N. M., and Boothroyd, B. (1965). *Clin. Orthop. Related Res.* **50,** 103.
Hastings, A. B., and Huggins, C. B. (1933). *Proc. Soc. Exp. Biol. Med.* **30,** 458.
Hirschmann, P. N., and Nichols, G., Jr. (1971). *Calcif. Tissue Res.* (in press).
Kashiwa, H. K. (1970). *Clin. Orthop. Related Res.* **70,** 200.
Martin, J. H., and Matthews, J. L. (1970). *Clin. Orthop. Related Res.* **68,** 273.
Nichols, G., Jr. (1967). Unpublished observations.
Nichols, G., Jr. (1970). *Calcif. Tissue Res.* **4,** Suppl., 61.
Nichols, G., Jr., and Rogers, P. (1971). *Pediatrics* **47,** 211.
Nichols, G., Jr., Flanagan, B., and van der Sluys Veer, J. (1969). *Arch. Intern. Med.* **124,** 530.
Peck, W. A., Birge, S. J., Jr., and Fedak, S. A. (1964). *Science* **146,** 1476.
Sampson, H. W., Matthews, J. L., Martin, J. H., and Kunin, A. S. (1970). *Calcif. Tissue Res.* **5,** 305.
Stern, P. H., and Austin, J. (1970). *Fed. Proc., Fed. Amer. Soc. Exp. Biol.* **29,** 566.
Woods, J. F., and Nichols, G., Jr. (1963). *Science* **142,** 386.

Discussion

Dr. Eisenberg: One of the things that disturbed me about Bill Neuman's presentation was the concept that the fluid in contact with the bone salt is in static equilibrium with the bone. It probably, it seems to me, is changing composition all the time in response to metabolic changes induced by the membrane. I was wondering if you had had occasion to expose your bone cells to a fluid resembling Dr. Neuman's so-called bone fluid and to determine what the metabolic activities are or what the efflux and influx rates of calcium are.

Dr. Nichols: No, we haven't. However, we have incubated whole bone fragments *in vitro* in a medium of the composition which he describes without producing any effect.

Dr. Rich: In the past, two other groups working in this area, Matthews and Kashiwa, have concentrated on morphological demonstrations of calcium and phosphate in cells without providing quantitative data, while until now, you primarily have had quantitative information. Therefore, it is interesting to see you combine your former approach with morphological studies.

It should be possible to measure the number and average size of the spherules which appear to contain calcium and phosphorus; there probably are several hundred per cell, perhaps with an average diameter of around 1 μ. You already have information from which you can calculate the amount of calcium per cell. I wonder, with full realization of the assumptions that would have to be made, whether you could decide on how much calcium phosphate would be in the average spherule. Although any such calculation would be only very approximate, it could be of some interest to know, within an order of magnitude, how many calcium atoms might be in each spherule. There would be a different significance in terms of concept if the amount of calcium could be accounted for on the basis of possible binding sites than if, for instance, there were enough calcium in the cell to account for 50% of the volume of the spherules.

The second point I want to ask about is whether your calculated influx rates are of the same order of magnitude as the mass transfer coefficients that André Borle has found in kidney cells, as he described earlier in the conference.

Dr. Nichols: I would have to do the calculations for the last question, but I suspect they are not terribly different from Dr. Borle's data. On the first question, I would have to get together with Herb Kashiwa and count granules, I think, in order to know whether we are really seeing the same thing. However, the calculation of the calcium content of a single spherule could be made if one knew how many sperules were present per cell, how many cells were present, and if one could assume (which seems a reasonable first approximation) that the calcium-rich fraction which Peter Hirschmann [P. N. Hirschmann and G. Nichols, Jr., *Fed. Proc., Fed. Amer. Soc. Exp. Biol.* **29**, 801 (1970)] has been isolating contains all the spherules present in the cell sample.

Dr. Bordier: Did you look at the morphological aspects of the cells that you have separated in the fractions? Do the osteoblasts and the osteocytes have different shapes, and do the osteocytes keep the extensions which they have *in vivo*? Could you also comment upon the coat in which calcium phosphate is embedded?

Dr. Nichols: Taking your question in reverse order, we don't really know for certain the nature of the coat. We would like to think that it contains lipid and protein. You will notice that we have a little bit of alkaline phosphatase hanging in it, which we put in there because Steve Doty some years ago had shown there was alkaline phosphatase associated with subcellular granules in osteocytes [S. B. Doty, B. H. Schofield, and R. A. Robinson, in "Parathyroid Hormone and Thyrocalcitonin (Calcitonin)" (R. V.

Talmage and L. Belanger, eds.), pp. 169–181. Excerpta Med. Found., Amsterdam, 1968]. As I remember, it was not magnesium-dependent. We thought that this alkaline phosphatase might be there as a sort of self-jettisoning mechanism, so that as pH and phosphate concentration changed at the periphery, coats broke up. Whether that is true or not, of course, is speculation but it is a nice idea. I would like to think that the coat material is the same material which Dr. Irving is finding at the calcification front [J. T. Irving and R. E. Wuthier, *Clin. Orthop. Related Res.* **56,** 237–260 (1968)] and which is missing in vitamin D deficiency, but the proof of that idea is still lacking.

Regarding cell processes, we have looked at the morphology of these cells only under the light microscope so far, and at that magnification, they all look round. There are no cell processes that we can see. Elizabeth Lloyd has looked at some of them under the electron microscope, and she would, I am sure, back me up in saying that they look pretty tattery at that level, but, whether their cell processes were broken off in the process of isolation or whether they may have retracted, I don't know. Either is possible.

Dr. Leonard: I don't happen to think that pH 6.5 is particularly ludicrous. What is the evidence?

Dr. Nichols: Yes, I thought it would be between 6.8 and 6.5 largely because of Chris Nordin's [B. E. C. Nordin, *J. Biol. Chem.* **227,** 551 (1957)] data and the thought that, at that pH, one might have reasonably high calcium phosphate concentrations in the fluid without having precipitation. As a matter of fact, in a way it sort of fits with Bill Neuman's views regarding the concentration of calcium in bone fluid (W. F. Neuman, this volume).

Dr. Leonard: Have you studied calcium uptake and efflux in the presence of magnesium ions?

Dr. Nichols: There is some magnesium in the medium we use. We have not varied the magnesium ion to see whether it affects it.

THE ROLE OF MITOCHONDRIA IN INTRACELLULAR CALCIUM REGULATION*

J. L. Matthews, J. H. Martin, C. Arsenis, R. Eisenstein, and K. Kuettner

The mechanism of initiation of mineralization and the mechanisms of calcium homeostasis are still a matter of investigation. Recently, more attention has been directed toward the evaluation of the role of the cell and its organelles in these processes. Kashiwa (1966) has studied cells at mineralization sites utilizing the Schiff base glyoxal bis(2-hydroxyanil) (GBHA) that produces a red deposit with calcium. Cells associated with mineralization stained positively. GBHA positive intracellular sperules of $\frac{1}{2}$–2 μ diameters were described in cartilage and bone cells. Incorporation of isotopic calcium by bone and cartilage cells has been reported by Johnston (1953), Salomon and Ray (1966), and Matthews et al. (1968). Localization of the total cell calcium has not been successful as preparative procedures have removed the ions of interest. Thus, the studies to date have dealt primarily with the localization of intracellular bound calcium and its relationship to mineralization and homeostasis. Nichols (1970), Sobel et al., (1960), Urist (1966), Kashiwa (1966), and Matthews et al. (1968) have all suggested an association between increased concentrations of bound cal-

---

* This work supported by Grants from the National Institutes of Health, Nos. DE224-03, AM13799-01, and AM09132.

cium and the onset of mineralization. Mineralization has been observed in the matrix immediately surrounding cell processes by Anderson (1969), Schenck *et al.* (1967), Bonnuchi (1969), and others.

Electron-dense particles have been described in the mitochondria of cells of bone and cartilage by Cameron *et al.* (1967), and Martin and Matthews (1970). The latter have reported that the granules vary in number and position as a consequence of vitamin D and parathormone and have proved the mitochondrial granules to be useful indices of intracellular bound calcium. This chapter will present additional studies on the number, distribution, and chemical nature of mitochondrial granules from cartilage, bone, gut, and calciphylactic skin.

Experimental Protocol

Rachitic Studies

Weanling Holtzman rats were pair-fed a phosphate-sufficient rachitogenic diet and a vitamin D_2-supplemented diet for 2 weeks. Control animals were fed Purina Lab Chow *ad libitum*. Two week rachitic rats were intubated with 10 IU vitamin D_2. Rats were killed with ether at 15, 30, 60, 120, 360, 720, 1200, and 2400 minutes post intubation. Specimens of bone, cartilaginous growth plate, and duodenum were prepared for electron microscope examination.

Calciphylactic Studies

Weanling rats were sensitized with dihydrotachysterol and were challenged 29 hours post sensitization with epilation and pinching of the skin. Rats were killed with ether at 15, 30, 60, 120, 360, 720, 1200, and 2400 minutes following challenge. Specimens of skin from the area challenged and the surrounding unchallenged area were prepared for electron microscope examination.

Parathormone Studies

Weanling rats were injected with 10 USP units of parathyroid extract. Rats were ether killed at 5, 15, 30, 60, 120, and 360 minutes, and specimens of tibial cortical bone were prepared for electron microscope examination.

Analysis of Subcellular Fractions and Mitochondrial Granules

The hypertrophic zone from 60–75 pound calf scapula and costochondral junctions were dissected immediately after sacrifice. The tissue was homogenized in a mixture of 0.15 M KCl, 0.015 M tris, and adjusted to pH 7.4 with HCl. Mitochondria were purified according to the method of Greenawalt et al. (1964) in a sucrose gradient.

Method

MICROSCOPE TECHNIQUES

Skin, growth plates, and metaphyseal bone from weaning rats and calf scapula were removed immediately after the animals were killed and fixed in 1.5% osmic acid buffered with s-collidine to which calcium chloride was added to give a 5 mmoles per-liter concentration. The specimens were allowed to fix for 1 hour and then were dehydrated in alcohol and embedded in Epon. Some specimens were fixed without the addition of calcium and mitochondrial granule counts were made from comparable specimen regions. No difference in granule number was found, but granules from tissues fixed in calcium fixative were more electron dense. One micron sections were cut and stained with Paragon and viewed with the light microscope for orientation. Ultrathin sections were made with an ultramicrotome and were picked up on silicon monoxide-coated grids prepared according to the technic described by Thomas and Greenawalt (1968). Specimens were viewed with a Phillips 300 electron microscope. No lead or uranium staining was used.

Following viewing with the electron microscope, ultrathin sections were incinerated to 500°C for 15 minutes in a muffle furnace and again viewed with the electron microscope. The same fixative procedures were used for examination of subcellular fractions. Low-viscosity epoxy was used as an embedding medium. Cell fractions were centrifuged in the epoxy and polymerized in centrifuged capsules. Some fractions were allowed to air dry on silicone films.

BIOCHEMICAL TECHNIQUES

Mitochondrial granules were separated by ultracentrifugation from mitochondria isolated from homogenized cartilage. The inorganic components were evaluated by ashing the granules in sulfuric acid. Calcium and magnesium were determined by atomic absorption spectrophotometry. Phosphate was determined by the method of Fisk and Subbarow. Organic components were evaluated for ribonucleic acids by the technique of Schneider (1955). Analysis for the presence of lysozyme was carried out after electrophoresis on cellulose acetate as previously described (Kuettner et al., 1968). Lipids were extracted for mitochondrial pellets.

Mitochondrial Lipid Extraction

The mitochondrial pellet was homogenized for 3 minutes under nitrogen in 20 ml chloroform–methanol 2:1 which contained 1 mg butylated hydroxytoluene (BHT) per liter of solvent. The suspension was filtered through a medium porosity sintered glass funnel under nitrogen, and the residue re-extracted with C/M 2:1 (10 ml). The extracts were pooled, the residue extracted with chloroform–methanol–HCl 200:100:1 (10 ml) for 12 hours at $-20°C$, the hydrochloric acid neutralized with sodium bicarbonate, the suspension filtered, and the extract added to the previous extracts.

Granule Lipid Extraction

The mitochondrial granule pellet was suspended in chloroform–methanol 2:1 with BHT for 12 hours at $-20°C$, the granule was centrifuged, the extract was placed in the freezer, and the pellet was resuspended in 0.2 M EDTA (pH 7.5) for 24 hours at 4°C. The granules were centrifuged, washed once with water, and resuspended in chloroform–methanol 2:1 for 24 hours at $-20°C$. The granules were centrifuged and resuspended in chloroform–methanol–HCl 200:100:1 for 24 hours at 4°C, the extract was neutralized with sodium bicarbonate, centrifuged, and the extracts pooled.

Solvent Evaporation

The pooled extracts were evaporated under nitrogen to near-dryness (drying extracted lipids results in breakdown of some phospholipids at the solid-air interface) and taken up in chloroform to a total volume of 100 μl.

Phospholipid Separation and Quantitation

To determine the total amount of lipid present, a 10 μl portion of the lipid extract was weighed on a Cahn microbalance and the lipid calculated (1). The total phospholipid present was determined by phosphorous analysis (see below) and the neutral lipid determined by difference.

The phospholipids were separated by two dimensional thin layer chromatography (TLC) using chloroform–methanol–ammonia (65:25:4) in the first dimension and chloroform–acetone–methanol–acetic acid–water (5:2:1:1:0.5) in the second dimension. The plates were charred, the spots aspirated, and the phosphorous quantitated. A neutral lipid profile was run but the neutral lipids were not quantitated.

EDTA Extract

To insure no lipid carry over into the EDTA extract, the extract was made 3 N with respect to HCl, flushed with nitrogen sealed, and heated at

100°C for 3 hours. The solution was extracted three times with hexane, the hexane was evaporated, and the residue was taken up in chloroform, the fatty acid solution was shaken with a calcium nitrate solution, the excess copper nitrate was removed, and the choloroform solution was analyzed for the fatty acid copper salt.

Results

The growth plate of rats fed a vitamin D-supplemented rachitic diet were examined for distribution of mitochondrial granules and were compared with the distribution previously reported from rats fed a Purina Chow diet. Growth plate widths of the two groups were similar. Both groups demonstrated a gradient of distribution of mitochondrial granules in the chondrocytes.

Small mitochondrial granule concentrations were found in the proliferative zone, but increased concentrations were found in the succeeding zones. The highest granule count was found in the hypertrophic cell zone (Fig. 1). Further, the number of mitochondria per cell also increases toward the junction with the calcifying zone. The observation is in agreement with the data of C. Arsenis, Table I, indicating that in calf cartilage, the activity of mitochondrial enzymes also increase in the same areas. Arsenis has also found that isolated mitochondria from calf costochondral junction cartilage can be separated according to the method of Greenawalt et al. (1964) into a light and heavy mitochondrial population. Preliminary data indicate that the heavy population is approximately two-thirds of the whole. These granules were absent in chondrocytes in the zone of provisional calcification, suggesting that the intracellular calcium was imparted to the matrix at this site. The dying chondrocytes below this zone did not show mitochondrial granules.

Growth plate of rachitic rats did not show this gradient of intracellular calcium concentration. Only the cells of the hypertrophic cell zone contained mitochondrial granules, indicating a reduction in the calcium binding capacity of chondrocytes in rachitic rats. Figure 2 is a chondrocyte from the hypertrophic zone of a rachitic rat. Intubation with vitamin D_2 restored the mitochondrial granule gradient in the growth plate within 24 hours. Granules were found inside the microvilli of rachitic rat duodenal lining cells but were not present in the mitochondria. Mitochondrial granule concentrations were high within 16 hours following administration of vitamin D. The microvillus granules were absent. Mitochondrial granule numbers were reduced 100% by 24 hours. Figure 3 is an electron micro-

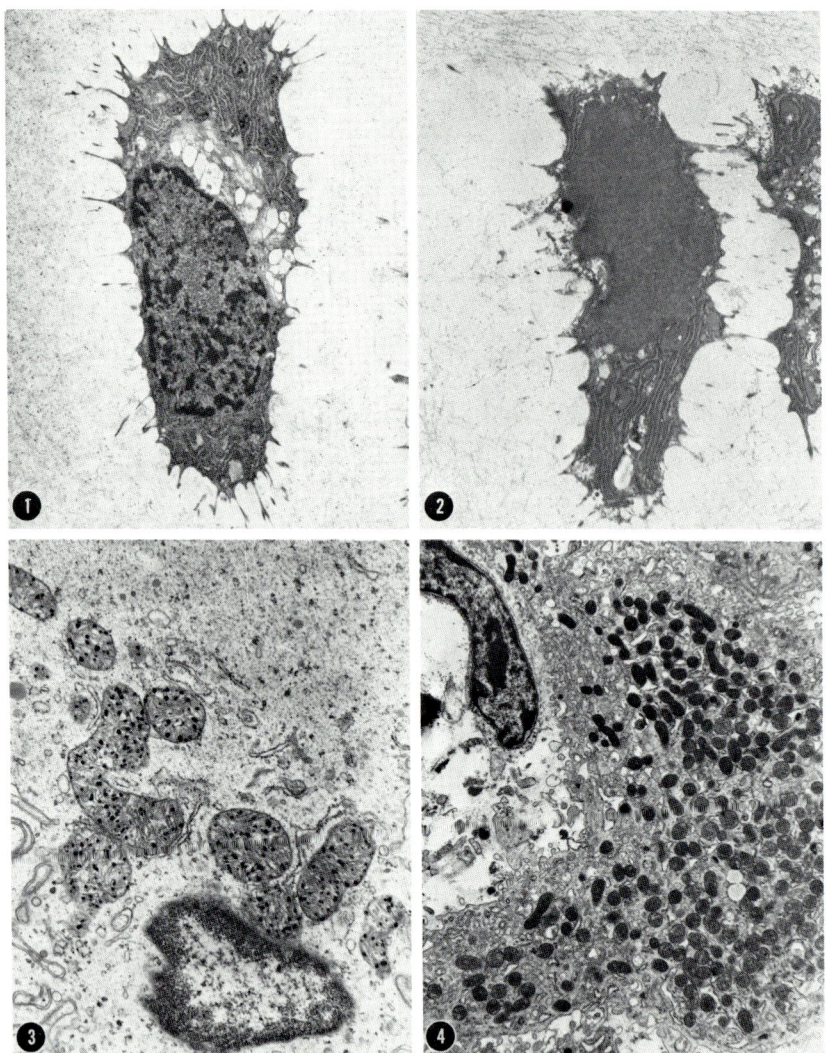

Fig. 1. Electron micrograph of chondrocyte showing electron dense granules in the mitochondria (× 6138)

Fig. 2. Electron micrograph of chondrocyte from 2 week rachitic rat. Mitochondrial granules are absent. (× 4125)

Fig. 3. Electron micrograph of mitochondria from duodenal epithelial cells of rachitic rats following intubation with vitamin D_2. (× 9570)

Fig. 4. Electron micrograph of osteoclast showing intracellular gradient of mitochondrial granule concentration. (× 5973)

graph of the mitochondria of a rachitic rat duodenal cell 16 hours following administration of vitamin D_2.

Osteoclasts, ostecocytes, and osteoblasts also show large numbers of mitochondrial granules. Figure 4 is an electron micrograph of an osteoclast showing mitochondrial granules. In these cells, the mitochondria located in the bone side of the cell cytoplasm have several granules. Mitochondria in the middle of the cell contain fewer granules, and those on the vascular side of the osteoclast have the least number of granules. This intracellular gradient of mitochondrial granule distribution indicates that high

TABLE I

Enzyme Activities (a) and Specific Activities (b) of Different Calf Cartilage Tissues[a]

Enzyme	Nasal septum		Scapula				Costochondral junction			
			Resting		Hypertrophic and Columnar		Resting		Hypertrophic and Columnar	
	a	b	a	b	a	b	a	b	a	b
Cytochrome oxidase	2.0	0.62	11.0	2.48	40	16.3	8.7	0.62	88.4	2.34
Malic acid dehydrogenase	100.0	4.6	190.0	19.3	507	166.0	96.0	6.8	910.0	24.0
Inorganic pyrophosphatase (acid)[b]	6.0	0.29	3.8	0.029	73	4.07	6.6	0.47	180.0	4.75
Inorganic pyrophosphatase (alk)[b]	1.0	0.12	2.0	0.12	83	1.87	2.6	0.19	161.0	4.23
Alkaline phosphatase[b]	0.8	0.35	2.0	0.35	160	32.2	42.0	3.04	1300.0	34.6
Inorganic phosphate	5.0	0.29	6.2	0.55	64	1.33	4.8	0.34	50.0	1.33

[a] Enzyme activity is expressed as micromoles/hour × grams of wet tissue; specific activity is expressed as micromoles/hour × milligrams of soluble protein.

[b] These enzymes are included in this table as this is evidence that they may be involved in calcification events.

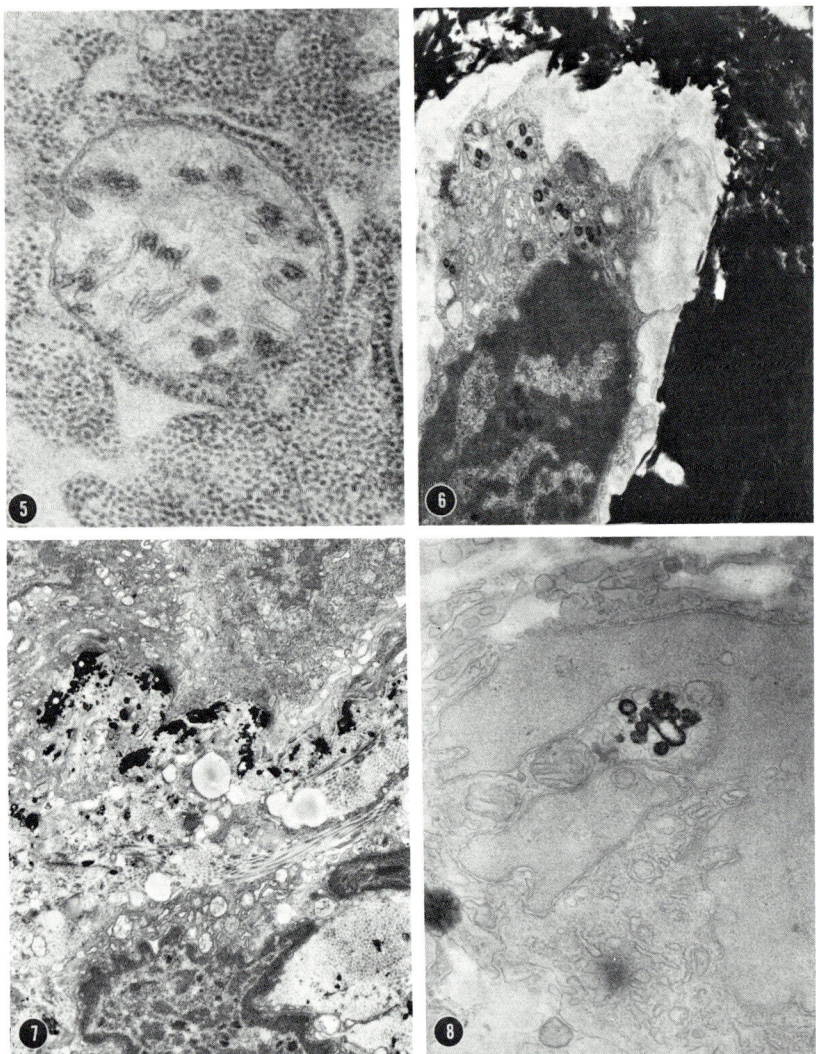

Fig. 5. Electron micrograph of mitochondrion of an osteocyte. Dense granules are associated with the cristae. The mitochondrion is surrounded by rough-surfaced endoplasmic reticulum. ($\times$ 56,430)

Fig. 6. Electron micrograph of osteocyte that contains several granules per mitochondrion. ($\times$ 12,375)

Fig. 7. Electron micrograph of fibrous connective tissue of skin showing deposition of mineral in the matrix following a calciphylactic challenge. ($\times$ 7,414)

Fig. 8. Electron micrograph of cytoplasm of a fibroblast that contains electron-dense spherules following a calciphylactic challenge. ($\times$ 17,050)

intracellular calcium concentractions are present at the resorbing surface but are reduced on the vascular side. The mitochondria presumably act as calcium reservoirs and prevent the entering ionic calcium from reaching toxic cytoplasmic levels. Osteoblasts contain a greater number of mitochondrial granules when engaged in matrix synthesis. Flat osteoblasts that do not appear to be engaged in synthesis as judged by the number of organelles, but which serve as lining cells, do not have large concentration of mitochondrial granules. Granules observed in the synthesizing cells may have contributed their bound calcium to the mineralizing matrix as was seen in the chondrocytes. Osteocytes contain zero to two granules per mitochondrion in the control bones. At 1 hour post parathormone administration, approximately 20% of the osteocytes show granule concentrations in excess of three granules per mitochondrion (Fig. 5 and 6).

Calciphylactic reactions were observed in the skin of rats sensitized with dihydrotachysterol and challenged with pinching and epilation of the skin of the back. A mineralized collagenous matrix was formed within 48 hours (Fig. 7). The first cellular response, seen as early as 1 hour, was the appearance of mitochondrial granules in the fibroblasts. This increase in intracellular mitochondrial granule content was followed by an increase in the number and size of Golgi complexes. Membrane-limited spherules were formed at the Golgi complex. These spherules increased in electron density, and at 6 hours, several electron dense spherules were present in the cell at the plasma membrane. Mitochondrial granules were reduced in number at this stage and were absent at 24 hours. Figure 8 is an electron micrograph of intracellular spherules. Figure 9 is an electron micrograph of the spherules of the preceding figure following ashing at 500°C for 15 minutes. A high mineral content is indicated by the residual ash. Spherules were subsequently released into the collagenous matrix. This event was accompanied by matrix mineralization.

Mitochondrial granules were thus found in cells preceding the onset of mineralization, were found to be vitamin D dependent, and they increased in concentration in osteoclasts, gut epithelial cells, and bone cells following parathormone administration. Thus, mitochondrial granules appear to play a significant role in transcellular movement of calcium and in initiation of mineralization.

The unique relationship between mitochondrial granules and intracellular calcium prompted a further evaluation of the chemical constituents of these granules. Figure 10 is an electron micrograph of a mitochondrion from an intact osteocyte. The granules appear to consist of electron-dense particles suspended in a less dense amorphous matrix. Isolation from homogenized cartilage yielded subcellular fractions including mitochondria. Figure 11 is an electron micrograph of an unstained mitochondrion contain-

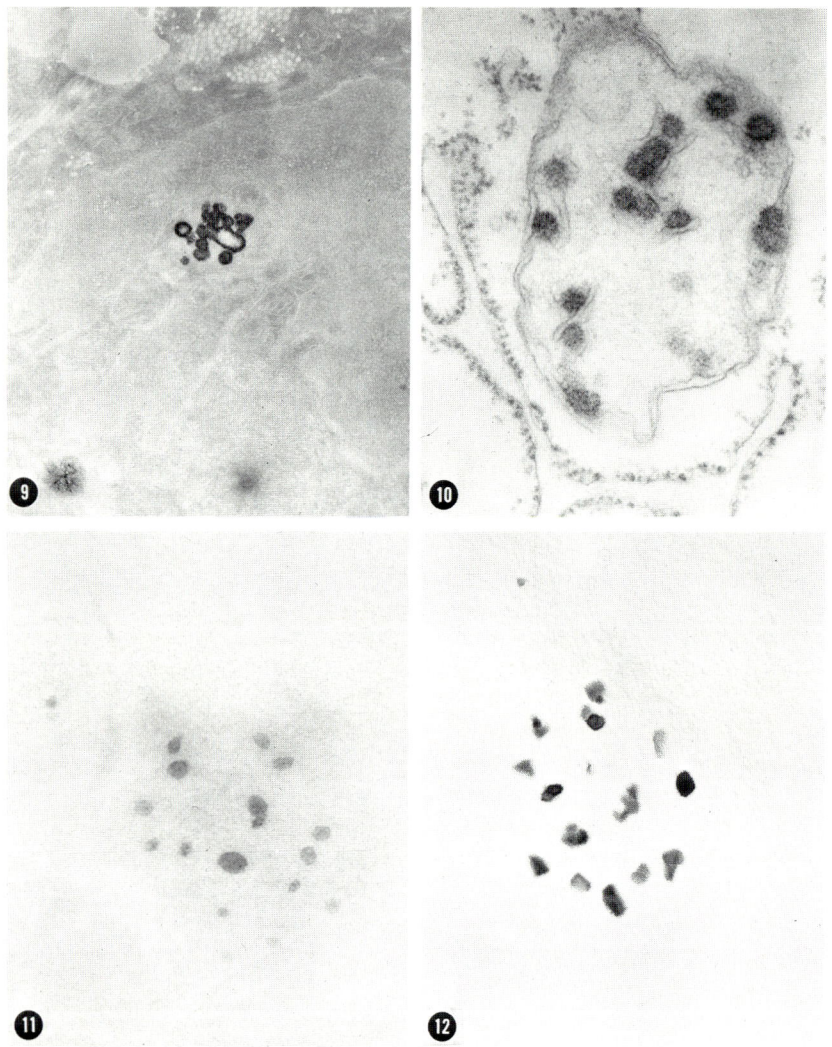

Fig. 9. Electron micrograph of microincinerated cell shown in Fig. 8. The electron-dense spherules persist following incineration at 450°C for 15 minutes. Outlines of cell membranes and organelles are negative images due to the loss of osmium. ($\times$ 17,050)

Fig. 10. Electron micrograph of mitochondrion showing electron-dense granules. This figure is typical of mitochondria in hypertrophic chondrocytes, parthyroid hormone-stimulated osteoblasts, osteoclasts, and osteocytes. The same configuration is seen in calcium-absorbing epithelial cells and fibroblasts preceding calcospherule formation in calciphylaxis. ($\times$ 56,430)

Fig. 11. Electron micrograph of unstained isolated mitochondrion. Electron-dense granules are contained within the mitochondrion. ($\times$ 33,550)

Fig. 12. Electron micrograph of an incinerated, unstained, mitochondrion. The granules persist following burning at 450°C for 15 minutes. ($\times$ 33,550)

ing electron-dense particles following isolation in calcium free media. Ultrasonication of purified mitochondria permitted the isolation of mitochondrial granules (Weinbach, 1967). Figure 12 is an electron micrograph of granules made following microincineration. The presence of inorganic material is confirmed. Preliminary analysis of the organic constituents indicate a high lipid content, protein and RNA measured by the presence of ribose and traces of lysozyme. It was found that essentially no lipid was lost in the EDTA treatment as less than 0.5% of the total lipid was present in the extract after hydrolyses as free fatty acids.

The phospholipid profile of the mitochondrial granules showed that approximately two-thirds of the phospholipids were present as phosphatidlycholine (lecithin). No phosphatidylserine was present in the granules, which would indicate little if any extramitochondrial contamination. Up to 25% of the total phospholipids was present as phosphatidylethanolamine. The presence of close to 5% of diphosphatidylglycerol (cardiolipin) indicates some contamination of the granules with mitochondrial material.

Preliminary data indicate that mitochondria from cartilage are different in their phospholipid profile from those derived from other tissues (liver, spleen, heart, muscle, brain, insect flight muscle). Also, lecithin seems to be the predominant phospholipid of cartilage mitochondria. Whether or not this is due to the large amount of granular material present in the tissue studied is under investigation.

Another unusual finding concerning the mitochondrial granules is what appears to be a high neutral lipid content. While the neutral lipids have not yet been quantitated, the profile showed the presence of cholesterol, cholesterol ester, free fatty acid, a trace of triglyceride, and four other neutral lipids, at present under investigation. If the conventional method of subtracting the weight of the phospholipids from the total lipid extract were applied, one-third of the lipid material would be present as phospholipids. However, due to the high mineral content of the granules, a statement that two-thirds of the total lipid material can be considered neutral lipids does not seem to be justifiable. Quantitative neutral lipid analysis is in progress

Summary

Binding of calcium by mitochondria has been established in liver (Greenawalt et al., 1964; Lehinger et al., 1963), kidney (Deluca and Engstrom, 1961; Engstrom and Deluca, 1964; Vasington and Murphy, 1962), bone and cartilage (Martin and Matthews, 1969, 1970), small intestine

(Cassidy *et al.*, 1969; Matthews *et al.*, 1970), nerve (Sampson *et al.*, 1970; Yates and Yates, 1968), and muscle, as well as avian shell gland (Elder and Schraer, 1969; Hohman and Schraer, 1966) and earthworm calciferous glands (Crang *et al.*, 1968). This uptake has been reported in liver and kidney to be, approximately, 2.7 $\mu\mu$ of calcium per milligram of mitochondrial protein and 1.6 $\mu\mu$ of phosphate per milligram mitochondrial protein (Rossi and Lehninger, 1963; Vasington and Murphy, 1962). Our values of mitochondrial granules showed calcium to be approximately three times in excess of total phosphorus in granules isolated from intact tissue mitochondria. Preliminary crystallographic studies of isolated mitochondrial granules derived from the hypertrophic cartilage zone proved to be up to 30% calcium phosphate with a definite crystalline apatite line by x-ray diffraction as well as infrared absorption. The finding that these absorption bands represent crystalline hydroxyapatite may not indicate that in the intact crystalline hydroxyapatite is present, since amorphous calcium phosphate in the presence of sucrose transforms into crystalline hydroxyapatite within 24 hours at 4°C (Termine, 1970).

The uptake of calcium by mitochondria requires ATP, Mg^{2+}, an oxidizable substrate such as succinate, citrate, or isocitrate, and phosphate and is accompanied by a lowering of pH (Brierley *et al.*, 1963; Lehninger *et al.*, 1963; Rossi and Lehninger, 1963; Vasington and Murphy, 1961, 1962; Wasserman, 1964). This magnesium requirement may account for the relatively high values of magnesium, approximately one-third of the calcium (approximately 3 atoms of Ca/Mg) we find in the isolated granule. Brierley *et al.* (1963) reports that the ratio of calcium to phosphate is approximately 1.5–1.0, whereas Rossi and Lehninger (1963) reported using a value of 1.67 $\pm$ 0.03 atoms of Ca^{2+} per molecule of phosphate. After comparing this value with values we found in the isolated granules from intact tissues, we concluded that not all of the calcium phosphate was apatite.

The uptake of calcium in mitochondria isolated *in vitro* is inhibited by inhibitors of electron transport and uncouplers of phosphorylation, but not by inhibitors of oxidative phosphorylation (Deluca and Engstrom, 1961; Mela, 1969; Rossi and Lehninger, 1963: Vasington and Murphy, 1961, 1962). Carafoli (1970), upon reviewing the literature of calcium binding, concluded that "low-affinity" and "high-affinity" binding sites exist that require no energy, in addition to the energy-linked binding sites. He believes these sites to be mitochondrial phospholipids. Our analyses have shown most of the granule phospholipid to be lecithin, a poor calcium binder at neutral pH. It has also been demonstrated that phosphate incorporation into mitochondrial phospholipids is dependent upon oxidative phosphorylation and that the omission of calcium has no effect upon incorporation of phosphate (Taylor, 1969). This latter observation has bearing on our hypothesis of the possible presence of a mitochondrial calcium binding site, which might account for the calcium to phosphate ratios reported here, calcium and phosphate being concentrated independently.

Investigators have reported that vitamin D causes mitochondrial swelling and a disruption of cristae organization (Deluca *et al.*, 1960a,b). Finkelstein and Schachter (1962) reported that vitamin D repleted rats bind more ^{47}Ca at 0°–5°C than a corresponding fraction from deficient animals, and Scarpelli *et al.* (1959) has shown that massive doses of vitamin D causes mitochondrial damage accompanied by the accumulation of citrate and calcium. In our experiments, vitamin D appears to be essential for calcium transport through the cell, an event which is signaled by a transient rise in mitochondrial granules. The precise role of the organic granule constitutuents remains to be established. Although a calcium-binding protein and phospholipid was anticipated, the ribonucleoproteins have not as yet been considered.

A large amount of calcium exists within the mitochondria in some aggregated, nonionic form. The function of this phenomenon is presently unknown. Some possible explanation might be that it acts as a body store or reservoir for calcium (Rasmussen *et al.*, 1963), as a regulator of intracellular calcium levels (Rasmussen, 1966; Wasserman, 1964; Matthews *et al.*, 1970), or as a shuttle system for the transcellular movement of ions across the cell (Hamilton and Holdsworth, 1969; Halstead, 1969; Rasmussen, 1966; Wasserman, 1964). Their dependence upon vitamin D; variation with parathormone; relation to calcium absorption, osteolysis, and bone resorption, calciphylaxis; and onset of mineralization strongly suggest a direct relationship to the homeostatic mechanism and mineralization. Additional work is necessary to establish the interrelationships between the mineral and organic constituents.

REFERENCES

Anderson, H. D. (1969). *J. Cell Biol.* **41**, 59.
Bonnuchi, E. (1969). *Calcif. Tissue Res.* **3**, 38.
Brierley, G. P., Murer, E., and Green, D. E. (1963). *Science* **140**, 60.
Cameron, D. A., Paschall, H. A., and Robinson, R. A. (1967). *J. Cell Biol.* **33**, 1.
Carafoli, E. (1970). *Biochem. J.* **116**, 2.
Cassidy, M. M., Galdner, A. M., and Tidball, C. S. (1969). *Amer. J. Physiol.* **217**, 680.
Crang, R. E., Holsen, R. C., and Hitt, J. B. (1968). *BioScience* **18**, 299.
Deluca, H. F., and Engstrom, G. W. (1961). *Proc. Nat. Acad. Sci. U.S.* **47**, 1744.

Deluca, H. F., Reiser, S., and Steenbock, H. (1960a). *Fed. Proc., Fed. Amer. Soc. Exp. Biol.* **19,** 419.
Deluca, H. F., Reiser, S., Steenbock, H., and Koesberg, P. (1960b). *Biochim. Biophys. Acta* **50,** 526.
Elder, J. A., and Schraer, H. (1969). *Fed. Proc., Fed. Amer. Soc. Exp. Biol.* **28,** 284.
Engstrom, G. W., and Deluca, H. F. (1964). *Biochemistry* **3,** 379.
Finkelstein, J. D., and Schachter, D. (1962). *Amer. J. Physiol.* **203,** 873.
Greenawalt, J. W., Rossi, C. S., and Lehninger, A. L. (1964). *J. Cell Biol.* **23,** 21.
Halstead, L. B. (1969). *Calcif. Tissue Res.* **3,** 103.
Hamilton, J. W., and Holdsworth, E. S. (1969). *Calcif. Tissue Res.* **4,** 284.
Hohman, W., and Schraer, H. (1966). *J. Cell Biol.* **30,** 317.
Johnston, D. M. (1953). *J. Biophys. Biochem. Cytol.* **4,** 163.
Kashiwa, H. K. (1966). *Stain Technol.* **41,** 49.
Kuettner, K. W., Guenther, H. L., Ray, R. D., and Schumacher, F. B. (1968). *Calcif. Tissue Res.* **1,** 298.
Lehninger, A. L., Rossi, C. S., and Greenawalt, J. W. (1963). *Biochem. Biophys. Res. Commun.* **10,** 444.
Martin, J. H., and Matthews, J. L. (1969). *Calcif. Tissue Res.* **3,** 184.
Martin, J. H., and Matthews, J. L. (1970). *Clin. Orthop.* **68,** 273.
Matthews, J. L., Martin, J. H., Lynn, J. A., and Collins, E. J. (1968). *Calcif. Tissue Res.* **1,** 330.
Matthews, J. L., Martin, J. H., Sampson, H. W., Kunin, A. S., and Roan, J. H. (1970). *Calcif. Tissue Res.* **5,** 91.
Mela, L. (1969). *Biochemistry* **8,** 2481.
Nichols, G. (1970). *Calcif. Tissue Res.* **4,** Suppl., 61.
Rasmussen, H. (1966). *Fed. Proc., Fed. Amer. Soc. Exp. Biol.* **25,** 903.
Rasmussen, H., Deluca, H., Arnaud, C., Hawker, C., and von Stedingk, M. (1963). *J. Clin. Invest.* **42,** 1940.
Rossi, C. S., and Lehninger, A. L. (1963). *Biochem. Z.* **338,** 698.
Salomon, C. D., and Ray, R. D. (1966). *J. Bone Joint Surg.*, **48A,** 1575.
Sampson, H. W., Dill, R. E., Matthews, J. L., and Martin, J. H. (1970). *Brain Res.* **22,** 157.
Scarpelli, D. G., Tremblay, G., and Pease, A. (1959). *Fed. Proc., Fed. Amer. Soc. Exp. Biol.* **18,** 504.
Schenk, R. K., Spiro, D., and Wiener, J. (1967). *J. Cell Biol.* **34,** 175.
Schnieder, W. (1955). *Methods Enzymol.* **3,** 680.
Sobel, A. E., Burger, P. A., and Laurence, P. A. (1960). *Trans. N. Y. Acad. Sci.* [2] **22,** 233.
Taylor, D. D. (1969). *Biochem. J.* **111,** 665.
Termine, J. (1970). Personal communication.
Thomas, R. S., and Greenawalt, J. E. (1968). *J. Cell Biol.* **39,** 55.
Urist, M. R. (1966). *Clin. Orthop. Related Res.* **44,** 13.
Vasington, F. D., and Murphy, J. V. (1961). *Fed. Proc., Fed. Amer. Soc. Exp. Biol.* **20,** 146.
Vasington, F. D., and Murphy, J. V. (1962). *J. Biol. Chem.* **237,** 2670.
Wasserman, R. H. (1964). *N. Y. State J. Med.* **64,** 1329.
Weinbach, E. C. (1967). *Biochim. Biophys. Acta* **148,** 256.
Yates, R. D., and Yates, J. C. (1968). *Z. Zellforsch. Mikrosk. Anat.* **91,** 388.

Discussion

Dr. Urist: The chemical morphology of the mitochondrial granules warrant some comment. The size and numbers of mitochondrial granules are clear, but some incorrect statements have been made about the histochemistry. Several speakers have mentioned the Kashiwa GBHA method as though it were a stain for calcium phosphate. The Kashiwa stain in the concentrations used on calcified tissues localizes protein-bound calcium, not apatitic calcium; it may stain protein–calcium–phosphate complexes, having a Ca/P ratio of 1.0; it does not stain inorganic apatite crystals at the concentrations of the dye used for histology. Indeed, this fact is the fundamental principle of the Kashiwa method of staining hypertrophic chondrocytes, osteoblasts, and osteocytes.

The GBHA reaction depends upon exposing a block of tissue to a stain-fixative solution. The fixative is alcohol in an alkaline solution at pH of about 10; the alcohol dehydrates and fixes the tissue while the high pH drives the reaction between calcium and intracellular protein toward formation of protein–calcium and protein–calcium–phosphate complexes. The stain, GBHA, hydroxyanil glyoxal bis, chelates calcium bound to protein. Brushite crystals may bind some dye *in vitro*, but tricalcium phosphates and apatites do not.

A different but related question is about the function of mitochondrial granules. Are the granules formed as a defense mechanism of the cell against unphysiological intracellular concentrations of the calcium ion? The quantity of intracellular calcium is normally very small, in general, less than 1.0 mmole per kilogram of soft tissue. Normally, the living cell has defense mechanisms against influx of concentrations of calcium which make mitochondrial granules *in vitro*. I think that we must try to answer the question of whether the mitochondrial granules are a defense mechanism against high intracellular calcium concentrations and whether mitochondria have something to do with calcification.

Dr. Matthews: I think that it depends on what you mean by "defense mechanism." I assume that you mean that you consider that there is some intracellular level which is toxic, and I would agree with that. Since mitochondrial granules increase with increased calcium loads, the mitochondria would be a "defense mechanism." But also, in that sense, granule counts appear to be a valid means of indexing the level of calcium within the cell.

Dr. Talmage: There is no reason why a process which teleologically began as a "defensive" mechanism for the cell cannot, through evolutionary processes, become an "offensive" mechanism.

Dr. Urist: The calcification mechanism controls the deposition of large quantities of calcium outside the cell membrane, in spaces in and between collagen fibrils. If the microcrystalites are at first subcrystalline, then crystalline, what are the dimensions of the granules, and are they subcrystalline or crystalline in the mitochondria in the intact tissue *in vivo*?

Dr. Matthews: We asked Dr. Termine the question about apatite in granules and sent him some of the lyophilized granule preparations as prepared by Drs. Arsenis and Kuettner. He reported to us that, of the mineral present, he found 30% apatite. But his procedure required some time and getting it to him required some time. The question was asked, how long would it take for the granules to convert from some amorphous bound form to the apatite form under the conditions imposed? He reported that, within the experimental period, 30% conversion to apatite would be anticipated.

Dr. DeLuca: First, I would like to offer a comment. I think that your results with the brush border particularly are interesting, because it seems to correlate well with a lot of data that have been obtained both in our laboratory and elsewhere, inasmuch as we feel that the primary site of vitamin D action is at the brush border surface. I was particularly confused by an early portion of your discussion in regard to the cartilage study in rickets in which you concluded that phosphate did not play a role.

Dr. Matthews: Let me clarify that. We used two situations. The first time I did the rachitic study on the growth plate, we used a diet which was deficient in both vitamin D and phosphate. When I first reported our findings, the question was posed, don't you have a diet that did not involve both a phosphate deficiency and vitamin D deficiency? We repeated the experiment with a diet that was vitamin D-deficient, but phosphate sufficient, and in that experiment we concluded that the effects observed earlier were not as dependent on phosphate deficiency as on vitamin D deficiency.

Dr. DeLuca: Does that mean that granules are not formed? Or are granules formed in the case of the diet that has normal amounts of phosphate, but deficient in vitamin D?

Dr. Talmage: Phosphate-rich animals showed the same picture as phosphate deficient?

Dr. Matthews: Yes, they did.

Dr. DeLuca: Then does this mean that you saw rachitic lesions in this diet or not?

Dr. Matthews: All we saw in rats fed this diet was elongation of the growth plate with reduction in mineralization below the hypertrophic area. I was told this is only possible with one strain of rats. With Holzman rats we succeeded in getting growth plate effects with phosphate-sufficient diets, whereas other rats require a phosphate deficiency.

Dr. Lloyd: I would like to ask about the granules which are not in mitochondria. Do I understand you to say that these other granules are Kashiwa-like granules, and are these granules in the Golgi apparatus, which suggests that they might be secreted? Second, if that is true, do you think that these granules could arise in and be associated with the lysosomes in the cells. The reason I ask this question is that a group in the biology division at Argonne have observed by activation analysis that minerals such as potassium, iron, and Zinc bind much more to lysosomal membranes than to mitochondrial membranes. Unfortunately, they have not so far looked at calcium binding. I wonder whether you think these other granules could be in the lysosomes.

Dr. Matthews: Not unless lysosomes bud off the Golgi and are then secreted. I can show you that these vesicles are budded off Golgi lamellae and are extruded intact from the cell. I think we would have to regard them as some sort of typical secretory-type vesicle, as opposed to lysosomes. Your first question was, did I think these were Kashiwa-type granules. I would have preferred to call them Matthew's granules, but in deference to Dr. Kashiwa's prior work, I have to say that I think that they correspond in size and number to the granules he described. I have not, however, used GHBA on the calciphylactic response to confirm this.

Dr. Kashiwa: As you know, Dr. Matthews, we use ultra thick, hand sectioned fresh bone. We were forced to use thick fresh bone sections because manipulation, such as fixation or dehydration, depleted the cells' calcium. If we fix the tissue with osmium, then we do indeed see something like mitochondrial calcium. Do you think that calcium is really present in the mitochondria in cells *in vivo*? We could not show such an insoluble form of calcium in osteoblasts or in chondrocytes stained fresh. Although you did not put calcium in your osmium, you do have a lot of tissue calcium around which could have diffused into the mitochondria.

Dr. Matthews: I think the only answer I can give is that if it were strictly a case of fixation, one would not expect to see the growth plate gradient distribution we have shown. Nor would you expect to see variations under other physiological conditions. I do believe it is quite possible that calcium could be added from cells or media in the preparation. I do believe, though, that mitochondrial granules have been seen in cells by Pease, who froze these in liquid nitrogen. This is a freeze-etching type technique and has produced some elegant configurations of granules.

Dr. Kashiwa: That is manipulation.

Dr. Talmage: This is one of the instances of uncertainty in electron microscopy, but unfortunately it is one of the problems we have to live with in order to use these techniques.

Dr. Nichols: You have shown us beautiful pictures of mitochondrial granules and you have shown that, in calciphylaxsis, there are Kashiwa granules or Matthews granules which seem to pass from cells into the matrix. But at the beginning, you specifically commented that you had never been able to show a mitochondrial granule or a mitochondrion going down a cell process. The really burning question is, have you been able to find in the natural process, the noncalciphylaxsis process, the granule in a bone or cartilage cell going down its process and popping out at the end?

Dr. Matthews: I haven't seen this either in cartilage cells or in bone cells. The only place I have seen what appeared to me to be secretory-type granules, as related to the onset of calcification, was in the calciphylactic response.

Several persons who have talked here in the past day or so have been looking at the tiny vesicles associated with the cells. If, as we observed in the calciphylactic response, the mitochondria unload as some type of secretory event occurs, then bone and cartilage cell mitochondria may also unload on some nongranular carrier. I have not seen mineral inside vesicles, however.

BONE FORMATION AND RESORPTION BY OSTEOCYTES*

D. Baylink and J. Wergedal

Introduction

During the past decade, there has been a renewed interest in osteocyte metabolism, because it now seems clear that these cells are not metabolically inactive. Bélanger and co-workers (1963) have demonstrated that osteocytes are capable of removing matrix as well as mineral from their perilacunar regions, and Baud has presented electron micrographic evidence for bone resorption by osteocytes (Baud, 1962). A number of recent studies utilizing such methods as electron microscopy (Baud, 1968), autoradiography (Young, 1963), and tetracycline labeling (Baylink and Bernstein, 1967; Vittali, 1968) have supplied indirect evidence for bone formation by osteocytes.

Bone functions as a mechanical support and as a mineral reservoir, and osteocytes may be involved in both these functions. Based on the assumption that osteocytes are capable of forming bone, it has been suggested that osteocytes might heal ultramicroscopic defects in bone and thus prevent the development of microfractures (Baylink and Bernstein, 1967) which would impair bone strength. In addition, the hypothesis has been advanced that osteocytes play an important role in serum calcium homeostasis (Vittali, 1968; Talmage, 1967). Osteocytes could effect calcium homeo-

---

* This study was supported in part by grants from the U.S. Public Health Service AM-09096, DE-02600, and HD-04872.

stasis through changes in formation and resorption, or as suggested by Marshall (1969), through exerting some control over long term exchange. Because the osteocyte population is huge, a small change in osteocyte metabolism could mediate the rapidly occurring effects of calcitonin and parathyroid hormone on bone.

Despite the considerable evidence that osteocytes are metabolically active, the specific functional role played by osteocytes in bone and mineral metabolism remains uncertain, mainly because there are almost no quantitative studies on osteocyte metabolism. Therefore, the present study was undertaken to quantitate one of the functional processes of osteocytic metabolism, that of bone formation. In this study we demonstrate that osteocytes actually do form bone and we compare the amount of bone formed by osteocytes to that formed by osteoblasts in a sampling site within the femoral diaphysis. In addition, we make an estimate of bone resorption by osteocytes.

Methods

Osteocytic bone formation was determined by measuring the increase in osteocyte perilacunar tetracycline label width and the decrease in osteocyte lacunar area in sections of bone from groups of rats sacrificed after having received daily tetracycline injections for varying periods up to 17 days. All rats in this study were fed a semisynthetic diet containing 0.6% calcium and 0.6% phosphorus (Wergedal, 1969), except for one group which was fed a calcium-free diet ($<0.01\%$ calcium) for 5 days in order to stimulate bone resorption (Stauffer et al., 1971).

Protocol

Twenty-four male Sprague–Dawley rats were divided into four groups of six animals each. At the beginning of the experimental period, when the rats were 31 days of age, the first group received a single intravenous injection of tetracycline, 20 mg per kilogram of body weight, and was sacrificed 2 hours later. At the same time that the first group was injected with tetracycline iv, the three remaining groups were started on daily ip injections of 20 mg/kg body weight of tetracycline. The second group was sacrificed after 3 days of tetracycline injections, the third group after 7 days, and the fourth group after 17 days. In addition, rats 55 days of age and older were sacrificed after receiving tetracycline for varying periods of time.

In a separate experiment, procion was used to evaluate perilacunar matrix formation. Thirty-one-day-old rats were given either a single iv injection or ip injections every third day for varying periods up to 17 days of procion H8BS, 100 mg/kg (Prescott et al., 1968).

Section Preparation

Preparation of Ground Sections for Microscopic Measurements

After sacrifice, the left femurs were removed, dissected free of soft tissues, and accurately bisected. Three consecutive transverse ground sections, about 30 μ thick, were then prepared from the distal end of the bisected femur from each rat. All sections were mounted in Abopon, a water-soluble nonfluorescent mounting medium. Many of the parameters which were measured on these sections are illustrated schematically in Fig. 1. For some studies, tibias were used, in which case sections were made from the proximal portion of the shaft after transection at the fibular junction (Baylink et al., 1970).

Demineralized Sections

H & E-stained paraffin sections were prepared from demineralized segments of the midfemoral diaphysis from the 38-day-old rats to measure the linear dimensions of osteoblasts. Unstained paraffin sections and ground

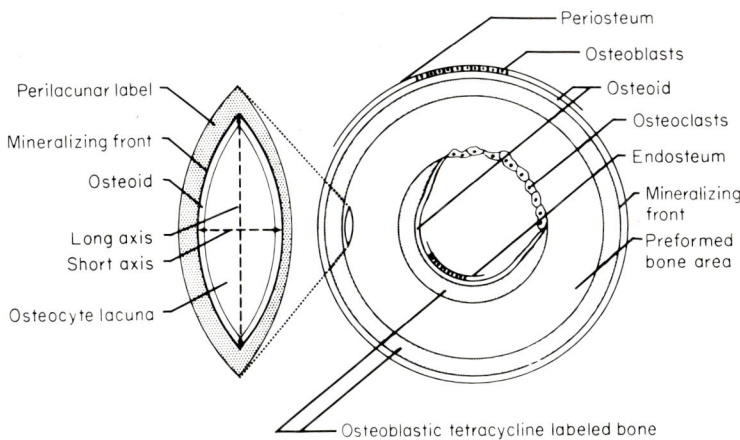

Fig. 1. Schema of measured parameters in femoral cross section. Since this section is considered to be 1 mm thick, measurements of those areas depicted on the right can be directly converted to volumes. For example, the preformed bone area in a 1 mm thick section is considered to be the preformed bone volume.

sections were prepared from the femurs of the procion-treated rats to evaluate perilacunar procion labels.

Histochemical Procedures

Intense acid phosphatase activity within lacunae was used to determine distribution of resorbing osteocytes in fresh, unfixed sawed sections by means of a previously described method using α-naphthol phosphate as the substrate (Wergedal and Baylink, 1969). Perilacunar osteoid was identified by its metachromatic reaction to toluidine blue (Baylink *et al.*, 1968); in order to avoid demineralization during staining, unfixed ground sections were stained in an aqueous solution of toluidine blue and for only 3 minutes. Perilacunar osteoid was also visualized, because of its relatively low refractive index, by interference-contrast microscopy.

Infiltration of Bone Pores with Fluorescent Plastic

Mineralized segments of the femur were infiltrated with Epon 812, which was doped with 0.8% (w/v) rhodamine B, by immersing the bone in doped Epon within a pressure bomb and subjecting the system to 10 atm of pressure. After polymerization, ground sections were made and viewed by fluorescence microscopy to evaluate the caliber of canaliculi.

Sampling Procedure for Microscopic Measurements

Measurements were made of about 100 osteocytes in the lateral-posterior half of the three diaphyseal cross sections from each rat femur. By measuring only osteocytes which were within 10 μ of the inner border of the periosteal appositional tetracycline label, the osteocytes sampled were of a specific age which could be readily calculated (Fig. 2; also see calculations). In this region all osteocytes, which had perilacunar tetracycline labels and whose lacunar dimensions enlarged as one focused in toward the center of the section, were measured.

Microscopic Measurements

Osteocyte Perilacunar Tetracycline Label Width and the Long and Short Axes of Osteocyte Lacunae

These three parameters, which are illustrated in Fig. 1, were measured on each labeled osteocyte using a filar micrometer and a magnification of 1250 ×. Fluorescence microscopy was used for measurements of perilacunar label width and bright field microscopy for measurements of the long and short axes of the lacunae. Measurements of lacunar axes were in the sampling site described above and also in osteocytes within 10 μ of the endosteal osteoclastic resorbing surface in group 3. The label was wider on one side of the lacunae than the other. Perilacunar label width was measured in the central third of the wider label in all groups. In group 3, both the narrow and wide label widths were measured and the ratio of these widths was used to estimate the narrow label width in the remaining groups.

Number of Osteocytes per Unit Volume of Bone

The number of osteocytes observed within the area of an ocular grid and throughout the depth of the section was counted using an objective with a depth of focus longer than the section thickness. All osteocyte lacunae, including those opening into the top and bottom of the section, were counted in two fields per quadrant of the cross section. Counts were made in "thin" ($\sim$ 30 μ) and in "thick" ($\sim$ 60 μ) sections. Section thickness was measured with a mechanical gauge* in the same four positions in which cell counts were made. The mean number of osteocytes per grid area in the thin section was subtracted from that in the thick section to obtain the number of osteocytes per grid area in the depth of bone equal to the difference in thickness between the two sections.

Area of Perilacunar Labeled Bone in the Preformed Bone Area

The preformed bone area is that area of bone located between the osteoblastic periosteal and endosteal appositional labels in a 1 mm thick section (Fig. 1). In group 3, the percentage area of perilacunar labeled bone within the preformed bone area was measured by the point counting method (Frost, 1962a).

Endosteal Tetracycline-Labeled Area, Periosteal Tetracycline-Labeled Width and Area, Bone Area, Medullary Area, and Preformed Bone Area

These areas were measured on a Grafacon tablet† from microscopic images formed on the tablet by means of camera lucida. The periosteal tetracycline label width in the lateral–posterior portion of the cortex was measured with a filar micrometer.

Dimensions of Osteoblasts

These measurements were made on H & E-stained paraffin sections using an ocular micrometer. Width and length of osteoblasts were measured in

* Mikrokator, C E J Gage Co., Dearborn, Michigan.
† Model 1010A Bolt Beranek, Newman, Inc., Santa Ana, California.

cross sections and depth in longitudinal sections. No correction was made for shrinkage, which was probably at least 26% (Baylink et al., 1970).

CALCULATIONS

Osteocyte Lacunar Area and Volume

In order to calculate osteocyte lacunar area from the measured lacunar axes, lacunar area was measured with a planimeter, and the long and short axes were measured with a vernier caliper on photographs of seventy-five osteocytes within the sampling site. When the formula for an ellipse was used to calculate lacunar area from the measured long and short axes, there was a strong correlation between the calculated and the measured lacunar areas ($r = 0.93$, $p < .001$). However, the calculated lacunar area was slightly overestimated by this formula, and therefore, the following emperical formula, which exactly predicted the lacunar area, was derived:

$$A = \pi SL/4.47, \qquad (1)$$

where A is the osteocyte lacunar area, S is the short axis, and L is the long axis of the osteocyte lacunae.

Osteocyte lacunar depth was measured in longitudinal rather than in cross sections and only in the first group of rats. Osteocyte lacunar volume was calculated from lacunar depth by substituting Eq. 1 into the formula for a sphere,

$$V = 2D/3 \, (\pi LS/4.47), \qquad (2)$$

where V is lacunar volume and D is lacunar depth.

Osteocyte Age

Considering that an osteoblast becomes an osteocyte when it becomes embedded in osteoid, the age of osteocytes in the sampling site was calculated by the following formula:

$$\text{Age} = N + D/R_a, \qquad (3)$$

where N is the number of days of tetracycline administration, R_a is the rate of periosteal osteoblastic bone apposition, and D is the distance of the osteocyte sampled from the osteoblastic-osteoid interface at the beginning of the tetracycline labeling period (Fig. 2). D was calculated by adding the periosteal osteoid width, the 2 hour periosteal osteoblastic label width,*

---

* This is essentially equivalent to the width of the mineralizing front (Baylink et al., 1970).

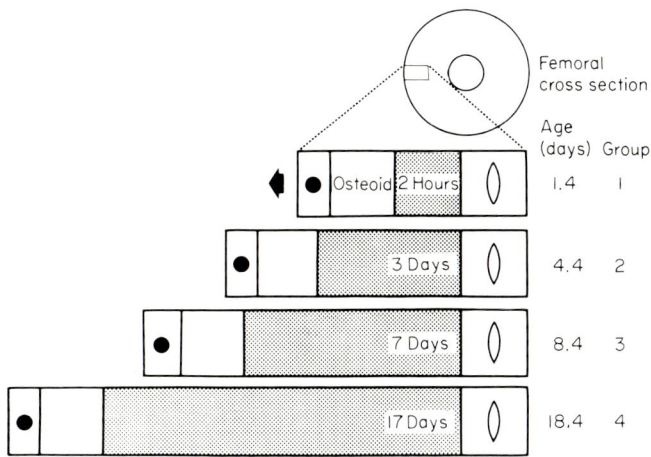

FIG. 2. Schema of the osteocyte sampling procedure. The enlarged bars represent segments of periosteal bone from each of the four groups of rats, the nucleated rectangles are osteoblasts, and the stippled areas are the bone areas labeled with tetracycline by osteoblastic bone formation. The length of the tetracycline labeling period is shown in the stippled area. The arrow indicates the direction of osteoblastic bone formation. Since all groups were injected with tetracycline at the same time, the inner border of the osteoblastic tetracycline label was in the same position in all rats at the beginning of the experiment. Therefore, the osteocytes sampled in all groups were of the same age at the beginning of the experiment. If one considers that an osteocyte is zero days old when it becomes embedded in osteoid, the age of the osteocytes sampled in each group is equivalent to the time required to form the width of bone between the osteoid surface and the osteocyte sampled. This width was measured and converted to time, as indicated at the right of each bar, from measurements of the periosteal osteoblastic bone apposition rate.

and the mean distance ($5\ \mu$) of the osteocytes from the periosteal osteoblastic tetracycline label.

Osteocytic Bone Formation Rate

This is the total volume of bone formed by osteocytes in the sampling site in a 1 mm thick section and was calculated for group 3 by adding the volume formed by osteocytes in newly formed bone (periosteal and endosteal tetracycline-labeled bone) to that formed by osteocytes in preformed bone.

The volume of bone formed by osteocytes in newly formed bone (i.e., by osteocytes 7 days or less in age) was calculated as follows. The mean lacunar volume at day zero was calculated from the measured axes using Eq. 2. Since the lacunar dimensions at day 7 (group 3) were not measured, they were calculated by subtracting the corrected wide and narrow perilacunar label widths in group 3 from each of the lacunar dimensions in group 1, and these values were used to calculate the mean lacunar volume at day 7. The difference between the mean lacunar volume on day zero and on day 7 is the mean volume of bone formed per osteocyte in those osteocytes 7 days of age. The volume of bone formed by osteocytes within the periosteal and endosteal osteoblastic appositional labels—i.e., by osteocytes 7 days of age or younger—was obtained by multiplying the total number of osteocytes in this labeled bone by half the amount of bone formed per osteocyte in 7 days. The number of osteocytes in this age range was calculated by multiplying the measured number of osteocytes per cubic millimeter of bone by the volume of periosteal and endosteal labeled bone in a 1 mm thick section.

The volume of bone formed by osteocytes in preformed bone (Fig. 1) (i.e., by osteocytes older than 7 days of age) was calculated as follows. The measured percentage area of perilacunar labeled bone in the preformed bone area was converted to specific volume, which is the percent volume in an infinitely thin section (Frost, 1962a), by correcting for the focal depth of the objective used. The specific volume of perilacunar labeled bone was multiplied by the preformed bone volume to obtain the volume of perilacunar labeled bone. To calculate the volume of bone formed from this labeled bone volume, it was necessary to correct for the volume of the perilacunar mineralizing front: the values obtained for the perilacunar labeled volume were multiplied by the factor 0.59, which was derived from the ratio between mineralizing front and label widths in group 3, assuming that this ratio was a mean value for osteocytes of different ages.

Rates of Periosteal Osteoblastic Bone Apposition and Total Osteoblastic Bone Formation

In group 3, the periosteal bone apposition rate, which is the width of new bone added per day (along the lateral–posterior portion of the femoral cortex), was calculated by dividing the 7 day periosteal label width minus the 2 hour label width (i. e., mineralizing front width) by 7 days. The total bone formation rate, which is the volume of bone formed per day at the periosteum and the endosteum in a 1 mm thick section, was calculated as previously described (Baylink *et al.*, 1970).

Endosteal Osteoclastic Bone Resorption Rate

This rate was calculated as previously described (Baylink *et al.*, 1970) for group 3 from measurements of medullary area in groups 1 and 3 and endosteal labeled area in group 3.

Pore Volume Measurements

Mercury porosimetry is a standard engineering method used in materials testing for determining pore volumes and pore radii in porous materials (Winslow and Shapiro, 1959). The porosimeter* used in this work was capable of pressures up to 15,000 pounds per square inch, thus permitting measurements of pores as small as 0.006 μ in radius. Because of the small size of the bone samples measured, it was necessary to construct a special small sample chamber with a volume of 0.37 cc in order to achieve adequate sensitivity.

Mercury porosimetry was used to measure lacunar–canalicular volume in the femoral diaphyses from five 31- and five 38-day-old rats. The results obtained were used in calculating the rate of osteocytic bone resorption. Measurements were made on 1 cm diaphyseal segments of the two femurs from each rat after noncollagenous protein had been removed by extraction with 0.1 N NaOH for 72 hours and fat had been removed by extraction with chloroform–methanol in a Soxhlet apparatus for 24 hours.

In this method, the volume of mercury forced into bone pores is determined as a function of the pressure applied. Because the caliber of the pores filled is a function of the pressure applied, one can calculate the radius as well as the volume of the various pores in bone (Winslow and Shapiro, 1959). Since canaliculi are circular to elliptical in cross section (Baud, 1969), their radii were calculated by the equation derived by Washburn which obtains for pores that are circular in shape (Washburn, 1921),

$$r = -2\sigma \cos \theta / P, \tag{4}$$

where σ is the surface tension of mercury, θ is the contact angle of mercury and bone, P is the pressure applied, and r the radius of the smallest canaliculi filled at pressure P. The surface tension of mercury used in this calculation was 473 dynes/cm (Winslow and Shapiro, 1959) and the contact angle of mercury and bone was 130°, a value obtained by direct measurement.

The distribution of pore volume as a function of pore radius was obtained by first calculating the distribution function, $D(r)$ by formula,

$$D(r) = dV/dr, \tag{5}$$

where dV is the total volume of all pores of radii between r and $r + dr$ (Ritter and Drake, 1945), and then plotting $D(r)$ against r. The application of this method to measurements of lacunar–canalicular pores is described in detail in a separate publication (Baylink et al., 1971).

* Model No. 5-7119, American Instrument Company, Inc., Silver Springs, Maryland.

Precision

When the various morphological measurements were made in duplicate, the measuring error ranged from $\pm 5\%$ to $\pm 14\%$. Because the changes in osteocytic bone formation with time were considerably larger than these measuring errors, we were able to quantitate satisfactorily these changes in formation.

Duplicate measurements on three bone samples by mercury porosimetry gave almost identical pore volume distribution curves for each sample. Before the second measurement, the mercury remaining in the bone from the first measurement was removed by heat (110°C) and vacuum (0.05 mm Hg).

Results

Location of Osteocytes Displaying Perilacunar Tetracycline Labels

Perilacunar tetracycline labeling was observed in all bones examined (calvaria, spine, femur, tibia, and other long bones), and was most prominent in the femoral diaphysis. In the femur and in other long bones, perilacunar labeling was most extensive adjacent to periosteal osteoblastic appositional tetracycline labels. In general, the number of osteocytes with perilacunar labels and the width of these labels were positively correlated with the rate of osteoblastic apposition and the degree of vascularity. Thus, the rate of periosteal osteoblastic apposition, the degree of vascularity, and the amount of perilacunar labeling were all greater in the lateral–posterior than in the medial–anterior portion of the femoral

TABLE I

WIDTH OF PERILACUNAR TETRACYCLINE LABELS

Group	Duration of tetracycline administration	Osteocyte age (days)	Perilacunar label width[a] (μ)
1	2 hours	1.4	$0.50 \pm .03$
2	3 days	4.4	$0.90 \pm .13$
3	7 days	8.4	$1.09 \pm .17$ $(0.91 \pm .15)$[b]
4	17 days	18.4	$1.30 \pm .14$

[a] Mean $\pm$ S.D.

[b] Labels were wider on one side of the lacuna than the other; only the wide label values are given except in group 3, where the narrow label value is shown in parenthesis.

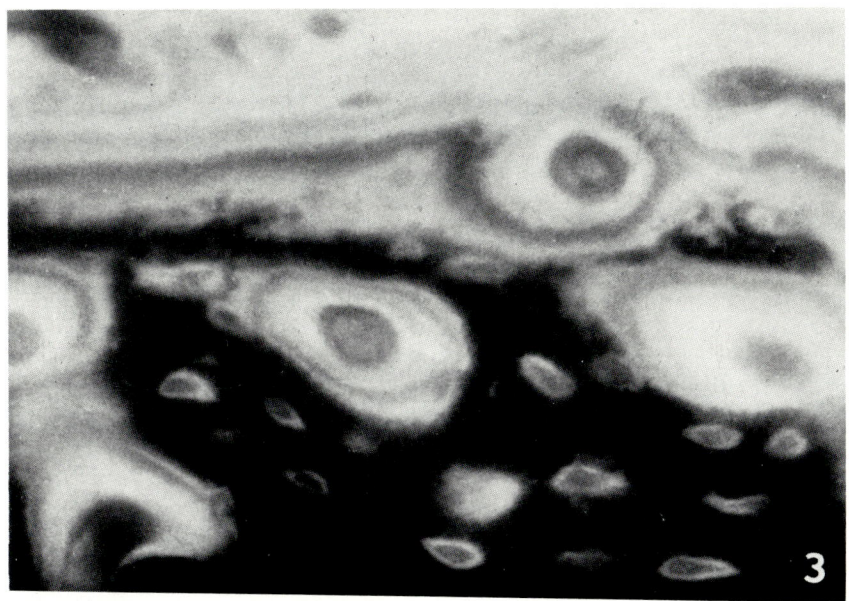

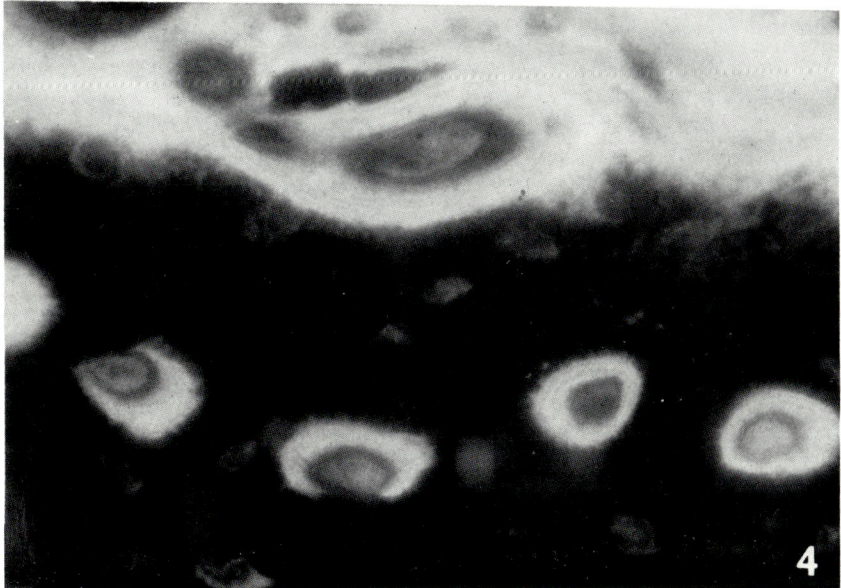

Figs. 3 and 4. Fluorescence photomicrographs of the periosteal region of the femur (Fig. 3) and the tibia (Fig. 4) from a rat in group 3 after 7 days of tetracycline administration showing that there are more labeled osteocytes near the periosteal osteoblastic appositional label in the femur than in the tibia. The bright bands at the top are the periosteal appositional labels. ($\times$ 580)

diaphysis. Also, perilacunar labeling was more prominent in the femoral than in the less vascular tibial diaphysis (Figs. 3 and 4). Finally, both periosteal osteoblastic apposition and perilacunar labeling were considerably less in rats over 55 days of age than in 31-day-old rats.

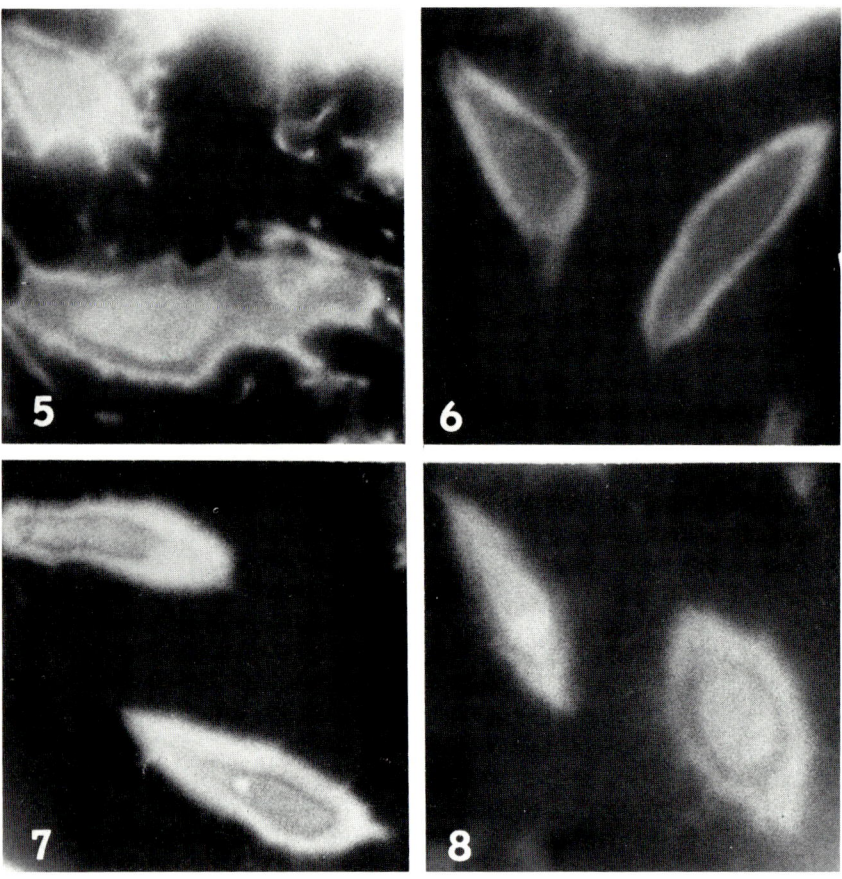

FIGS. 5–8. Fluorescence photomicrographs after 2 hours (Fig. 5), 7 days (Fig. 6), and 17 days (Fig. 7) of tetracycline administration and after 17 days (Fig. 8) of procion administration. The tetracycline labels are located in the mineralized bone surrounding each lacuna, and the procion labels extend from perilacunar osteoid into mineralized bone. Perilacunar label width in Fig. 5 represents the width of the mineralizing front, since essentially no bone apposition occurred in 2 hours. Thereafter, as a result of perilacunar bone apposition, there is a progressive increase in perilacunar tetracycline label width as a function of osteocyte age which is about 4.4 and 18.4 days for Figs. 6 and 7, respectively. Intralacunar fluorescence is due to autofluorescence of cellular material and to intracellular tetracycline or procion fluorescence. ($\times$ 3080)

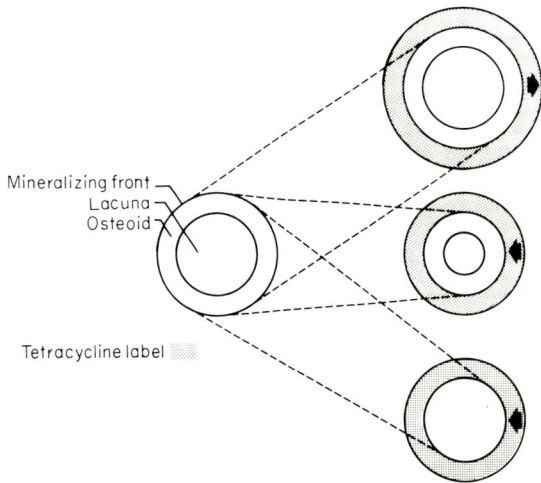

FIG. 9. Possible mechanisms that could account for the observed increase in perilacunar tetracycline label width. The circle on the left represents a young osteocyte at the beginning of the experiment before tetracycline was administered. The three circles on the right represent mature osteocytes after 17 days of tetracycline administration, and each illustrates a different mechanism that could account for the increase in label width. Broken lines connect the borders of lacunar areas to facilitate comparisons of these areas. In the first osteocyte (at the top), label width increases as a result of progressive diffusion of tetracycline into preexisting perilacunar mineral in the direction indicated by the arrow, and consequently there is no change in lacunar area with osteocyte age. Lacunar area decreases with osteocyte age in the second osteocyte as a result of bone apposition, and in the third osteocyte as a result of mineral deposition in preexisting osteoid. Since no new matrix is formed in the third osteocyte, no osteoid is seen around this lacuna.

Width of Perilacunar Tetracycline Labels as a Function of Osteocyte Age

Over the 17 day experimental period there was a progressive increase in perilacunar label width as a function of osteocyte age (Figs. 5–7, Table I). This increase in label width could have resulted from perilacunar bone apposition, the deposition of mineral in perilacunar osteoid, or the progressive diffusion of tetracycline further into the perilacunar mineral phase. These three possible mechanisms are schematically illustrated in Fig. 9.

If diffusion of tetracycline into the perilacunar mineral phase were responsible for the increase in perilacunar label width, one would not expect to find a change in lacunar area with osteocyte age. However, as

TABLE II

Lacunar Axes and Calculated Lacunar Areas[a]

Osteocyte age (days)	Short axis (μ)	Long axis (μ)	Lacunar area (μ^2)
1.4	4.12 ± 0.44	11.08 ± 1.17	32.1 ± 6.39
18.4	3.44 ± 0.29	8.57 ± 1.00	20.7 ± 3.11

[a] In order to calculate lacunar volume, it was necessary to measure lacunar depth, which was 21.3 ± 4.7 μ in osteocytes 1.4 days of age. Data are given as mean ± S.D.

shown in Table II, lacunar area was 35% less in osteocytes 18.4 days old (group 4) than in osteocytes 1.4 days old (group 1), and in group 4 the calculated value for lacunar area, based on the increase in perilacunar label width, was 17.9 μ^2, which is reasonably close to the measured value of 20.7 μ^2.

The maximum width of perilacunar osteoid for osteocytes of any age was about 0.8 μ, and the maximum perilacunar label width (group 4) was 1.3 μ. Therefore, if the decrease in lacunar area with osteocyte age were entirely due to the deposition of mineral in preexisting osteoid without any new matrix formation, one would not expect to see osteoid around older osteocytes. However, as shown in Figs. 10 and 11, osteoid was seen around old as well as young osteocytes suggesting that during the experimental period, matrix formation did not cease and that the volume of matrix mineralized and the volume of matrix formed were about equal.

Perilacunar matrix formation was also evaluated by labeling perilacunar matrix *in vivo* with procion. Whereas tetracycline is taken up in the perilacunar mineral phase, we found that procion, which is a fluorescent dye (Prescott *et al.*, 1968), is taken up in perilacunar osteoid and thus can be used to evaluate perilacunar matrix formation. Twenty-four hours after an injection of procion, the fluorescent label was found in perilacunar osteoid, and as with tetracycline, the longer procion was administered the wider the perilacunar procion labels (Fig. 8). After 17 days of procion administration, a portion of this label was located in mineralized perilacunar bone as would be expected if matrix were being formed and mineralized. These two findings of a progressive increase in procion label width with time and of perilacunar osteoid around old osteocytes indicate that the progressive increase in perilacunar tetracycline label width was not simply due to deposition of mineral in preexisting perilacunar osteoid, but rather to the coordinated processes of formation and mineralization of matrix.

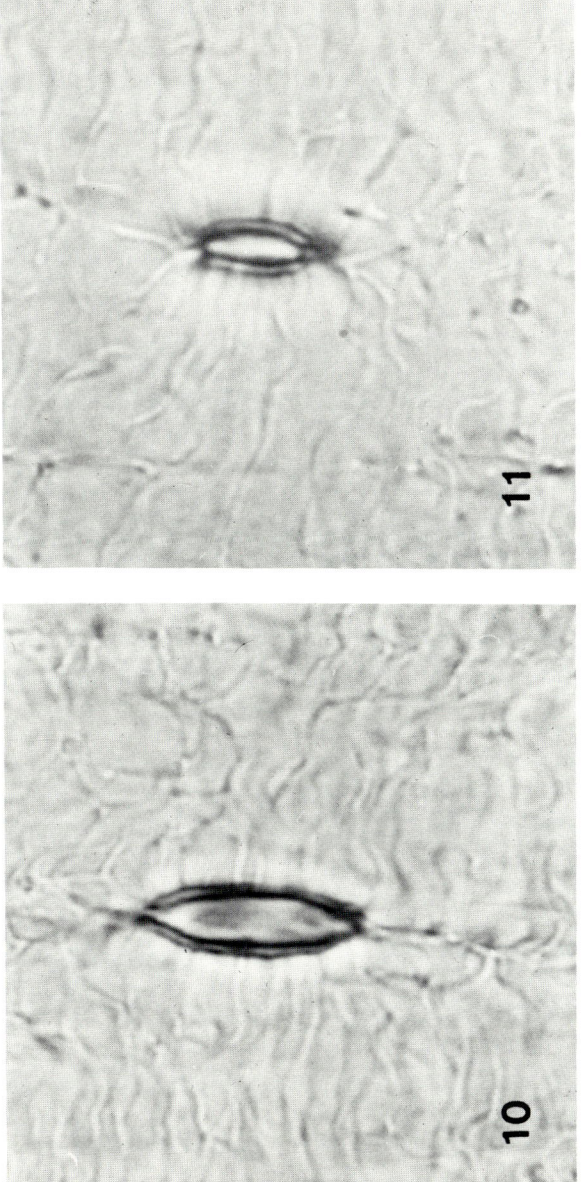

FIGS. 10 and 11. Bright field photomicrographs of an unstained ground section demonstrating perilacunar osteoid. Lining the lacuna of a young (Fig. 10) and also an old (Fig. 11) osteocyte is a narrow band of osteoid which is outlined by dark borders. Perilacunar osteoid is visualized here by virtue of the fact that it has a lower refractive index than mineralized bone. When ground sections were stained with aqueous toluidine blue, these bands of perilacunar osteoid stained metachromatically. (× 2490)

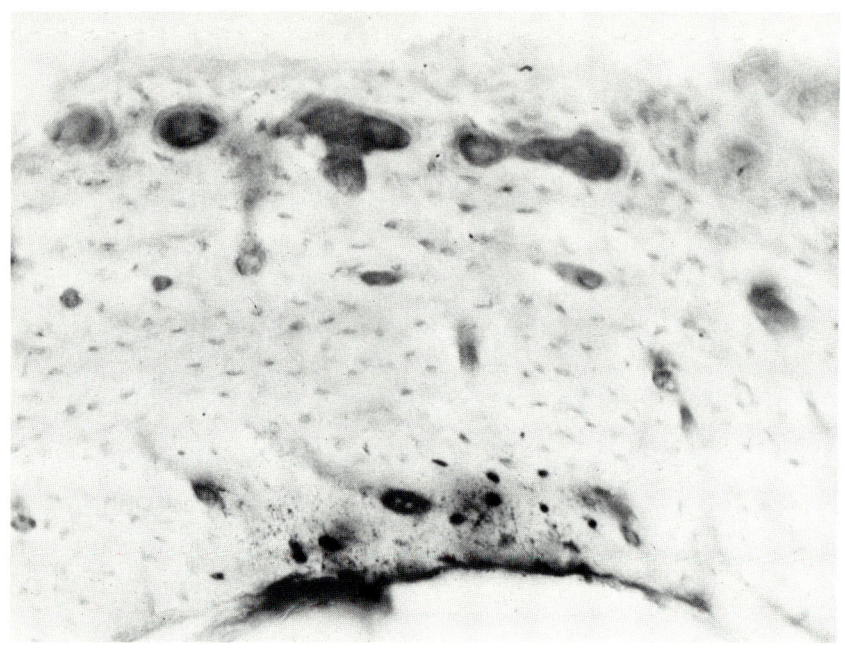

Fig. 12.

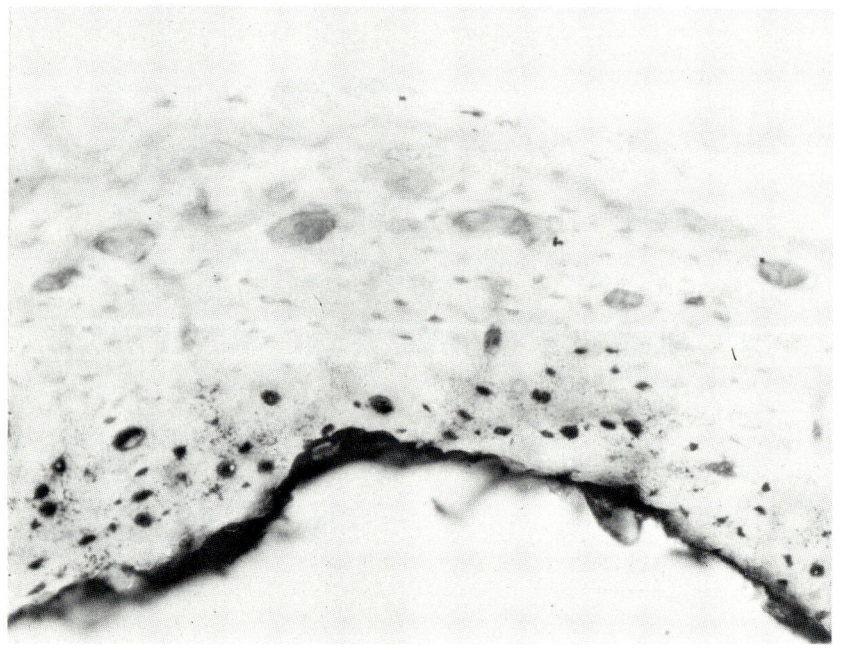

Fig. 13. For legend see facing page.

Location of Resorbing Osteocytes

Although the findings thus far indicate that the increase in perilacunar label width was due to bone apposition, they do not necessarily indicate that the process of bone apposition was continuous over the 17 day experimental period. For example, there is the possibility that in young osteocytes there are alternating short periods of perilacunar formation and resorption and that what we measured was not continuous formation but net formation.

Studies of the distribution of acid phosphatase activity in osteocytes suggest otherwise. We, as well as others, have shown that there is an association of intense acid phosphatase activity with sites of active osteoclastic resorption (Wergedal and Baylink, 1969). Some osteocytes also exhibit an intense intralacunar acid phosphatase activity which distinguishes them from remaining less active osteocytes. These active osteocytes are nearly always located in the vicinity of endosteal osteoclastic resorbing surfaces or the resorbing surfaces of nearby vascular canals, suggesting that these active osteocytes were resorbing bone (Fig. 12).

This conclusion is supported by the results of a study in which resorption was stimulated. In rats fed a calcium-free diet for 5 days, a treatment which increases the rate of endosteal osteoclastic resorption (Stauffer et al., 1971), there was increased acid phosphatase activity at endosteal osteoclastic resorbing sites, and as well, a definite increase in the number of these strongly acid phosphatase-positive osteocytes. Even under this strong stimulus, these resorbing osteocytes were still confined to the vicinity of sites of endosteal osteoclastic resorption (Fig. 13).

From these results it seems very probable that intense intralacunar acid phosphatase activity is a marker for resorbing osteocytes. Therefore, because we found that subperiosteal osteocytes less than 18 days of age, though active, did not display intense intralacunar acid phosphatase activity, it is probable that what we measured was continuous bone formation by osteocytes.

FIGS. 12 and 13. Bright field photomicrographs showing the distribution of intense intralacunar acid phosphatase activity in ground sections from a normal rat (Fig. 12) and from a rat fed a calcium-free diet for 5 days (Fig. 13). The endosteal resorbing surface and nearby osteocytes and canaliculi are all stained intensely for acid phosphatase activity. Although more osteocytes displaying intense intralacunar acid phosphatase activity are seen in bone from the calcium-deficient rat than in normal bone, in both they are located near endosteal osteoclastic resorbing surfaces, and none are seen in recently formed bone near the periosteum which is located at the top of each photomicrograph. ($\times$ 218)

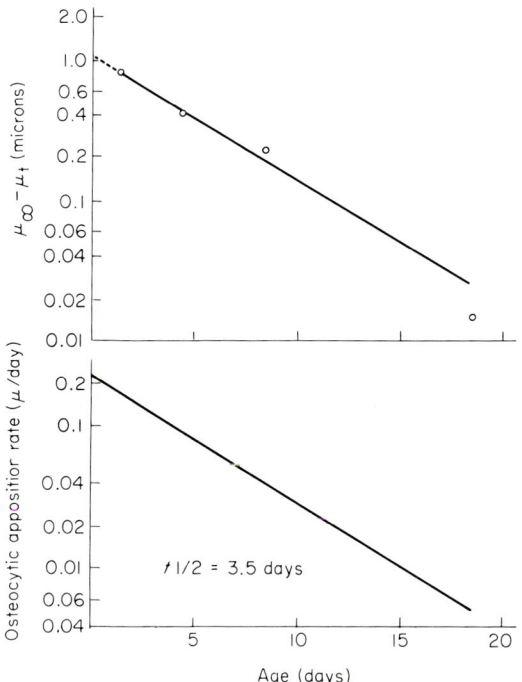

FIG. 14. Top, the difference between maximum perilacunar label width (μ_∞) and perilacunar label width (μ_t) versus time. Bottom, the osteocytic bone apposition rate calculated from Eq. 7 using the values derived from the relationship illustrated above.

Osteocytic Bone Apposition as a Function of Osteocyte Age

Since essentially no apposition occurred in 2 hours, the perilacunar label width in group 1 represents the width of incompletely mineralized bone in the perilacunar region into which tetracycline rapidly diffuses. This same phenomenon occurs at sites of osteoblastic matrix formation and mineralization (Baylink et al., 1970). This interpretation was confirmed by the finding that the width of perilacunar tetracycline labels in ground sections stained with tetracycline *in vitro* was about the same as that found for the 2 hour *in vivo* label. Therefore, in order to obtain the width of the perilacunar label due to bone apposition, the mean width of the 2 hour label was subtracted from each of the measured values of perilacunar width in groups 2–4.

The increase in this corrected label width with time appeared to be a logarithmic function. Therefore, the quantity $\mu_\infty - \mu_t$ was plotted on a log scale as a function of osteocyte age (Fig. 14, Top), where μ is the corrected perilacunar label width. Because the points fall on a straight line on a log scale, the label width can be described by:

$$\mu = A(1 - e^{-k(t-1.4)}), \tag{6}$$

where A is the asymtotic value for label width and t is time. The formula for the apposition rate, $d\mu/dt$, then becomes:

$$d\mu/dt = Ake^{-k(t-1.4)}. \tag{7}$$

Since label width due to bone apposition was zero in osteocytes 1.4 days rather than 0 days of age, 1.4 was subtracted from known values of t. Equation 6 was solved for k and A using the method of least squares and known values of μ and t. The values of k (0.204) and A (0.815) were then substituted into Eq. 7 to obtain the perilacunar bone apposition rate.

As shown in Fig. 14, Bottom, there was a logarithmic decrease in the perilacunar bone apposition rate as a function of osteocyte age. Assuming this relationship, which was determined for osteocytes in mineralized bone, holds while osteocytes are still in osteoid, the maximum perilacunar apposition rate, which occurred at time zero, was 0.22 μ per day (Fig. 14, Bottom).

Pericanalicular Tetracycline Deposition

As illustrated in Fig. 15, pericanalicular tetracycline labeling was greatest at sites immediately adjacent to periosteal osteoblastic appositional tetracycline labels. These pericanalicular labels were found to persist for long periods after the serum tetracycline level had dropped, suggesting that mineral deposition occurs in pericanalicular regions. If this were true, one might expect to find larger canaliculi in young bone than in mature bone.

It is difficult to evaluate the caliber of canaliculi on either stained or unstained sections because one sees canalicular borders, which are relatively broad, rather than the lumen of canaliculi. Therefore, the caliber of canaliculi was evaluated by infiltrating bone with plastic containing a fluorescent dye. In such specimens, there appeared to be a progressive decrease in the volume of canaliculi as indicated by the amount of fluorescent plastic within canaliculi with bone age (Fig. 16). A better resolution of canaliculi is seen in Fig. 17 in which some of the canaliculi at the mineralizing front are obviously larger in caliber than those in more mature bone. It is also possible that some of the increased fluorescence in young bone could have been due to an increased number of canaliculi.

These two findings, of permanent pericanalicular tetracycline fluorescence and of decreasing canalicular caliber with bone age, are both consistent with pericanalicular mineral deposition in young bone. However, these findings do not necessarily indicate that new pericanalicular matrix was

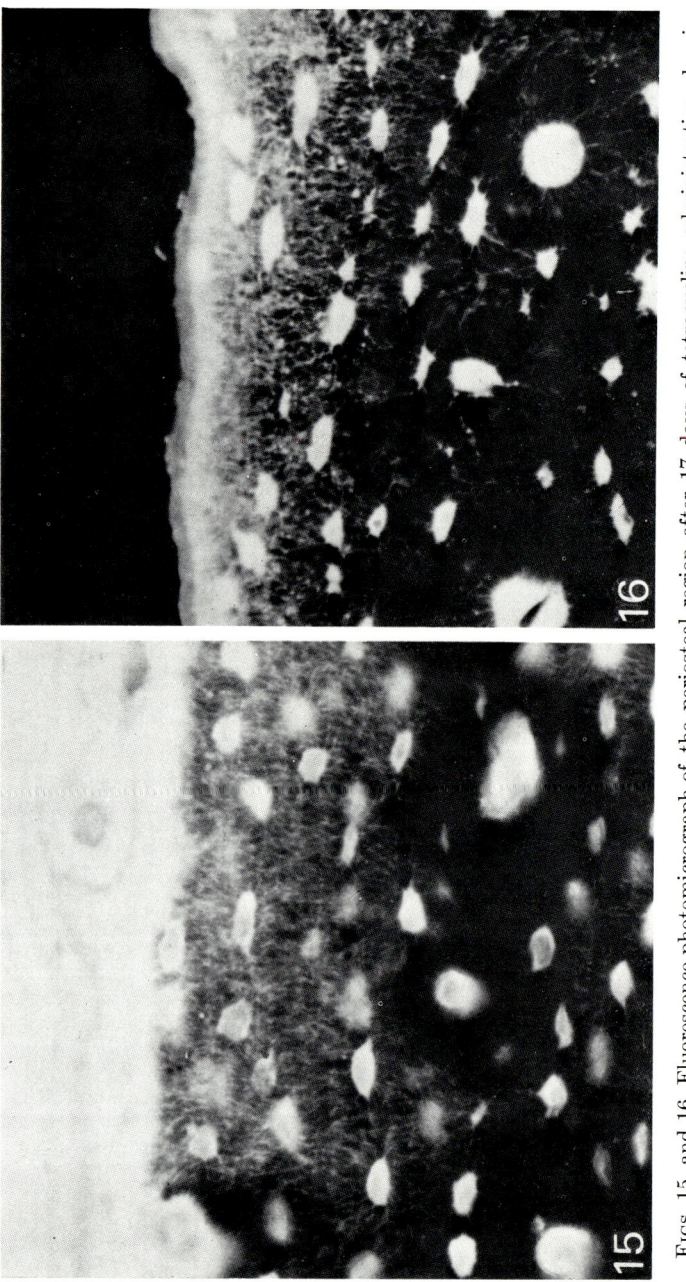

FIGS. 15. and 16. Fluorescence photomicrograph of the periosteal region after 17 days of tetracycline administration showing pericanalicular tetracycline labeling in bone beneath the periosteal osteoblastic appositional tetracycline label. (× 580) (Figure 15). Fluorescence photomicrograph of a bone infiltrated with Epon doped with rhodamine B showing that the volume of canaliculi, as indicated by the amount of fluorescent plastic within canaliculi, progressively decreases from the mineralizing front at the top of the photomicrograph toward more mature bone below. (× 580) (Figure 16).

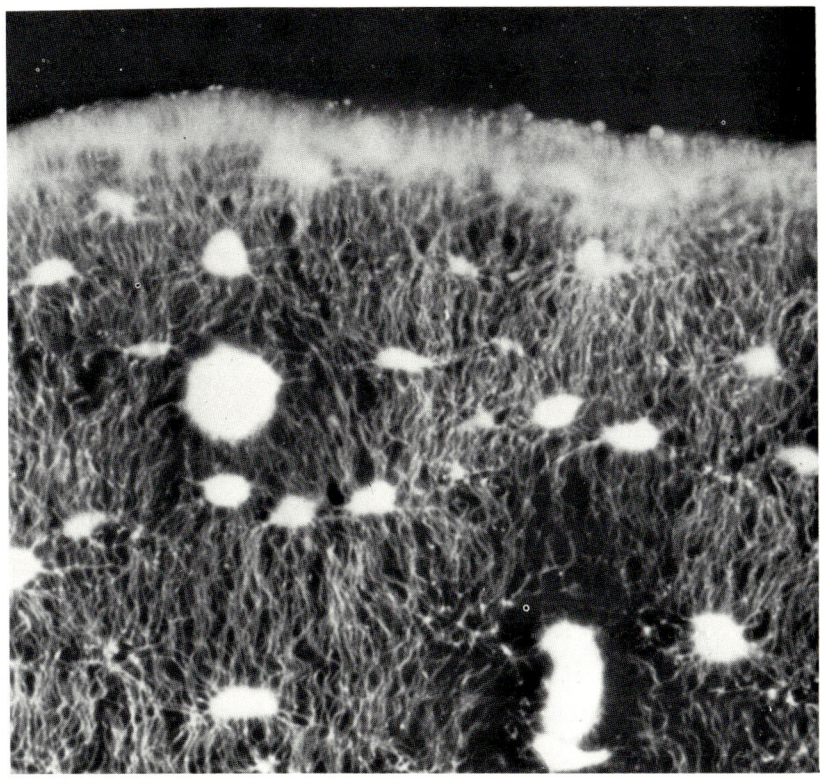

FIG. 17. Photomicrograph of specimen similar to that shown in Fig. 16 showing that the caliber of some canaliculi at the mineralizing front at the top are obviously larger than in more mature bone below. (× 1053)

formed, because the mineral may have been deposited in preexisting pericanalicular osteoid. In any case, our findings indicate that mineral deposition occurs around canaliculi as well as around lacunae in young bone.

Osteoblastic versus Osteocytic Bone Formation

Table III gives measured and Table IV calculated data dealing with bone formation and resorption by osteoblasts, osteocytes, and osteoclasts. In group 3, over the 7 day measuring period in a 1 mm thick section, the total volume of bone formed by periosteal and endosteal osteoblasts was 0.088 mm^3 per day, whereas that formed by osteocytes was only 0.0012 mm^3 per day. The value obtained for osteocytic formation is somewhat too high because we assumed that subperiosteal osteocytic formation in the

TABLE III

MEASURED PARAMETERS RELATED TO BONE FORMATION AND RESORPTION BY OSTEOBLASTS, OSTEOCLASTS, AND OSTEOCYTES IN 38-DAY-OLD RATS (GROUP 3) AFTER 7 DAYS OF TETRACYCLINE ADMINISTRATION

Parameter	Mean ± S.D.
Periosteal labeled area (mm^2)	0.47 ± 0.27
Endosteal labeled area (mm^2)	0.18 ± 0.10
Preformed bone area (mm^2)	2.07 ± 0.29
Basal medullary area (mm^2)[a]	3.07 ± 0.44
Final medullary area (mm^2)	3.16 ± 0.28
Periosteal label width (μ)	83.3 ± 17.8
Periosteal osteoid width (μ)	5.3 ± 0.3
Periosteal mineralizing front width (μ)[a]	5.5 ± 0.6
Length of osteoblasts (μ)	10.5
Depth of osteoblasts (μ)	15.4
Width of osteoblasts (μ)	4.6
Osteocytes (number/mm^3)	23,450
Specific volume of perilacunar labels in preformed bone area (%)	0.33 ± 0.08

[a] Measured in group 1.

medial–anterior portion of the femoral diaphysis was the same as that in the lateral–posterior portion, whereas it appeared to be substantially less.

Lacunar–Canalicular Volume

In order to calculate the rate of osteocytic bone resorption (as described in the next section), it was necessary to determine the change in lacunar–

TABLE IV

RATES OF BONE FORMATION AND RESORPTION BY OSTEOBLASTS, OSTEOCYTES, AND OSTEOCLASTS[a]

Rate	Osteoblasts	Osteocytes	Osteoclasts
Bone formation (mm^3/day)	0.088[b]	0.0012	—
Bone apposition (μ/day)	11.1[c]	0.22[d]	—
Bone resorption (mm^3/day)	—	0.0015[d]	0.013[e]

[a] All values apply to a 1 mm thick section from the femoral diaphysis.
[b] At the periosteum and endosteum.
[c] At the periosteum.
[d] Maximum value.
[e] At the endosteum.

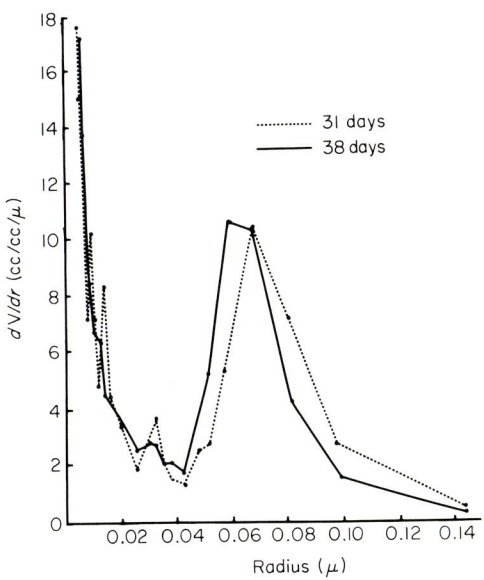

FIG. 18. Distribution of pore volume as a function of pore radius. The lacunar–canalicular volume probably lies between pore radii of about 0.04–0.14 μ; the pores smaller than about 0.006 μ in radius represent what we term microcanaliculi. Thus, the area under the large peak represents the lacunar–canalicular volume. Each point for both curves represents a mean value obtained from five rats.

canalicular volume in the femoral diaphyses from 31- as compared with 38-day-old rats. Lacunar–canalicular volume measurements were made by means of mercury porosimetry.

As previously indicated, in this method the volume of mercury forced into bone pores was determined as a function of the pressure applied. Because bone is not wetted by mercury, pressure must be applied to cause mercury to enter bone pores, and the pressure required to fill the pores progressively increases as the caliber of the pores intruded becomes smaller. For example, the pressure required to fill pores 0.14 μ in radius is 800 pounds per square inch, whereas the pressure required to fill pores 0.006 μ in radius is 15,000 pounds per square inch (Fig. 18). Once the mercury penetrates into a canaliculus, no further pressure change is required to fill the corresponding osteocyte lacuna. Therefore, the volume registered in the region of canalicular radii includes lacunar as well as canalicular volume. Since the maximum radius found microscopically for canaliculi was about 0.14 μ, the lacunar–canalicular volume probably lies between pore radii of about 0.14 and 0.04

TABLE V

LACUNAR–CANALICULAR VOLUME OF THE RAT FEMORAL DIAPHYSIS

Rat age (days)	Lacunar–canalicular volume (cc/cc of bone) (mean ± S.D.)
31	0.0348 ± .0063
38	0.0347 ± .0032

μ (Fig. 18); the pores smaller than about 0.04 μ in radius represent what we term microcanaliculi (Voss and Baylink, 1970). Thus, the area under the large peak in Fig. 19 represents the combined lacunar–canalicular volume. The lacunar–canalicular volume was essentially the same in 31- and 38-day-old rats, as shown in Table V.

Rate of Osteocytic Bone Resorption

If one knows the volume of bone formed by osteocytes, and in addition, the net change in lacunar–canalicular volume over the same time period, it is possible to estimate osteocytic bone resorption. Osteocytic bone formation was measured in group 3 over a 7 day period in rats sacrificed at 38 days of age, and lacunar canalicular volume was measured in the femurs of 31- and 38-day-old rats. If no osteocytes had been added or lost during the 7 day experimental period, the change in lacunar–canalicular volume would have been equal to the volume of bone resorbed minus the volume of bone formed by osteocytes. However, during the 7 day period, there was a gain in young forming osteocytes through osteoblastic bone formation and a loss of resorbing osteocytes through osteoclastic bone resorption. Accordingly, the change in lacunar volume is given by:

$$\Delta LV = R - F + A_{lv} - L_{lv}, \qquad (8)$$

where ΔLV is the change in lacunar volume, R is the volume of bone resorbed by osteocytes, F is the volume of bone formed by osteocytes, A_{lv} is the lacunar volume added, and L_{lv} is the lacunar volume lost. By rearranging, we obtain the formula for osteocytic bone resorption:

$$R = \Delta LV + F - A_{lv} + L_{lv}. \qquad (9)$$

The lacunar volume added was calculated by multiplying the mean volume of a young osteocyte, the number of osteocytes per unit volume of bone, and the volume of bone formed by osteoblasts. Similarly, the lacunar volume lost was calculated by multiplying the mean volume of a resorbing osteocyte, the number of osteocytes per unit volume of bone, and the volume of bone resorbed by osteoclasts. The lacunar volume of resorbing osteocytes was obtained by substituting calculated values for lacunar area and lacunar depth into Eq. 2. The lacunar area of resorbing osteocytes was calculated from the measured lacunar axes using Eq. 1. Lacunar depth of resorbing osteocytes was calculated by assuming that the ratio between lacunar long axis and lacunar depth was the same in resorbing as in forming osteocytes.

The values of the parameters used to calculate osteocytic bone resorption are shown in Table VI. In order to set an upper limit for osteocytic bone resorption, the maximum increase which could have occurred in canalicular volume, within the uncertainty of the determination, was used instead of the actual measured change given in Table V. The statistical uncertainty was about ±10% of the lacunar-canalicular volume, and on this basis, the maximum increase which could have occurred in this volume is given in Table VI. When the values given in Table VI were substituted into Eq. 9, the osteocytic bone resorption rate in a 1 mm thick section from our sampling site was 0.0015 mm³ per day (Table IV).

In calculating osteocytic bone resorption, we used lacunar volume in some instances and lacunar-canalicular volume in others. The ultimate effect of this should be such that our value for osteocytic resorption is an overestimation of this rate. Because of this and because we used the maximum increase which could have occurred in lacunar-canalicular volume, it seems likely that our value represents the maximum osteocytic bone resorption rate. Although these results indicate that the rates of osteocytic bone resorption and osteocytic bone formation were about the same (Table IV), it should be emphasized that our measure of osteocytic bone resorption must be considered an estimate.

TABLE VI

VALUES USED TO CALCULATE THE RATE OF OSTEOCYTIC BONE RESORPTION

Parameter	(mm³/day)[a]
Change in lacunar-canalicular volume	0.0014
Osteocytic bone formation	0.0012
Lacunar volume added	0.0013
Lacunar volume lost	0.0002[b]

[a] In a 1 mm thick section.
[b] The measured lacunar area used in this calculation was 24.6 μ^2.

Discussion

This study clearly demonstrates that in rapidly growing rats young osteocytes form bone (i.e., they form matrix which subsequently becomes mineralized). As with many other growth functions (Laird, 1965), osteocytic function, as indicated by the perilacunar bone apposition rate, decreases exponentially as a function of cell age.

In the femoral cortex, forming osteocytes were primarily seen in young subperiosteal bone, whereas resorbing osteocytes, as indicated by intense intralacunar acid phosphatase activity, were primarily seen near the endosteum adjacent to sites of osteoclastic resorption. Even when the number of resorbing osteocytes was increased by feeding a calcium-free diet, such cells were still primarily located near the endosteum and none were seen in young subperiosteal bone. Thus, it appears that young osteocytes continue the bone formation initiated when these same cells were osteoblasts, that during this period of formation no perilacunar resorption occurs, and that only after these cells have completed a forming phase are they capable of responding to a resorptive stimulus. This interpretation is consistent with the findings of Talmage and Elliott (1958), who demonstrated that the maximum resorptive response following parathyroid extract administration occurs in those areas containing bone mineral which was deposited 2–3 weeks prior to the resorptive stimulus (Talmage and Elliott, 1958).

In a previous study, we demonstrated that in the tibial diaphysis, periosteal and endosteal osteoblastic formation composed 90% of the total osteoblastic formation, only 10% occurring at vascular canals (Baylink et al., 1969). Therefore, it was of interest in the present study to compare the volume of bone formed by osteocytes to that formed by osteoblasts at the periosteum and endosteum in the femur. Although the amount of osteoblastic bone formation occurring at vascular canals is greater in the femur than in the tibia, the majority of osteoblastic formation in the femur also occurs at the periosteum and endosteum. In the femur we found that the volume of bone formed by osteocytes was only 1.3% of that formed by osteoblasts (Table IV).

A comparison can also be made of the amount of bone formed per cell by osteoblasts and osteocytes. Although the osteoblastic bone apposition rate was 11.1 μ per day, according to our measurements, osteoblasts formed bone around only 29% of their surface. Therefore, if formation were spread over the entire surface of osteoblasts, as occurs for osteocytes, the osteoblastic bone apposition rate would be 3.2 μ per day, whereas the maximum apposition rate for osteocytes was only 0.22 μ per day. This suggests that there is a sharp decrease in matrix formation by osteoblasts at the time that they become embedded in osteoid matrix.

According to our calculation, the maximum rate of osteocytic bone resorption was about the same as the rate of osteocytic bone formation and was about an order of magnitude less than the rate of osteoclastic bone resorption (Table IV). That the osteocytic bone resorption rate in rapidly growing rats is relatively low is further supported by the finding that the number of resorbing osteocytes in our sampling site was considerably less than the number of forming osteocytes.

In different skeletal sites, wide variations were found in both osteocytic and osteoblastic bone formation, and osteocytic bone formation appeared to be highest in those areas where osteoblastic bone formation was highest. Also, resorbing osteocytes were almost always located in the vicinity of sites of osteoclastic bone resorption, and when osteoclastic bone resorption was increased by feeding a calcium-free diet, it was accompanied by an increase in the number of resorbing osteocytes. Furthermore, in a previous study on the distribution of alkaline and acid phosphatases in bone cells, we found that young osteocytes resembled osteoblasts and that old osteocytes resembled osteoclasts (Wergedal and Baylink, 1969). These observations lead to the interpretation that in the rapidly growing rat not only osteocytic and osteoblastic bone formation, but also osteocytic and osteoclastic bone resorption are closely linked and probably share common control mechanisms.

Since we measured total osteocytic and total osteoblastic bone formation in a unit volume of the skeleton, we can make, by extrapolating these rates to the entire skeleton, a rough estimate of the effects that a change in either of these two rates could have on the serum calcium concentration. By extrapolating the rate of osteocytic bone formation found in the femur (0.0004 mm^3 per cubic millimeter of bone) to the entire skeleton, which contained about 920 mg of calcium in our 113 gm rats (group 3),* and by considering that the extracellular fluid is 260 ml per kilogram of body weight (Wilde, 1945) and that bone calcium concentration is 27% of the dry weight (by electron microprobe analysis), one finds that a 5% change in osteocytic bone formation for 24 hours could result in only a 0.7% change in serum calcium. In contrast, a 5% change in osteoblastic bone formation for the same period of time could result in a 50% change in serum calcium. Accordingly, if osteocytic bone formation ceased for 1 hour, this could raise the serum calcium by only 0.06 mg per 100 ml, and in order for osteocytic bone formation to decrease the serum calcium by 1 mg per 100 ml in 1 hour, it would have to increase by 1600%. Therefore, on a quantitative basis, it

---

* Based on the finding that the skeleton of 170 gm rats contains 1400 mg of calcium (Bernhart et al., 1969).

seems unlikely that osteocytic bone formation plays a major role in the regulation of the serum calcium concentration in the rapidly growing rat.

It should be emphasized that our results, showing that osteocytic bone formation is only a small fraction of the total formation, do not rule out the possibility that osteocytes are involved in calcium homeostasis. There are at least three reasons to suspect that osteocytes might be capable of mediating rapid changes in the rate of calcium transfer between bone and blood. First, bulk flow through the lacunar–canalicular system is fairly rapid, as indicated by our finding that all lacunar–canalicular surfaces are labeled with tetracycline within about 30 minutes after an intravenous injection of tetracycline. Second, the lacunar–canalicular surface area, which we found to be about 1480 m² per liter of bone,* is about two thousand times greater than the osteoclastic Howship's lacunar surface area (Frost, 1962b; Robinson, 1964). Third, we previously demonstrated that the solubility of perilacunar mineral was substantially greater than that of interlacunar mineral (Baylink *et al.*, 1968). Thus, the mineral adjacent to osteocyte lacunae and canaliculi may represent a specialized mineral phase with a turnover which is relatively rapid compared to mineral turnover as a result of formation and resorption on major bone surfaces. However, this mechanism would have to be of limited capacity, otherwise one would expect to find changes in the mineral concentration of mature bone, whereas mineral concentration in mature bone appears to be relatively stable (Marshall, 1969).

Long-term exchange is another mechanism whereby osteocytes could participate in calcium homeostasis. Marshall has demonstrated that in adult dogs the rates of augmentation and diminution, which together represent long-term exchange, are at least equivalent to the rates of accretion and resorption and turn over an amount of calcium equal to that in blood every day. Because the rates of augmentation and diminution are not constant, it was suggested that long-term exchange is at least partially under cellular control, the most likely cell candidate being the osteocyte (Marshall, 1969).

Despite our finding that osteocytic bone resorption is relatively low in normal rats, this process could still be significantly involved in calcium homeostasis. For example, Bélanger and co-workers have demonstrated in experimental animals that treatment with parathyroid extract causes large increases in lacunar area as a result of osteocytic osteolysis (Bélanger *et al.*,

---

* This figure was calculated by assuming that the total canalicular volume is 40% of the lacunar–canalicular volume (Frost, 1962b). Although our value for lacunar–canalicular surface area is similar to that found for human bone, 1500 m²/liter, by Robinson (1964), our value includes microcanalicular surface area whereas his does not.

1963). Before this mechanism or the other mechanisms mentioned above can be assigned a specific role in serum calcium regulation, further quantitative studies will be necessary.

Conclusions

The data from the present study are consistent with the following conclusions: (1) osteocytes form bone, (2) the rate of osteocytic bone apposition decreases exponentially as a function of osteocyte age, (3) osteocytic bone formation is only about 1.3% of osteoblastic bone formation, (4) osteocytic bone resorption is probably similar in magnitude to osteocytic bone formation, and (5) in rapidly growing rats it is unlikely that osteocytic bone formation plays an important role in serum calcium homeostasis.

Acknowledgments

We are grateful to Professor O. J. Whittemore, Professor of Ceramic Engineering, University of Washington, for assistance with the mercury porosimeter measurements; Dr. Clayton Rich for helpful criticism; Dr. N. Maloney for taking the photomicrographs; Mrs. L. Thompson, Mr. G. Perez, Miss E. Yee, and Mr. E. Feist for their invaluable technical assistance; and to Mrs. D. Herold for typing the manuscript.

References

Baud, C. A. (1962). *Acta Anat.* **51,** 209.
Baud, C. A. (1968). *Clin. Orthop.* **56,** 227.
Baud, C. A. (1969). Personal communication.
Baylink, D. J., and Bernstein, D. S. (1967). *Clin. Orthop.* **55,** 51.
Baylink, D. J., Morey, E., and Rich, C. (1968). *In* "Parathyroid Hormone and Thyrocalcitonin (Calcitonin)" (R. V. Talmage and L. Bélanger, eds.), p. 196. Excerpta Med. Found., Amsterdam.
Baylink, D. J., Morey, E., and Rich, C. (1969). *Endocrinology* **84,** 261.
Baylink, D. J., Stauffer, M., Wergedal, J., and Rich, C. (1970). *J. Clin. Invest.* **49,** 1122.
Baylink, D. J., Whittemore, O., and Wergedal, J. (1971). Manuscript in preparation.
Bélanger, L. F., Robichon, J., Migicovsky, B. B., Copp, D. H., and Vincent, J. (1963). *In* "Mechanisms of Hard Tissue Destruction," Publ. No. 75, p. 531. Amer. Ass. Advance. Sci., Washington, D.C.
Bernhart, F. W., Savini, S., and Tomarelli, R. M. (1969). *J. Nutr.* **98,** 443.
Frost, H. M. (1962a). *Henry Ford Hosp. Med. Bull.* **10,** 267.
Frost, H. M. (1962b). *Henry Ford Hosp. Med. Bull.* **10,** 35.
Laird, A. K. (1965). *Growth* **29,** 249.
Marshall, J. H. (1969). *In* "Mineral Metabolism" (C. Comar and F. Bronner, eds.), Vol. III, p. 2. Academic Press, New York.
Prescott, G. H., Mitchell, D. F., and Fahmy, H. (1968). *Amer. J. Phys. Anthropol.* **29,** 219.

Ritter, H. L., and Drake, L. C. (1945). *Ind. Eng. Chem., Anal. Ed.* **17,** 782.
Robinson, R. A. (1964). *In* "Bone Biodynamics" (H. M. Frost, ed.), p. 423. Little, Brown, Boston, Massachusetts.
Stauffer, M., Baylink, D., Wergedal, J., and Rich, C. (1971). Manuscript submitted for publication.
Talmage, R. V. (1967). *Clin. Orthop.* **54,** 163.
Talmage, R. V., and Elliott, J. R. (1958). *Endocrinology* **62,** 717.
Vittali, P. H. (1968). *Clin. Orthop.* **66,** 213.
Vose, G. P., and Baylink, D. J. (1970). *Anat. Rec.* **166,** 239.
Washburn, E. W. (1921). *Proc. Nat. Acad. Sci. U.S.* **7,** 115.
Wergedal, J. E. (1969). *Calcif. Tissue Res.* **3,** 55.
Wergedal, J. E., and Baylink, D. J. (1969). *J. Histochem. Cytochem.* **17,** 799.
Wilde, W. S. (1945). *Amer. J. Physiol.* **143,** 666.
Winslow, N. M., and Shapiro, J. J. (1959). *Amer. Soc. Testing Mater., Proc.* **236,** 39.
Young, R. W. (1963). *In* "Mechanisms of Hard Tissue Destruction," Publ. No. 75, p. 471. Amer. Ass. Advance. Sci., Washington, D.C.

Discussion

Dr. Heaney: I have two questions. One, what you have demonstrated are osteocytes participating in the completion of the process which they had initiated as osteoblasts. Do you have any observations which would relate to the possibility of repair of osteocytic osteolysis after, for example, parathyroid stimulation?

My second question relates to your measurement of osteocytic bone formation relative to osteoblastic bone formation. Were these values rates or were they total contributions per osteocyte relative to total contribution of an osteoblast, and did they take into consideration only the peripheral ring of osteocytes that were just outside of your labeled area, or all of the osteocytes which had been included for the duration of the tetracycline labeling period, which in some cases was 7 days?

Dr. Baylink: With respect to your first question, I have not studied repair of osteocytic osteolysis in rat bone. However, in bone biopsies from human subjects, I have made observations which are consistent with such a repair process. For example, in old bone, one sometimes sees osteocytes with very large lacunae, and since lacunae of young osteocytes normally tend to be larger than those of old mature osteocytes, it is reasonable to assume that these large older osteocytes were resorbing bone sometime in the past. Surrounding some of these large older osteocytes, I have observed collagen bundles which did not conform to the original alternating lamellar pattern, but rather were oriented parallel to the long axis of the lacunae. In addition, these collagen bundles were more intensely birefringent and smaller in caliber than those in the remainder of bone. Thus, it would appear that such osteocytes, after maturation, had gone through a phase of bone resorption and subsequently a phase of bone formation.

In answer to your second question, the osteocytic bone formation rate is the total volume of bone formed per day by all osteocytes in a 1 mm thick section from the femoral diaphysis.

Dr. Goldhaber: We, too, have observations indicating that osteocytes can lay down new osteoid, but I think the question that Dr. Heaney raised is pertinent to this observation. That is, the osteocytes seem to be early in their stage of development when this happens. Have you done any more direct studies? That is, have you injected tritiated proline to see whether or not the isotope appears in a layer around the osteocyte during any portion of your study on rats? That would be more definite proof. I am a little worried about the tetracycline, which might be confused with the mineral in the area. Have you done any studies on osteoid per se?

Dr. Baylink: I have not used tritiated proline to evaluate matrix formation by osteocytes. However, I consider the demonstration of a progressive increase in perilacunar tetracycline label width with osteocyte age, of a decrease in lacunar area with osteocyte age, and of osteoid surrounding old as well as young osteocytes to be direct evidence of matrix formation and mineralization in the perilacunar region of osteocytes.

Dr. Goldhaber: To put it another way, if the hypothesis is correct, would you expect that labeled proline would appear in that perilacunar area?

Dr. Baylink: Very definitely.

Dr. Bélanger: Dr. Baylink, you estimate the time of survival of your osteocytes by the fact that they are labeled with tetracycline, don't you, as far as they can go after the onset of your experiment? Is that the way you estimate the time of survival of your cells?

Dr. Baylink: Osteocyte age was calculated by first measuring the distance of the osteocyte from the periosteal osteoblastic-osteoid interface and then converting this distance to time from measurements of the periosteal-osteoblastic bone formation rate. For this calculation, an osteoblast was considered to have become an osteocyte when it became surrounded by bone matrix. Accordingly, an osteocyte was zero days old when it was at least half surrounded by bone matrix. Our measurements of bone formation were done on osteocytes between 1.4 and 18.4 days of age.

Dr. Bélanger: You assume that at this age the osteocyte is still alive just by looking at it; is that it?

Dr. Baylink: Since they were forming new bone, I presume that they were alive.

Dr. Bélanger: In our own work years ago, with Dr. Migicovsky, we labeled the cell with DNA precursors and, in the trabecular bone of young rats of about the same age as yours, we couldn't see any more of this label after 4 days. We assumed that the cells are dead after that time, or that the DNA has left the cell, at any rate. In this sort of material, it is difficult to understand that bone formation would go on after that time. The total turnover time of trabecula was 4 days.

Dr. Baylink: In my sampling site, osteocytes older than 4 days of age represent a huge fraction of the total number of osteocytes. If all osteocytes older than 4 days of age were dead, more than 80% of the osteocytes in the femoral diaphysis would be dead.

Dr. Bélanger: Our work, as mentioned, was on trabecular bone. The main point I want to bring up is that the younger the bone, the more rapid are these events. I just question whether the type of material that you are using now is the material most representative of physiological activity as related to homeostasis.

Dr. Baylink: The technique of measuring osteocytic bone formation was such that the higher the rate, the greater the accuracy of the measurement. Accordingly, this process was measured in the femoral diaphysis because, in this site, osteocytic bone formation was greater than in all other sites that I examined. Furthermore, in the femur, osteocytic bone formation did not appear to be greater in the metaphysis than in the diaphysis. Therefore, the value which I obtained for the osteocytic bone formation rate should be higher than the mean value for the entire skeleton.

Dr. Urist: Dr. Baylink presents the problem of interpretation of the locus of the tetracycline label. When tetracycline is administered to an intact animal, it is deposited on the bone mineral crystal surfaces in approximately the same location as citrate would be. The molecule is too large to fit anywhere inside crystal surfaces. Tetracycline also labels collagen and other organic materials *in vitro*, but not any large quantity in the concentrations that are non-toxic to mammals. In any case, 99.9% of the tetracycline deposited *in vivo* is removable with the mineral phase.

In an electron micrograph of an osteocyte, you see an envelope of uncalcified collagen in the pericellular intralacunar position. The younger the cell, the thicker the envelope of uncalcified collagen. It is important in this connection to note that for technical reasons, electron microscope studies are done only on young tissues in order to section the tissues; but young or old, osteocytes are always surrounded by an envelope of collagen which is not calcified. This envelope is about 0.5 μ in thickness. The place new mineral could go in the course of aging of an osteocyte would be in a sacred area of the intralacunar uncalcified collagen. The question, therefore, is, are you seeing calcification of preformed pericellular collagen?

Dr. Baylink: If I understand your question correctly, you would like to know how I distinguish tetracycline uptake in perilacunar mineral from that in perilacunar matrix. It is true that if the blood level of tetracycline is high at the time of sacrifice, one sees faint tetracycline fluorescence in perilacunar matrix. However, it is not difficult to distinguish this from tetracycline fluorescence in perilacunar mineral, because in the latter the fluorescence is much brighter. This interpretation was confirmed by the finding that the region with the brighter fluorescence had a higher refractive index, as would be expected, since mineralized bone has a higher refractive index than bone matrix.

Dr. Urist: Does tetracycline label mineralization of the preformed collagen in space between the cell wall and metachromatic zone?

Dr. Baylink: The combined demonstration of an increase in perilacunar tetracycline label width and a decrease in lacunar area are indicative of perilacunar mineral deposition. This mineral deposition could have occurred in preexisting osteoid, or it could have occurred in conjunction with the coordinated processes of matrix formation and mineralization. Since the maximum osteoid width was 0.8μ, and since the mean width of the perilacunar tetracycline label due to bone apposition was 0.8μ if no new matrix had been formed, one would not expect to see osteoid surrounding older osteocytes. However, as illustrated, osteoid was seen around old osteocytes as well as young osteocytes. These results are consistent with the conclusion that young osteocytes form new bone matrix.

Our results using procion to label newly formed matrix substantiate this conclusion. Procion is a fluorescent dye which is taken up in bone matrix. Twenty-four hours after an injection of procion, this dye was found in perilacunar osteoid, and the longer procion was given, the wider the perilacunar procion labels. After 17 days of procion administration, the perilacunar procion label was similar in width to the 17 day perilacunar tetracycline label. Thus, the coordinated processes of new matrix formation and subsequent mineralization occur in the perilacunar region of young osteocytes, a finding analogous to that seen at sites of osteoblastic matrix formation and mineralization.

Dr. Urist: Do you assume that the osteocyte is producing new collagen?

Dr. Baylink: No, I am not assuming it, I am demonstrating it.

Dr. Bordier: In human hyperparathyroidism, osteolysis is markedly increased. But the release of mineral around the osteocytic lacunae is not always associated with removal of the matrix. In this occasion, would not the tetracycline label also leave the matrix? If so, it would not indicate matrix formed at the time of the labeling.

Dr. Baylink: From my experience, it is more likely that the tetracycline label in the perilacunar region of resorbing osteocytes in bone from patients with hyperparathyroidism is located in the perilacunar mineral phase rather than in perilacunar matrix. If so, this could be either indicative of perilacunar mineral deposition, or more likely, indicative of a low concentration of mineral in the perilacunar mineral phase. Because the mineral concentration in the perilacunar mineral phase of resorbing osteocytes is frequently lower than that in interlacunar bone, tetracycline can diffuse into and label this low mineral content bone in the same way that tetracycline labels the low mineral content bone at the mineralizing front. Additional information, such as a change in tetracycline fluorescence with time, would be necessary to determine which of these two processes was operative.

Dr. Simmons: I think that our experiences with tracers, such as tritiated glycine and proline [D. J. Simmons, *Proc. Soc. Exp. Biol. Med.* **121,** 1165 (1966); D. J. Simmons and A. S. Kunin, *Clin. Orthop.* **68,** 261 (1970)], permit us to say that osteocytes can form bone matrix, but only when they are very young. Autoradiographs of bone sections from rats sacrificed 1 hour after an ip injection of proline-^{3}H show silver grains over young osteocytes. These labeled cells are still present in front of the line of silver grains marking labeled bone matrix after 3 days, long after the effective labeling time has passed. If young osteocytes did not form bone matrix, it would be difficult to understand why the mature osteocytes have smaller lacunae.

Dr. Raisz: Could we draw the conclusion that osteocytic bone resorption is quantitatively of the order of one hundredth of osteoclastic resorption comparable to the relation between osteocytic and osteoblastic bone formation? Did you make any calculations on the basis of the maximal volume for osteocytic bone resorption and what contribution that makes to total bone resorption in your system?

Dr. Baylink: The endosteal osteoclastic bone resorption rate was an order of magnitude higher than the total (maximum) osteocytic bone resorption rate. In the mid-diaphysis, about 10% of osteoclastic bone resorption occurs around vascular canals and the remaining 90% at the endosteum. Therefore, the total osteoclastic bone resorption rate is at least an order of magnitude higher than the total (maximum) osteocytic bone resorption rate in the femoral diaphysis.

V. Calcium Transfer across Epithelial Tissues

INTESTINAL CALCIUM ABSORPTION, VITAMIN D, ADAPTATION, AND THE CALCIUM-BINDING PROTEIN*

R. H. Wasserman, R. A. Corradino, A. N. Taylor, and R. L. Morrissey†

The absorption of calcium by the intestinal tract occurs by at least two processes, one being active transport and the other diffusional in nature. The existence of an active transport mechanism was initially shown by Schachter and Rosen in 1959 and has been confirmed repeatedly by others. The active transport mechanism is characterized by saturability, inhibition by metabolic poisons, and some degree of specificity. The diffusional mechanism is characterized by being nonsaturable over a relatively wide range of calcium concentrations and being noninhibitable by metabolic poisons (Wasserman and Taylor, 1969).

One of the most important factors affecting calcium absorption in several animal species is vitamin D. The initial studies by Schachter and Rosen (1959) clearly showed that uphill calcium transport by the intestinal sac derived from a vitamin D-replete animal was greater than that from vitamin D-deficient animals. Harrison and Harrison (1960), at about the

---

* These studies were supported by NIH Grant AM-04652 and U.S.A.E.C. Contract AT(30-1)-4039.
† Present address: U.S. Army Medical Research and Nutrition Laboratory, Fitzsimmons General Hospital, Denver, Colorado.

same time, showed that the movement of calcium across gut sacs *in vitro* was accelerated by vitamin D, but by a nonmetabolically dependent mechanism. Our studies (Wasserman and Kallfelz, 1962; Wasserman *et al.*, 1966) tended to suggest that one aspect of vitamin D action was to increase transfer of calcium in both directions across the intestinal tract *in vivo*, which indicated that vitamin D affected the permeability characteristics of the membrane. The apparent effect of vitamin D on both a diffusional and active transport process was explained on the basis that the limiting step in the transport reaction was the rate at which calcium interacted with a transport system. Thus, in this simplified conceptualization, vitamin D was not required for the constitution of a component of the active transport complex, but functioned primarily on a diffusional barrier. Although this unifying hypothesis has merit, it is also plausible that vitamin D exerts two diversive and, perhaps, complimentary effects. Some evidence for this is given below, followed by a brief discussion of the relation of the vitamin D-induced calcium-binding protein (CaBP) to the adaptation mechanism, and finally, a description of an *in vitro* intestinal system amenable to the investigation of vitamin D action and calcium transport.

A Dual Effect of Vitamin D

The finding that the vitamin D-mediated absorption of calcium was inhibited or depressed by actinomycin D, puromycin, and cycloheximide (Schachter and Kowarski, 1965; Zull *et al.*, 1966; Norman, 1966) added another dimension to our knowledge of vitamin D mechanisms. These observations indicated that the effect of vitamin D was not due to the direct action of the steroid molecule on membranes, but to the synthesis of a "transport" protein for which the vitamin was required. At about the same time, a vitamin D-induced calcium-binding protein (CaBP) was identified (Wasserman and Taylor, 1966) and isolated (Wasserman *et al.*, 1968), and its behavior under various circumstances (A. N. Taylor and Wasserman, 1967; Wasserman and Taylor, 1968; Corradino and Wasserman, 1970; Wasserman, 1970) and its tissue localization were later investigated (A. N. Taylor and Wasserman, 1970a). The synthesis of CaBP was found to be inhibited by actinomycin D (Corradino and Wasserman, 1968). Complicating matters was the observation recorded by Zull *et al.* (1966) that when a large amount of vitamin D was given to a rat, the transfer of calcium across an everted duodenal sac under anaerobic conditions was not inhibitable by the concomitant administration of actinomycin D to the donor animal. This observation accentuated a hypothesis that has been long standing but which has yet no substantial basis and

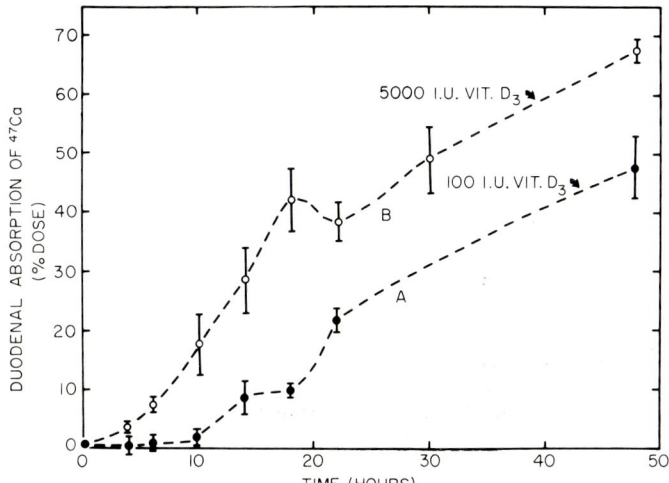

FIG. 1. Duodenal absorption of ^{47}Ca by rachitic chicks as a function of time after vitamin D_3 administration. At zero time, groups of rachitic chicks were given either 5000 IU vitamin D_3 (*upper curve*) or 100 IU vitamin D_3 (*lower curve*) by intramuscular injection in propyleneglycol. At the times designated in the figure, the duodenal absorption of ^{47}Ca over a period of 30 minutes was determined. Each point represents the mean of 5-6 chicks ±S.E.M. (Modified from Ebel et al., 1969.)

unequivocal explanation at the molecular level, that vitamin D can play more than one role in calcium absorption.

Data from our laboratory also suggest that vitamin D might have more than one effect on the intestinal absorption of calcium. Experiments in which the response of a rachitic animal to vitamin D with time is assessed often show two phases—an initial increase in absorption followed by a peak or plateau and then a subsequent rise (Fig. 1). The same pattern is also observed with 25-hydroxycholecalciferol (Fig. 2). These curves do not necessarily have to be interpreted on the basis of a dual mechanism but could be explained on the basis of the same molecular event separated in time by the transient limitation of an essential precursor, or perhaps a limitation in the conversion of vitamin D to a more active form.

A multiple mechanism of vitamin D, however, is also suggested from curves in which the absorption of calcium is measured as a function of the amount of vitamin D_3 given to the vitamin D-deficient animal at a standard time. As shown in Fig. 3, the resulting curves are bi- or possibly triphasic in character. This type of curve is less likely to be explained on the basis of a limiting precursor.

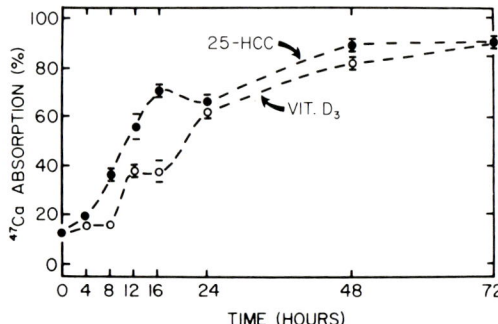

FIG. 2. Duodenal absorption of ^{47}Ca as a function of time after vitamin D_3 or 25-hydroxycholecalciferol (25-HCC) administration. Experimental protocol as in Fig. 1 except that 100 IU vitamin D_3 (*lower curve*) or its molecular equivalent of 25-hydroxycholecalciferol (*upper curve*) was given. Each point represents the mean of 6 chicks ±S.E.M. (Corradino, 1970, unpublished data.)

Although it might be tempting to suggest that one of the time-related phases is dependent on protein synthesis and the other is a direct membrane alteration by vitamin D_3 or 25-hydroxycholecalciferol (25-HCC), Norman (1965) demonstrated that actinomycin D blocked the total absorptive effect of 100 IU vitamin D_3 in the chick, the same level of vitamin D_3 used in experiments depicted in Figs. 1 and 2. Thus, both of these phases appear to be dependent on protein synthesis. One phase is undoubtedly associated with the formation of CaBP. The meaning of the other protein synthetic step can only be speculated upon at this time, but some possibilities can be offered. This step might be related to a calcium-sensitive adenosine triphosphatase (Melancon and DeLuca, 1970, see below) and an alkaline phosphatase (Norman *et al.*, 1970) associated with intestinal brush borders. The activity of each of these enzymes is enhanced by vitamin D and could constitute part of the calcium translocation system. Another possibility might be related to the conversion of vitamin D_3 and/or 25-HCC to other vitamin D metabolities in the intestine. An inducible enzyme for converting 25-HCC to another metabolite (peak V) is discussed in this volume by DeLuca. If this (peak V) or another metabolite has special membrane-altering properties (a highly speculative proposal), one of the actinomycin D-sensitive steps could be explained. Assuming this to be the case, an important problem would be to determine whether the hypothetical "membrane" steriod precedes or accompanies the synthesis of the "transport" protein. Since CaBP can be detected at the same time that a physiolgical effect of vitamin D_3 in rachitic chicks can be observed (Ebel *et al.*,

1969), it seems unlikely that the formation of the "membrane" steroid is a prerequisite for CaBP synthesis.

The observation of Zull *et al.* (1966) that actinomycin D does not inhibit the effect of large doses of vitamin D_3 (when given together) might be due merely to the arrival of the vitamin D at the target site before the antibiotic becomes effective. It might also represent a direct membrane effect, and act in a fashion similar to that of vitamin D_3 on the calcium permeability of the membranes of isolated mitochondria (DeLuca *et al.*, 1962). Taken together with the above information, it is suggested that vitamin D might exert not two but three effects, corresponding to the three phases noted in Fig. 3, two of which are actinomycin D-sensitive and one which is not.

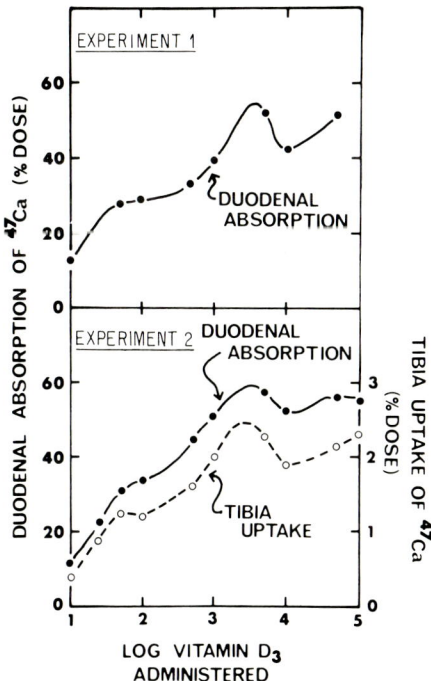

FIG. 3. Duodenal absorption of ^{47}Ca by rachitic chicks as a function of vitamin D_3 level. At 24 hours after dosing (chicks given doses of vitamin D_3) indicated in the figure were anesthetized and the degree of ^{47}Ca absorption by a ligated segment of duodenum *in situ* was determined. The period of absorption was 30 minutes. The upper curve is modified from Ebel *et al.* (1969) and the lower curves are the results of a replicate experiment. In experiment 2, the uptake of absorbed ^{47}Ca by the tibia was also measured. Each point is the mean of 5–10 chicks.

These studies are mentioned to point out the complexities of the problem in understanding vitamin D mechanisms and to raise questions that require additional systematic study. However, recognizing more explicitly the possible existence of multiple actions of vitamin D may aid in resolving discrepancies in interpretation of observations made by different groups.

Adaptation

Attention by our group has been given over past years, with varying degrees of vigor, to the problem of adaptation. As used in this context, adaptation refers to the process by which an animal can alter its efficiency of calcium absorption in response to the dietary intake of calcium. This phenomenon has been regonized for many years and has been studied in some detail by Nicolaysen and his group (1953) who made three prominent observations: (a) the process of adaptation is vitamin D-dependent, (b) the rapidity of adaptation varies inversely with the age of the animal, and (c) the degree of absorption of calcium is inversely related to the degree of mineralization of the skeleton. Nicolaysen also proposed that the skeleton can elaborate a factor which affects calcium absorption. Significant experimental observations were also made by Kimberg et al. (1961), using the in vitro everted gut sac and intestinal slice procedures. They showed again that adaptation is a vitamin D-dependent process, and that the rat retains the potential to adapt, despite the removal of the parathyroid glands, the hypophysis, and the adrenal glands. This information immediately tends to eliminate the parathyroid glands as the mediator of adaptation. Another significant study, also done several years ago, was that by Carlsson (1953) who investigated the effect of phosphate deficiency on the absorption of calcium by rats. The idea behind this experiment was that if it is the undermineralized skeleton that elaborates the adaptation factor, such a factor should be secreted whether the diet is deficient in calcium or in another mineral required for bone formation. The data showed that rats on a phosphate-deficient diet absorbed calcium to a greater degree than those on a normal phosphate intake. As had other investigators, such at Stanbury (1968) and Benson et al. (1969), Carlsson arrived at the conclusion that the skeleton plays a significant role in determining the extent of calcium absorption and that the parathyroid glands are not directly involved.

We had previously shown that the amount of vitamin D-dependent CaBP was greater in animals adapted to low calcium diets than in those raised on normal calcium intakes (Wasserman and Taylor, 1968). More recently, detailed investigations were undertaken to assess the effects of

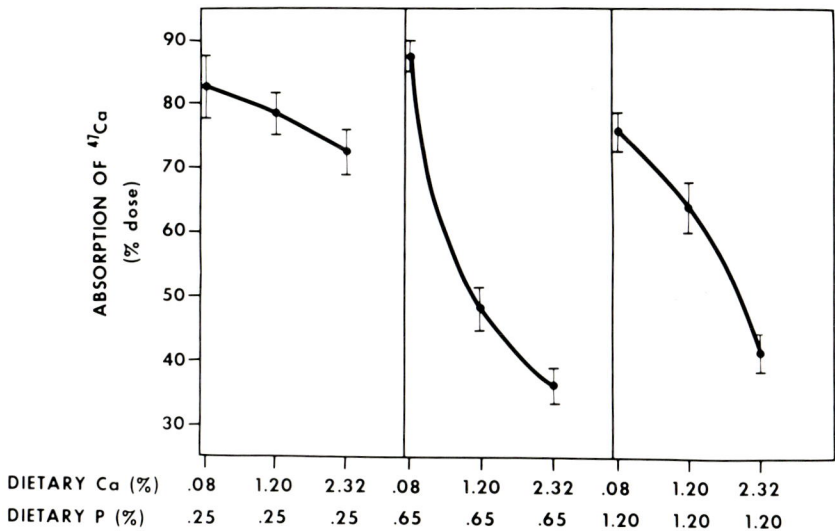

FIG. 4. Effect of dietary calcium and phosphorus on the duodenal absorption of ^{47}Ca. The chicks fed a normal diet were transferred to diets with varying calcium and phosphorus contents at age 17 days. At 10 days, absorption was measured. The various diets are given in the above figure. Each point represents the mean plus or minus standard error of the mean of 6 chicks per group. (From Morrissey and Wasserman, 1971.)

various calcium and phosphate intakes in chicks on both calcium absorption by the duodenum *in situ* and the CaBP concentration in these same segments (Morrissey and Wasserman, 1971). In this study, nine diets were compounded to yield diets containing deficient, normal, or high calcium concentrations and deficient, normal, or high phosphorus concentrations. As shown in Fig. 4, it is clear that the type of diet ingested by the animal had a significant effect on the efficiency of absorption of calcium from the duodenum. In general, the efficiency of calcium absorption was inversely related to the calcium content of the diet, particularly in those groups receiving either the normal or high phosphorus diets. A significant aspect of these studies was the verification of the observation of Carlsson that a phosphate-deficient diet, containing either a normal or high calcium level, resulted in a high rate of calcium absorption.

The CaBP concentration in the duodenum of the chicks in these various groups was closely correlated with the degree of absorption. The rate constant of absorption was estimated from the data, and a plot of this value versus CaBP concentration (Fig. 5) demonstrates this point; the

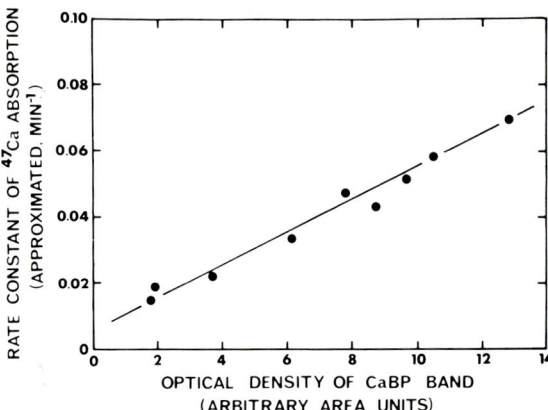

FIG. 5. Correlation between the rate constant of ^{47}Ca absorption and CaBP concentration. The rate constant of absorption was estimated from the data given in Fig. 4. The correlation coefficient was 0.99. CaBP concentration was quantitated by determining the optical density of the characteristic CaBP band on an acrylamide gel. (From Morrissey and Wasserman, 1971.)

correlation coefficient was calculated to be 0.99. In this same study, the ash content of the tibia (percent ash per fat-free dry weight) was also determined and, in Fig. 6, these data are plotted against the rate constant of calcium absorption. An inverse correlation between these two parameters is readily discernable, and the correlation coefficient was −0.94, indicating a possible interdependency of these two variables. As part of the same study, plasma calcium levels were also measured and, perhaps most revealing, were the values of the low phosphorus group. Those chicks receiving the low phosphorus–high calcium diet were hypercalcemic. As previously suggested by Mueller et al. (1970), the chick seems to be highly dependent on intestinal absorption of calcium for maintaining blood calcium levels and is less prone to the action of endogenous calcitonin as compared to other species. Thus, despite a high calcium level in the diet and a hypercalcemic state (in terms of total plasma calcium), the animals maintained a high rate of calcium absorption. Like the suggestions of others, these data indicate that the parathyroid gland most likely does not play a primary role in the process of adaptation, but that adaptation is more related to the degree of mineralization of the skeleton. However, a role of parathyroid hormone in conjunction with some other factor, or a secondary role, cannot be discounted.

Additional investigations were undertaken to obtain information on the intestinal site or sites altered during the process of adaptation (Morrissey and Wasserman, 1970). For this purpose, procedures previously used to assess the effect of vitamin D on calcium transport were employed (Wasserman and Taylor, 1969). Chicks on a calcium-deficient or calcium-adequate diet were anesthetized, and a 1 ml test dose of radio-calcium (with 1 mg ^{40}Ca in 0.15 M NaCl) was placed in a ligated loop of duodenum. At various time intervals thereafter, the absorption of radiocalcium from the lumen, the uptake of radiocalcium and stable calcium by the mucosa, and the appearance of radiocalcium in blood were measured. With similarly prepared animals, radiocalcium (at tracer levels only) was injected into a wing vein and the uptake of radiocalcium by the mucosal tissue and the radiocalcium transferred into the intestinal lumen were determined. In the latter case, the duodenum was ligated as in the absorption study and loaded with stable calcium only. Figure 7 shows that, at the shortest sampling period (2½ minutes), a significant difference in the absorption of calcium occurred. At this same time period, no difference in the uptake of radiocalcium by the mucosal tissue was noted, while at later time periods, there was a greater retention of radiocalcium in the mucosa of the calcium-replete group than in that of the calcium-deficient group (Fig. 8). These data suggest that in the adapted animal, the transfer of calcium from lumen to mucosal tissue was less affected. Studies on the transfer of ^{47}Ca in the opposite direction indicated that the uptake of plasma ^{47}Ca by the mucosal tissue and the transfer of ^{47}Ca into the duodenal lumen were

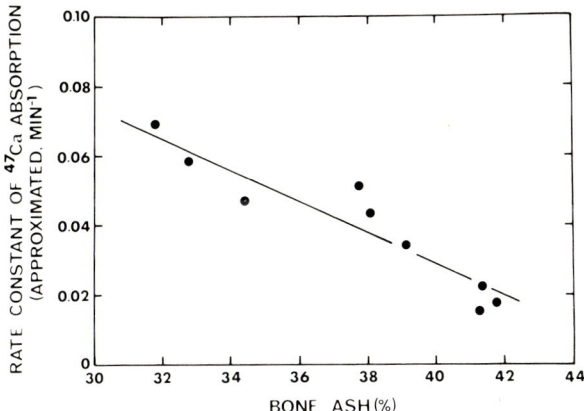

FIG. 6. Correlation between the rate constant of absorption of ^{47}Ca and bone ash (percent ash of tibia per unit fat-free, dry weight). The correlation coefficient was −0.94. (From Morrissey and Wasserman, 1971.)

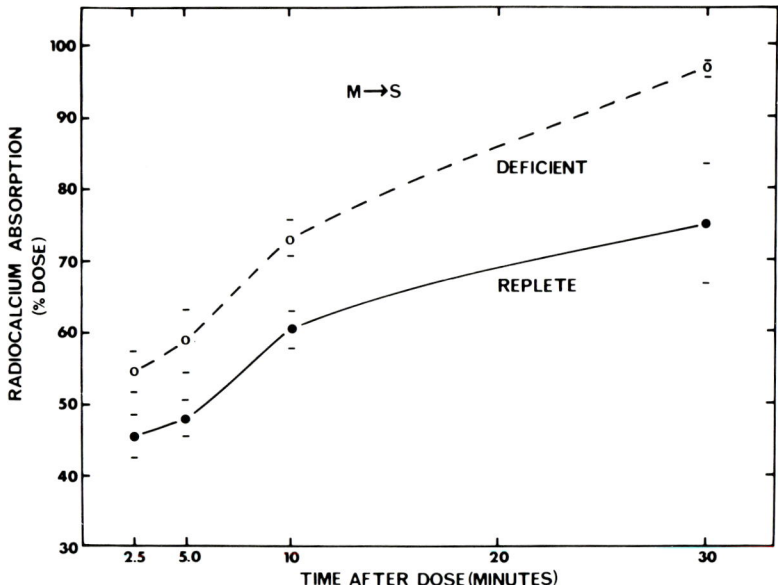

Fig. 7. Duodenal absorption of ^{47}Ca in calcium-deficient and calcium-replete chicks. The *in situ* duodenal loop procedure was used, as in Fig. 1. The chicks were handled similarly to those described in Fig. 4. Dietary phosphorus was 0.65%, and the calcium content was either 0.08% (deficient) or 1.2% (replete). Each point represents the mean plus or minus standard error of the mean of 5–6 chicks. (From Morrissey and Wasserman, 1970.)

greater in the adapted than in the normal chick. Again, as in the absorption study, the permeability of the basal and/or lateral borders of the intestinal cell seems to be affected by the process of adaptation. Whether the greater transfer of ^{47}Ca from plasma to lumen reflects only the increased passage of radionuclide into the mucosal tissue, or is due to an additional effect on the brush border, cannot be differentiated.

Two prominent differences might be mentioned between the flux patterns noted in the vitamin D-replete, calcium-deficient chick and vitamin D-deficient chick. In the vitamin D-deficient chick, the entry of luminal ^{47}Ca into the mucosal tissue was depressed, whereas no difference was observed at this step between the calcium-deficient and calcium-replete animal. In the vitamin D-deficient chick, no difference was noted in the transfer of ^{47}Ca from plasma to mucosal tissue, whereas in the calcium-deficient chick, this flux was increased. Thus, it appears that the intestinal sites affected by adaptation differ, in some respects, from those altered by vitamin D. Most revealing would be a knowledge of the distribution of CaBP at the subcellular level in these different situations.

Melancon and DeLuca (1970) recently showed that a calcium-sensitive adenosine triphosphatase (CaATPase) of brush borders was increased by vitamin D in rachitic animals. We confirmed this finding (A. N. Taylor and Wasserman, 1970b) but could not show a change in this enzyme until after CaBP was detectable and until after vitamin D had altered calcium absorption. Also, as shown in Table I, no differences were observed between the CaATPase associated with the brush borders in the calcium-deficient and calcium-replete animal.

Overall, these studies on adaptation accentuate the possible role of the skeleton in the control of calcium absorption by the intestine and tend to support the Nicolaysen hypothesis on the elaboration of a message from bone to intestine, with the size of the message being related to the degree of mineralization of the skeleton. To date, of course, no unique factor has been discovered that could be considered the endogenous factor of Nicolaysen.

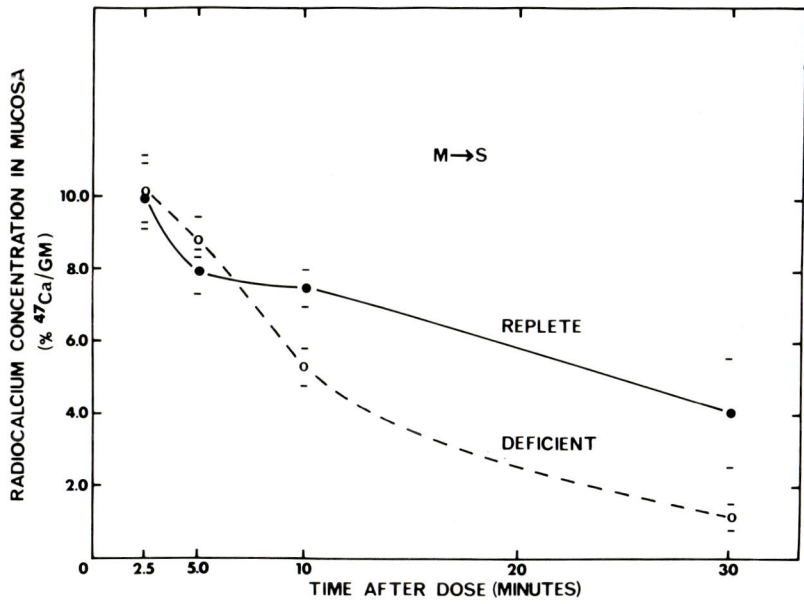

FIG. 8. Uptake of ^{47}Ca by duodenal mucosa as a function of time in calcium-deficient and calcium-replete chicks. This was part of the same study given in Fig. 7. The measurement of mucosal ^{47}Ca was as described elsewhere (Wasserman and Taylor, 1969). (From Morrissey and Wasserman, 1970.)

TABLE I

Adaptation, CaBP, and CaATPase[a]

Activity measured	Adequate calcium	Deficient calcium
CaBP[b]	7.8 ± 0.2	11.4 ± 0.5
ATPase[c]	72.1 ± 7.1	65.1 ± 3.7
CaATPase[c]	299 ± 32	331 ± 46

[a] Taylor and Wasserman, unpublished data.

[b] The calcium-binding activity (percent ^{45}Ca per milligram of protein) of supernates from mucosal cell homogenates was determined by the Chelex resin assay (Wasserman and Taylor, 1966).

[c] The ATPase activity associated with the isolated brush border fraction of intestinal cells (Forstner et al., 1968) was determined in the absence of added calcium (ATPase) and in the presence of 10 mM calcium (this value minus basal ATPase equals CaATPase) by the method of C. B. Taylor (1962). The assay period was 15 minutes in the presence of 2.5 mM ATP, and the values represent micrograms of liberated P_i per milligram of brush border protein.

Until a specific bone factor has been found, this remains an area of speculation.

Mention might also be made of two related questions in regard to control mechanisms. As indicated before, the evidence indicates that the process of adaptation requires the presence of vitamin D. What aspect of this process might be dependent thereon? We had noted previously that when vitamin D is given to a rachitic animal, there is an "overshoot" in the production of CaBP and the degree of absorption of calcium. Although these observations may be explained in several ways, they might indicate that the so-called endogenous factor is already present and accessible in the rachitic animal and the administration of vitamin D then allows the hypothetical factor to manifest its effect. If this is true, then the vitamin D-dependent process is at the end organ—namely, the intestine—and would not be required for the elaboration of the hypothetical factor from bone. It is also conceivable that the conversion of vitamin D_3 or 25-HCC to a more active form might be the critical step in the control of calcium absorption. This would mean that the conversion mechanism would have to respond to altered calcium states, a situation not yet shown. Then, too, the overshoot effect might, in the vitamin D-deficient state, be due to the suppression of enzymes that accelerate the degradation of 25-HCC or to the enhancement of enzymes that result in the more rapid conversion of vitamin D_3 to 25-HCC or other metabolites.

The second question concerns the effect of other physiological variables, such as the growth, lactation, pregnancy, and egg-laying, on the efficiency of calcium absorption. Is the increase in calcium absorption under these conditions controlled by the same mechanism as in adaptation? In all these situations, the metabolism of bone is greater than in the quiescent adult state. Are these relationships mediated by the factor proposed by Nicolaysen some 30 years ago?

Synthesis of CaBP in Organ Culture

In the progress of research on the problem of calcium absorption and vitamin D effects, we seem to cycle between *in vitro* and *in vivo* studies, hopefully using the approach best suited to the purpose at hand. Some of our initial investigations had been with the everted sac and intestinal slices. In an effort to assess the physiological significance of the data obtained, we then began to resort to *in situ* and *in vivo* experiments designed to obtain the same type of information derivable from the *in vitro* approach. Hopefully, the former would have more meaning and better simulate the state of affairs in the animal under normal circumstances. The cycle, however, has taken us back to an *in vitro* approach, initiated specifically for the reason that one does employ such systems: to have the capacity to control (to a certain extent) the environment of the tissue under observation and to impose certain variables at will. The particular problem under investigation was the study of the mechanisms and variables controlling the amount of CaBP synthesized by the intestinal mucosa.

It was noted earlier by Corradino *et al.*, (1969) that embryonic intestine was devoid of CaBP up until the day of hatching, at which time its presence could be readily demonstrated. Using this information, Dr. Corradino investigated the possibility of using this sterile, CaBP-less tissue in organ culture, with interesting results (Corradino and Wasserman, 1971a). The initial question asked of this system was whether or not it would respond in a predictable manner to the inclusion in the medium of vitamin D and related steroids, particularly with regard to the synthesis of CaBP and enhancement of calcium transport. By including vitamin D_3 at levels as low as 25 IU per milliliter in the incubating medium, the formation of CaBP occurred after a 48 hour period of incubation (Table II). It was also shown that the ability of the tissue to accumulate calcium was enhanced by vitamin D treatment (Table II). Additional experiments showed that 25-HCC was also capable of inducing the synthesis of CaBP and was two to three times more potent than vitamin D_3 itself. Thus, the system showed three characteristics expected of the *in vivo* situation: (a) induction

TABLE II

CaBP Induction and Enhancement of ^{47}Ca Uptake in Cultured Embryonic Chick Intestine by Vitamin D_3[a,b]

Vitamin D_3 in medium (IU/ml)	CaBP content[c] (μg/100 mg tissue wet weight)	^{47}Ca uptake[d] (percent dose/100 mg tissue wet weight)
0	0	13.14 ± 0.22
400	1.35	16.73 ± 0.67

[a] Corradino and Wasserman (1971a).

[b] Duodenal loops from 20-day-old chick embryos were incubated in organ culture in 70% McCoy's 5A (modified)—30% fetal bovine serum plus 100 units per milligram of nystatin. Incubation at 37.5°C for 48 hours.

[c] CaBP measured by radial immunoassay.

[d] ^{47}Ca uptake determined by incubating tissue (at 48 hours) in a buffer solution (pH 7.2) containing ^{47}Ca for 30 minutes.

of the synthesis of CaBP, (b) an increased uptake of calcium due to treatment, and (c) a positive response to 25-HCC and other vitamin D-related steroids. Studies with radioactively labeled leucine showed that newly synthesized CaBP had a much higher specific activity than the balance of the intestinal proteins. Although this is indicative of *de novo* synthesis, it is still possible that a precursor protein with as high a specific activity as CaBP may go undetected with the procedures used.

What was somewhat puzzling was the fact that vitamin D_3 itself was effective, particularly in view of the proposed concept that vitamin D_3 is first transformed into an active metabolite before it can exhibit biological activity (DeLuca, 1969). A primary site of transformation of vitamin D_3 to 25-hydroxycholecalciferol was suggested to be the liver (DeLuca, 1969). Since liver was absent from the organ culture preparation, it is apparent that the necessary transformation either can occur in the intestine itself or need not occur at all for biological effectiveness.

Unequivocal criteria necessary to state that CaBP participates in some transport function would require that calcium transport be inhibited by a specific inhibitor of CaBP (such as a specific antibody) or that the transport function of a CaBP-less tissue could be elevated by incorporating the protein into the tissue. Recent experiments have shown that, indeed, the latter was achievable with the *in vitro* embryonic intestinal system. Intestinal tissue, after incubation with CaBP for a period of 18 hours under the usual organ culture conditions, was found to translocate calcium more rapidly into and across the intestinal epithelium by the everted sac technique (Corradino and Wasserman, 1971b). Importantly, these data give substantive support to the idea that the vitamin D-induced CaBP has a prominent role in calcium translocation and, in some way, directly participates in the reaction.

Concluding Remarks

The calcium absorptive system has been under intensive investigation for several years, and knowledge of some of its characteristics has greatly expanded. It appears, for example, that vitamin D action requires the synthesis of a vitamin D-induced transport protein involved in calcium translocation. It also appears that a prominent cellular site of vitamin D action is the mucosal border. Associated with the brush border is CaBP, as shown by immunofluorescent antibody studies (Taylor and Wasserman, 1970). Also associated with the brush border is a vitamin D-stimulated, calcium-sensitive adenosine triphosphatase, a significant finding by Melancon and DeLuca (1970). If the CaATPase is equated with a calcium pump, the localization of this enzyme on the brush border is difficult to understand in view of the concept of Schachter et al. (1966) and a model given previously (Wasserman, 1968). In this model, permeation across the brush border is by a passive mechanism and that across the lateral and/or serosal border by active transport. Vitamin D was thought to alter primarily the permeability properties of the brush border, affecting the calcium pump directly or indirectly via the greater rate of calcium influx into the cell. Bar and Hurwitz (1969), in their elegant studies with the laying hen, also suggest that the entrance step is primarily downhill thermodynamically. Also, Adams et al. (1969) observed that filipin could elevate calcium transport across chick intestine *in vitro* and almost to the level seen in the vitamin D-replete animal. Filipin, a polyene antibiotic known to alter permeability properties of cholesterol-containing membranes, might increase the rate of passive transfer of calcium across the mucosal border and, in this way, duplicate vitamin D action in accordance with the model (alternate explanations for filipin action were given by Adams et al., 1969).

The intestinal CaATPase has also been studied by Parkinson and Radde (1970a,b) and they suggest that the vitamin D effect might be due to a difference in the retention of lateral membrane "tags" by the two different brush border preparations. Parkinson and Radde (1970a,b) also indicated that the level of CaATPase in non-brush border intestinal membrane fractions was not altered by vitamin D.

The role of CaBP in calcium absorption is unknown, but accumulated evidence as given herein and reviewed elsewhere (Wasserman and Taylor, 1969; A. N. Taylor and Wasserman, 1969), supports the hypothesis that it is intimately involved with the calcium absorptive process. The enhancement of calcium translocation in embryonic chick intestine *in vitro* directly by CaBP provides further substantial evidence for such a role. Whether it acts as a carrier, as a modifier of the calcium permeability characteristics of membranes, or in some other way cannot yet be stated. The observations that the calcium binding affinity of CaBP for calcium can be altered reversibly by urea (Ingersoll and Wasserman, 1971) or lysolecithin (Wasserman, 1970) might bear on its function.

Summary

Assessment of the pattern of response of the intestinal absorptive system of rachitic chicks to varying levels of vitamin D, and the temporal response to a single dose of vitamin D_3, supports the contention that the steroid might elicit its effect in more than one way. Tentatively, it is speculated that two responses appear to be actinomycin D-sensitive and one actinomycin D-insensitive. The synthesis of CaBP is probably associated with the first type. The nature of the other actinomycin D-sensitive process is unknown. The actinomycin D-insensitive process might represent a direct effect of vitamin D_3 on the intestinal membrane, and because of this, there is a change in its cation permeability.

Adaptation of chicks to low calcium diets results in the increased formation of CaBP and an increased absorption of calcium. From the results of experiments described herein, it appears that the calcium absorptive system responds to the degree of mineralization of the skeleton by a mechanism not necessarily mediated by the parathyroid glands. Also, CaBP is the first macromolecule associated with the calcium absorptive process shown to change in response to this dietary alteration.

The cellular site of the intestinal tissue which changes during adaptation appears to differ from that which is altered when vitamin D_3 is given to a rachitic animal. Whereas vitamin D_3 affects the transfer of calcium from intestinal lumen to mucosal tissue and, possibly secondarily, from mucosal tissue to blood, adaptation seems not to affect mucosal tissue uptake of calcium, but primarily the passage of calcium from mucosal tissue to blood.

An *in vitro* organ culture system was recently developed using embryonic intestinal tissue that does not contain CaBP. Incubation of the tissue in the presence of vitamin D_3 or 25-hydroxycholecalciferol induces the formation of CaBP and increases calcium uptake by the tissue. Incubation of the tissue with purified CaBP in the absence of vitamin D_3 increases the rate of transfer of calcium across the intestine; this provides direct evidence that CaBP is involved in the calcium translocation process and represents the first demonstration of reconstitution of a transport process by a binding protein in a higher organism.

REFERENCES

Adams, T. H., Wang, R. G., and Norman, A. W. (1969). *Fed. Proc., Fed. Amer. Soc. Exp. Biol.* **28,** 759.
Bar, A., and Hurwitz, S. (1969). *Biochim. Biophys. Acta* **183,** 591.
Benson, J. D., Emery, R. S., and Thomas, J. W. (1969). *J. Nutr.* **97,** 53.
Carlsson, A. (1953). *Acta Pharmacol. Toxicol.* **9,** 32.
Corradino, R. A., and Wasserman, R. H. (1968). *Arch. Biochem. Biophys.* **126,** 957.
Corradino, R. A., and Wasserman, R. H. (1970). *Proc. Soc. Exp. Biol. Med.* **133,** 960.
Corradino, R. A., and Wasserman, R. H. (1971a). *Science* **172,** 731.
Corradino, R. A., and Wasserman, R. H. (1971b). *Biophys. Soc. Abst.* **11,** 276a.
Corradino, R. A., Taylor, A. N., and Wasserman, R. H. (1969). *Fed. Proc., Fed. Amer. Soc. Exp. Biol.* **28,** 760.
DeLuca, H. F. (1969). *Fed. Proc., Fed. Amer. Soc. Exp. Biol.* **28,** 1678.
DeLuca, H. F., Engstrom, G. W., and Rasmussen, H. (1962). *Biochemistry* **48,** 1604.
Ebel, J. G., Taylor, A. N., and Wasserman, R. H. (1969). *Amer. J. Clin. Nutr.* **22,** 431.
Forstner, G. G., Sabesin, S. M., and Isselbacher, K. J. (1968). *Biochem. J.* **106,** 381.
Harrison, H. E., and Harrison, H. C. (1960). *Amer. J. Physiol.* **199,** 265.
Ingersoll, R. J., and Wasserman, R. H. (1971). *J. Biol. Chem.* **246,** 2808.
Kimberg, D. V., Schachter, D., and Schenker, H. (1961). *Amer. J. Physiol.* **200,** 1256.
Melancon, M. J., Jr., and DeLuca, H. F. (1970). *Biochemistry* **9,** 1658.
Morrissey, R. L., and Wasserman, R. H. (1970). Unpublished data.
Morrissey, R. L., and Wasserman, R. H. (1971). *Amer. J. Physiol.* **220,** 1509.
Mueller, G. L., Anast, C. S., and Breitenbach, R. P. (1970). *Amer. J. Physiol.* **218,** 1718.
Nicolaysen, R., Eeg-Larsen, N., and Malm, O. J. (1953). *Physiol. Rev.* **33,** 424.
Norman, A. W. (1965). *Science* **149,** 184.
Norman, A. W. (1966). *Amer. J. Physiol.* **211,** 829.
Norman, A. W., Mircheff, A. K., Adams, T. H., and Spielvogel, A. (1970). *Biochim. Biophys. Acta* **215,** 348.
Parkinson, D. K., and Radde, I. C. (1970a). *McLean Conf. Cell Mech. Calcium Transfer Homeostasis,* 1970.
Parkinson, D. K., and Radde, I. C. (1970b). Private communication.
Schachter, D., and Kowarski, S. (1965). *Bull. N.Y. Acad. Med.* [2] **41,** 241.
Schachter, D., and Rosen, S. M. (1959). *Amer. J. Physiol.* **196,** 357.
Schachter, D., Kowarski, S., Finkelstein, J. D., and Ma, R.-I. W. (1966). *Amer. J. Physiol.* **211,** 1131.
Stanbury, S. W. (1968). *In* "Nutrition in Renal Disease" (G. M. Berlyne, ed.), Livingstone, Edinburgh.
Taylor, A. N., and Wasserman, R. H. (1967). *Arch. Biochem. Biophys.* **119,** 536.
Taylor, A. N., and Wasserman, R. H. (1969). *Fed. Proc., Fed. Amer. Soc. Exp. Biol.* **28,** 1834.

Taylor, A. N., and Wasserman, R. H. (1970a). *J. Histochem. Cytochem.* **18**, 107.
Taylor, A. N., and Wasserman, R. H. (1970b). *Fed. Proc., Fed. Amer. Soc. Exp. Biol.* **29**, 368.
Taylor, C. B. (1962). *Biochim. Biophys. Acta* **60**, 437.
Wasserman, R. H. (1968). *Calcif. Tissue Res.* **2**, 301.
Wasserman, R. H. (1970). *Biochim. Biophys. Acta* **203**, 176.
Wasserman, R. H., and Kallfelz, F. A. (1962). *Amer. J. Physiol.* **203**, 221.
Wasserman, R. H., and Taylor, A. N. (1966). *Science* **152**, 791.
Wasserman, R. H., and Taylor, A. N. (1968). *J. Biol. Chem.* **243**, 3987.
Wasserman, R. H., and Taylor, A. N. (1969). *Miner. Metab.* **3**, 321.
Wasserman, R. H., Taylor, A. N., and Kallfelz, F. A. (1966). *Amer. J. Physiol.* **211**, 419.
Wasserman, R. H., Corradino, R. A., and Taylor, A. N. (1968). *J. Biol. Chem.* **243**, 3978.
Zull, J. E., Czarnowska-Misztal, E., and DeLuca, H. F. (1966). *Proc. Nat. Acad. Sci. U.S.* **55**, 177.

Discussion

Dr. Barzel: Do you have evidence that calcium binding protein forms in response to vitamin D in the adult animal, or is all your information based on studies in young, growing animals?

Dr. Wasserman: Most of our studies have been on the growing chick, but we know that the young animal has a greater concentration of intestinal CaBP than mature animals. Also, adult animals (roosters) respond to low calcium diets by an elevation in CaBP levels. However, we have not administered vitamin D to a vitamin D-deficient mature animal, so your question cannot be answered directly.

Dr. DeLuca: Bob, I wasn't quite clear on the time correlation experiment. I gather that those measurements of calcium binding protein were done with the immunoassay. Do you find that as time goes on following vitamin D and after detecting the small amount by immunoassay (which we cannot do), there is a very large increase in calcium binding protein after you get a crowning over of absorption? That is, Can you say that there is a direct quantitative correlation between binding protein and calcium absorption capacity?

Dr. Wasserman: In the steady state situation, as exemplified in the adaptation studies described in this chapter, there is a fairly good correlation between CaBP and the capacity of the intestine to absorb calcium. Several other such correlations have been documented. It is also quite true that CaBP can be detected by the immunoassay at the same time that a significant physiological response to vitamin D is seen after vitamin D is given to a rachitic animal. However, by the ion exchange assay, the correlation between absorption and CaBP levels is not that great. By this assay, there appears to be a time differential between these two parameters. This may be explained on the basis of assay sensitivity. And one must also recognize that CaBP occurs in at least two sites with perhaps only one of these sites (brush border) being concerned with calcium absorption. If we knew what proportion of the total CaBP is located at the functional site, the correlation might be considerably better during the short period after vitamin D administration. Also, in the studies of MacGregor *et al.* [*Biochim. Biophys. Acta.* (1970) **222**, 482, it was shown that in chicks given a subminimal level of vitamin D, the incorporation of leucine-^{14}C into CaBP after a supplemental dose of vitamin D increases dramatically before the physiological response occurs.

Dr. Goldhaber: If you add the vitamin D to the chorioallantoic membrane of the chick embryo, would you stimulate calcium binding protein in the intestine before it hatched?

Dr. Wasserman: No. I think you are putting your finger on one of the puzzling and interesting aspects of the system. The fact is there is no inadequacy of vitamin D in the egg. Yet, in the normal state of affairs, CaBP in intestinal tissue is not detectable until the day of hatch. But, under organ culture conditions, CaBP does not appear unless vitamin D_3 is present in the culture fluid. This is an important problem in terms of developmental biology. Dr. Corradino did inject vitamin D_3 and no effect was observed. However, by injecting cortisone, there was a stimulation of precocious synthesis of CaBP prior to the time of hatching.

Dr. Decker: Have you, utilizing the fluorescent antibody technique, looked for CaBP in other tissues besides intestine?

Dr. Wasserman: I'd like to refer this to Dr. Alan Taylor.

Dr. Taylor: The kidney and shell gland were examined with the fluorescent antibody technique. However, because of the low levels of CaBP in these tissues and the titer of the antiserum used, the localization of CaBP was not achieved.

Dr. Cohn: Your data, which compare the stability constants of the complexes of CaBP with several ions to the transport of these ions across the intestine, suggests to me that you believe that CaBP plays a role in the transport across the intestine of a variety of ions. Am I right in making this assumption, and if so, do you have some other data to support that idea?

Dr. Wasserman: There is a considerable body of evidence implicating CaBP in the absorption of calcium. We have no such evidence with regard to the absorption of other alkaline earths. We had merely pointed out the correlation between the relative binding affinities of CaBP with Ca^{2+}, Sr^{2+}, Ba^{2+}, and Mg^{2+} and the relative absorption of these cations under vitamin D stimulation, that is all. One certainly could not conclude from those data that CaBP is involved in the absorption of each of these ions.

Dr. Nichols: Bob, I was intrigued by your comment that the only tissues in which you find CaBP are of epithelial origin. This made me wonder whether you had been able to discover this material in any tissue which was of nonepithelial origin. Bone certainly is a mesothelial tissue, and perhaps this is the reason that the CaBP isn't there. Would you like to comment?

Dr. Wasserman: Yes. That is a possibility, George. The evidence is reasonably convincing that vitamin D does have a direct effect on bone, and if there is a mechanism similar to that in the intestine, then we would suspect the existence there of a vitamin D-dependent calcium-binding protein. However, there may be a different manifestation of vitamin D action at that site or an immunologically different CaBP may be present.

Dr. Posner: When the CaBP takes the calcium across a membrane, does it pass through the membrane itself with the calcium or does it release the calcium in some way and let it pass through by itself?

Dr. Wasserman: We really have no evidence on mechanism, if and how it is acting in this sort of carrier-like fashion, or if it is interacting with the membrane as part of the mechanism. Only shaky hypotheses are now available.

Dr. Dirksen: You have shown some nice data regarding high, low, and normal levels of calcium and phosphorus. Have you similar data regarding magnesium as related to CaBP levels in the intestine?

Dr. Wasserman: We have yet to show any significant effect of dietary magnesium on CaBP formation. Chicks on low calcium diet synthesize more CaBP than those on normal level. If the amount of calcium used to supplement the low calcium diet is replaced by an equivalent amount of strontium, CaBP synthesis is inhibited. If the dietary calcium is instead replaced by magnesium, CaBP levels are the same as in the low calcium group; i.e., magnesium elicited no detectable effect.

Dr. Wuthier: We have done a recent study on vitamin D deficiency in chicks. One of the things that impressed us in the vitamin D deficiency state was a remarkably higher serum magnesium [R. E. Wuthier, *Calcif. Tissue Res.* (1971) (in press)]. I wondered if anyone, particularly you, would care to comment as to how this mechanism might come about, because it is quite in contrast to what one finds in the pig or some other species where a decrease in serum magnesium is observed.

Dr. Wasserman: No, I have nothing to offer as to the mechanism to explain your observation on vitamin D-deficient chicks. We have not, ourselves, studied magnesium metabolism in rachitic and vitamin D-replete chicks in any detail.

Dr. Hitchman: Does the lysolecithin complex of CaBP disassociate during solvent extraction or Sephadex gel filtration? We would be interested in any other information.

Dr. Wasserman: The degree of disassociation of the lysolecithin–CaBP complex in aqueous solvents (and on the gel filtration column) depends on several factors, including the intrinsic binding constant of the reaction. We also have not studied this matter in any detail, but certainly, if one homogenizes in buffers containing taurocholate (and probably other detergents), the complex will be broken.

Dr. Vincenzi: Am I correct in assuming that no enzymic activities have been defined?

Dr. Wasserman: It has no ATPase activity, calcium dependent or otherwise.

Dr. Vincenzi: Have any other enzymic activities been explored?

Dr. Wasserman: We really haven't gone through the whole spectrum of possible enzymic activities, but it also is not associated with alkaline phosphatase.

VAGARIES IN THE USE OF ISOLATED INTESTINAL MUCOSAL CELL PREPARATIONS WITH PARTICULAR EMPHASIS ON CALCIUM UPTAKE*

Richard C. Bray and Irwin Clark

Introduction†

Studies *in vivo* of calcium absorption by the intestine often yield results at variance with those obtained from studies *in vitro*. For example, results from isolated preparations suggest that magnesium ions (Schachter and Rosen, 1959; Hendrix *et al.*, 1963) or parathyroidectomy (Rasmussen, 1959) inhibit calcium transport, while net absorption studies *in vivo* clearly show that magnesium ions increase calcium absorption (Clark, 1965; Clark and Belanger, 1967; Clark, 1969) and that parathyroidectomy is without any significant effect (Gran, 1960; Wasserman and Comar, 1961; Clark and Smith, 1964, Sammon *et al.*, 1970). On the other hand, the action

---

* This work was supported by U.S.P.H.S. Grant Nos. AM 04071 and TIAM 5408 and Atomic Energy Commission Contract No. AT (30-1) 2530.

† Abbreviations used in this paper: TCA = trichloroacetic acid, PCA = perchloric acid, DNA = deoxyribonucleic acid, BSA = bovine serum albumin, ATP = adenosine triphosphate, EDTA = ethylenediaminetetraacetic acid, HEPES = N-2-hydroxylipiperazine-N-2-ethane sulfuric acid neutralized with sodium hydroxide.

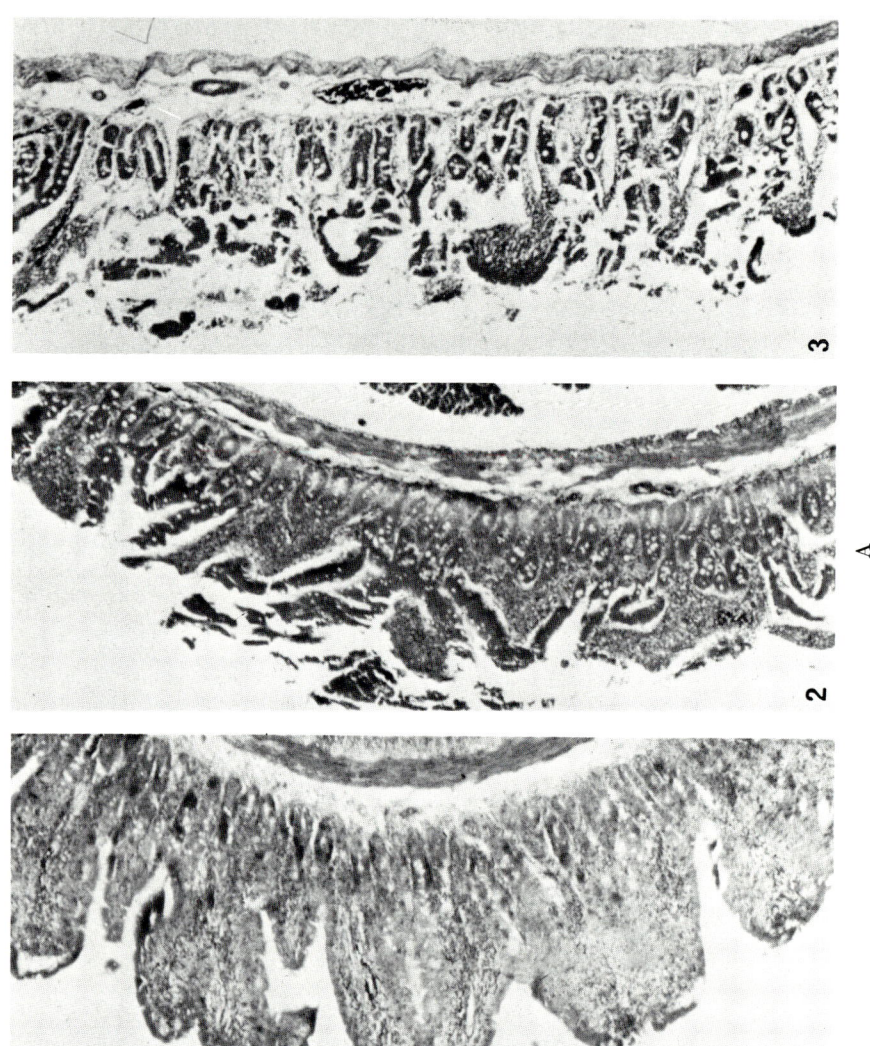

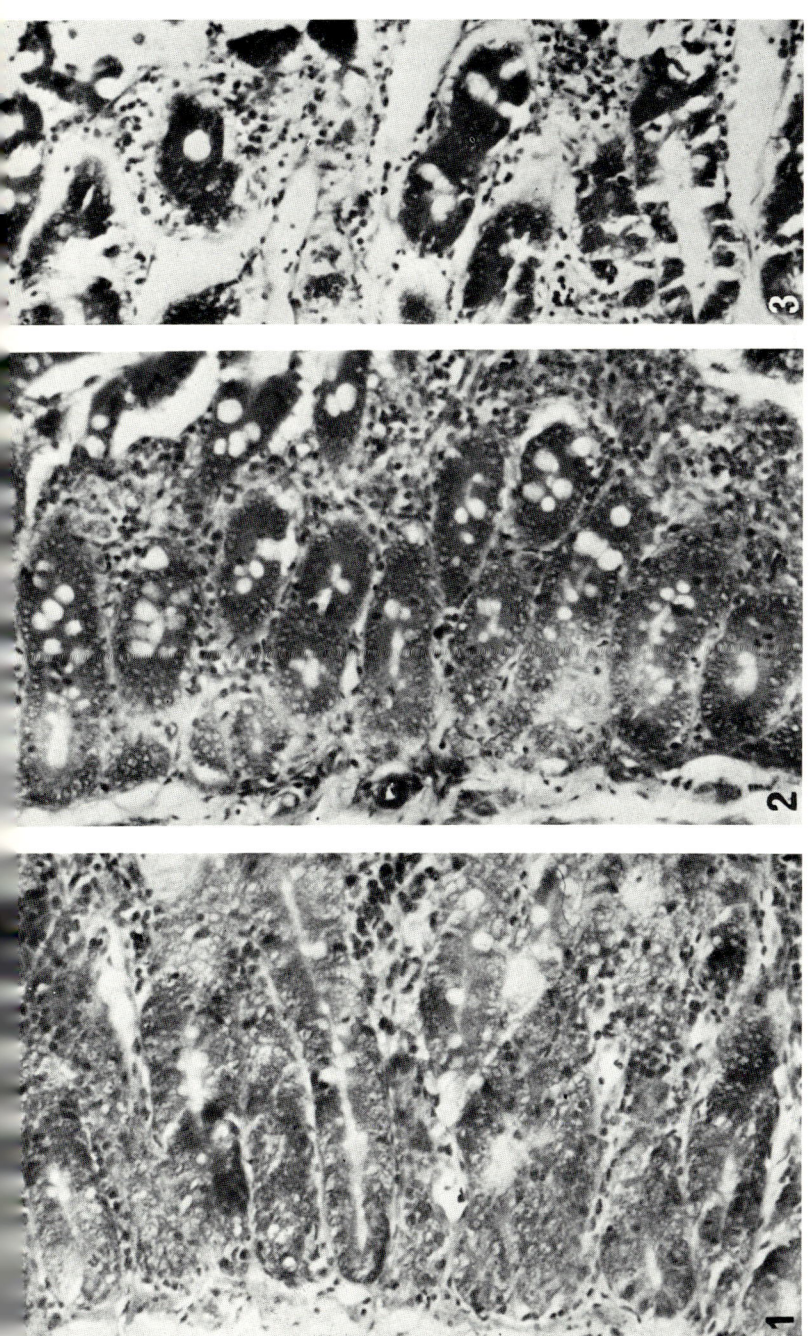

FIG. 1. Everted gut sac preparations prepared and incubated by the procedure of Schachter et al. (1966). A. Sections of serosal wall and villi (1) freshly made, (2) incubated 30 minutes, (3) incubated 60 minutes (× 40). B. Details of basal cell structure of villi at same intervals (× 240).

of vitamin D to increase calcium absorption or transport is observed in both types of studies (Dowdle *et al.*, 1960; Harris and Innes, 1931). What accounts for these discrepancies?

Measurements of calcium transport *in vitro* by the intestine have been done in two general ways: (a) using whole sections of the gut (Schachter *et al.*, 1960, 1966; Martin and DeLuca, 1969) and (b) using isolated cells or villi obtained from the intestinal mucosa by various means (Hashim and Clark, 1969; Perris, 1966; Kimmich, 1970; Rasmussen *et al.*, 1963). In the everted gut sac, an example of the first kind, the tissues remain approximately in their normal highly organized state, and overall transport of calcium against a concentration gradient has definitely been demonstrated. However, this transport occurs in a nonphysiological mode through underlying muscle layers and serosal membranes into a place which would be equivalent topologically to the peritoneal cavity. One must therefore have reservations in equating the process to absorption as it occurs *in vivo*. In addition, since there are changes in the appearance of mucosal cells (Fig. 1), transport by these cells may be altered. Indeed, active transport as measured may be through cells other than columnar cells.

Isolated cell preparations are also nonphysiological and interpretation of results is complicated by the following considerations.

1. A mucosal cell, once removed from its locus in the tissue and placed in an incubation medium, in principle may absorb materials from all sides. Cell surfaces other than the brush border, which is its normal working side, may take up calcium. If entry of calcium occurs through surfaces other than the brush border, it is clearly nonphysiological.

2. Calcium entering the cells *in vivo* is rapidly transferred from the cell into the vascular system. In the isolated cell preparation this process cannot occur; all that can be determined is net uptake of calcium by the cells.

3. In most systems *in vitro*, the concentration of the external calcium is much higher than the normal calcium level in the cell, which is of the order of 10^{-5} M. Incubation media often have concentrations ranging from 10^{-4} M to 10^{-2} M calcium. There is always present a potential for purely passive entry of calcium into the cells, a situation which also commonly prevails *in vivo*. Differentiation between active and passive transport is almost impossible, since the final calcium concentration in the cell may never reach or exceed that of the medium in a typical brief experiment.

4. It is impossible to obtain a preparation of pure intestinal mucosal cells uncontaminated by other types of cells and substances such as mucins. Furthermore, these impurities are not necessarily constant either qual-

itatively or quantitatively from one preparation to another. The assumption has genererally been made, but not proven, that only mucosal cells take up calcium. In addition, although such preparations contain considerable numbers of single cells, the majority are in groups which tend to agglomerate during incubations into stringy, mucoid-looking masses. These difficulties exist both with cells obtained by scraping and cells isolated by the hyaluronidase procedure of Perris (1966) as modified by Kimmich (1970).

5. Interpretation of the significance of radioactive calcium taken up depends upon the number of cells involved, and it is not possible to know how many of the total cells present actually take up calcium.

6. Another problem in all work *in vitro* is that of cell stability during the experiment. It is well known that cells taken from an animal degenerate rapidly and as we shall see, this is very much a problem in work involving intestinal preparations.

7. A potential difficulty of a different kind, frequently overlooked, is the insolubility of calcium biphosphate. This salt dissolves to the extent of less than 1 mM at pH 7.4. Combinations of calcium and HPO_4^{2-}, ions which exceed the implied solubility product occur in many experiments. While obvious precipitation usually does not take place, the potential for adsorption of calcium phosphate salts or complexes cannot be ignored. We have encountered instances where this clearly occurred. Calcium studies in physiological bicarbonate buffer systems entail the risk of calcium carbonate precipitation as well.

The following studies were undertaken to examine the behavior of isolated intestinal cell preparations in more detail to achieve a better understanding of the processes involved in calcium uptake and to evaluate whether experiments of this type offered any possibility of supplying valid data relevant to calcium uptake *in vivo*.

Materials and Methods

Male albino rats of Holtzman or other standard laboratory strains weighing from 170 to 350 gm were used. Weights of animals were nearly the same in any given experiment. Strain and size of the rats did not appear to influence results. All animals were deprived of food for 16–20 hours before use. High specific activity ^{45}Ca and galactose-U-^{14}C were obtained from International Nuclear Corporation. Radiochemical purity exceeded 99%. The enzymes and other reagents used were obtained from usual commercial sources and were of the best quality. Calcium was released from cells by treatment with a solution 0.1 M in cadmium chloride* and 0.02 N in HCl at 47°C for 10 minutes followed by vigorous mixing by Vortex mixer. In some cases, cells were extracted with 10% TCA at room temperature or with 0.5 N PCA at 70°C, depending on subsequent intentions. Release of calcium is achieved fully by all methods. Two extractions of 2 ml each were made, combined, and made to a known volume. Radioactivity was measured by placing suitable portions of extracts in 10 ml of Bray's solution (Bray, 1960) and counting in a Packard Tri Carb Model No. 3003 with efficiency of about 85%. All samples were prepared in duplicate and counted at least twice. Quenching, estimated by channel ratios, was always minor and was constant in each experiment. Calcium and magnesium were determined by atomic absorption spectrophotometry.

DNA was extracted from the cells by heating 15–20 minutes at 70°C in 0.5 N PCA. Two extractions were combined and portions assayed by the method of Dische (1930) as modified by Burton (1956). Similarly treated high molecular weight DNA was used as a standard. To determine protein, the residues were dissolved in 1 M NaOH and assayed either by the method of Lowry et al. (1951) or biuret. BSA was the standard.

Incubation Media

Experiments were run in either Krebs–Ringer–bicarbonate (Umbreit et al., 1957) or HEPES buffer systems. Details of the ions present were varied and are noted with individual experiments. Ionic strength was always close to that of 0.15 M NaCl. The pH was 7.4 ± 0.1 in all cases. Calcium = 45 was at 1 μCi/ml in almost all cases. As different total calcium concentrations were used, the specific activity varied, but it was constant in any given experiment. In some experiments the medium was supplemented with 0.25 M sucrose and 0.020 M glucose or fructose, but these were not found to improve the results and in later experiments were omitted.

Preparation of Cells

The procedure, an adaptation of that of Dickens (1941) was similar to that described previously (Hashim and Clark, 1969) with slight changes. Rats were decapitated, and the entire small intestine was quickly removed, flushed through with 50 ml of cold saline, and placed on ice. It was then cut into segments 8–10 cm long, each of which was run through with a small, blunt glass rod and slit with a scalpel to give an open sheet. Sheets were

---

* Hatcher and Goldstein (1969) have shown that cadmium improves quantitative precipitation of DNA.

placed on a chilled plate of glass, mucosal side up, and the edge of a glass slide was drawn lightly across the surface. Material collected was dropped into 5 ml of cold saline in a conical plastic centrifuge tube. After dispersal by brief use of a Vortex mixer, the suspended cells were forced through nylon cloth. They were then sedimented for 3–4 minutes at 500 g and washed twice in the same way with 7 ml portions of cold saline. This procedure removes most fine subcellular debris. Microscopic examination indicates that such preparations are predominantly clumps of surface cells with some free cells and contain relatively little material from deep layers. Cells from several rats were then combined, resuspended in saline, and pipetted into flasks containing the incubation medium at 0°C. Usually 1 ml of suspended cells was added to 4 ml of medium. Five to eight samples were obtained per rat and typically contained about 5 mg protein and 400 µg DNA.

Experimental Procedure

Incubation of cells was conducted in silicone-coated 25 ml Erlenmeyer flasks on a Dubnoff type shaker. In early experiments, a gas mixture of 95% oxygen-5% carbon dioxide was continuously pumped over the cells, but this was not found necessary and the flasks were usually simply stoppered after being thoroughly gassed with the oxygen and carbon dioxide mixture. The pH was still approximately 7.4 even after long incubations. At the end of incubation, the flasks were chilled and the cell suspension was poured into 10 ml conical glass screw-capped centrifuge tubes set in ice. Three to four minutes of centrifugation at 500 g yielded a pellet of the order of 0.15 ml. The cells were then washed twice with 8 ml portions of medium containing no ^{45}Ca or with buffered saline containing unlabeled calcium at a concentration equal to or somewhat greater than that used during the incubation using the same low speed centrifugation. Free and readily exchangeable ^{45}Ca is almost entirely removed by this procedure, as shown by analysis of the successive supernates and by the fact that the amount of ^{45}Ca extractable from the cells declined only very slowly with subsequent washings. Material washed in this manner should be largely or entirely freed of mitochondria, ribosomes, other subcellular debris smaller than nuclei, as well as of bacteria.

Results

Relation of Calcium Uptake to Calcium Concentration

In an effort to obtain some indication of the nature of the uptake process in experiments of this kind, we measured the amount of ^{45}Ca in the cells as a

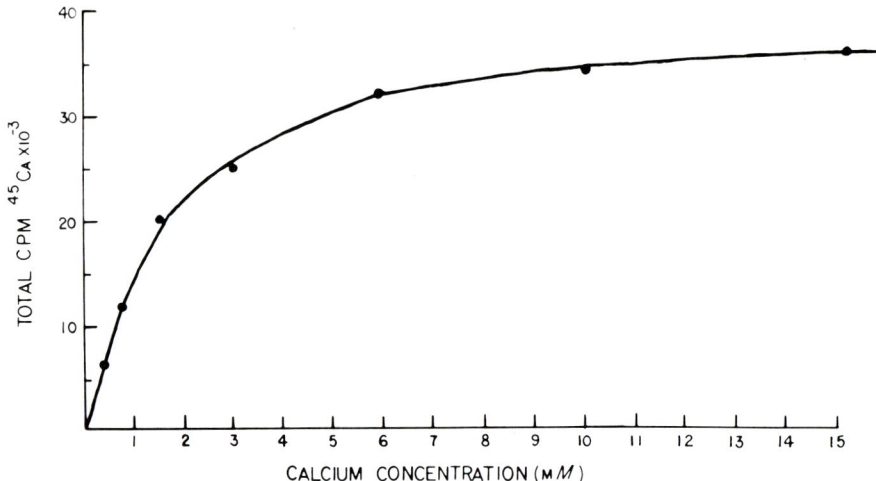

Fig. 2. Relation of calcium uptake by intestinal cells to calcium concentration. Cells were incubated in 0.12 M HEPES buffer, pH 7.4, containing 16 mM glucose and 0.25 mM K_2HPO_4 for 20 minutes at 34°C. Specific activity of all ^{45}Ca was 3 μCi per micromole.

function of the calcium concentration of the medium, the specific activity of the calcium being the same in all incubations. Figure 2 shows that a smooth plot is obtained which is nonlinear and biphasic. This could be interpreted as indicating that passive entry of calcium predominates at high concentrations, while there is active uptake at low concentrations.

EFFECTS OF METABOLIC INHIBITORS

In search of confirmation of this indication of active uptake at low concentrations, we tested the effects of a number of common metabolic inhibitors on the ^{45}Ca taken in by cells at 1 mM near the shift point of the curve in Fig. 2. The results are shown in Fig. 3. Surprisingly, none of these agents cause significant inhibition. In particular, it was found that a high concentration of cyanide ion, which would stop all electron transport to oxygen, seems to increase the uptake. This unexpected effect has been observed previously, though at lower concentration. Mercuric ion, which has the strongest effect, could well be acting in a gross, nonspecific manner, since p-chloromercuribenzoate, a more specific agent against sulfhydryl enzymes, is less effective. Ouabain, which commonly interferes with active transport, is without effect as are inhibitors of glycolysis. The lack of effect of warfarin argues against the involvement of mitochondria. In addition,

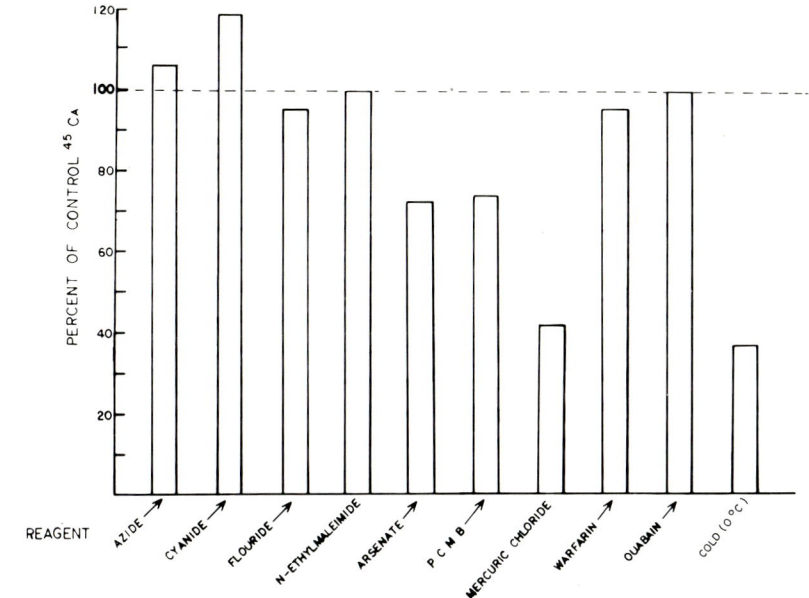

Fig. 3. Influence of metabolic inhibitors on calcium uptake by intestinal cells. Inhibitors were included in incubation medium at following concentrations: NaN_3 10 mM, NaCN 20 mM, NaF 1 mM, N-ethylmaleimide 0.8 mM, potassium arsenate 40 mM, PCMB (p-chloromercuribenzoate) 0.3 mM, $HgCl_2$ 0.3 mM, warfarin 0.5 mM, ouabain 0.5 mM. Medium was Ringer–bicarbonate plus 20 mM glucose in most cases. Incubation in 1 mM Ca^{2+} was for 15 minutes at 35°C.

we have been unable to reproduce the stimulation of calcium uptake by glucose which we reported previously using a calculation based on DNA recoveries (Hashim and Clark, 1969).

Relation of Calcium Uptake to Cellular Integrity

The inhibitor studies gave little support for the idea that an active process was being observed. Nonetheless, we felt that the results might have some physiological relevance, since much calcium absorption *in vivo* is undoubtedly passive, and even passive entry to the cell could in principle be subject to regulation. However, before drawing any further conclusions we thought it necessary to examine the relation between calcium uptake and cellular integrity more thoroughly.

During work done with this system, an abiding problem has been decline of DNA in the preparation during the course of incubation, frequently to

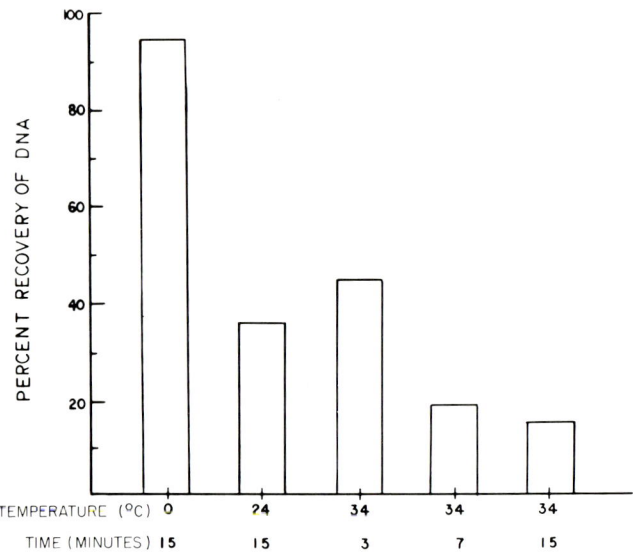

FIG. 4. DNA in isolated product as compared to a like cell sample at zero time and 0°C. Incubation was in Krebs–Ringer–bicarbonate with 0.25 M sucrose and 10 mM Ca^{2+} (1.2 mM Mg^{2+}).

less than 40% of the initial amount. This phenomenon had been noted earlier by others but not clarified in detail (Stewart and Zbarsky, 1963). For a long time this was accepted as representing normal breakdown of cells, and calculations of calcium uptake were simply based on final DNA values. However, we were always uneasy about this situation, particularly because small DNA recoveries magnify the implied uptake per cell. We persistently noted that high ratios of calcium uptake per cell at 38°C compared to 0°C controls were almost always associated with low DNA recoveries in the 38°C samples rather than with really large differences in the absolute radioactivities. We have examined this matter further, with interesting results. Figure 4 shows that in an experiment with poor DNA recovery, the bulk of the DNA disappeared very quickly in the first few minutes of incubation and that sizeable loss of DNA occurs even on brief incubation at the lower temperature of 24°C. In marked contrast, DNA is quite stable at 0°C. In fact, samples kept at 0°C for periods of up to 3 hours usually show very little decrease in DNA. Whether DNA is lost by simple cell breakdown or in some other way, the process has a very high temperature coefficient. This suggested that some complex enzymic process might be involved. If DNA can vanish this rapidly, it is possible, if not likely, that at least some of it is being broken down inside the nuclei of cells before the cell as a whole breaks down. This is also suggested by the fact that histological observations at end of incubation still show whole cells or clumps but with significantly less nuclear material.

A basic assumption necessary for any calculation based on uptake/DNA is that essentially whole cells containing nuclei are centrifuged down at low speeds. Another assumption is that broken cells would release their DNA into the medium and that this DNA would not be centrifuged down at low speeds. To check these assumptions, a preparation of cells was homogenized for 2 minutes either before or after the incubation. While this might possibly have failed to break every cell, it could reasonably be expected to rupture the great majority of them. Figure 5 shows that DNA in ground cells was only a modest amount lower than in normally handled ones. Clearly, the DNA in ground cells was not released and dispersed in such a way that it was lost from our final low-speed sedimenting fraction. The main effect of DNA recovery was not the disruption of the cells but the subjection of

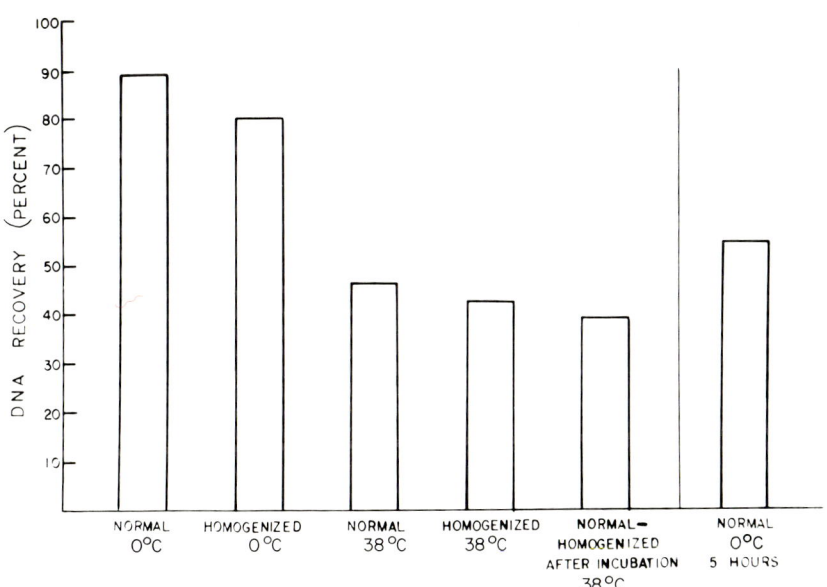

FIG. 5. DNA recoveries from normal and homogenized mucosal cells. Cells prepared normally or like portion of cells previously homogenized for 2 minutes in a Potter–Elvejhem device were incubated for 13 minutes in 0.12 M HEPES buffer containing 1.2 mM Ca^{2+} and 1.1 mM Mg^{2+}. Recoveries of DNA were compared to nonincubated samples.

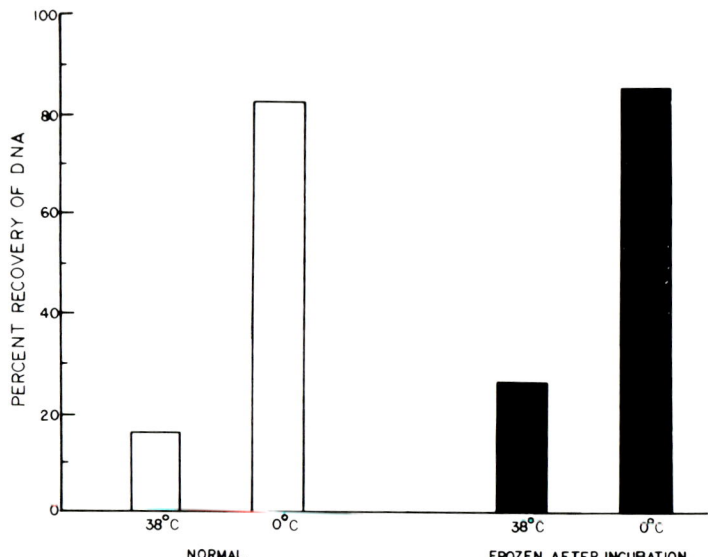

Fig. 6. DNA recovery in normal and frozen cell samples. Identical aliquots of cells were incubated for 15 minutes with 2 mM Ca^{2+} and 1.2 mM Mg^{2+} in Ringer–bicarbonate buffer, pH 7.4, either at 0°C or 38°C. Some samples were frozen five times at −80°C before washing and isolation.

them to room temperature for a few minutes. Note that cells held 5 hours at 0°C still retained more DNA than those warmed to 38°C for only 13 minutes—a phenomenon which we have now observed regularly.

As a check on the validity of the grinding procedure, cells were subjected to several cycles of freezing and thawing. Thawing was conducted at 5–10°C followed by immediate refreezing at −80°C. Microscopic examination of smears of this material confirmed that this procedure totally disrupted the cells. Nonetheless, DNA values on the washed debris were about as high as on normal, nonabused samples (Fig. 6).

Clearly, the method of estimating the relative number of intact cells by determination of DNA in the final washed product is unsound. In fortunate cases, experiments analyzed on this basis may appear to give reasonable results which could well be roughly correct. However, in view of the above findings, this type of calculation must be abandoned, and earlier results based on it must be viewed with reservation. We now feel that any uptake reported is best calculated on the basis of gross counts per portion of cells, at least in experiments where factors causing sizeable differences in recovery of material are absent.

In attempts to improve DNA recovery, we investigated the effects of ions other than Na^+, Cl^- and HCO_3^-, which had been shown previously to be noncritical. Figure 7 illustrates a striking result, namely that the large loss of DNA did not occur if magnesium was omitted (or its concentration reduced below 0.3 mM). However, cellular integrity was not improved, since microscopic examination of each preparation showed a singular lack of cellular detail and stringy masses of material which stained as nucleic acids. Although lack of magnesium prevented DNA breakdown, it did not maintain the cells in a normal state. Possible interpretations of the preservation of DNA might be that these cells contain a potent DNase which requires magnesium; or perhaps in the absence of magnesium the DNA is denatured, rendering it impervious to attack by DNase.

Another assumption in studies of this kind is that those cells which take up calcium either remain intact during incubation, or, if they break down, their calcium is released into the medium. It is also necessary to assume that broken or dead cells and large noncellular debris do not take up calcium significantly. If they do, interpretation of uptake data is rendered virtually impossible. Some types of intestinal cell debris do exhibit calcium binding under some conditions as has been noted by Wasserman and Taylor (1963). However, the important binding factor which he has characterized

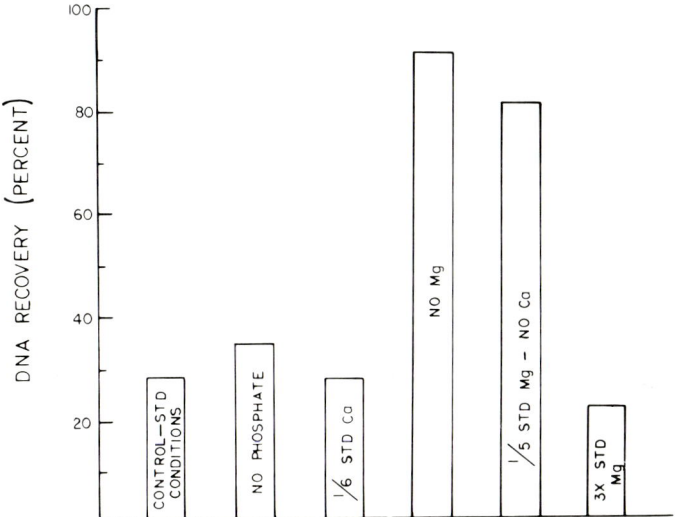

Fig. 7. Influence of magnesium, calcium, and phosphate on DNA recovery. Cells were incubated for 15 minutes at 35°C in Ringer-bicarbonate buffer. The "standard" calcium concentration was 8 mM and standard magnesium 1.2 mM.

(Wasserman et al., 1968) is a soluble protein which appears in the high speed supernatant fraction once cells are broken. This binding protein should not be present in such broken cells as might be recovered in our experiments. We noted, however, a disturbing tendency for the total recovered counts of ^{45}Ca to vary relatively little in experiments, although cell degeneration as indicated by the DNA recovery varied a great deal. Eventually we asked the question: if the incubation period is prolonged until the vast majority of the cells have degenerated and DNA almost vanished, is it still possible to recover material which contains a lot of calcium? The answer is shown in Table I. A pellet of not much reduced size was recovered even after 6 hours at 38°C. DNA, while not totally gone, was down to the order of 2%. Nonetheless, there was a relatively large amount of ^{45}Ca in the pellet (roughly eight times that found after the usual short incubation and up to the order of 1% calcium by weight). Also, 80% or more of these counts were still attached to the isolated material if it was frozen and thawed five times before the washing steps. Clearly, the bulk of the counts taken up, at least during the extended phase of the incubation, became attached in such a way that they were not released to the medium when cells degenerated, but remained bound to easily sedimentable debris.

TABLE I

DNA RECOVERY AND CALCIUM-45 UPTAKE IN MUCOSAL CELL PREPARATIONS[a]

Buffer	Time at 38°C	Approximate DNA recovery (%)	^{45}Ca (cpm)	µg calcium
Experiment A				
Ringer–bicarbonate system	15 minutes	21	39,000	1.45
	6 hours	1[b]	325,000	13.6
	6 hours, then frozen[c]	2[b]	265,000	9.9
Experiment B				
HEPES System	15 minutes	29	27,000	1.0
	6 hours	1.3[b]	230,000	8.5
	6 hours, then frozen[c]	3.3	224,000	8.3

[a] Calcium concentration 2 mM in all cases.

[b] The lowest DNA values were at margin of measureability.

[c] Cells were frozen and thawed 5 times at the end of incubation, but before the washing steps.

TABLE II
Calcium Uptake and Retention by Normal and Broken Cells[a]

Experiment	Conditions	Total ^{45}Ca in washed product (cpm)
1	Normal Procedure	27,000
	Cells frozen five times after incubation	28,000
2	Normal Procedure	29,000
	Cells homogenized before incubation	26,600
	Cells homogenized after incubation	23,000

[a] In both experiments cells were incubated 15 minutes at 38°C in 0.12 M HEPES, pH 7.4, containing 2 mM Ca^{2+} and 0.25 mM Mg^{2+} and K$_2$HPO$_4$. Cell breaking procedures were performed before washing steps.

Also, ^{45}Ca recovery in cell samples frozen and thawed several times after a normal 15 minute incubation but before the washing steps was esentially the same as in samples handled in the conventional way (Table II). Further, cells homogenized either after or before incubation yielded a pellet containing almost as much ^{45}Ca as one from cells used in the normal gentle way. Thus, cellular integrity had no significant effect on calcium binding.

Time Course of Calcium Binding

We should emphasize that this binding of calcium by intestinal cellular debris differs from the more or less immediate reaction characteristic of most chemical binding situations, since it has the property of progressing in a steady manner with time, as shown by Fig. 8. There is a trace of binding at zero time, but calcium then continues to accumulate in the material for several hours, typically at a roughly linear rate at 38°C. The process is quite strongly temperature dependent, as shown by Fig. 9, and seems to fall off more with time at 0°C.

This property of intestinal cells, whatever interest it may possess in itself, seems to destroy any last hope of useful interpretation of studies of this kind in terms of normal calcium absorption processes. The relationship of calcium in the samples to calcium in the medium must reflect primarily a complex binding process.

While these results could also be imagined to reflect the gradual formation of an inorganic precipitate containing calcium, this is contraindicated by the fact that the binding is seen equally when neither phosphate nor any source of carbonate are present, as well as by the fact that it is decreased by low temperature. We are also confident that bacterial contamination is not the cause for several reasons: (1) Bacterial growth proceeds exponentially after an initial lag phase when the number of bacteria present is negligible; the time course of calcium binding is not of this form. (2) High concentrations of chloramphenicol did not decrease the binding. (3) The method of washing the samples after incubation should remove most bacteria.

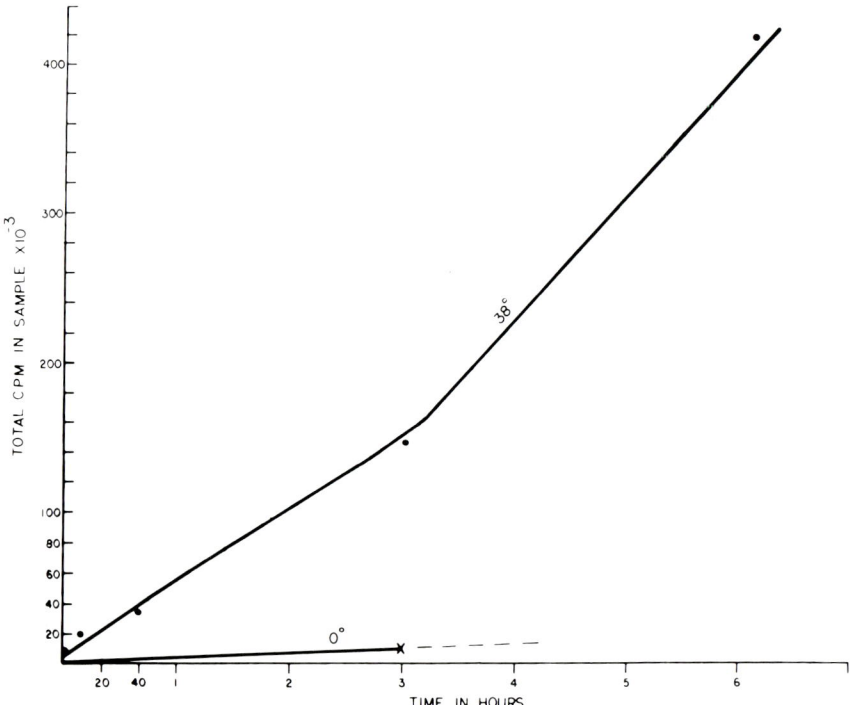

FIG. 8. Time dependence of binding of calcium to intestinal cells broken by freezing. Mucosal cells, which had been prepared as usual and then subjected to nine cycles of rapid freezing, were incubated in a Ringer–bicarbonate buffer containing 6 mM ^{45}Ca but no other salts. The large amount of cellular debris which was recovered by low speed washing (see Section II) was assayed for ^{45}Ca.

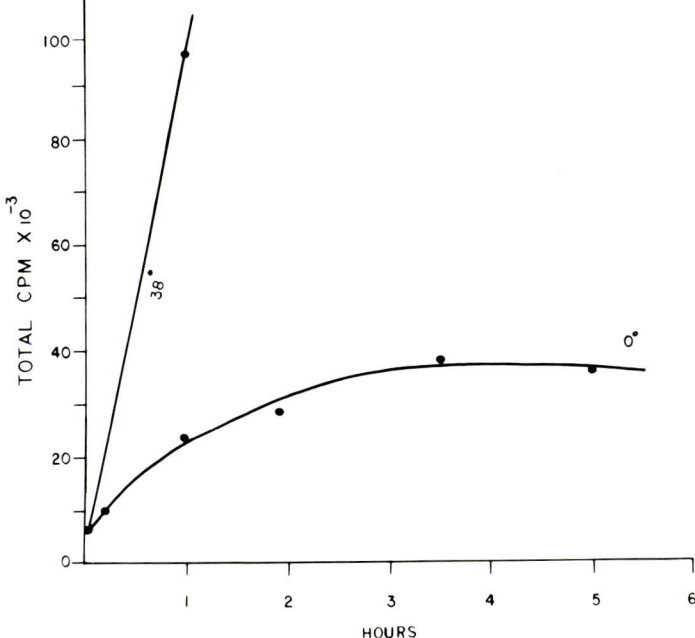

FIG. 9. Time course of calcium binding by frozen cells at low and high temperature. Mucosal cells prepared as in Fig. 8 were incubated in simple 0.12 M HEPES buffer containing 1 mM ^{45}Ca and no phosphate.

TABLE III

BINDING OF CALCIUM IN THE PRESENCE OF HIGHER CONCENTRATIONS OF OTHER IONS[a]

Competing ion	Factor of excess over calcium	^{45}Ca bound (% of control)
Mg^{2+}	10	81
Sr^{2+}	4	65
Ba^{2+}	4	64
Be^{2+}	3	100
Li^{2+}	15	100
K^+	40	100
HPO_4^{2-}	36	100

[a] Frozen intestinal cells were incubated 1 hour at 38°C in Ringer–bicarbonate buffer, pH 7.4, with Ca^{2+} concentration of 1 or 2 mM and added ions at concentrations exceeding Ca^{2+} by factor indicated.

Specificity of Binding for Calcium

To determine the specificity of this binding, we tested the effects of various closely related ions at concentrations severalfold in excess of the calcium present in the medium. If any of these ions is bound to the same site with the same order of effectiveness, the competition should greatly reduce the amount of ^{45}Ca in the isolated product. Table III shows that while the closely related ions strontium and barium do compete to some extent, their affinity for the site is considerably less than that of calcium. Magnesium competes very little and alkali ions not at all. Sodium was not tested directly, since all media and washes contain a large excess of sodium over calcium. These data suffice to show that the binding process is sufficiently oriented specifically toward calcium that one may reasonably regard it as a calcium-specific reaction.

Nature of the Binding Substance

In an attempt to obtain some information about the general class of substances involved in the binding, we tested the effect of a variety of enzymes and other relevant reagents. Only large, clear cut effects are likely to be significant in crude experiments of this nature. Also, many of these

TABLE IV

Influence of Enzymes on Calcium Binding to Intestinal Debris[a]

Enzyme	Concentration (μg/ml)	^{45}Ca bound (% of control)	Protein recovered (% of control)
RNAase	100	100	100
DNAase	24	100	100
Lysozyme	400	115	125
Hyaluronidase	400	100	90
Neuraminidase	15 (units)	95	100
Lipase	600	120	130
Phospholipase C	500	220	100
Phospholipase D	500	100	130
Acid phosphatase	400	76	85
Collagenase	500	200	100
Chymotrypsin	200	75	66
Trypsin	200	48	44
Pronase	360	36	28

[a] Freeze-ruptured mucosal cells were incubated in Ringer–bicarbonate buffer containing 2 mM ^{45}Ca at 38°C for 60 minutes in presence of enzymes, and the material isolated as usual.

TABLE V
INFLUENCE OF REAGENTS AND OTHER FACTORS ON CALCIUM BINDING BY INTESTINAL CELL DEBRIS[a]

Reagent	Concentration	^{45}Ca bound (% of control)	Protein recovery (% of control)
p-Chloromercuribenozoate	2 mM	74	100
N-Ethylmaleimide	3 mM	58	86
Iodoacetate	3 mM	62	93
Mersalyl	2 mM	65	120
HgCl$_2$	1 mM	69	180[b]
Mercaptoethanol	20 mM	100	72
ATP (+Mg)	2 mM	60	100
Cyclic AMP (derivative)	0.5 mM	95	100
Citrate	2× Ca	47	100
Sodium dodecylsulphate	0.3%	58	29
Triton X-100	0.3%	15	76
Sodium deoxycholate	0.3%	15	73
Sodium deoxycholate	1.0%	<1%	33
Formaldehyde	3.6%	67	108
pH lowered to 5.5[b]	—	<5%	116
EDTA in last wash only	20 mM	4	100

[a] Frost-ruptured cells incubated 60 minutes at 38°C in Ringer–bicarbonate medium. Calcium at 2 mM.

[b] Protein recovery raised by denaturation of soluble protein.

[c] By addition of acetate buffer.

agents lead to sizeable changes in overall recovery of material as indicated by protein values or visual estimation of the pellet. In these cases, a correction should doubtless be applied, but it is not possible to know its exact nature.

Table IV shows the effects of high concentrations of enzymes which attack the main types of biological macromolecules. Some allowance must be made for fact that not all of these enzymes are optimally active at pH 7.4, but it could be expected that all would show at least some activity under the experimental conditions. It appears that calcium is almost certainly not attaching to a nucleic acid, and probably not to a mucopolysaccharide, a phospholipid, or collagen. Results with all proteolytic enzymes tested are inconclusive, since the natural reduction in recovery of protein is similar to the reduction of ^{45}Ca. It is reasonable to speculate that calcium might be bound to a protein; this matter is left open.

Table V shows the effect of some chemical reagents on the calcium binding process. The most striking and probably most significant effects were seen with agents which are primarily detergents. Inclusion of 1% sodium deoxycholate in the incubation medium caused almost total suppression of calcium binding; it also solublized about two-thirds of the protein. Lower concentrations of sodium deoxycholate or Triton X-100 also reduced calcium binding markedly with only slight reduction in protein recovery. We have also found that most of the ^{45}Ca was removed from the residue by washing once with chloroform–methanol, whereas aqueous washes have little effect, ruling out calcium present as an inorganic precipitate. All sulfhydryl-binding reagents had a modest inhibitory effect, but the levels tested were higher than normally used, and as with whole cells, none was as effective as mercuric ion. These results suggest strongly that the site of calcium binding may be a membrane or some other lipid-rich structure. Further conclusions cannot be reached from present data.

COMPARATIVE BEHAVIOR OF UPTAKE IN OTHER SYSTEMS

It seemed wise to check whether calcium binding is specific for intestinal cells, since other cells might behave the same way with respect to calcium. Further, the uptake of a nonionic substance was examined to see

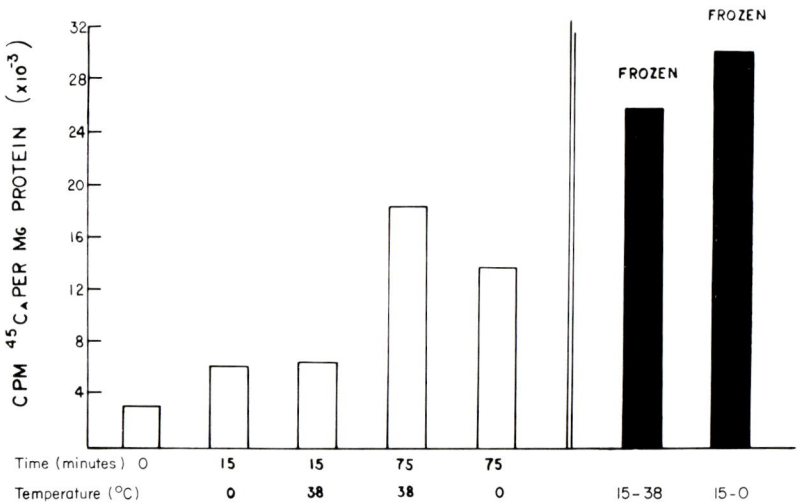

FIG. 10. Uptake of ^{45}Ca by thymocytes. Thymic cells were isolated by teasing glands of young rats in saline and washing and resuspending as with intestinal cells (see Section II). Portions of cells were incubated in simple 0.12 M HEPES buffer (pH 7.4) containing ^{45}Ca at 4 mM as only additive for 15 or 75 minutes. In a similar experiment, cells first frozen three times were used.

Calcium Binding by Isolated Intestinal Cells 333

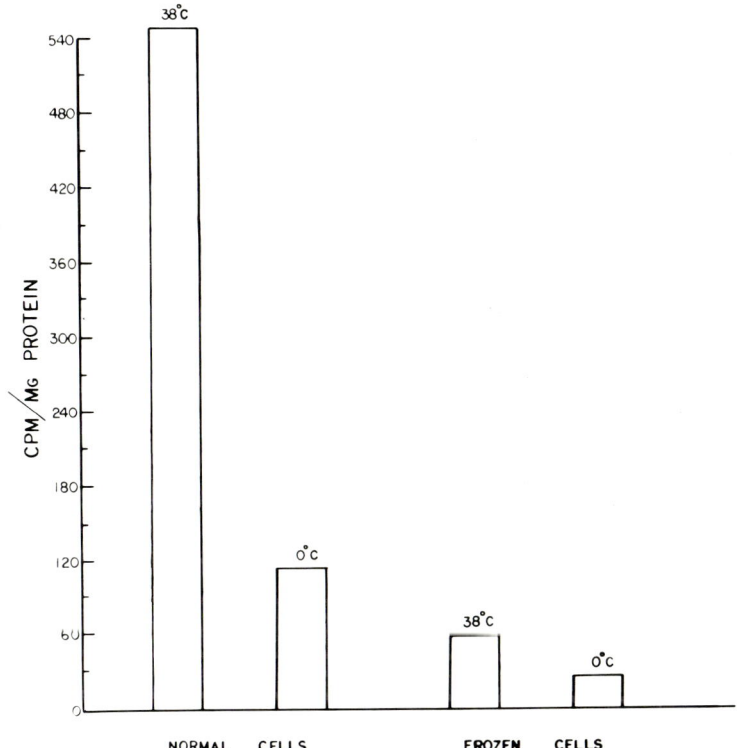

FIG. 11. Uptake of galactose-¹⁴C by intestinal mucosal cells. Mucosal cells were prepared by the procedure used by Kimmich (in press) and incubated for 8 minutes at 0° or 38°C in medium similar to his—tris-buffered saline pH 7.4—supplemented with 1 mg/ml BSA and containing 4 mM D-galactose-¹⁴C. They were then isolated by our procedure (see Section II) and the cells were broken with TCA to extract radioactivity for counting.

if it also was associated with binding. In view of the different types of cell being used, results are given as counts per milligram of protein for better comparison. Figure 10 shows preliminary results of incubating thymic cells in our incubation system. Thymic cells also exhibit calcium uptake and binding, though less than intestinal cells at the time periods tested. However, this experiment reveals three differences in detail: (1) temperature dependence is almost nil; (2) frozen thymic cells bind more calcium than intact cells; (3) the counts taken up do not increase as much with time as is the case with intestinal cells. While calcium binding can clearly occur in this completely different type of cell, it is evidently a different type of reaction than is seen in intestinal cells.

The properties of galactose uptake by intestinal cells, which has been studied in other aspects by Kimmich (1970), were examined briefly using his method of cell preparation, but our method of incubation and workup. Figure 11 shows that in this short experiment frozen cells bound very little galactose compared to that taken up by normal cells and that the system behaved reasonably otherwise. While the physiological significance of this observation is not known, it does show that not all materials taken up by intestinal cells are handled in the same way as calcium.

Summary and Conclusions

The experiments reported here show that the bulk of calcium taken up by intestinal mucosal cell preparations is in fact simply bound to some cellular component. It is immaterial whether the cells are intact or completely disrupted, calcium binding occurs to about the same extent. The time and temperature dependence of calcium binding suggest a progressive unmasking of binding sites as the struture of the materials involved changes during the general degeneration which accompanies incubation. The efficacy of detergents in inhibiting calcium binding and of chloroform–methanol in removing the bound calcium are strongly suggestive of a lipid component being involved. Further, the parallel loss of protein and decreased ^{45}Ca uptake suggest the involvement of protein also. Taken together, these imply that binding might be to a lipoprotein either on the cell membrane or within the cell. While it is not impossible that this calcium-binding property of mucosal cells may play some role in uptake and transport *in vivo*, it can only be regarded as an artifact where transport studies *in vitro* are concerned.

The rapid degradation of DNA with temperature and time in isolated mucosal cell preparations clearly show the danger of using DNA as an index of cell numbers for calcium uptake and the advisability of short term and low temperature incubations periods. If the nucleus in the cell breaks down, the possibility of degeneration of other cell constitutents is a likely one and raises the question of the physiological significance of cellular uptake of substances of any kind by isolated intestinal cell preparations. The binding of calcium to thymic cells not normally involved in calcium uptake implies the existence in this type of cell of some sort of calcium-binding material also. The different behavior of galactose as compared to calcium indicates a different mode of uptake by muscosal cells. The data with galactose suggests active transport (Kimmich, 1970), while those with calcium demonstrate some form of binding.

Finally, all work using isolated intestinal cell preparations for calcium uptake studies reported from our laboratory as well as from other should be viewed with caution in light of the present results. Further, it should be apparent that extrapolation of data from isolated intestinal cell preparations to absorption as it occurs *in vivo*, at least in the case of calcium, should not be made without confirmation by experiments *in vivo*.

REFERENCES

Bray, G. A. (1960). *Anal. Biochem.* **1,** 279.
Burton, K. (1956). *Biochem. J.* **62,** 315.
Clark, I. (1965). *Nature (London)* **207,** 982.
Clark, I. (1969). *Endocrinology* **85,** 1103.
Clark, I., and Bélanger, L. (1967). *Calcif. Tissue Res.* **1,** 204.
Clark, I., and Smith, M. R. (1964). *Endocrinology* **74,** 421.
Dickens, F., and Weil-Malherbe, H. (1941). *Biochem. J.* **35,** 7.
Dische, Z. (1930). *Mikrochemie* **8,** 4.
Dowdle, E. B., Schachter, D., and Schenker, H. (1960). *Amer. J. Physiol.* **198,** 269.
Gran, F. C. (1960). *Acta Physiol. Scand.* **49,** 211.
Harris, L. J., and Innes, J. R. M. (1931). *Biochem. J.* **25,** 367.
Hashim, G., and Clark, I. (1969). *Biochem. J.* **112,** 275.
Hatcher, D. W., and Goldstein, G. (1969). *Anal. Biochem.* **31,** 42.
Hendrix, J. Z., Alcock, N. E., and Archibald, R. M. (1963). *Clin. Chem.* **9,** 734.
Kimmich, G. A. (1970). *Biochemistry* **9,** 3659.
Lowry, O. H., Rosebrough, N. H., and Randall, R. J. (1951). *J. Biol. Chem.* **193,** 205.
Martin, D. L., and DeLuca, H. F. (1969). *Arch. Biochem. Biophys.* **134,** 139.
Perris, A. D. (1966). *Can. J. Biochem.* **44,** 687.
Rasmussen, H. (1959). *Endocrinology* **65,** 517.
Rasmussen, H., Waldorf, A., Dziewiatkowski, D., and DeLuca, H. (1963). *Biochim. Biophys. Acta* **75,** 250.
Sammon, P. J., Stacey, R. E., and Bronner, F. (1970). *Amer. J. Physiol.* **218,** 479.
Schachter, D., and Rosen, S. M. (1959). *Amer. J. Physiol.* **196,** 357.
Schachter, D., Dowdle, E. B., and Schenker, H. (1960). *Amer. J. Physiol.* **198,** 263.
Schachter, D., Kowarski, S., Finkelstein, J. D., and Ma, R.-I. W. (1966). *Amer. J. Physiol.* **211,** 1131.
Stewart, B. E., and Zbarsky, S. H. (1963). *Can. J. Biochem. Physiol.* **41,** 1483.
Umbreit, W. W., Burris, R. H., and Stauffer, J. F. (1957). "Manometric Techniques," p. 149. Burgess, Minneapolis, Minnesota.
Wasserman, R. H., and Comar, C. L. (1961). *Endocrinology* **69,** 1074.
Wasserman, R. H., and Taylor, A. N. (1963). *Nature (London)* **198,** 30.
Wasserman, R. H., Corradino, R. A., and Taylor, A. N. (1968). *J. Biol. Chem.* **243,** 3978.

Discussion

Dr. Hurwitz: Intestinal cells are by nature asymmetric, and by isolating them in a solution where they lose their asymmetry, you may be also causing a loss of integrity. I may add that we, as well as others, have studied the uptake of calcium by mucosa by perfusing the whole intestine. This would be on the side of the brush border, and we have done this without disrupting or without taking the cells off the underlying tissues. The results thus obtained are quite different than yours. For example, uptake of calcium as a function of time increased toward equilibrium, and bile salts actually enhanced calcium uptake. Sodium, potassium, lithium, or the absence of those monovalent ions increased uptake, unlike your case. And so, all in all, I think that intestinal cells floating in solution may result in a somewhat unfortunate preparation.

Dr. Clark: I agree.

Dr. Borle: I would like to qualify your last statement. One may have valid reservations about the viability of isolated cell systems, except when the cells are grown in culture. I don't want to feel I am out of business.

Dr. Clark: I am sorry, but I am not trying to put you out of business. I agree with Dr. Hurwitz that when a cell is removed from its site *in vivo* and put into an abnormal situation *in vitro*, where it can change its shape, that is now quite a different cell. But, individual cells, such as blood, thymic, or other cultured cells, are perfectly valid systems to use.

Dr. Harrison: The everted gut sac system doesn't need defending, but I want to make a few points. The everted gut sac system can be used for the study of transport over short periods; one can study calcium transport not over an hour or 90 minutes, as was done originally, but in periods of a few minutes, or at the most 15 minutes, and find the same results. These systems are obviously functioning and the cells are still intact. I think Dr. Hurwitz very well pointed out that, in intestinal mucosa, once one loses the structural organization, the oriented transport is lost.

We also tried working with isolated intestinal cells and were not able to demonstrate a vitamin D effect. That isn't surprising, because we assume that the vitamin D effect is only or primarily at one border of the cell, and we are losing that kind of asymmetric or oriented organization in the cell suspension.

I have just one other point of disagreement. I think there is ample evidence *in vivo* that parathyroid hormone does increase calcium transport in a variety of studies, both in man and in animal.

Dr. Clark: In reply to the everted gut sac technique, I think it does what it is supposed to do: it measures active transport and it does that very well. My objection is that many investigators equate active transport *in vitro* with absorption as it occurs *in vivo*. I think these are two completely different phenomena.

With reference to the last point, we have studies (unpublished), and there is also a paper by S. J. Birge, W. A. Peek, M. Berman, and G. D. Whedoll [*J. Clin. Invest.* **48**, 1705 (1969)] which shows equivocal results with respect to parathyroid hormone and parathyroidectomy on calcium absorption. However, they point out that the area distal to the duodenum is of greater importance for calcium absorption than the duodenum where active transport is most prominent. Again it depends on what one means by calcium absorption. If it is net absorption, i.e., intake of calcium minus fecal calcium, I don't think any good experimental studies have clearly shown parathyroid hormone increases calcium absorption.

Dr. Irving: In view of Dr. Wasserman's paper, have you tried your experiment on tissues from rachitic animals?

Dr. Clark: No, I haven't. We published some results on the effect of vitamin D on isolated cell preparations [G. Hashim and I. Clark, *Biochem. J.* **112**, 275 (1969)], and unfortunately, I don't think any of the uptake studies now reported are valid. I think the release studies are all right.

Dr. Irving: Is Dr. Wasserman's calcium binding protein doing the binding that you are describing?

Dr. Clark: We shouldn't have any of Dr. Wasserman's binding protein in our preparation. I should have explained that we scrape the cells from the mucosal or use the hyaluronidase procedure to release them. We then spin the preparation at very low speeds (500 g) for about 2–3 minutes, wash twice, and each time discard the supernate. Dr. Wasserman's binding factor is in the supernate. We probably would have only traces in our preparation. Don't you agree, Dr. Wasserman?

Dr. Wasserman: I'm not sure. If the cell is broken by conventional homogenization, calcium-binding protein is released. But, under your conditions, Dr. Clark, it may still be associated with the preparation.

Dr. Bronner: I agree with most of the things that Harold Harrison said, but I don't want to leave this audience with the impression that parathyroid hormone has any clear-cut effects on calcium absorption, at least in the rat. Bob Wasserman pointed out that he, too, has been unable to show any effects on absorption *in vivo* and *in vitro*. *In vivo*, we have been unable to demonstrate a significant effect of parathyroidectomy on calcium absorption [P. J. Sammon, R. E. Stacey, and F. Bronner, *Amer. J. Physiol.* **218**, 479 (1970)]. *In vitro*, studying the effects of low and high calcium diets on what appears to be the synthesis of a calcium-binding protein, we have shown [F. Bronner, *in* "Membrane Proteins. Proceedings of a Symposium Sponsored by the New York Heart Association," pp. 134–135. Little, Brown, Boston, Massachusetts, 1969] that when you shift animals from a high- to a low-calcium diet, there is an increase in calcium-binding protein in the intestine within 24 hours. This increase was totally unaffected by parathyroidectomy. In other words, the synthesis of calcium-binding protein in the rat appears to be parathyroid hormone-independent. This is not unexpected, because from the viewpoint of overall regulation, it would be surprising for all calcium regulation to depend on a single feedback loop.

Dr. Hastings: I have been trying for some time to interest people who work with everted gut sacs in using appropriate incubation fluids. Some years ago we made a quite thorough study of the acid–base balance of jejunal juice. You might think that that is something that varies very easily. It doesn't; its pH is about 6.2, its bicarbonate is about 10 mM, and its carbon dioxide tension is about 100 mm. This is the environment which these mucosal cells are used to. Krebs–Ringer solution, whether it has bicarbonate or not, is a very pathological solution in which to study what is going on. I would like to see investigators really know what part of the gut they are everting and what the usual environment is that those mucosal cells are used to before they draw conclusions on calcium, DNA, or anything else.

ACTIVE TRANSPORT OF CALCIUM ACROSS PLACENTA AND MAMMARY GLAND MEASURED *IN VIVO*

D. S. Kronfeld, C. F. Ramberg, Jr., and Maria Delivoria-Papadopoulos

Introduction

The rate of transport of calcium and other materials across or through epithelial membranes has been measured most commonly in *in vitro* systems designed to allow sampling on both sides of the membrane, e.g., the frog skin or the everted gut sac. The most acceptable measurements are made when conditions force the transport to maximum velocity if active transport is involved (Dietschy, 1970). *In vitro* studies have increased greatly our understanding of the properties of membranes and the ways membranes handle various substances. It would be useful, also, to measure transport rates *in vivo*, which often may proceed at less than maximum velocity.

In vivo studies usually deal with transport across multiple layers of cells. We started looking at transport through maximal multilayers in cows by means of nutritional balances. Combining these with a tracer kinetic analysis, following Bronner and others, we measured calcium transport from gut and bone to blood and from blood to gut, bone, urine, and milk (Ramberg *et al.*, 1971). The limitations of this approach, especially when applied to parturient cows, brought home to us the need for finer discrimination in regard to both time and site. We have turned to the use of two tracers administrered simultaneously at two different sites, sampling at both sites, and analysis of the data by a combination of deconvolution and compartmental analysis.

Calcium absorption has been studied by deconvolution (Hart and Spencer, 1967) and by a combination of deconvolution and compartmental analysis, with a tracer being given at one time into the blood and another into the gut (Birge et al., 1969). We have done similar experiments on absorption in cows, except that two tracers have been used simultaneously. Then we proceeded to study maternal–placental–fetal transfers of calcium in sheep. In this work, we have made two advances; we have defined the placental components, and we have differentiated active from passive transport. We have also begun to study the active transport of calcium across the mammary epithelium, i.e., from blood into milk.

Placental Calcium Transport

The studies of plasma calcium in maternal and fetal blood by Delivoria-Papadopoulos et al. (1967) suggested the presence of active transport across the placenta (Table I). The sudden cessation of this source of calcium may contribute to the development of hypocalcemia in the neonate, a condition too common in human neonates, but strangely unreported in animals. Also, the placental outflow of calcium from the blood may con-

TABLE I

Plasma Calcium and pH in Maternal and Fetal Blood[a]

Parameter	Human (22 pairs)[b]		Sheep (12 pairs)[b]	
	Maternal	Fetal	Maternal	Fetal
Total calcium (mEq/kg water)	5.7 ± 0.4	6.5 ± 0.5	4.5 ± 0.6	7.3 ± 0.8
Diffusible calcium (mEq/kg water)	2.9 ± 0.5	3.8 ± 0.4	2.8 ± 0.2	4.9 ± 0.4
pH	7.38	7.28	7.32	7.28

[a] Data from Delivoria-Papadopoulos et al. (1967).
[b] Mean ± S.D.

tribute to hypocalcemia developing prepartum in cows or more commonly, in sheep. We are performing experiments on sheep, but our model of the maternal–placental–fetal calcium system was built first on data published by MacDonald et al. (1965).

The animals were anesthetized, plastic catheters were inserted into umbilical (fetal) and uterine vessels, and ^{47}Ca was injected into the maternal bloodstream and ^{45}Ca into the fetal bloodstream. A series of blood samples were taken for 2 hours in monkeys or 4–6 hours in sheep and analysed for calcium content and radioactivity. Thus, four curves were obtained: ^{45}Ca and ^{47}Ca in maternal and in fetal blood.

The ^{47}Ca curve in the mother and the ^{45}Ca curve in the fetus each require the sum of at least two exponential terms in monkey or three terms in sheep for a good fit, so the maternal and fetal systems each have at least two or three components in monkey and sheep, as observed, respectively. These multiexponential equations are also used as the weighting functions in the deconvolution procedure. The ^{45}Ca curve in the mother represents a response in the mother to the input from the placenta of the tracer injected into the fetus. The ^{47}Ca curve in the fetus, similarly, represents the response in the fetus to the input from the placenta of the tracer injected into the mother. Given these responses, the inputs may be derived in terms of the weighting functions. Assuming that the system is linear, once the response to one input is known, the response to any other input may be calculated by convolution, and the input corresponding to any other response (output) may be calculated by deconvolution. Examples of this procedure are described in detail by Hart and Spencer (1967) and Birge et al. (1969), and the mathematical procedures are described by Rescigno and Segre (1966).

$$R(t) = \int_0^t I(\theta) \, W(t - \theta) \, d\theta,$$

where $R(t)$ is the response, $I(t)$ the input, $W(t)$ the weighting function, i.e., the response to an instantaneous injection, and θ is a dummy variable of integration.

By sampling the blood bathing both sides of the placental tissue, we are able to mathematically dissect the responses of the placenta (transfer functions) from those of the maternal and fetal calcium systems (weighting functions). From the placental transfer functions, we are able to formulate a model of placental calcium transfers, recouple it to the models of the maternal and fetal calcium systems, then test it against the original data. The simultaneous fit to all four curves constrains the model parameters and increases its uniqueness. The steady state solution of the model yields the tracer calcium flows.

At this point, the model had five compartments for the monkey and seven for the sheep. Steady state solutions yield a (net) transport rate of calcium from mother to fetus of 47 mg/day for MacDonald's monkey and 880 mg/day for our sheep. MacDonald *et al.* (1965) used only the initial slopes of their curves to estimate transport rates. For the monkey fetus, which we have restudied, their estimates were 118 mg/day from mother to fetus and 334 mg/day from fetus to mother, a net gain of −216 mg/day by the fetus.

With the aid of several assumptions, we can build a model which will differentiate between diffusional flows and active transport across the placenta.

1. Assume there are two placental compartments.
2. Assume that one placental compartment subserves active transport in the form of two flows, one from maternal compartment one, the other to fetal compartment one.
3. Assume that the other placental compartment subserves passive transport, i.e., four diffusional flows: to and from maternal compartment one and to and from placental compartment one.
4. Assume that the diffusional flows out of the placenta equal one another.
5. Assume that the diffusional flows into the placenta from the mother and the fetus are proportional to the plasma Ca^{2+} concentrations in the mother and fetus, respectively.

The model now has six compartments in the monkey and eight in the sheep, with two compartments in the placenta in each case. Steady state solutions give values for active transport of 75 mg/day in the monkey and 873 mg/day in the sheep, with corresponding net fetal losses by diffusion of 28 mg/day in the monkey and 3 mg/day in the sheep (Fig. 1). The monkey fetus weighed 0.45 kg and the sheep fetus 4.3 kg, so the active transport rates were 167 and 203 mg/day/kg body weight, respectively, i.e., fairly similar. In contrast, net diffusion from fetus to mother was much greater in the monkey than in the sheep, 62 compared to 0.7 mg/day/kg body weight, respectively. This difference brings to mind the fact that the sheep placenta is syndesmochorial, a much thicker barrier to diffusion than the homochorial placenta of the monkey.

It may seem to workers experienced in the analysis of a single tracer dilution curve that we have claimed to extract an extraordinary, perhaps incredible, amount of information from these experiments. The crucial gain is obtained when there are four curves to fit instead of just a single curve.

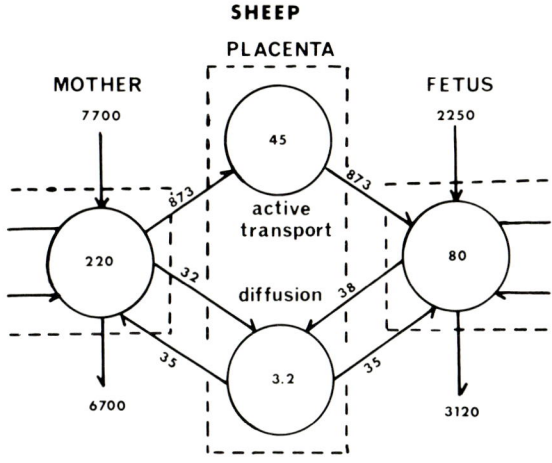

Fig. 1. A comparison of calcium transport across the placenta in a sheep (top) and a monkey (bottom). The monkey fetus was about one-tenth the weight of the sheep fetus, so the active placental transport of calcium was about the same in both species when expressed in terms of body weight. Placental diffusion of calcium in the sheep is about one one-hundredth that in the monkey.

The limitation in this work so far has been the use of anesthesia and the consequent short period of observation. We now can maintain chronically implanted catheters in the sheep fetus and therefore plan to perform experiments with observational periods of 24 hours or more on unanesthetized sheep.

Mammary Calcium Transport

The onset of lactation is the major condition predisposing to the development of parturient hypocalcemia. This does not develop in mastectomized cows. Moreover, if a cow starts to lactate prior to parturition, she develops hypocalcemia at the onset of lactation rather than at parturition. The colostrum output and its calcium content (0.20%), however, are no greater in cows which develop severe hypocalcemia and paresis than in those which remain mildly hypocalcemic and clinically normal (Hibbs et al., 1951). So other factors which tend to compensate for the colostral drain of calcium must help determine the degree of hypocalcemia.

The above hypothesis is usually taken to be a conclusive fact. Yet it has a weakness. The crucial transport may be that from blood into mammary gland tissue rather than that into milk, i.e., there may be a calcium resevoir in the mammary cells (Marshak, 1957). Sometimes cows develop hypocalcemia prepartum without milking. This phenomenon is more common in sheep. Indeed ewes usually develop hypocalcemia and a paretic syndrome a week or two prepartum without lactating. This may be due to calcium flow to the fetus, but it may also be a calcium flow into a mammary resevoir.

The presence of a calcium delay in the udder is supported by the finding of a high specific activity in milk calcium than in plasma calcium in a cow injected with ^{45}Ca 20 days prepartum (Visek et al., 1953) and by the time lag between equal specific activities of calcium in plasma then milk (Swanson et al., 1956) (Fig. 2).

We have tried to measure the mammary uptake of calcium from the blood by means of arteriovenous difference and blood flow experiments (Kronfeld and Ramberg, 1970). These efforts were not successful, mainly because the mammary arteriovenous difference of calcium is continually changing and mean values tend to be very small. The antipyrine absorption method for estimating mammary bloodflow is likely to be unreliable in recumbent or parturient cows, because the mammary vein blood may not be representative of the total mammary effluent under these conditions.

There are greater prospects of success in measuring the calcium flow into a mammary compartment, and the mass of calcium in that compartment, by means of the experimental approach described above regarding the placenta (Figs. 2 and 3). There are difficulties. The tracer injected into the udder gives a jumbled curve in the milk and a curve with a peculiar bump in the blood (Fig. 3). This was not anticipated, because we find smooth curves in both milk and blood following antipyrine infusion into the teat cistern. The curve in blood following mammary infusion of ^{45}Ca

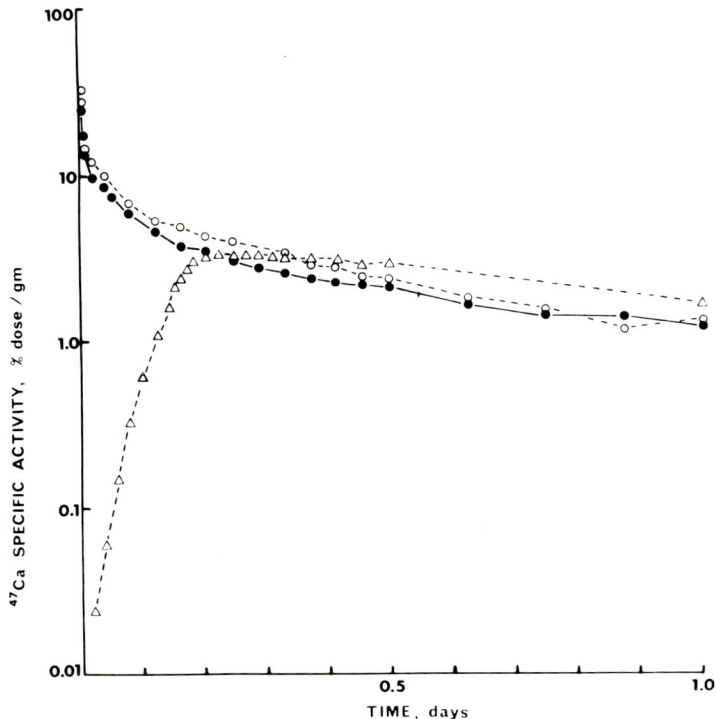

FIG. 2. The specific activity of calcium determined in plasma [pulmonary artery (●) and left mammary vein (○)] and milk (△) after an intravenous injection of ^{47}Ca. The rising phase of the milk curve indicates a delay in the mammary transfer of calcium from blood to milk. The peak in this curve at 4–6 hours reflects the turnover rate of the mammary component. This suggests the presence of a mammary calcium component equivalent in size to about 20–25% of the daily lactational calcium loss in addition to the milk calcium stored within the udder.

solution suggests that some tracer enters the blood very rapidly, while the remainder enters from a more slowly exchanging compartment, perhaps the resevoir postulated by Marshak and others.

We have found recently that the calcium ion concentration in milk is 8.1 ± 1.2 mEq/liter (mean ± S.D., 29 observations), i.e., four times as high as the plasma ion concentration, 2.02 ± 0.25 mEq/liter. This comparison indicates the presence of active calcium transport across the mammary gland.

At this stage, we have most of the information needed to build a mam-

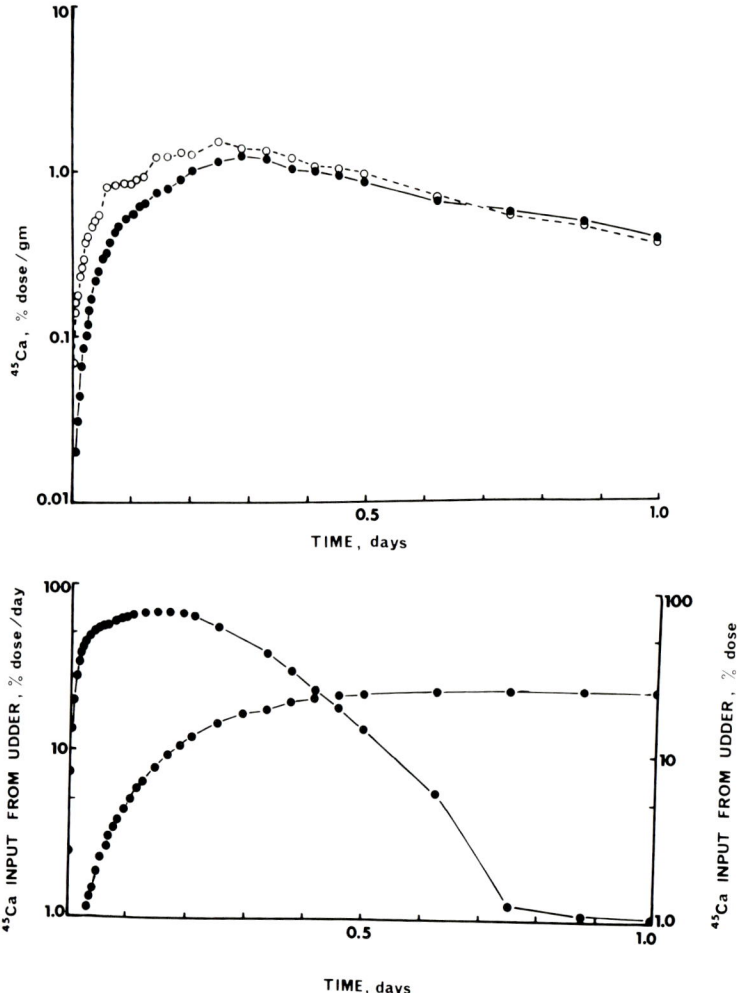

Fig. 3. The appearance of ^{45}Ca in the left mammary vein and pulmonary artery following its injection into the teat cisterns of the two right quarters of the udder (● = pulmonary artery; ○ = left mammary vein). Using the plasma calcium-specific activity obtained following a single injection of ^{47}Ca (made at the same time as the intramammary administration of ^{45}Ca) as a weighting function (see Fig. 2), an input function is obtained by deconvolution which represents the progressive input of ^{47}Ca into the circulation from the udder (bottom). This may be thought of as a nonconstant infusion of tracer into the blood from the udder. The integral of this input function is the cumulative amount of tracer delivered from the udder to the blood from the time of injection to time t. The asymptote of this curve was 25% of the dose of the ^{45}Ca. The remaining 75% of the tracer was largely removed when the cow was milked 12 hours after the tracer injection. The two peaks on the input curve indicate that at least two absorption processes are involved.

mary model like that for the placenta. We do not feel secure about the milk–mammary components, however. Perhaps measuring the radioactivity of calcium in diffusible and protein-bound fractions will clarify the situation. Meanwhile, a few tentative estimates may be made. The calcium transport into the mammary gland must equal the calcium loss in milk (1.0–1.2 gm/kg, i.e., 20–50 gm/day, in good cows) plus about 25%, the calcium flow back into blood may be attributed to diffusion, and the opposing diffusional flow into the gland from the blood will be two-eigths of this, in proportion to the calcium ion concentrations. It is clear that active transport of calcium from the blood to the gland cells is greater than the calcium loss in milk and that a mammary reservoir of calcium does exist.

Further work is needed to define the mammary calcium system. We are especially keen to study it in parturient cows. Does the active transport mechanism continue to decalcify the blood while the cow is dying of hypocalcemia?

ACKNOWLEDGMENTS

This work is supported in part by the USPHS (grants AM12112 and AM31380) and by the USAEC (contract AT 30-1-3360). The calcium ion assays on cow's blood and milk were performed by Dr. Jurg Blum and Mrs. Kaye Johnson using an Orion electrode. The mathematical procedures were performed by means of the SAAM25 computer program with help from Dr. Mones Berman and Mrs. Marjorie Weiss.

REFERENCES

Birge, S. J., Peck, W. A., Berman, M., and Whedon, G. D. (1969). *J. Clin. Invest.* **48,** 1705.
Delivoria-Papadopoulos, M., Battaglia, F. C., Bruns, P. D., and Meschia, G. (1967). *Amer. J. Physiol.* **213,** 363.
Dietschy, J. M. (1970). *Gastroenterology* **58,** 863.
Hart, H., and Spencer, H. (1967). *Proc. Soc. Exp. Biol. Med.* **126,** 365.
Hibbs, J. W., Pounden, W. D., and Krauss, W. E. (1951). *J. Dairy Sci.* **34,** 855.
Kronfeld, D. S., and Ramberg, C. F. (1970). In "Parturient Hypocalcemia" (J. J. B. Anderson, ed.), pp. 107–117. Academic Press, New York.
MacDonald, N. S., Hutchinson, D. L., Hepler, M., and Flynn, E. (1965). *Proc. Soc. Exp. Biol. Med.* **119,** 476.
Marshak, R. R. (1957). *Penn. Vet. Ext. Quart.* **146,** 104.
Ramberg, C. F., Mayer, G. P., Kronfeld, D. S., Phang, J. M., and Berman, M. (1970). *Amer. J. Physiol.* **219,** 1166.
Rescigno, A., and Segre, G. (1966). "Drug and Tracer Kinetics." Ginn (Blaisdell), Boston, Massachusetts
Swanson, E. W., Monroe, R. A., Zilversmit, D. B., Visek, W. J., and Comar, C. (1956). *J. Dairy Sci.* **39,** 1594.
Visek, W. J., Monroe, R. A., Swanson, E. W., and Comar, C. L. (1953). *J. Dairy Sci.* **36,** 373.

Discussion

Dr. Radde: Some data on the pH and Ca content of maternal and human plasma are shown in the following tabulation:

MATERNAL AND NEONATAL CALCIUM ION ACTIVITY

Plasma	pH	Ca^{2+} (mEq/liter)	Total calcium (mEq/liter)
Maternal	7.44 ± 0.01	1.97 ± 0.08	4.33 ± 0.15
Fetal	7.25 ± 0.04	2.43 ± 0.04	5.39 ± 0.16

You see that the ionized calcium in the maternal plasma is significantly lower than fetal ionized calcium. Similarly, total calcium levels are also lower in the maternal than in the fetal plasma. The pH values show similar differences, as Dr. Kronfeld described. I have one question, Dr. Kronfeld: How do you picture the active transport process for calcium across the placenta?

Dr. Kronfeld: We have pictured active transport loosely. I have no enzyme or protein to offer you on this active transport.

Dr. Assali: Having spent fifteen years trying to understand how oxygen is transferred from mother to fetus, I can assure you that you will have many years to work on this particular field, particularly in dealing with such substances as calcium, which are a lot more complex than oxygen. I assume that you are concluding that calcium crosses the placenta in two ways, part by active transport and part by diffusion. The transport of most substances across the placenta are flow limiting. My first question is, did you change in any way the flow of blood on either the maternal side or the fetal side and see whether this change influences the shape of your curves?

Second, if you settle on the assumption that transfer is by diffusion, how did you try to quantitate the net amount that goes from one side to another? How did you assess the influence of the many factors which affect diffusion, like the surface area of the placenta, the shunting mechanism, the thickness of the placenta, the electrochemical gradient and the pattern of blood flow on both sides of the placenta? All of these factors influence even the simple diffusion process.

Dr. Kronfeld: Thank you for the encouragement, Dr. Assali. We believe that calcium transfer is diffusion-dependent rather than flow-dependent for two reasons. The earliest rate constant obtained by kinetic analysis is much slower than one would expect with a flow-dependent system. Second, we cannot detect arteriovenous differences of calcium concentration or specific activity in the umbilical or uterine arteriovenous systems. We want to study placental blood flow, but have not done so yet. We have used antipyrine extensively to study mammary blood flow. There, of course, we can pick up big arteriovenous differences.

Dr. Assali, we would like to study to all the factors you mentioned as Ussing did so beautifully in the flux ratio idea. He put them all in a bracket and cancelled them out. We want to relate placental calcium transport in opposite directions to the calcium activities, just as Ussing did in the flux ratio, but we have not measured activities yet.

Dr. Barzell: In light of Dr. Melman's discussion, I wish to bring to your attention the fact that in milk, be it human, cow, or goat milk, potassium, like calcium, is highly concentrated as compared to the blood level. For instance, cow milk, which contains 118 mg% (59 mEq/liter) calcium, contains 114 mg% (36.9 mEq/liter) potassium [*U.S., Dep. Agr., Agr. Handb.* No. 8, p. 39 (1963)]. It is possible, then, that in milk, too, the potassium influences the calcium content. Do you know of any studies of transport of electrolytes other than calcium into milk?

Dr. Kronfeld: There have been studies of strontium, iodine, and cesium transfer into milk. I agree that potassium may be involved in calcium transport. There is a disease in cows like the one mentioned by Dr. Harrison in humans, which is a variant of parturient hypocalcemia. If hypocalcemia becomes protracted, calcium injections no longer cure the disease, and we infer that hypocalcemia is no longer the dominant problem. In some cases it appears that potassium depletion interferes with calcium transport.

CALCIUM TRANSFER ACROSS THE AVIAN SHELL GLAND*

Harald Schraer and Rosemary Schraer

Introduction

We have employed the shell gland of the domestic hen as a model system for studying calcium translocation because it is capable of moving large quantities of this element in defined periods of time and because the site of the final deposition of the calcium carbonate shell is separate and distinct from the cells that transport the calcium. It has recently been estimated that the eggshell, which contains about 2 gm of calcium, is formed in approximately 14 hours (Mongin, 1970). This amounts to moving 2.4 mg of calcium across the shell gland mucosa in 1 minute. For the sake of perspective, it is interesting to compare this value with that of a champion lactating dairy cow which weighs about 400 kg. Such an animal is capable of secreting 43 gm of calcium per day (Kleiber and Luick, 1956), or 108 mg/kg/day. The hen, which weighs about 2 kg, secretes calcium at the rate of 1000 mg/kg/day. If one can assume that the biological mechanisms that are concerned in translocating large amounts of calcium in the avian shell gland are based on amplifications of generalized processes, then this tissue is a logical choice for investigating calcium translocation. I shall take this

---

* These investigations were supported by research grants DE01764 and AM05970 from the U. S. Public Health Service.

opportunity to review some of our past work with this tissue and studies now in progress.

Anatomical Considerations

The shell gland is the thick-walled pouchlike portion of the oviduct, which is greatly distended and thin-walled when it contains an egg with a calcified eggshell. In addition to secreting the calcium carbonate for the eggshell, it also secretes other materials, such as shell matrix, fluids, and other mineral ions (Mongin and Sauveur, 1970). The organ has a rich blood supply which increases in vascular volume when it is forming a shell (Hodges, 1965). The walls of the shell gland consist of a mucosal layer, which is composed of an inner columnar epithelium and a layer of tubular gland cells. Layers of smooth muscle and connective tissue surround the mucosa, and a sheet of serosal cells lies outside the muscle. The columnar epithelium consists of two types of cells, those with apically positioned nuclei and those with basally positioned nuclei. Occasionally, goblet cells are dispersed among the apical and basal cells. The apical cells contain cilia and microvilli; the basal cells have microvilli only. Both cell types contain secretory granules. The tubular gland cells contain microvilli on the luminal surface. More detailed observations of the anatomy and fine structure are contained in several recent reports (Freedman and Sturkie, 1963; Hodges, 1965; Johnston et al., 1963; Nevalainen, 1969; Breen and DeBruyn, 1969; Schraer and Schraer, 1970). It is revealing to compare the histological features of a shell gland from which the egg was removed before fixation (Fig. 1) with one in which the tissue was fixed while the shelled egg remained in place (Fig. 2). In the first case, the mucosa is characterized by having a thick layer of tubular glands. This is due to the mucosa being thrown into deep folds. In the second case, the tubular gland layer is relatively thin with shallow folds. The smooth muscle layer lies close to the mucosa in sections prepared in the first manner, which is not the the case when the shell gland is allowed to contract by removing the egg prior to fixation as in the second type of fixation.

Note that the capillaries in Fig. 2 are distributed mainly between the layer of tubular glands and the columnar epithelium. This differs from the capillary distribution in Fig. 1, where they appear to be distributed among the tubular gland cells and underneath the columnar epithelium. In order for the calcium to reach the oviduct lumen upon leaving the capillaries, it can move to the interstitial space from which it can move into the tubular gland cells, the columnar cells, or the intercellular spaces of either. The junctional complexes which occur in both groups of cells would probably

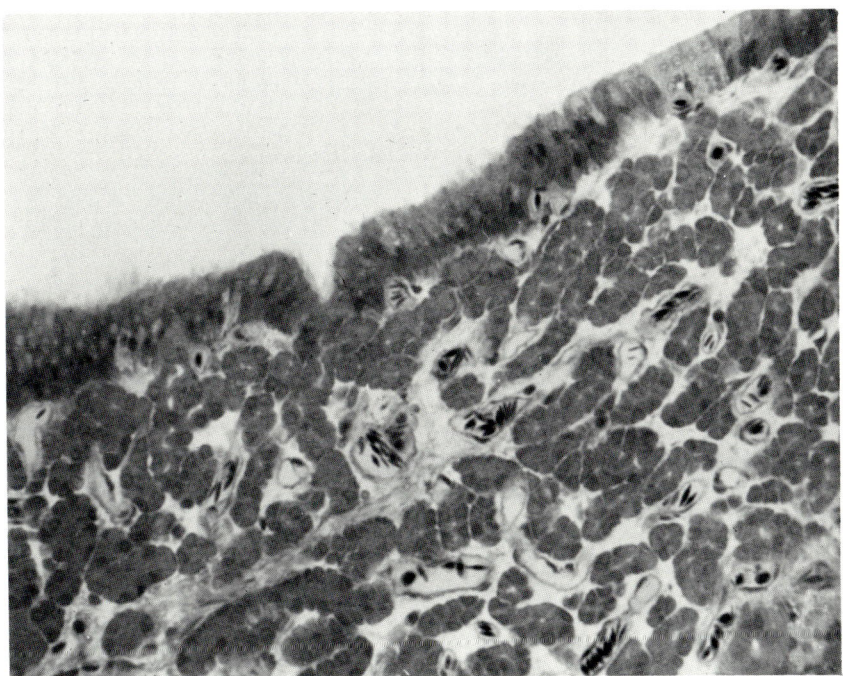

Fig. 1. Photomicrograph of shell gland mucosa. A hard-shelled egg was removed from the shell gland before tissue was taken for fixation in 3% glutaraldehyde followed by 1% osmium tetroxide. s-Collidine was used as a buffer. (× 190)

impede or stop movement of calcium between the cells. It seems probable that calcium moves into both types of cells, and the problem lies in determining which cell type, if not both, plays the major role in transporting this ion. The site of production for the carbonate ion has been assigned to the tubular glands (Diamantstein and Schlüns, 1964). Histochemical tests have revealed no significant quantities of calcium in either cell type; however, microincineration studies at the light and electron microscope levels show a higher ash content in the columnar cells (Turchini, 1924; Richardson, 1935; Hohman and Schraer, 1967). It should be pointed out that the high ash could be due to other metallic ions than calcium. An electron micrograph of the ash pattern of a thin section of the columnar cells is shown in Fig. 3. A plasma of excited oxygen was used to remove the organic constitutents from Epon-embedded sections which had been fixed in s-collidine-buffered glutaraldehyde. No metal-containing com-

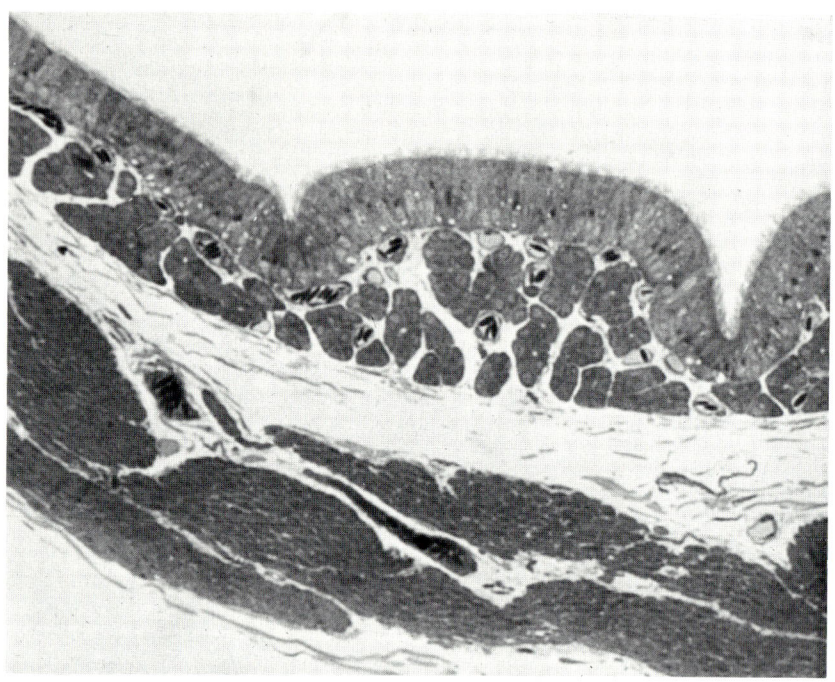

FIG. 2. Photomicrograph of shell gland fixed while a hard-shelled egg was in the shell gland. The fixatives were the same as in Fig. 1. (× 190)

ponents were used in fixation, and stains were omitted. A review of the application of this technique has been described by Thomas (1969). The spodograms of the columnar cells frequently show granules with residues near the lumen (Fig. 3) and in the nuclear region. Other features of the columnar cells, such as cilia and microvilli, are also evident. The tubular gland cells also show a characteristic ash pattern and do not contain the discrete granular ash deposits observed in the columnar cells.

Chemical analysis of oviduct tissue has shown a relationship between the position of the egg in the oviduct and the amount of calcium in the tissue (Schraer and Schraer, 1965). When the different functional segments of the oviduct were compared, the shell gland showed changes in calcium levels which appeared to be associated with the location of the egg in the oviduct. There was least calcium in the shell gland when it contained an egg, and the most when the egg entered the oviduct. The isthmus tissue, which forms the shell membranes, had twice as much calcium. The tissue samples in this earlier study contained the muscle and mucosal layers. A question

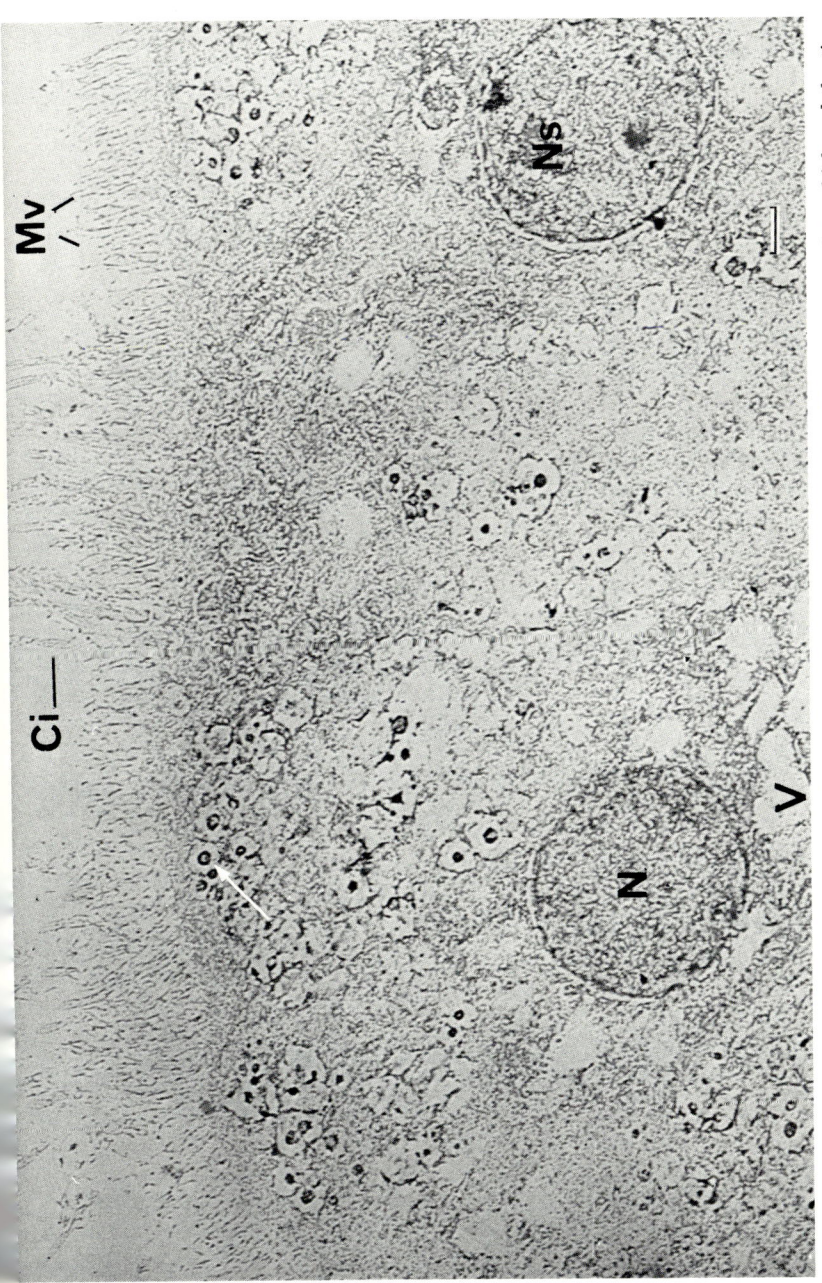

FIG. 3. Electron micrograph of columnar epithelium after low temperature ashing. The section was 0.5 μ thick and the tissue was fixed in collidine-buffered glutaraldehyde. Ash deposits from cilia (Ci) and microvilli (Mv) are seen on the apical borders. Dense deposits with less dense centers (arrow) are frequent near apical border. Ash residues of the nucleus (N) and nucleolus (Ns) can be identified and vacuolated (V) areas are free of ash deposits. (× 5900) (Hohman, 1967.)

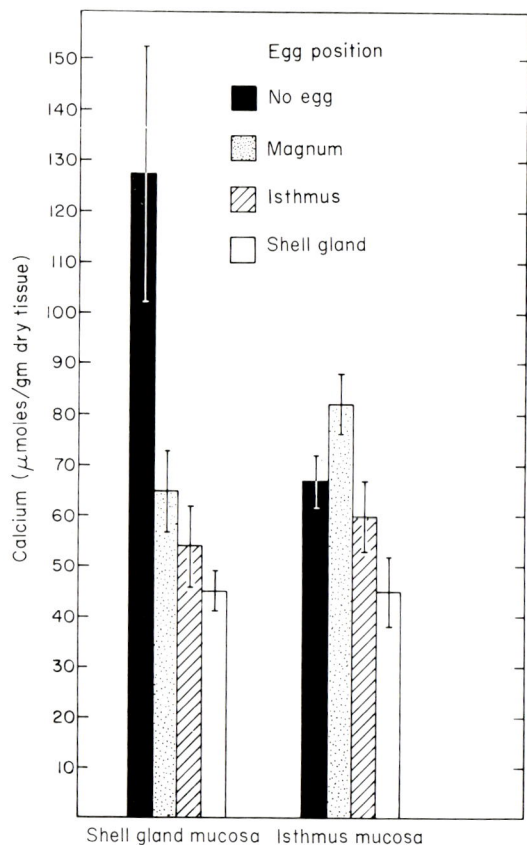

FIG. 4. The calcium content of the shell gland and isthmus mucosae when an egg is in different parts of the oviduct. Standard errors are indicated.

posed by the work centered around the contribution of the muscle component to the calcium values.

Recent work on the calcium content of the shell gland mucosa is shown in Fig. 4 along with comparable data for the isthmus mucosa. The data show that both tissues are equally high in calcium, and both show similar changes with different egg positions in the oviduct. The singular exception is the unusually high value found in the shell gland mucosa from oviducts that did not contain an egg anywhere in the tract. The low calcium value in the shell gland when a shell was being formed and the higher values found when the oviduct was empty or contained an egg elsewhere parallels the finding for shell gland mitochondria (Hohman and Schraer, 1966), in which case the mitochondria in ^{45}Ca-treated hens had more ^{45}Ca per milligram of nitrogen when no egg was in the oviduct than when an egg was present in the shell gland.

Autoradiographic Localization of Calcium

We have employed the technique of autoradiography with ^{45}Ca in an effort to determine which cells of the mucosa may serve as the route of calcium transport (Gay and Schraer, 1971). Hens where given 5 mCi of ^{45}Ca intravenously and were sampled 5 minutes later for pieces of mucosa from the shell gland, isthmus, and magnum. The tissues were processed by freeze-substitution (Feder and Sidman, 1958) to retain the easily diffusible calcium in the tissue. Fixation was accomplished in 1% osmium tetioxide in methanol and the tissues were embedded in butylmethacrylate. Tissue samples were also set aside before processing and prepared for ^{45}Ca determination by counting in the Geiger region. For grain counting, sections 2 μ thick were used with Ilford K-5 Nuclear Research Emulsion (Caro and van Tubergen, 1962). Comparison of the two methods for determining the radioactivity (Fig. 5) shows very good agreement between grain counts and cpm per milligram dry weight. The shell gland contained about two to five times more radioactivity than did the isthmus and magnum. Grain counts of the different segments given in Table I show that the columnar cells of the shell gland had the highest count when compared to tubular glands

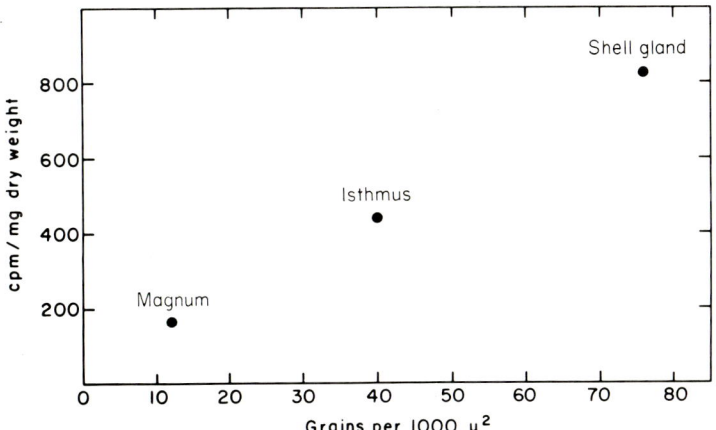

FIG. 5. Comparison of grain counts with level of radioactivity in unprocessed tissue from four birds given ^{45}Ca intravenously (Gay and Schraer, 1971).

TABLE I

MEAN GRAIN COUNTS OF AUTORADIOGRAPHS OF TISSUE CONTAINING INTRAVENOUSLY ADMINISTERED CALCIUM-45[a]

Tissue[b]	Grain count[c] (mean ± S.E.)	
	Columnar epithelium	Tubular glands
A. All birds regardless of egg position (4)		
Shell gland	47.0±6.3	29.0±2.4
Isthmus	19.4±6.1	20.7±5.3
Magnum	6.8±0.7	4.7±0.5
B. Calcifying a shell (2)		
Shell gland	59.0±2.0	27.0±2.0
Isthmus	30.6±5.2	31.0±4.8
Magnum	7.8±2.4	4.8±1.1
C. Noncalcifying (2)		
Shell gland	35.1±1.4	30.9±1.9
Isthmus	8.2±0.9	10.4±0.9
Magnum	5.1±0.6	4.6±0.5

[a] From Gay and Schraer (1971).
[b] Number of animals is in parentheses.
[c] Grain counts of 50 microscopic fields.

from the same tissue and from both cell types of the isthmus and magnum. When the shell gland data are separated according to egg position, the differences between the cell types are greater. During shell deposition, the shell gland columnar cells may have a relatively higher proportion of radioactivity than at other times. In the noncalcifying condition, the difference in grain counts between the columnar epithelium and tubular glands for each segment was negligible; the shell gland, however, showed the highest values. The results of these experiments show that the shell gland mucosa has a higher affinity for administered ^{45}Ca than the other tissues studied. The higher concentration of grains over the columar cells, which may vary with the physiological state of the shell gland, supports the view that the columnar cells may play a larger role in calcium movement than do the tubular glands.

Calcium Transport Studies

We have previously demonstrated that calcium translocation to the mucosal side from the serosal side of the isolated shell gland occurred without an external transmural concentration gradient, depended on the presence of an egg in the shell gland at the time of excision, and required energy derived from oxidative metabolism (Ehrenspeck *et al.*, 1967). More recently, we have studied the transmural potential difference (PD), membrane conductance, calcium fluxes, and their response to the carbonic anhydrase inhibitor acetazolamide (Ehrenspeck *et al.*, 1971). The electrical measurements were made in an apparatus modeled after that developed by Ussing and Zerahn (1951). The PD generated by the membranes of active shell glands after about 40 minutes of incubation was of the order of 1 mV, with the mucosal surface always negative. In preparations with shell glands that were engaged in shell formation, ^{45}Ca influx (calcium movement from serosa to mucosa) continued unchanged when the transmural potential difference was reduced to zero (Fig. 6). On the other hand, small changes in PD did affect ^{45}Ca efflux (mucosa to serosa), increasing it by 46 ± 9% (Fig. 7). Cyanide (5 mM) abolishes the transmural potential. The relationship between calcium movement and PD was examined by comparing quiescent shell glands with those actively secreting calcium at the time of sacrifice. As shown in Table II, the stable PD's of shell glands in two secretory phases were the same.

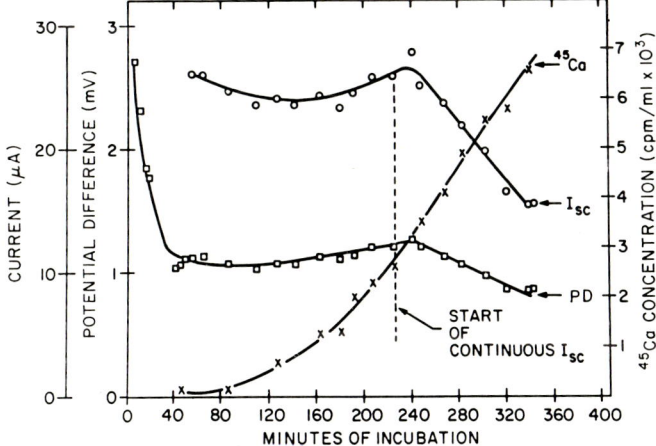

FIG. 6. The time course of transmural PD and the effect of short-circuit (I$_{sc}$) conditions on ^{45}Ca movement *in vitro* from serosa to mucosa. The graph represents data of one experiment. Key: ○ = I$_{sc}$ profile with direction from mucosa to serosa; □ = corresponding PD profile with the serosa positive relative to the mucosa; × = the change in ^{45}Ca concentration in the sampling compartment with time. During the continuous measurement of I$_{sc}$ to the right of the vertical dashed line, the shunting circuit was temporarily interrupted for an open-circuit PD measurement. (Ehrenspeck *et al.*, 1971.)

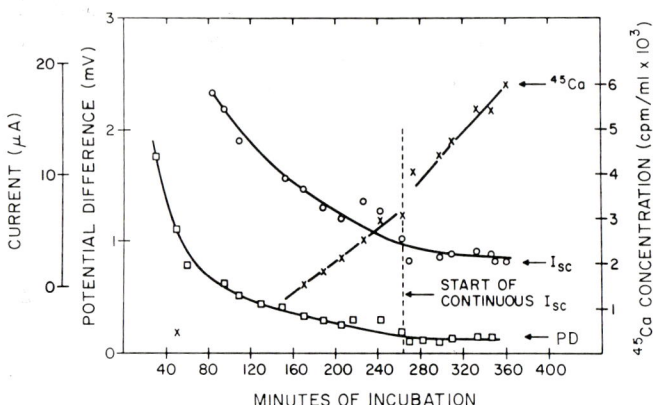

FIG. 7. The effect of short-circuit conditions on ^{45}Ca movement *in vitro* from mucosa to serosa. The graph represents data of one experiment. For explanation of symbols and procedural details, see Fig. 6. (Ehrenspeck *et al.*, 1971.)

Membrane conductance (G) which may be defined as the reciprocal of resistance (R), $G = 1/R$ (Scheie, 1967), was also calculated from the electrical data. Table II shows that active shell glands had twice the conductance of quiescent shell glands, which fact could be interpreted to mean that there is a net increase in permeability to ions for shell glands which were actively secreting shell minerals.

A second incubation system, which was described in an earlier publication (Ehrenspeck *et al.*, 1967), was used to study the net flux of the tissue to changes in the incubation medium. Table III shows that the unidirectional fluxes of untreated paired membranes from active shell glands resulted in a

TABLE II

TRANSMURAL POTENTIAL DIFFERENCE AND CONDUCTANCE OF ISOLATED SHELL GLAND[a]

Reproductive phase	PD (mV)	Conductance (mmhos/cm²)
Active[b] (5)	0.75±0.13	16±1
Quiescent[c] (6)	0.76±0.18	7±2

[a] Values are means ± S.E. Number of preparations is given in parentheses.

[b] Shell gland contained an egg and was depositing shell. From Ehrenspeck *et al.*, (1971).

[c] No egg in shell gland. In four cases, the oviduct did not contain an egg; in one case an egg was in the magnum, and in another it was in the isthmus.

TABLE III

CALCIUM FLUXES ACROSS ISOLATED ACTIVE SHELL GLAND[a]

Calcium flux (neq/cm²/hour)			Flux ratio[b]
Influx	Efflux	Net influx	(influx/efflux)
83±4	33±4	50±6	3.1±0.5

[a] Values are means ± SE of fourteen observations. Shell gland contained an egg and was depositing shell at the time of excision. From Ehrenspeck et al. (1971).

[b] Mean was computed from the flux ratios of individual paired membrane preparations and not from the data shown.

flux ratio of 3.1 ± 0.5. There was a net transmural movement of calcium from serosa to mucosa. It is important to note that the application of Ussing's equation for passive ion transport (Ussing and Zerahn, 1951) indicates that the magnitude of the PD, which was one mV, is too small to account for the calcium flux ratios observed. For flux ratios of 2.5–3.5, a PD of 12–17 mV would be expected.

The effect of actazolamide (50 mM) on unidirectional calcium flux was to increase influx by 47 ± 18% and efflux by 58 ± 18% (Table IV). The flux

TABLE IV

EFFECT OF ACETAZOLAMIDE AND POTASSIUM CYANIDE ON CALCIUM FLUXES OF ACTIVE SHELL GLAND[a]

Treatment	Calcium flux (neq/cm²/hour)		Flux ratio[b]
	Influx	Efflux	(influx/efflux)
Group A (7)			
Control[c]	82±7	39±6	2.5±0.6
Acetazolamide	114±8	57±8	2.1±0.2

[a] Values are means ± SE. Number of preparations is given in parentheses. Shell gland contained an egg and was depositing shell at the time of excision. From Ehrenspeck et al. (1971).

[b] Means were computed from the flux ratios of individual paired membrane preparations in each group.

[c] Each paired membrane was used as its own control.

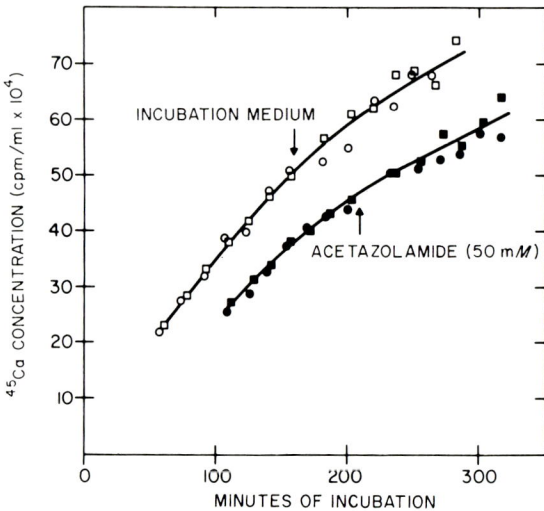

FIG. 8. Effect of acetazolamide on ^{45}Ca movement through stripped membranes. Each curve represents data of one paired membrane preparation from a different experimental animal. Upper curve depicts a control in which incubation medium in the amount usually added with the dissolved drug was introduced. Circles indicate influx, and squares indicate efflux; arrows denote initiation of treatments. (Ehrenspeck et al., 1971.)

ratio, however, was not significantly altered from control values. The effect of acetazolamide was to inhibit carbonic anhydrase in the mucosal layer, since acetazolamide had no effect if the mucosa was scraped from the preparation. The unidirectional calcium fluxes in such scraped preparations, however, were ten times higher than those observed in intact membranes (Fig. 8), and movement of ^{45}Ca in both directions was identical in magnitude. The effect of the acetazolamide suggests that electrolyte accumulation and transfer mediated by carbonic anhydrase in the mucosal cells plays a role in the generation of PD. The enzyme has been identified in the mucosal tissue by Bernstein et al. (1968), who observed that carbonic anhydrase was found in the supernatant fraction following cell fractionation of mucosal cells. Little or no enzyme was observed in the mitochondrial fraction. The enzymic hydration of metabolic carbon dioxide is thought to be catalyzed by the enzyme in mucosal cells. Concomitant with calcium ion translocation, the bicarbonate anion is thus made available to supply a counterion for calcite precipitation in the lumen of the oviduct.

Since membrane potential did not change with egg location in the oviduct, it appears that H^+ and HCO_3^- concentration remain relatively constant in the mucosa. This brief review of our work on transport characteristics of the excised shell gland supports the view that at least part of the calcium translocation by the shell gland may be active. The data indicate that the mucosa limits and controls the rate of calcium movement and that net calcium flux to the lumen-facing side of the shell gland occurs in the absence of a chemical potential difference.

Mitochondria and Metal Ion Translocation

The function of mitochondira in metal ion translocation has been documented since the early 1950's. Much of the published work has been performed on isolated mitochondria and has led to an historical, generalized concept that mitochondria from various tissue sources are similar, if not identical, in function. The generalization is undoubtedly due to the fundamental role of all mitochondria in energy metabolism. However, in our emerging understanding of their role in ion movement through cells it appears that some mitochondria from tissues involved in the translocation of large quantities of calcium may demonstrate specialization in both uptake and release of that metal ion.

Our early work with mitochondria from the mucosa of the hen's shell gland showed that when hens were dosed with ^{45}Ca during the laying cycle, the ^{45}Ca entered the mitochondria of both liver and shell gland (Hohman and Schraer, 1966). The distribution of the ^{45}Ca in the subcellular fractions from cells of both tissues showed that the greatest quantities occurred in the mitochondrial fraction of the shell gland mucosa. Liver mitochondria and nuclei were about equal (Fig. 9). Shell gland mitochondria accumulated significantly higher ^{45}Ca per milligram of nitrogen than did those from liver cells and the mitochondrial fraction of the shell gland cells accumulated more than a proportional amount of the ^{45}Ca. Quantitative data from studies of the subcellular fractions demonstrated that when shell glands were not actively calcifying, a greater proportion of the radionuclide accumulated in the mitochondria (Fig. 10). This data supports the thesis that while the mitochondria of both tissues take up calcium, mitochondria from tissues involved in extensive calcium translocation appear to have some specialization, whether qualitative or quantitative, to handle the ion translocation.

Since our previous experimental approaches demonstrated that the shell gland mucosal tissue varied in calcium content during specific phases of the ovulatory cycle, a comparative study of isolated shell gland mitochondria from this tissue was undertaken. Liver was chosen again as a source of control mitochondria, and the endogenous calcium content of mitochondria derived from both tissues were compared. Figure 11 indicates that the iso-

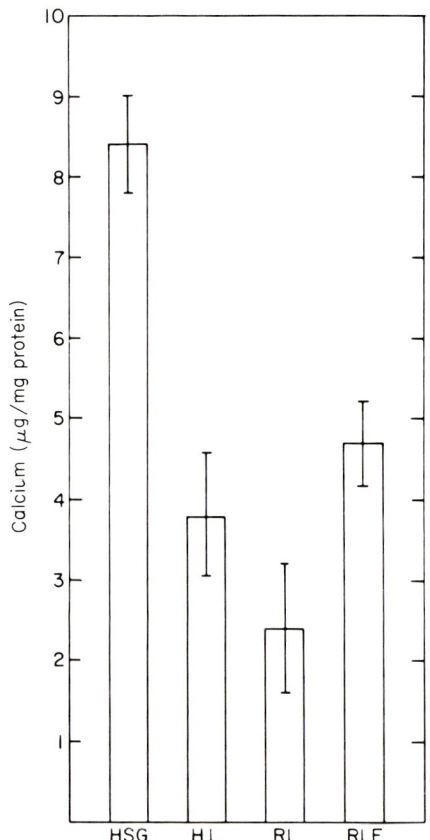

FIG. 11. The calcium content of mitochondria isolated from shell gland mucosae and livers of hens and roosters. HSG = hen shell gland; HL = hen liver; RL = rooster liver; RLE = liver from roosters treated with 10 mg estradiol valerate (Squibb) weekly for 6 weeks. $N = 6$ for each treatment; standard errors are indicated.

mitochondria under *in vitro* conditions (Elder, 1970). Isolated mitochondria from actively laying hens were incubated *in vitro* in the presence of a medium, containing 10 mM tris, 3 mM ATP, 10 mM succinate, 4 mM P$_i$, 10 mM magnesium, and 4 mM calcium labeled with ^{45}Ca at pH 6.2 and 25°C; the patterns of uptake and release of calcium in the mitochondria were observed, and the data are shown in Fig. 12. Under such conditions, shell gland uptake is more rapid than that shown for liver mitochondria. After 20 minutes of incubation, shell gland mitochondria begin to release the cation; a similar release was not observed in the liver mitochondria. At this

Transfer Across the Avian Shell Gland

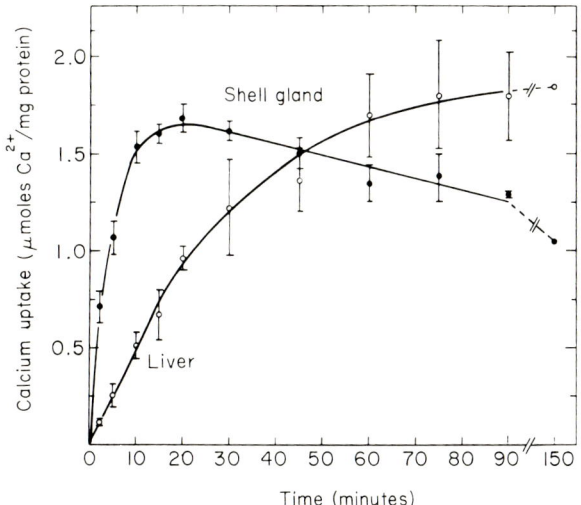

FIG. 12. Calcium uptake with time by isolated mitochondria of shell gland mucosae and livers of two laying hens. The bars represent the range. (Elder, 1970.)

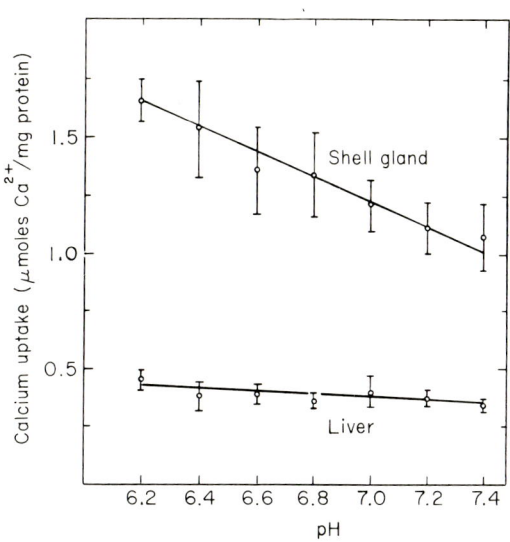

FIG. 13. Calcium uptake by isolated mitochondria of shell gland mucosae and livers of two laying hens as a function of pH. (Elder, 1970.)

It is interesting that Dr. Schraer claims binding of calcium occurs even at the pH of his system *in vivo*. The explanation may lie in the large quantity of protein produced by the shell gland system. The calcium leaves the blood, not only because of a unique system of transporting ions, but more remarkably because of an enormous sink, i.e., the shell gland matrix, which removes calcium and carbonate ions. The calcium is secreted in a restricted area circumscribed by tissue hyperemia, including a high rate of blood flow. Nearly everyone working on the problem of calcification of the shell matrix investigates carbonic anhydrase. The reason, of course, is that the hen's eggshell mineral is not calcium phosphate, but calcium carbonate. Carbonic anhydrase inhibitors, e.g., sulfanilimide, do not elucidate the mechanism of calcification. We fed sulfanilimide to laying hens and obtained soft-shelled eggs, but found that sulfanilimide also increased the rate of transport of the egg through the oviduct. The drug increased the rate of peristalsis and caused premature laying of the eggs, irrespective of its effect as an enzyme inhibitor. Have any other carbonic anhydrase inhibitors been tested in the laying hen?

Dr. Schraer: We only tried acetazolamide. We have some other information on this subject. Carbonic anhydrase has been reported to fall in birds that have been given DDT. Birds treated this way lay eggs with chalky or thinner shells. However, the amount of carbonic anhydrase, which is thought to be present in the shell gland mucosa, is probably greater than is needed for supplying carbonate ions for shell formation. A drop of only 16% of the carbonic anhydrase activity has been reported to cause thinner egg shells in Japanese quail. The DDT effect on carbonic anhydrase may be indirect, since we have some preliminary data which indicates that DDT and DDE do not inhibit hen carbonic anhydrase activity at the molecular level [R. S. Bernstein and R. Schraer, personal communication (1970)].

Dr. Matthews: I was very interested in your demonstration of the selective difference between the two mitochondria from the two sources. I was going to report that in our fractionation of the growth plate, the hypertrophic growth plate mitochondria were actually two classes of mitochondria, one that was heavy and one that was light. There isn't much difference between the two. Even in those two cells that have mitochondria possibly specialized to be reactive to calcium transport, I think there are other classes of mitochondria that have other functions.

Dr. Schraer: We never saw calcium phosphate or carbonate granules in any of the mitochondria as they appeared in the sections of normal shell gland or liver.

Dr. Matthews: I have never seen them in mammary glands either.

ACTIVE TRANSCELLULAR TRANSPORT OF CALCIUM BY EMBRYONIC CHICK CHORIOALLANTOIC MEMBRANE

A. Raymond Terepka, James R. Coleman, James C. Garrison, and Robert F. Spataro

A freshly laid fertile hen's egg contains 25 mg of calcium, all but a few milligrams of which are present in the egg yolk. After 21 days of incubation, the newly hatched chick contains almost six times this amount (Romanoff, 1967). All this additional calcium accumulated by the embryo is supplied by the egg shell.

Johnston and Comar (1955) determined the total calcium content of chick embryos throughout their entire incubation period, and their results, which we have confirmed, are replotted in Fig. 1. Clearly, the rapid accumulation of calcium by the embryo for bone formation occurs between the thirteenth or fourteenth day of incubation and hatching. Over this period, calcium is liberated from the shell, diffuses down through the noncellular shell membranes, and gains entrance to the chick's circulation via the chorioallantoic membrane.

The chorioallantoic (C-A) membrane is formed by the progressive fusion of the allantois, an outgrowth of the embryonic hind-gut, and the chorion, an ectodermal derivative (Romanoff, 1960). The relationship between the C-A membrane from a 16-day egg and the shell membranes and eggshell are shown in Fig. 2. The fused membrane consists of three layers: (1) an inner

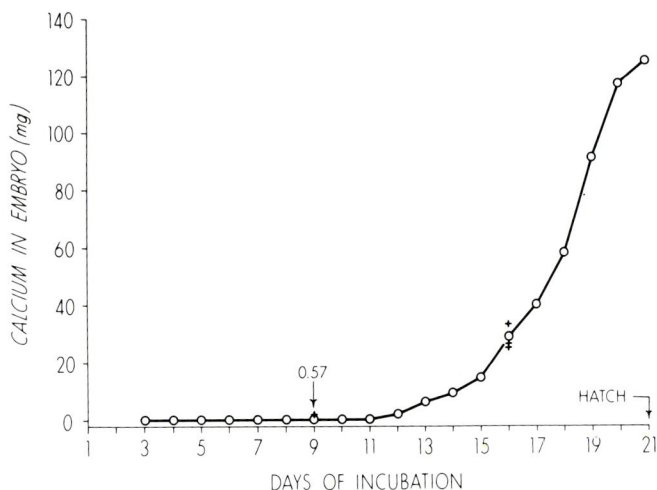

FIG. 1. Calcium content of chick embryos as a function of the days of incubation replotted (○) from the data of Johnston and Comar (1955). Isolated points (+) are unpublished values by this author.

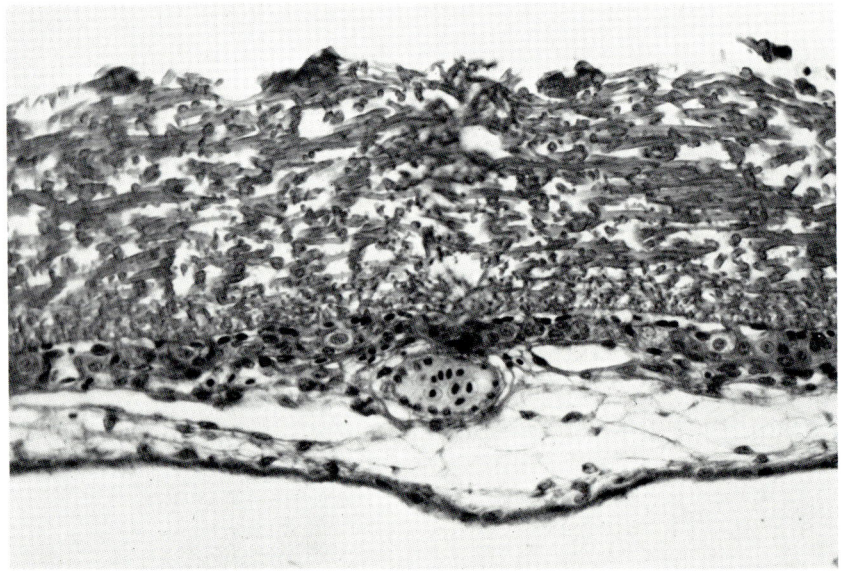

FIG. 2. Cross section of the C-A membrane and shell membrane from a 16-day-old chick embryo. (About 385 ×)

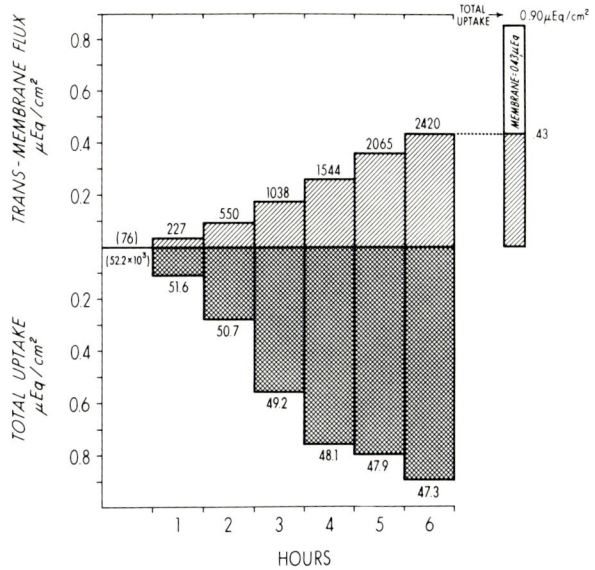

Fig. 3. Control Ussing chamber experiment with 1 mM calcium on both sides of the C-A membrane and ⁴⁵Ca only on the outside. The disappearance of calcium from the outside solution (total uptake) is plotted below the zero base line and the appearance of calcium in the inside solution (TMF) is plotted above. The numbers above and below each bar indicate the counts per minute of ⁴⁵Ca in the two solutions in this experiment. The small bar graph on the right compares total uptake with TMF and tissue ⁴⁵Ca retention in this experiment. (Terepka et al., 1969.)

endodermal cell layer in contact with the allantoic fluid, an embryonic excretory product, (2) a mesodermal layer containing scattered fibroblasts, collagen fibers, and small to medium sized blood vessels, and (3) an outer ectodermal cell layer supporting and surrounding the extraembryonic respiratory capillaries. The ectoderm at this stage is firmly attached to the inner shell membrane, which is fused, in turn, to the outer shell membrane. The egg shell proper, which is composed of almost pure calcium carbonate in the form of calcite, is attached to the outer shell membrane.

It is a simple procedure to remove 3–4 cm² of the C-A membrane from under the air space of the egg (where it is covered only by the inner shell membrane) and mount this in an Ussing type transport chamber. In such a preparation, it can be shown that calcium is actively transported by the ectodermal cell layer (Terepka et al., 1969). Figure 3 illustrates the results obtained with Krebs–Ringers bicarbonate solution containing 1 mM calcium on both sides of the membranes and aerated with 5% carbon dioxide in oxygen. Calcium-45 was added only to the outside (ectodermal) solution.

The uptake of outside solution ^{45}Ca by the membrane is plotted below the zero base line. Based on the initial solution count and the counts that disappeared, approximately 0.90 μEq of calcium per square centimeter of membrane left the outside solution in 6 hours. The cumulative appearance of ^{45}Ca in the inside solution, plotted above the abscissa, indicates a transmembrane flux (TMF) of 0.43 μEq/cm^2, about half the amount taken up by the membrane from the outside. The difference between total uptake and TMF was accounted for by the ^{45}Ca still remaining in the membrane at the end of the experiment. This is shown diagramatically in the small bar graph on the right in Fig. 3. Characteristically, the membrane contains one-half to two-thirds of the calcium that leaves the outside solution. There is also a parallel decrease in stable calcium concentration in the outside solution and a corresponding increase in the inside solution and in the membrane at the end of the 6 hours.

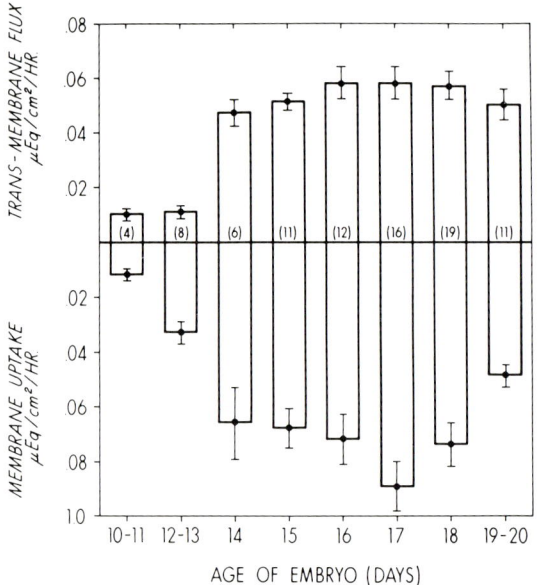

FIG. 4. Transport of calcium by C-A membranes of different embryonic age. TMF is plotted above, and membrane uptake is plotted below the zero base line so that length of the bar also represents total transported calcium from the outside solution. Number of experiments is in parentheses within each bar, and the S.E. of the mean is shown. (Terepka et al., 1969.)

Since the accumulation of calcium by the embryo begins at a rather precise time (13–14 days of incubation), we ran a series of control experiments with C-A membranes from embryos of various ages. The results are shown in Fig. 4. Plotted above the zero baseline is the mean TMF in $\mu Eq/cm^2$/hour for the 6 hour experiment. The tissue uptake (based on the ^{45}Ca counts recovered in the membrane) is plotted below so that the total length of each bar is equivalent to the amount of calcium transported from the outside solution. After incubation day 13, the capability of the membrane to transport calcium is significantly increased, correlating well with the movement of calcium into the embryo (Fig. 1).

In the older transporting membranes, any interference with energy production markedly affects the calcium transport process. Decreased temperature, uncouplers of oxidative phosphorylation (such as dinitrophenol and Dicoumarol), oligomycin (an inhibitor of ATP regeneration), and lack of oxygen are all strongly inhibitory. The C-A membrane will transport calcium under short-circuit conditions, against small applied (5–10 mV) electrical gradients (Moriarty, 1968; Moriarty and Terepka, 1969) and against substantial (50:1) uphill chemical gradients (Terepka et al., 1969). The transport system is saturated at about 1.0 mM calcium in the outside bathing solution, while back flux, even at large downhill gradients, is characteristically small, less than 5% of forward flux. With this published data as a background, we can now turn to three aspects of the calcium transport mechanism currently under investigation in our laboratory.

Electron Probe Investigations

A correlated electron microscope and electron probe analysis of the tissue was prompted by our observation that the calcium transported across the C-A membrane was apparently sequestered or compartmentalized (Terepka et al., 1969). Even after 6 hours exposure to 1.0 mM calcium, which saturates the ectodermal active transport system, the specific activity of calcium in the membrane was only about two-thirds that of the calcium in the solution outside the membrane. On the other hand, the specific activity of the calcium transported to the inside solution was nearly equivalent to the specific activity present on the outside.

In the electron microscope, three different ectodermal cell types are identifiable, in addition to the extraembryonic respiratory capillaries (Leeson and Leeson, 1963; Coleman et al., 1970). The calcium sequestering compartments could exist within every cell or could be restricted to just one cell type. To help distinguish between these two alternatives, Dr. James

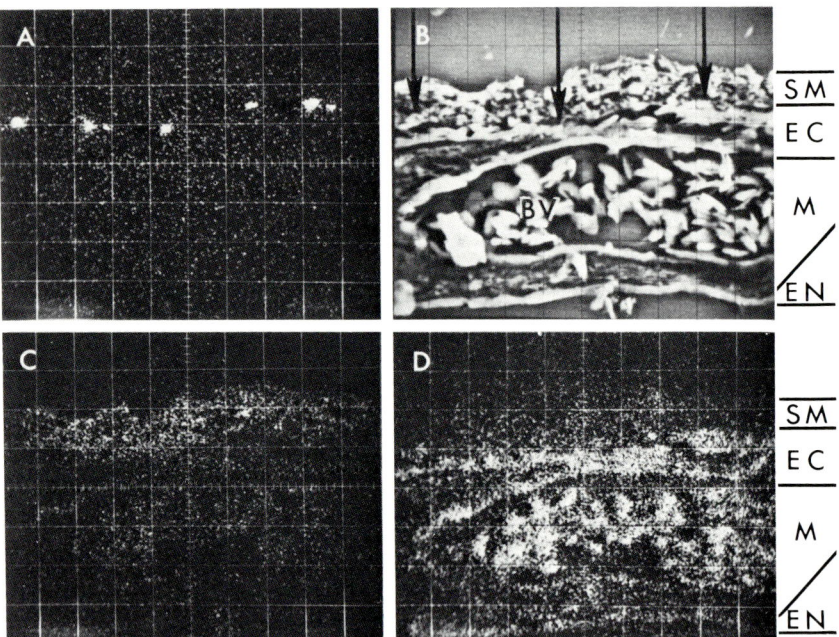

Fig. 5. Electron probe images of a 5 μ thick section of the C-A membrane at a magnification of 10 μ² per oscilloscope grid square.   A. Calcium x-ray image.   B. Total sample current image showing shell membrane (SM), ectodermal cell layer (EC), a large blood vessel (BV) in the mesoderm (M) and the thin endodermal cell layer (EN). Three sites of calcium localization are located just beneath the arrows; the others can be determined from coordinates of grid lines in the calcium x-ray image shown in A. C. Sulfur x-ray image.   D. Phosphorus x-ray image. (Coleman et al., 1970.)

Coleman in our Department used the electron probe x-ray microanalyzer to determine whether the calcium in transit across the membrane was localized or uniformly distributed. The electron probe revealed that calcium was restricted to certain characteristic sites within the ectoderm, and the correlated electron microscopy suggested that specialized cells within the membrane were responsible for active calcium transport.

Transporting membranes from the Ussing chambers were immediately fixed in buffered acrolein containing 1% sodium oxalate, which preserved cell structure and prevented loss and redistribution of calcium (Coleman et al., 1970). The tissues were dehydrated, embedded and sectioned without exposure to water, and then examined in the electron probe. Adjacent sections were examined by conventional electron microscopy.

The electron probe specimen current image of a 5 μ section is shown in Fig. 5B. Each large oscilloscope screen division is 10 μ. The resolving power of such total sample current images is comparable to light microscopy, and these oscilloscope images are used primarily for orientation and identification purposes. In Fig. 5B, one can distinguish the shell membrane (SM) above the respiratory capillaries which appear as dark areas in the ectodermal cell layer (EC). A large blood vessel (BV) containing erythrocytes is in the mesoderm (M) and the thin endodermal cell layer (EN) is seen near the bottom of the figure.

The calcium, sulfur, and phosphorus x-ray images of this specimen are seen in Figs. 5A, C, and D, respectively. Because of the low concentration of minerals in biological soft tissues, specific x-ray images require long photographic integrations (about 40 minutes). Signals not associated with tissue components and randomly distributed are due to electronic noise and cannot be ascribed to any particular element. Figure 5D, the phosphorus X-ray image, shows a generalized distribution, outlining the two cellular layers of the membrane and the nucleated red blood cells in the blood vessel. Shell membranes are very rich in sulfur and this is shown well in Fig. 5C, the sulfur scan. Figure 5A, the calcium x-ray image, is quite distinctive. The calcium signals are located at discrete sites only along the ectodermal surface of the membrane. The exact location of any of the calcium-containing sites in Fig. 5A can be determined by referring to the oscilloscope grid coordinates. Three of these sites lie just beneath the arrows in Fig. 5B, the corresponding sample current image. No such sites are found in young, nontransporting, membranes or in metabolically inhibited membranes. Membranes examined after exposure to strontium showed both strontium and calcium occupying similar sites.

After examining many such sections, Dr. Coleman concluded that these calcium concentrations visualized with the electron probe were located within the ectodermal cell layer and, more importantly, appeared to be limited to a certain type of ectodermal cell easily identifiable in the electron microscope. These cells, shown in Fig. 6C, were found immediately adjacent to respiratory capillaries (CAP in the figure) and always had long cytoplasmic processes bonding the capillaries to the shell membrane (SM). Such a cell can be distinguished in higher resolution specimen current images. In Fig. 6A, each grid square is 5 μ^2, and portions of the shell membrane (SM), ectoderm (E), and mesoderm (M) are visible. Directly beneath the junction of the shell membrane and the ectoderm are two respiratory capillaries which appear as dark spaces, and these contain three bright, roughly disk-shaped erythrocytes, one of which is labeled R. Between the two capillaries is an ectodermal cell of the type seen between the two capillaries in the electron microscope (Fig. 6C). It extends from the

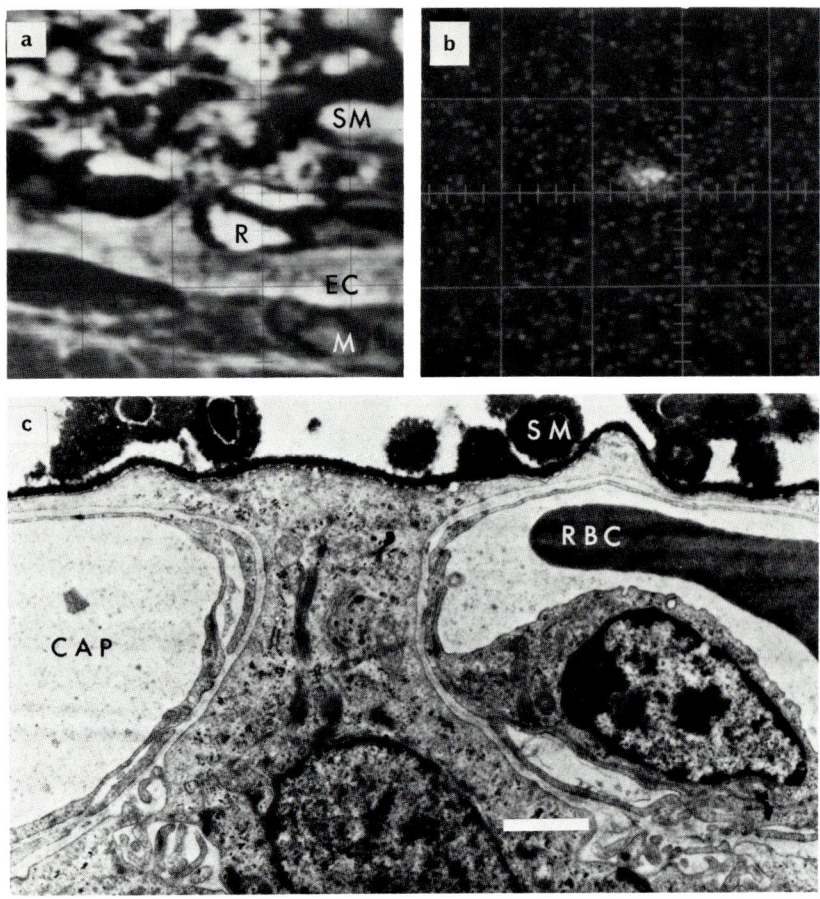

Fig. 6. A. Sample current image of C-A membrane at a magnification of 5 μ^2 per oscilliscope grid square. Portions of the shell membrane (SM), ectoderm (EC), and mesoderm (M) are visible. One erythrocyte in the respiratory capillaries is labeled R. B. Calcium X-ray image of specimen shown in A. C. Electron micrograph of thin section of C-A membrane in a region similar to that seen in A, showing the type of ectodermal cell seen between two capillaries. The ectodermal cell has long thin cytoplasmic processes that extend between the noncellular shell membrane (SM) and the endothelial cells of the capillaries (CAP). These ectodermal cells are the sites of calcium concentration as determined by electron probe analysis. (Bar represents 1 μ.) (Coleman et al., 1970.)

base of the ectodermal layer to the shell membrane. The calcium x-ray image of this section is shown in Fig. 6B. Only a small discrete region gives evidence of calcium signals above background levels. It can be determined from the grid coordinates that the calcium-rich region is located precisely between the two capillaries in the corresponding specimen current image (Fig. 6A), and just beneath the shell membrane–ectodermal cell junction.

The calcium-containing cells of the C-A membrane are quite distinctive. High resolution electron micrographs of the long cytoplasmic processes seen in Fig. 6C extending between the capillaries and the shell membrane, characteristically have a "fuzzy coat" (glycocalyx) and contain 400–1000 Å diameter vesicles. We have tentatively postulated (Terepka *et al.*, 1969) that these vesicles might be directly involved with calcium transport, but this still remains to be established. Interestingly, mitochondria are not particularly numerous in these cells, and those that are present tend to cluster around the nucleus which is usually located near the cell's basal surface, some distance from the calcium-containing cytoplasmic processes above the blood capillaries.

These preliminary observations suggest that transcellular transport of calcium by this epithelial membrane involves calcium compartmentation, and only certain cells are specifically involved in this process. The juxtaposition of calcium transporting sites and blood capillaries in the C-A membrane may facilitate the movement of egg shell calcium into the embryo's circulation when rapid skeletal calcification begins.

Oxygen Consumption and Active Calcium Transport

A second area of our current interest concerns the bioenergetics of the active transport mechanism. As a first step, we investigated the respiratory characteristics of the C-A membrane using conventional manometric techniques (Gilson Differential Respirometer). Calcium has a unique and very specific effect on the oxygen consumption of this membrane. The experiments graphed in Fig. 7 illustrate total oxygen consumption of the tissue as the content of calcium, magnesium, and strontium (indicated below the abscissa) is varied in the solution bathing the membrane.

The first two bars show the uptake of oxygen by the membrane in a bathing solution to which no calcium was added. With or without 0.5 mM magnesium in the medium, membrane oxygen uptake was about 9 μl/cm^2/hour. The second set of bars shows the significant stimulating effect of 1.0 mM Ca^{2+}, with or without Mg^{2+}, in the medium. Uptake of oxygen in-

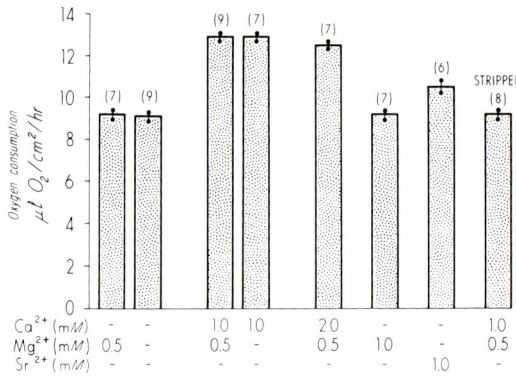

FIG. 7. Oxygen consumption of the C-A membrane, measured manometrically, as a function of calcium, magnesium, and strontium content in the bathing medium. Dash indicates that electrolyte was not added.

creased 45% to about 13 µl/cm²/hour. With 2 mM calcium (the next bar), there was no further stimulation of oxygen consumption, which agrees with our previous observation that the transport mechanism for calcium is saturated at a calcium concentration of 1.0 mM. The next two bars show that magnesium, in the absence of calcium, did not stimulate oxygen consumption above the basal rate, while strontium, which is transported by the membrane at a rate about one-third that of calcium, did cause a significant increase in oxygen uptake. Finally, the last bar shows the effect of stripping the inner shell membrane away from the underlying C-A membrane. Chamber experiments have shown that this procedure causes a profound inhibition of active calcium transport and it can be seen that the oxygen consumption in such stripped membranes is equivalent to oxygen consumption of membranes placed in Ca^{2+} free media (the first bar).

Is this effect of calcium on oxygen consumption specific to the ectodermal cell layer of the membrane, i.e., to those cells that are responsible for active transport, *in vivo*? To answer this question Mr. James Garrison, one of our graduate students, designed an Ussing chamber which contained, on one side, an oxygen-specific electrode (Garrison and Ford, 1970). The membrane could be mounted with either the ectodermal or endodermal surface facing the oxygen electrode. Through an electronic feedback circuit, the oxygen consumption of the cell layer facing the electrode could be monitored by recording the amount of an oxygen-rich solution required to main a constant pO_2 in the solution bathing the membrane surface. Some of his experiments are shown in Fig. 8.

With the endodermal side of the membrane facing the oxygen electrode, there was no effect of 1.0 mM calcium on oxygen consumption as shown in the first two horizontally hatched bars in the figure. The next three diagonally hatched bars show the effect of calcium and stripping on the oxygen consumption of the ectodermal cell layer. The addition of 1.0 mM calcium to the medium causes a significant increase of ectodermal oxygen consumption. The stripped membrane loses its ability to transport calcium and has an oxygen consumption which is very close to that of the membrane placed in a calcium-free medium.

That the O_2-stat apparatus is able to separate accurately the ectodermal and endodermal oxygen consumption is shown by the fact that addition of the individual ectodermal and endodermal values obtained in the O_2-stat agree very closely with the value obtained for total oxygen consumption by standard manometry. This is shown by the three sets of bar graphs on the right side of Fig. 8.

If the calcium-stimulated oxygen consumption in these experiments is combined with estimates of the amount of calcium actively transported during the same interval, a calcium/oxygen ratio for transport can be calculated. Considering the many assumptions involved, such calculations should only be regarded as rough approximations. Our data suggest that something of the order of one calcium atom is transported for each additional oxygen molecule consumed above the basal oxygen uptake level. In contrast, recent values given for active sodium transport by toad and turtle bladders (Nellans and Finn, 1970; LeFevre et al., 1970) indicate that

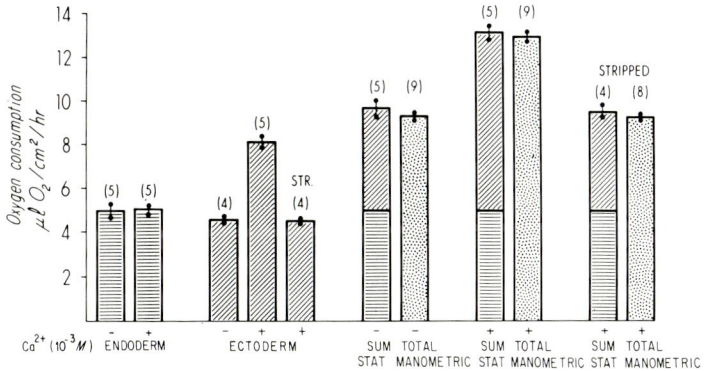

FIG. 8. Oxygen consumption of the endodermal and ectodermal cell layers of the C-A membrane in the presence (+) or absence (−) of 1.0 mM calcium as determined in the O_2-stat apparatus (see text). Dotted bars are total manometric values for oxygen uptake from Fig. 7. Horizontally hatched bars indicate endodermal values; diagonally hatched bars indicate ectodermal values.

approximately fifteen to twenty atoms of this monovalent ion are transported per oxygen molecule utilized. If our calculated Ca^{2+}/O_2 ratio is reasonably correct, it suggests to us that transcellular transport of a divalent ion such as calcium is not only metabolically quite expensive, but may involve a type of cellular pump activity entirely different from that involved in monovalent ion regulations.

Sulfhydryl Groups and Calcium Transport

The last area to be considered is the significance of sulfhydryl groups in the active calcium transport process and in the general maintenance of epithelial cellular integrity. In the course of our studies of the effects of metabolic inhibitors on active calcium transport by the membrane (Terepka et al., 1969), it was quite clear that any inhibitor affecting ATP regeneration markedly affected the transport process. In an attempt to evaluate the importance of anaerobic glycolysis on calcium transport, we used iodoacetate, a widely employed glycolytic blocking agent. A series of experiments were conducted with various concentrations of the inhibitor, and it was concluded that iodoacetate and other sulfhydryl-binding agents made the membrane leaky to calcium.

The three representative experiments in Fig. 9 will be used to summarize the findings. Data from a normally transporting C-A membrane is shown in A on the left. The broken line shows the progressive uptake of ^{45}Ca from the outside solution with time, and the solid line shows the progressive appearance of ^{45}Ca in the inside solution. The difference between the two lines represents the amount of calcium retained by the membrane. Characteristically, uptake of calcium from the outside solution precedes and is always greater than TMF. With 10^{-4} M iodoacetate added to the bathing media (B), entirely different results were obtained. Uptake of ^{45}Ca from the outside solution and TMF were virtually identical with little, if any, tissue retention.

Since iodoacetate's inhibitory action on enzyme function is related to its ability to bind to sulfhydryl groups, we tested the effect of a known potent sulfhydryl-binding agent, the organic mercurial mersalyl. As seen in Fig. 9C, the effect produced by 10^{-4} M mersalyl on the relationship between TMF and tissue uptake was similar to that observed with iodoacetate, but much more profound.

That the transfer of calcium across the membrane in the presence of these sulfhydryl-binding agents was a leak rather than active transport was confirmed in several ways. Even with large accumulations of ^{45}Ca counts in the inside solutions there was no detectable change in stable calcium

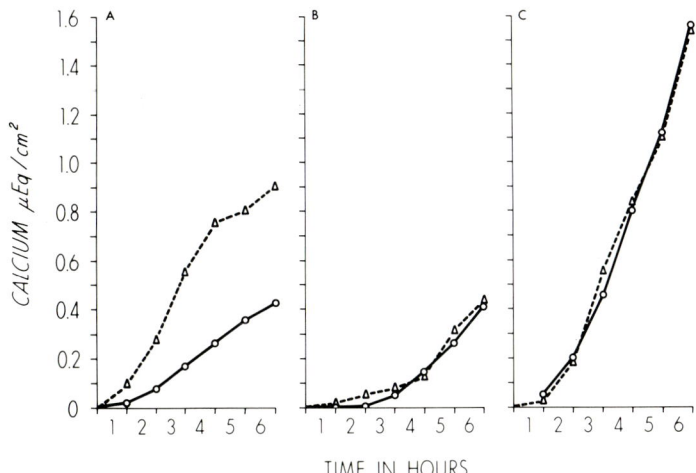

Fig. 9. Representative experiments showing the progressive uptake of labeled calcium from the outside solution ($\triangle\text{----}\triangle$) and its progressive appearance in the inside solution ($\bigcirc\text{—}\bigcirc$) in Ussing chamber experiments with the C-A membrane. In A, a normal control, the difference between the two values is accounted for by membrane retention. B and C show the effects of two sulfhydryl-binding agents (10^{-4} M iodoacetate and 10^{-4} M mersalyl, respectively) on these parameters. Even though the mechanism of transfer of label is different (see text), the ordinates are expressed in μEq Ca^{2+}/cm^2 for comparison to the control.

concentration in the two bathing solutions. Also, substitution of a nitrogen atmosphere for the normal oxygen atmosphere (thereby markedly depressing active calcium transport in control membranes) did not affect the rapid transfer of ^{45}Ca to the inside solution. Finally, in the presence of these agents, back flux of calcium, which in control membranes is very small relative to forward flux, was increased to values which were almost identical to forward flux.

Mechanically stripping the tightly bound inner shell membrane from the C-A membrane completely abolishes active calcium transport. Even though this procedure removes the external plasmalemma of the calcium transporting cells, it does not cause a calcium leak. The undamaged areas are still able to prevent ^{45}Ca movement across the membrane. It would seem, therefore, that this epithelial tissue is ordinarily impermeable to calcium except through its active transport mechanism, and the impermeability of the membrane is somehow dependent upon the presence of free sulfhydryl groups. It has been postulated (Farquhar and Palade, 1963) that the tight junction complexes observable by electron microscopy are the intercellular barriers preventing indiscriminate movement of ions across epithelial cellular membranes. If so, we would suggest that free sulfhydryl groups are an important component in the maintenance of these intercellular structures.

The experiments with iodoacetate and mersalyl led to another perhaps more significant observation. Note in Fig. 9B that during the first 3–4 hours, before the leak occurred, movement of labeled calcium into the membrane from the outside solution (broken line) was almost completely supressed, in distinct contrast to uptake of calcium by the normal membrane (A). Since active transport is initiated by tissue uptake of calcium, this suggested that a very early effect of the sulfhydryl-binding agents was an inhibition of the transport mechanism.

To investigate this effect further, Mr. Robert Spataro, a first year medical student, utilized a variety of sulfhydryl-binding agents whose reactivities are fairly well established from work on red blood cells (van Steveninck *et al.*, 1965; Shapiro *et al.*, 1970). By adjusting concentrations and duration of treatment with these agents, he was able to induce complete or partial inhibition of transport, as well as variations in the time of onset and magnitude of the calcium leak. Experiments with *p*-chlor-

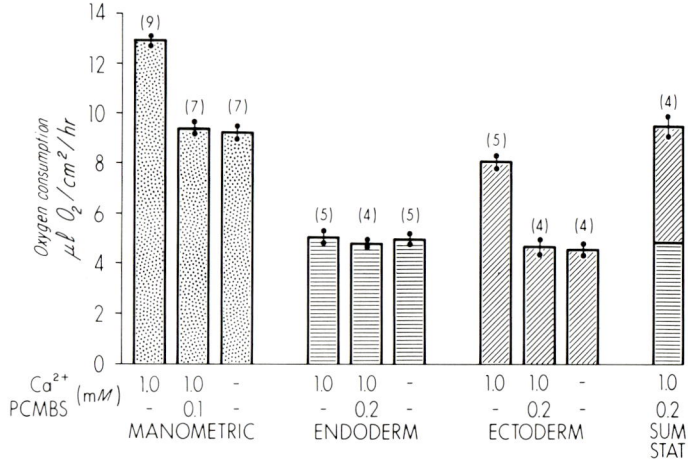

FIG. 10. Oxygen consumption of the C-A membrane as affected by a 15 minute pretreatment with 0.1–0.2 mM PCMBS on the presence (+) or absence (−) of 1.0 mM calcium in the bathing test medium. Dotted bars are total tissue manometric determinations. Endodermal (horizonatal hatching) and ectodermal (diagonal hatching) values were obtained with the O_2-stat apparatus.

mercuribenezenesulfonate (PCMBS), which only slowly penetrates the membrane, clearly separated transport inhibition from the leak effect. When the oxygen consumption of PCMBS-treated membranes was measured, the results shown in Fig. 10 were obtained.

Membranes were exposed to PCMBS for 15 minutes, rinsed briefly, and their total oxygen uptake was measured manometrically. As illustrated in the three dotted bars on the left, oxygen uptake falls almost exactly to the level observed when the membrane has no calcium to transport. Using the O_2-stat apparatus, it could be established that this effect of PCMBS was quite specific. Oxygen uptake in the endodermal cells (Fig. 10) was not affected by PCMBS pretreatment or by the removal of calcium. On the other hand, PCMBS pretreatment of the ectoderm was associated with a decrease in oxygen uptake which was almost exactly equivalent to the decrease in the calcium-deficient media. The last bar in Fig. 10 is simply the sum of the individual endodermal and ectodermal values obtained in the O_2-stat, which again show good agreement with the values for total oxygen uptake obtained by manometry.

These data suggest that a sulfhydryl-containing component on, or very close to, the external plasmalemma of calcium-transporting cells is directly involved with the active transport process. Specific calcium ATPases, which are also inhibited by sulfhydryl-binding agents, have been implicated in the transport of calcium across the plasma membranes of erythrocytes and muscle sarcoplasmic vesicles (Vincenzi and Schatzmann, 1967; Hasselbach and Seraydarian, 1966). Such an ATPase may also be essential for the initial entry of calcium into epithelial membranes. General cellular integrity seems to be dependent upon other, more deeply situated, sulfhydryl-containing components.

Concluding Remarks

In conclusion, we would like to suggest that, at least in this epithelial membrane, specialized calcium transporting cells are responsible for the transcellular transport of calcium. We have postulated previously that the initial entry of calcium into these cells constitutes the first active transport step and that a specialized form of endocytosis might be involved. It appears that this first step is dependent upon a cell membrane component, perhaps an enzymic function such as a calcium-activated ATPase, which is very sensitive to sulfhydryl-binding agents. Uninhibited C-A membranes in the presence of 1.0 mM calcium are maximally stimulated to transport calcium and in the process utilize a large amount of oxygen, apparently for

ATP regeneration. While the reason for this high Ca^{2+}/O_2 stoichiometry is not clear at present, one possibility we suggest is that stimulation of the calcium pump may involve the synthesis of a complex organic molecule. This could be a calcium-binding protein carrier, a specific calcium-activated enzyme, or new plasma membrane.

ACKNOWLEDGMENTS

The authors are particularly indebted to Dr. Margaret W. Neuman for critical help in the preparation of the manuscript. Miss Mary Pat Pauly, an undergraduate summer student fellow, contributed enthusiastically. Secretarial assistance was provided by Mrs. Jane Leadbeter.

This work was supported in part by USPHS grants 5 RO1 AM 08271, CA 03589, and 1 T1 DE 175 and in part under contract with the USAEC at the University of Rochester Atomic Energy Project and has been assigned Report No. UR-49-1340. Dr. Terepka is recipient of a USPHS Career Development Award, 9-K-AM-7876.

REFERENCES

Coleman, J. R., DeWitt, S. M., Batt, P. and Terepka, A. R. (1970). *Exp. Cell Res.* **63,** 216.
Farquhar, M. G., and Palade, G. E. (1963). *J. Cell Biol.* **17,** 375.
Garrison, J. C., and Ford, G. D. (1970). *J. Appl. Physiol.* **28,** 685.
Hasselbach, W., and Seraydarian, K. (1966). *Biochem. Z.* **345,** 159.
Johnston, P. M., and Comar, C. L. (1955). *Amer. J. Physiol.* **183,** 365.
Leeson, T. S., and Leeson, C. R. (1963). *J. Anat.* **97,** 585.
LeFevre, M., Gennaro, J., Cronkite, C., and Brodsky, W. (1970). *Biophys. J.* **10,** 198a (abstr.).
Moriarty, C. M. (1968). Ph.D. Thesis, University of Rochester (UR-49-989).
Moriarty, C. M., and Terepka, A. R. (1969). *Arch Biochem. Biophys.* **135,** 160.
Nellans, H., and Finn, A. (1970). *Biophys. J.* **10,** 196a (abstr.).
Romanoff, A. L. (1960). "The Avian Embryo." Macmillan, New York.
Romanoff, A. L. (1967). "Biochemistry of the Avian Embryo." Wiley, New York.
Shapiro, B., Kollmann, G., and Martin, D. (1970). *J. Cell Physiol.* **75,** 281.
Stewart, M. E., and Terepka, A. R. (1969). *Exp. Cell Res.* **58,** 93
Terepka, A. R., Stewart, M. E., and Merkel, N. (1969). *Exp. Cell Res.* **58,** 107.
van Steveninck, J., Weed, R. I., and Rothstein, A. (1965) *J. Gen. Physiol.* **48,** 617.
Vincenzi, F. F., and Schatzmann, H. J. (1967). *Helv. Physiol. Pharmacol. Acta* **25,** 233.

Discussion

Dr. Nichols: Dr. Terepka, I was intrigued by your cells and particularly by the fuzzy border which you showed. I wondered whether your concept was that this fuzzy border is involved somehow in uptake. Second, you showed us the locale of the calcium very well in your scans, but I wasn't sure what form you thought it was in, or where you thought it was in the cells, except that I believe you didn't think it was in mitochondria.

Dr. Terepka: We do see a fuzzy coat on the outer surface of the ectodermal cells, and some morphologists think this coat is very important for cellular function [S. Ito, *Fed. Proc., Fed. Amer. Soc. Exp. Biol.* **28,** 12 (1969)]. What it does exactly is not known, but I think it might be important for the initial binding step in all active transport processes. We have tentatively postulated that pinocytosis or endocytosis is involved in active calcium transport in the C-A membrane. It is possible that specialized areas of the fuzzy coat may also be involved in the initiation of such a mechanism, so we would like to be able to isolate some of this material for study. Perhaps PCMBS blocks calcium transport by affecting some enzyme function on, or just beneath, the coat.

Regarding your second question, all we can say is that with high resolution electron microscopy we do not see crystals or mitochondria in the area where the calcium x-ray signals originate. The calcium could be protein bound, perhaps to a special protein, such as Dr. Wasserman has described. We would like to have the resolving power in the electron probe to see whether the calcium is within vesicles, but we do not have this at the present time.

Dr. Borle: I wonder if the increased oxygen consumption that you see with calcium transport is not due to the uncoupling of mitochondria. When calcium enters the cells, I gather that some of it will be picked up by mitochondria. It is known that whenever small amounts of calcium are taken up by mitochondria, there is a small burst of respiration. I wonder if the increased oxygen consumption that you observed might be the consequence of calcium entry into the cell and of its uptake by mitochondria, rather than being the source of energy for the transport process that you postulate. The fact that you see no crystal or granules in mitochondria doesn't mean that there is no mitochondria able to pick up calcium.

Dr. Terepka: I only wanted to point out that the calcium-containing cells were not rich in mitochondria, and those that were present were not located where we see the calcium signals in the electron probe.

Dr. Borle: Dr. Schraer showed us that some mitochondria were heavily loaded with calcium without necessarily showing dark granules on electron micrographs.

Dr. Terepka: I think if all the calcium seen in our cells were available to the mitochondria, they would be fully uncoupled. In the respiration experiments, oxygen uptake was linear for 1-2 hours in the presence of 1.0 mM calcium, yet if dinitrophenol is added to such preparations, we see a rapid and marked stimulation of oxygen uptake. Also, in isolated mitochondria, oligomycin does not prevent calcium uncoupling, but in the C-A membrane, it blocks both oxygen uptake and calcium transport.

Dr. Neuman: You didn't have time to present the compartmentalization data which showed that the calcium that had been transported from the outside to the inside does so without a change in specific activity. Therefore, calcium in transport does not mix with the general calcium in the cells. This being the case, it seems unlikely that the calcium being transported would be accessible to the mitochondria.

Dr. Terepka: I did mention that calcium seems to be compartmentalized by the C-A membrane during its active transport. This conclusion was based on specific activity comparisons of the membrane with both the outside and inside bathing solutions [A. R. Terepka, M. E. Stewart, and N. Merkel, *Exp. Cell Res.* **58,** 107 (1969)]. We found that the calcium that appeared on the inside had a specific activity near that of the outside solution, while the specific activity of the membranes was always much lower, about one-third the outside solution specific activity. This compartmentation phenomenon suggested the electron probe work.

Dr. Urist: Let us look at the system that you have presented so ably from the beginning of development. When the egg is laid, the yolk contains about 30 mg of calcium.

This has been transported in the blood of the hen from the liver to the egg yolk granules. Thus, the embryo is provided with a supply of calcium, and there is no need for calcium transfer from the outside for embryonic development to get started.

As I understand Dr. Terepka's thesis, the embryo obtains an additional supply of calcium from the inside of the eggshell, but it is necessary to develop a tissue which is differentiated to do this work. Seeing Dr. Terepka's data on oxygen consumption suggests that the difference between the C-A membrane and other membranes is that the former is a highly differentiated tissue specializing in transport of calcium. Other membranes may not respond as dramatically to the same metabolic inhibitors by a reduction of calcium transport.

Dr. Terepka: As I indicated in the paper, the yolk only contains about 25 mg of calcium. However, the embryo at hatching contains about 160 mg and the remaining "spare" yolk, in fact, has more calcium than was present initially. This additional calcium is supplied by the shell, but to gain entrance to the embryo's circulation, it evidently must be pumped up hill to the plasma. Even at about 9 days of incubation, the embryo has a serum calcium of about 9 mg% [M. E. Stewart and A. R. Terepka, *Exp. Cell Res.* **58**, 93 (1969)]. Although we do not know what the calcium activity is outside the C-A membrane, I suspect it is very low. The active transport mechanism is there simply to get this calcium into the chick's circulation for transfer to the calcifying skeleton which acts as a calcium sink.

Dr. Urist: Your demonstration of a C-A membrane specialization in calcium transport is excellent. Now, can you tell us what puts the calcium carbonate in solution so it gets in the cell? How is the calcium carbonate on the inside of the shell put into solution? Why is the calcium accumulated in the C-A membrane cells? If one atom of calcium exits from the cell while another crosses the C-A membrane and enters the plasma, why is calcium accumulated? A protein specializing in transcellular transport of calcium could act as a bucket brigade, passing calcium from one protein molecule to the next, and so out of the cell. Only a very small rise in concentration of ionic calcium is tolerated in the cell, and if the system is anything like the plasma protein–calcium regulating system of the laying hen, the ionic calcium is in equilibrium with a specialized phosphoprotein having a high binding capacity but a low affinity constant (log K = about 2.3).

Dr. Terepka: Actually, your first question initially stimulated our interest in the C-A membrane. I still don't know the answer, but the solubility of calcium carbonate is so sensitive to pH, that I would suspect that hydrogen ions are involved. Exactly where they come from is another question, but the beauty of such a mechanism is clear. Metabolically produced acid could be neutralized as the calcium carbonate is converted to bicarbonate. This, in the presence of carbonic anhydrase, would escape as carbon dioxide and the embryo gains the calcium and some much needed water in the process.

In vitro, the accumulation of calcium in the membranes occurs because we have artifically closed the system by clamping the membrane in a transport chamber. Since this calcium was localized to particular cells, we are suggesting that these cells are the ones normally responsible for actively transporting the shell calcium *in vivo*.

Dr. Copp: Have you used this system to study the possible effect of parathyroid hormone and calcitonin?

Dr. Terepka: Yes, but with very impure preparations of each and they had no effect. The negative result with the parathyroid preparation doesn't bother me, even if the hormone was active and actually got into the cells. I suspect that the C-A membrane at the transporting stage has already been fully prepared by vitamin D and all the necessary hormones so that in 1 mM Ca^{2+} it is working at maximal capacity and cannot be stimulated any further. If we could get membranes from vitamin D or parathyroid hormone-depleted eggs, and we can't, these agents might then be stimulatory.

Dr. Raisz: In the shell membrane, I gather that the sulfate is probably some kind of acid mucopolysaccharide that can bind calcium. If that is true, would you expect a very low ionic calcium in the adjacent fluid?

Dr. Terepka: The electron microscope pictures show some very dense structures which are the actual shell membrane fibers. Between them is a very hydrated glycoprotein material. We don't have any information on their binding properties except that the calcium content of the whole shell membrane is very low.

VI. Sites and Modes of Action of Humoral Factors

CHEMISTRY OF PARATHYROID HORMONE

J. T. Potts, Jr., H. D. Niall, H. T. Keutmann, G. W. Tregear, R. Sauer, M. L. Hogan, B. Dawson, and G. D. Aurbach

Detailed studies of the chemistry of parathyroid hormone have long been hindered by the difficulties in obtaining the hormone in pure form in quantities sufficient for structural analysis. Nonetheless, during this time, work on the biological properties, mode of action, immunoassay, and metabolic fate of the hormone have been progressing. In each of these areas, important questions have now arisen which cannot be fully resolved without a better knowledge of the chemical structure of the active parathyroid hormone molecule.

For example, there are indications that the hormone in blood is not a single molecular entity (Berson and Yalow, 1968), but more likely consists of a mixture of the native hormone synthesized in the parathyroid gland with one or more smaller fragments of the polypeptide (Potts et al., 1971b). There have been speculations that the native eighty-four amino acid polypeptide is a prohormone and that the product from the gland is partially degraded prior to or concomitant with release (Sherwood et al., 1970; Arnaud et. al., 1970). Alternatively, the smaller fragments of the original biosynthesized polypeptide may arise from degradation of the hormone that occurs in peripheral organs after release from the gland (Potts et al., 1971b). The biological and immunological properties of any of such circulating fragments are of course presently unknown.

Similar complexities are found in attempting to analyze the mode of action of the hormone *in vivo* or *in vitro*. Recent advances in the chemistry of parathyroid hormone may help to improve this situation. Methods have been developed in our laboratory for isolation of completely pure parathyroid hormone free of contaminating proteins and of hormonal variants (Keutmann et al., 1971a). The complete covalent sequence of the major form (PTH-I) has been established independently by two groups (Niall et al., 1970; Brewer and Ronan, 1970). We have prepared (Potts et al., 1971a) a biologically active tetratriacontapeptide by solid phase synthesis; the synthetic peptide possesses all the known biological effects of parathyroid hormone on bone and kidney, in vivo and in vitro. The structural information required for biological activity has been more recently found to lie within the amino terminal twenty-nine residues (Keutmann et al., 1971b); however, the precise biological role of the carboxyl terminal two-thirds of the molecule remains unclear. This work will now be summarized and its potential significance briefly discussed.

Isolation

Numerous previous attempts have been made to isolate completely homogeneous parathyroid hormone. Methods used included standard gel filtration, ion exchange chromatography under a variety of conditions, preparative acrylamide gel electrophoresis, countercurrent distribution,

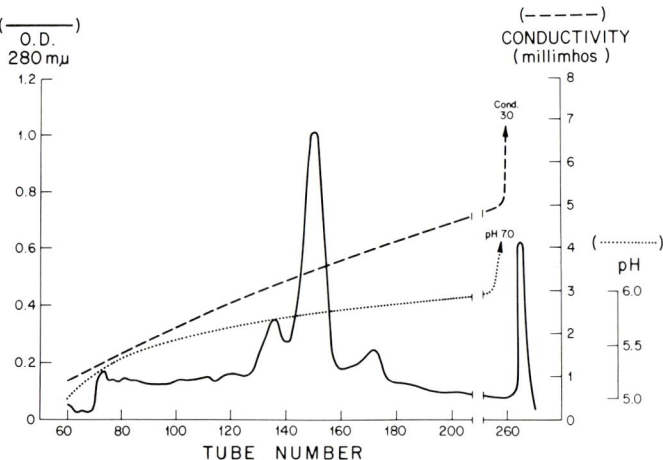

FIG. 1. Purification of bovine parathyroid hormone on a carboxymethylcellulose column in the presence of urea. The major component (PTH-I) eluted in tubes 145–155. The smaller peaks eluting earlier and later than the main peak represent minor hormonal variants (II and III) differing in amino acid composition from PTH-I.

adsorption chromatography on hydroxylapatite, gel filtration at low ionic strength, isoelectric precipitation, and partition chromatography. Of these approaches, only those using preparative disk gel electrophoresis or countercurrent distribution were successful in producing hormone of adequate purity. Neither method was ideal for large-scale purification.

Recently, we have developed a purification step employing ion exchange chromatography in the presence of 8 M urea (Keutmann et al., 1971a). This appears to result in disruption of noncovalent forces binding the hormone to contaminating peptides; it has the additional advantage that it also resolves molecular variants of the parathyroid hormone itself, which differ in amino acid composition from the major hormonal peptide. The separation obtained is shown in Fig. 1. The major peak seen represents the parathyroid hormone used in the structural analysis.

Sequence Analysis

The amino acid sequence of the major form of bovine parathyroid hormone was established by a combination of automated and manual degradation by the phenylisothiocyanate procedure. The complete sequence was determined in two runs on the protein/peptide sequenator. In the first run, fifty-four cycles of degradation were carried out using the protein methodology developed by Edman and Begg (Edman and Begg, 1967). This established the sequence from the amino terminus including the region known from earlier work (Potts et al., 1968) to contain the structural requirements for biological activity. The sequence of this region was in agreement with data obtained by amino acid analysis of peptides isolated after cleavage of the whole molecule with trypsin and cyanogen bromide. Confirmatory automated Edman degradations were carried out on the fragments comprising residues 19–84 obtained from cyanogen bromide cleavage and on the peptide 45–52 obtained from tryptic digestion.

The results of these experiments suggested the approach for completion of the sequence. The positions of all five arginines in the molecule were established in the long sequenator run on intact hormone. The most carboxyl-terminal arginine was found to be at position 52. This indicated that tryptic digestion of hormone in which the ϵ-amino groups of the lysines had been modified should produce a fragment extending from residues 53–84, since no tryptic-sensitive site would remain in this region. This approach was successful; the fragment consisting of residues 53–84 was isolated in high yield both from succinylated and from maleoylated hormone. The sequence of this fragment was established by a second sequenator run of thirty-one cycles. The C-terminal glutamine residue was

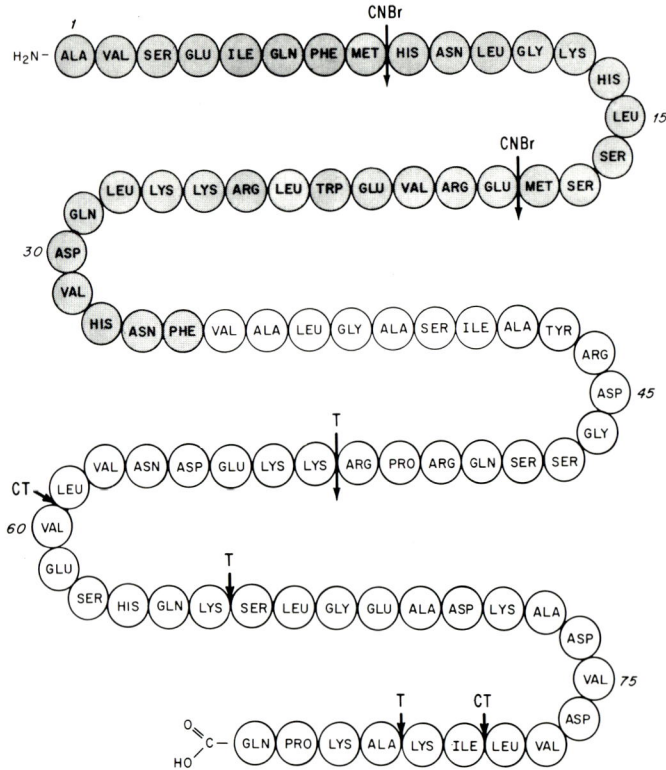

FIG. 2. The complete amino acid sequence of bovine parathyroid hormone-I. The arrows represent the positions of specific cleavages by cyanogen bromide (CNBr), trypsin (T), and chymotrypsin (CT) used during the structural analysis. The longer arrows represent primary cleavages of the native molecule; shorter arrows indicate cleavages achieved during subdigestion of the isolated carboxyl terminal fragment (residues 53–84). The sequence of the biologically active synthetic tetratriacontapeptide is shaded.

identified as the free amino acid. Confirmatory manual degradations were carried out on subfragments of the carboxyl terminal region generated by tryptic and chymotryptic digestion. Compositional data from these peptides and from others produced by dilute acid cleavage provided further confirmation. The complete sequence established by these procedures is being reported elsewhere (Niall *et al.*, 1970; Keutmann *et al.*, 1971b). The complete sequence and the site of limited cleavages important in the strategy of sequence analysis are shown in Fig. 2.

Synthesis: Properties of the Synthetic Peptide

Prior to the completion of the sequence of the carboxyl end of the molecule, synthesis of an amino terminal fragment representing residues 1–34 was initiated (Fig. 2). This fragment was chosen because earlier work suggested it should be biologically active. As stated above, studies since the synthesis was completed have shown that the sequence 1-29 is adequate for biological activity.

The method used for the synthesis was a modification of the solid phase procedure (Merrifield, 1963), using a new series of graft copolymers developed for applications in peptide chemistry (Battaerd and Tregear, 1967; Tregear, 1969). The details of the synthesis have been outlined elsewhere (Potts et al., 1971a).

The product after cleavage from the resin and purification by ion exchange chromatography and gel filtration was found to be biologically active. The biological activity of the synthetic tetratriacontapeptide was shown to be qualitatively identical to that of the native eighty-four amino acid polypeptide in each of the six presently available tests of the biological and immunological properties of parathyroid hormone: (1) elevation of serum calcium in dogs and rats; (2) increased excretion of phosphate in urine; (3) increased excretion of 3′, 5′-cyclic AMP in urine that precedes in time the observed phosphaturia; (4) stimulation of adenyl cyclase activity in bone cells *in vitro*; (5) stimulation of adenyl cyclase activity in kidney cell suspensions *in vitro*; (6) competitive displacement of ^{125}I-labeled-native parathyroid hormone binding to antibody.

Conclusion

Synthesis of a biologically active parathyroid polypeptide marks the culmination of an investigation begun by Collip in 1925 (Collip and Clark, 1925). Analysis of the structure of parathyroid hormone makes it clear that extracts made by Collip's method (hot dilute acid) must contain active fragments of the native molecule similar to the tetratriacontapeptide that we have synthesized. Recent investigations (Chase and Aurbach, 1967, 1970; Marcus and Aurbach, 1969) have shown that the earliest effect of parathyroid hormone in each receptor tissue (bone and kidney) is specific activation of adenyl cyclase and a consequent rise in the intracellular concentration of 3′, 5′-AMP within each tissue. The synthetic tetratriacontapeptide shows all of the specific properties of the native molecule; thus, it is clear that hormonal effects on both kidney and bone are the expression of the same limited region of the hormone molecule, a sequence of thirty-four amino acids or less at the amino terminus.

Study of the relative potency of the synthetic product, native hormone, and biologically active fragments of the native hormone that correspond in size to the synthetic tetratriacontapeptide indicate that the synthetic product is, if anything, more active *in vitro* than the natural fragments (residues 1–29) and has one-quarter to one-third of the potency of native hormone. The latter comparison does not take into consideration the finding that exposure of the native hormone to reagents used to remove the synthetic peptide from the resin results in significant loss of biological activity. Hence, it seems possible that the activity of the synthetic product may prove to closely approximate that of the native eighty-four amino acid peptide *in vitro*. Comparison of the potency of the synthetic fragment and the native hormone in the rat bioassay suggests that the synthetic fragment is relatively less active *in vivo* than *in vitro*. The activity of the synthetic tetratriacontapeptide *in vitro* in the kidney cyclase system is 400–600 units compared to 1600 units for the native peptide. *In vivo*, the activity of the synthetic peptide is only 100–150 units per milligram. This finding suggests that the carboxyl terminal portion of the molecule may protect the hormone against metabolic degradation during circulation from the parathyroids to receptors in kidney and bone. It will be possible to test the hypothesis by determining if the synthetic fragment is cleared more rapidly from blood than the native hormone.

However, detailed study of the amino terminal region is of greatest interest; such study should result in definition of the minimum structure required for biological activity and resolve the question as to whether receptor binding requirements are identical in kidney and bone. It will be important to study additional synthetic peptides shortened by successive deletion of amino acids from either the amino or carboxyl end of the 1–34 sequence. Analogues of the 1–34 sequence will also be of interest; choices for substitution will be guided by the comparative structural studies now in progress in our laboratory on the other bovine hormone molecules and the porcine hormone. We have found that in the closely similar sequence of the porcine peptide, several substitutions are found, some within the region of the active fragment sequence (Potts *et al.*, 1971c). There is only a single methionine residue in the porcine hormone (located at position 8), and the porcine peptide lacks tyrosine entirely.

Neither the natural bovine fragment (residues 1–29) nor the synthetic fragment (residues 1–34) displaced more than 50% of labeled intact bovine hormone from the antibody used in our clinical studies. This finding indicates that antibodies must be present in this antiserum that recognize portions of the sequence outside the biologically active 1–34 region. The recent findings in several laboratories (Sherwood *et al.*, 1970; Arnaud *et al.*, 1970) that suggest the presence of parathyroid hormone in blood differing in immunochemical properties and apparently in molecular size and metabolic fate from the native hormone can now be tested by use of antibodies specific for the biologically active region of the hormone and/or the biologically inactive carboxyl terminal portion. Such studies may clarify the nature of hormone biosynthesis, release, and peripheral degradation and should improve the precision and therefore clinical usefulness of immunoassays used to study primary and secondary disorders of parathyroid secretion in man.

REFERENCES

Arnaud, C. D., Tsao, H. S., and Oldham, S. B. (1970). *Proc. Nat. Acad. Sci. U.S.* **67,** 415.
Battaerd, H. A. J., and Tregear, G. W. (1967). "Graft Copolymers." Wiley (Interscience), New York.
Berson, S. A., and Yalow, R. S. (1968). *J. Clin. Endocrinol. Metab.* **28,** 1037.
Brewer, H. B., Jr. and Ronan, R. (1970). *Proc. Nat. Acad. Sci. U.S.* **67,** 1862.
Chase, L. R., and Aurbach, G. D. (1967). *Proc. Nat. Acad. Sci. U.S.* **58,** 518.
Chase, L. R., and Aurbach, G. D. (1970). *J. Biol. Chem.* **245,** 1520.
Collip, J. B., and Clark, E. P. (1925). *J. Biol. Chem.* **64,** 485.
Edman, P., and Begg, G. (1967). *Eur. J. Biochem.* **1,** 80.
Keutmann, H. T., Aurbach, G. D., Dawson, B. F., Niall, H. D., Deftos, L. J., and Potts, J. T., Jr. (1971a). *Biochemistry* **10,** 2779.
Keutmann, H. T., Niall, H. D., Sauer, R., Aurbach, G. D., and Potts, J. T., Jr. (1971b). *Biochemistry* (submitted for publication).
Marcus, R., and Aurbach, G. D. (1969). *Endocrinology* **85,** 801.
Merrifield, R. B. (1963). *J. Amer. Chem. Soc.* **85,** 2149.
Niall, H. D., Keutmann, H. T., Sauer, R., Hogan, M. H., Dawson, B. F., Aurbach, G. D., Potts, J. T., Jr. (1970). *Hoppe-Seyler's Z. Physiol. Chem.* **351,** 1586.
Potts, J. T., Jr., Keutmann, H. T., Niall, H. D., Deftos, L. J., Brewer, H. B., and Aurbach, G. D. (1968). *In* "Parathyroid Hormone and Thyrocalcitonin (Calcitonin)" (R. V. Talmage and L. F. Bélanger, eds.), p. 407. Excerpta Med. Found., Amsterdam.
Potts, J. T., Jr., Tregear, G. W., Keutmann, H. T., Niall, H. D., Sauer, R., Deftos, L. J., Dawson, B. F., Hogan, M. L., and Aurbach, G. D. (1971a). *Proc. Nat. Acad. Sci. U.S.* **68,** 63.
Potts, J. T., Jr., Murray, T. M., Peacock, M., Niall, H. D., Tregear, G. W., Keutmann, H. T., Powell, D., and Deftos, L. J. (1971b) *Amer. J. Med.* **50,** 639.
Potts, J. T., Jr., Keutmann, H. T., Niall, H. D., Habener, J. F., Tregear, G. W., Deftos, L. J., O'Riordan, J. L. M., and Aurbach, G. D. (1971c). *In* "Proceedings of the Fourth Parathyroid Conference." (R. V. Talmage, ed.) Excerpta Med. Found., Amsterdam (in press).
Sherwood, L. M., Rodman, J. S., and Lundberg, W. B. (1970). *Proc. Nat. Acad. Sci. U. S.* **67,** 1631.
Tregear, G. W. (1969). Ph.D. Thesis, Monash University, Australia.

Discussion

Dr. Bordier: Dr. Potts, did you measure the levels of parathyroid hormone in the plasma of vitamin D-deficient patients, and what happened to that level when vitamin D was given to the patients? Was it negatively related to serum calcium levels?
Dr. Potts: We have done a bit. Others have also, and might have some comments

to make. All I would be prepared to say, because the studies are limited so far, is that in vitamin D deficiency, there is evidence to support the thesis that there is secondary hyperparathyroidism. This view has been that vitamin D deficiency causes resistance to parathyroid hormone action. This, in turn, it was felt, would lead to hyperplasia of the parathyroids. Measurements of parathyroid hormone in a number of patients with vitamin D resistance of deficiency—I don't know how many patients altogether among the various labs have been studied—suggest that there is secondary hyperparathyroidism and high circulating concentrations of PTH.

I am not aware of a great deal of study with refeeding. However, Michael Kaye in a collaborative study with our group is trying to reverse the bony changes of osteodystrophy in patients with chronic renal failure. In treatment with dehydrotachysterol, he has achieved this. We are looking at parathyroid hormone levels after vitamin D repletion, but we don't have any definite data yet.

Dr. O'Riordan: Dr. Potts mentioned that we have isolated porcine parathyroid hormone (Woodhead, J. S., O'Riordan, J. L. H., Keutmann, H. T., Stoltz, M. L., Dawson, B. F., Niall, H. D., Robinson, G. T., and Potts, J. T., Jr. (1971) *Biochemistry* **10,** 2787. The reasons for doing this included the difficulty of achieving the final purification of bovine parathyroid hormone. I think, in fact, that we have been lucky in that it has come out in a very clean form with very much less difficulty than in the case of bovine parathyroid hormone. The preparation was homogeneous by several criteria including end-group analysis. The physical properties of bovine parathyroid hormone and porcine parathyroid hormone are very similar; thus their molecular size and charge properties are indistinguishable. They differ, however, in their amino acid composition. The composition of porcine parathyroid hormone is:

Asp_8, Ser_8, Glu_{11}, Pro_2, Gly_5, Ala_6, Val_9, Met_1, $Ileu_3$, Leu_{10}, Phe_1,

Lys_9, His_5, Arg_5, Trp_1,

The calculated molecular weight is 9423.

Littledike and Hawker [Endocrinology **81,** 261, (1967)] reported on partial characterization of the porcine hormone. One of the notable features of their preparation was the presence of threonine, but it is not present in the porcine hormone as we have isolated it. The porcine hormone has some very interesting characteristics. For example, it does not contain tyrosine. Despite this, it can be labeled with radioiodine. I presume, though we have not yet established it, that we are producing iodohistidyl residues. Another interesting feature of the porcine hormone is that it contains one rather than two methionine residues. Dr. Potts and his group have shown that the methionine residues of bovine hormone are of the 8 and 18 position, and it will obviously be fascinating to find out from which of these positions there is a deletion of a methionine in the porcine hormone. What we have established so far is that oxidation of the single methionine of porcine parathyroid hormone almost destroys biological activity; the potency goes down from 4000 units per milligram to 75 units per milligram; so the single methionine residue is essential for biological activity. However, oxidation of it does not affect immunological activity.

We have shown that the porcine hormone is immunologically different from both human and bovine parathyroid hormones [J. S. Woodhead and J. L. H. O'Riordan, *J. Endocrinol.* **49,** 79 (1971)]. This was done using a radioactive immunoassay system with labeled bovine and anti-bovine parathyroid hormone antisera. In addition, by using labeled porcine parathyroid hormone we showed with these antisera that there are almost certainly regions of immunological competence that are extremely similar in the hormones from the two species. Finally as Dr. Potts has said, he and his group have been studying the amino acid sequence of our preparation of porcine parathyroid hormone. It is going to be exciting to see where the differences in sequence between porcine and bovine parathyroid hormone are located.

Dr. Nichols: I would like to make a comment about Dr. Potts' observations regarding that very early fall in serum calcium after a dose of parathyroid hormone. He thought the calcium went into the bone cells, and I would like to echo that thought. We have two pieces of evidence to support this view. First, we can show an increased ^{45}Ca uptake into the cells *in vitro* after a dose of parathyroid hormone *in vivo*. Second, bone cell calcium has been found to be high in three patients with hypoparathyroidism and low in one with hyperparathyroidism.

If the model that we proposed is correct and the effect of parathyroid hormone is on cell uptake, and calcium exit from cells is controlled by phosphate and calcitonin, then in a patient with hypoparathyroidism who has a high phosphate, one might expect to see quite a lot of calcium inside the cells. Indeed, this is what we find in our three patients with this condition. In hyperparathyroidism the serum phosphate is low and the serum calcium is high and, although the parathyroid hormone effect is at its maximum, these patients would have a low cell calcium because of the removal of both the inhibitors of calcium efflux.

Dr. Hamilton: Dr. Potts, with respect to these nonhormonal peptides that you have eliminated through the modified procedure, what percentage contamination do they represent in the Sephadex-purified parathyroid hormone?

Dr. Potts: A rather significant percentage that varies from preparation to preparation. At times, with the best fractionation of material on conventional carboxymethylcellulose chromatography, you might have 25% contamination distributed between two nonhormonal peptides, say 15% and 10%, respectively, of the valine terminal versus the leucine terminal contaminant. We know they are nonhormonal, since if you do sequential degradation, three different sequences are read out at each step in degradation. It is impossible to work with such materials using new, sensitive sequence methods. Also, one does not want to have these in the material when doing definitive work.

PHYSIOLOGICAL IMPORTANCE OF THYROCALCITONIN*

Paul L. Munson, Cary W. Cooper, T. Kenney Gray, James D. Hundley, and Ahmed M. Mahgoub

Dr. Potts, in his paper, dealt with parathyroid hormone, which is essential for health and life. Dr. DeLuca discusses vitamin D, an equally essential vitamin or hormone. If an animal lacks either parathyroid hormone or Vitamin D there are indisputable serious pathological consequences. In contrast, at least in the usual laboratory situation, an animal can be deprived of thyrocalcitonin by removal of the thyroid gland without any obvious adverse effect.

It has often been suggested that thyrocalcitonin is an important adjunct to parathyroid hormone in the regulation of the level of blood calcium (Hirsch and Munson, 1969). Yet when the thyroid gland is removed from a rat or other animal, the blood calcium level appears to remain unchanged (Cooper *et al.*, 1970), quite in contrast to the dramatic fall in blood calcium after removal of the parathyroid glands. It is certainly true that the thyroid gland, by secreting thyrocalcitonin, is capable of very effectively combatting experimentally induced hypercalcemia, as

---

* Supported in part by a research grant from the National Institute of Arthritis and Metabolic Diseases (AM-10558) and a USPHS General Research Support Award (FR-5406). Dr. Cooper was the recipient of a Merck Sharp and Dohme Faculty Development Award, 1969; Dr. Gray was a USPHS Special Research Fellow, 1968–70.

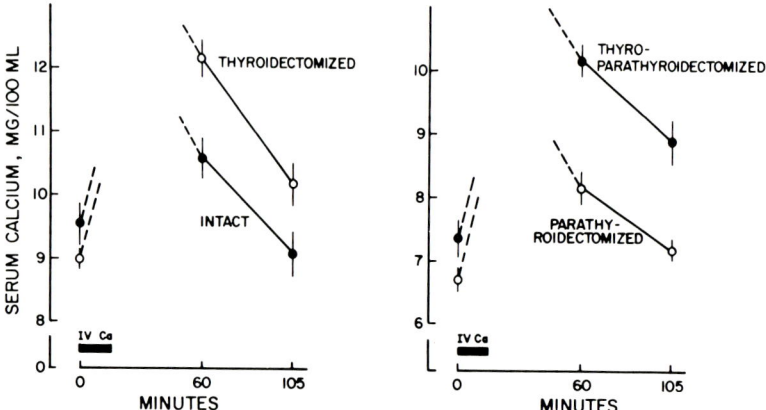

Fig. 1. Retarded return of serum calcium to normal after infusion of calcium chloride into thyroidectomized rats (with parathyroid transplants) and thyroparathyroidectomized rats as compared with intact and parathyroidectomized rats. Redrawn from Talmage et al. (1965).

shown some years ago for the first time by Talmage et al. (1965) (Fig. 1). In a similar manner, the thyroid gland can protect against hypercalcemia produced by injection of parathyroid hormone, as shown by Hirsch and Munson (1966) and others (Baghdiantz et al., 1965; Gittes and Irvin, 1965), or by excessive vitamin D, as shown by DeLuca et al. (1968) and Bugnon et al. (1967).

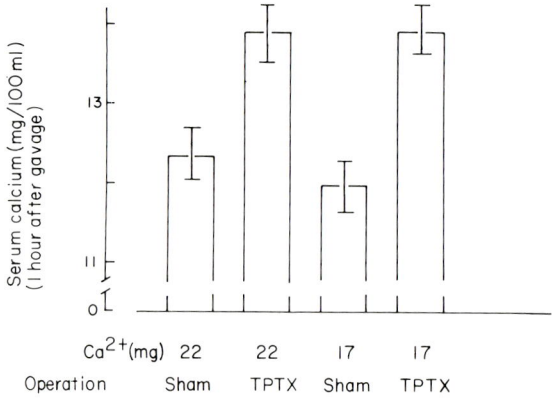

Fig. 2. Effect of thyroparathyroidectomy (TPTX) on serum calcium response of rats fasted 48 hours to moderate amounts of calcium chloride by stomach tube (Gray and Munson, 1970). Vertical lines or I-bars in this and succeeding figures represent standard errors.

However, these three types of experimental hypercalcemia are never encountered in normal life. Therefore, Dr. Gray and I sought a laboratory situation that might serve as a better model for an animal's actual experience; that is, one involving the oral ingestion of calcium. In our experiments (Gray and Munson, 1969; Munson and Gray, 1970), the responses of thyroidectomized and thyroid-intact rats to an oral calcium load were compared. The operations were performed 5 minutes before administration of calcium chloride by stomach tube and blood was drawn for calcium analysis 60 minutes later. In some of the experiments the rats had parathyroid autotransplants, so that the thyroid gland could be removed without disturbing the parathyroid glands, but in most of the experiments the simpler procedure of thyroparathyroidectomy was used. During the interval of 60 minutes the effect of parathyroidectomy is minimal. The results of illustrative experiments are shown in Figs. 2–4.

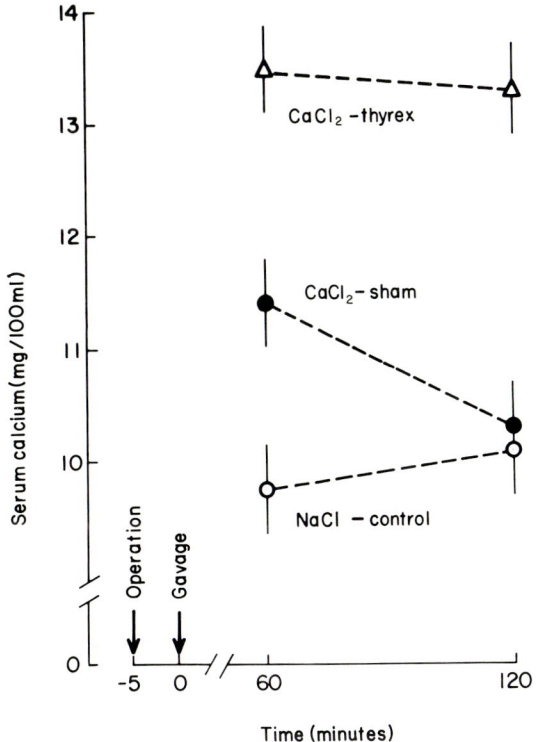

FIG. 3. Prolonged hypercalcemia in thyroidectomized rats (with parathyroid transplants) given 10 mg of calcium as calcium chloride by gavage after fasting, as compared with sham-operated rats and control rats given sodium chloride (Gray and Munson, 1969).

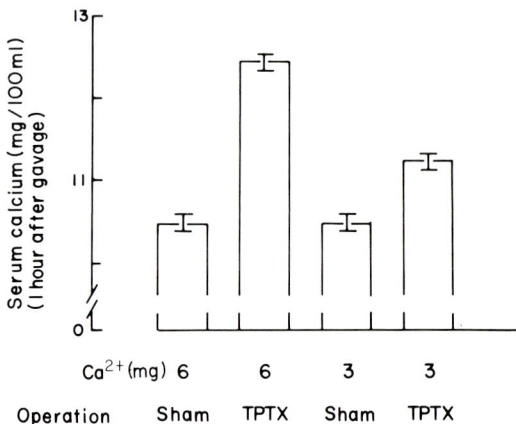

FIG. 4. Effect of thyroparathyroidectomy (TPTX) on serum calcium response of rats fasted 48 hours to small amounts of calcium chloride by stomach tube (Munson and Gray, 1970).

When a moderate amount of calcium was given by gavage (Fig. 2), hypercalcemia was produced even in rats with an intact thyroid gland. But the hypercalcemia was considerably more severe in the absence of the thyroid gland. The duration of the hypercalcemia was as long as 2 hours (Fig. 3). The protective effect of the thyroid gland was clear even when as little as 3 mg of calcium was given by mouth (Fig. 4). This is only about one-twentieth as much calcium as is consumed in a 1% calcium diet by a fasted rat during a similar time interval. These experiments demonstrated that the thyroid gland protects against hypercalcemia resulting from calcium administered by the natural oral route. Therefore, we developed the following hypothesis.

1. Calcium introduced into the gastrointestinal tract stimulates increased secretion of thyrocalcitonin in some manner if the thyroid gland is present.
2. Most likely this occurs because of rapid absorption of calcium from the intestine into the systemic circulation, resulting in an increase in the blood calcium level, which promotes release of thyrocalcitonin by direct action on the thyroidal thyrocalcitonin-secreting cells.
3. The resulting increase in blood thyrocalcitonin concentration acts on bone to inhibit resorption, thus reducing the blood calcium level back to normal.

We have tested various aspects of this hypothesis.

Physiological Importance of Thyrocalcitonin

To determine whether or not thyrocalcitonin secretion is actually increased when calcium is introduced into the gut we turned to the pig as the experimental animal because of the availability of the radioimmunoassay method for plasma thyrocalcitonin in this species (Deftos et al., 1968). This phase of the research was led by Dr. Cary W. Cooper.

Calcium chloride at varying dose levels was administered rapidly through a stomach tube to anesthetized pigs and peripheral blood and thyroid venous blood were collected at frequent intervals for calcium analyses. Thyrocalcitonin secretion was measured by radioimmunoassay of thyroid venous plasma. Figures 5–7 show the results of three illustrative experiments (Cooper et al., 1971b). After intragastric administration of calcium, the thyrocalcitonin concentration in thyroid venous plasma increased substantially in all cases. We assume that the same was true in our experiments in rats.

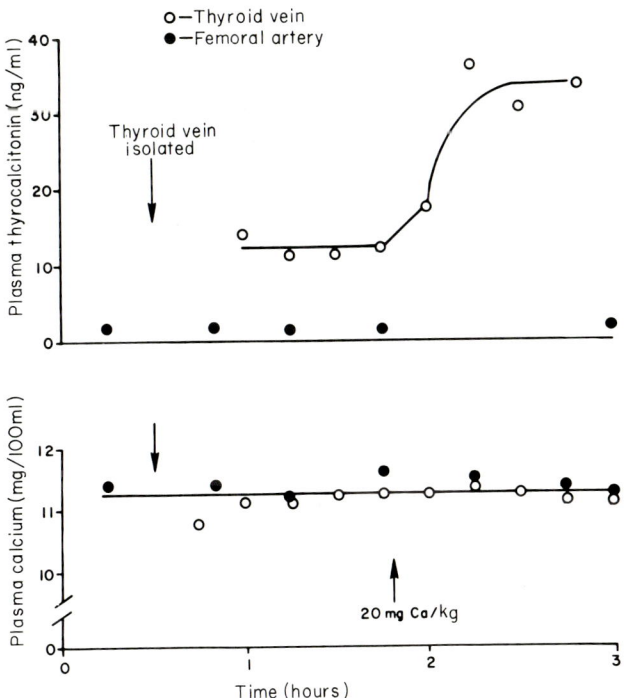

FIG. 5. Increase in concentration of thyrocalcitonin in thyroid venous plasma of a fasted pig after intragastric administration of calcium. A volume of 2% calcium chloride sufficient to deliver 20 mg calcium per kilogram of body weight was given rapidly via a feeding tube at the time indicated by the vertical arrow. (Cooper et al., 1971b.)

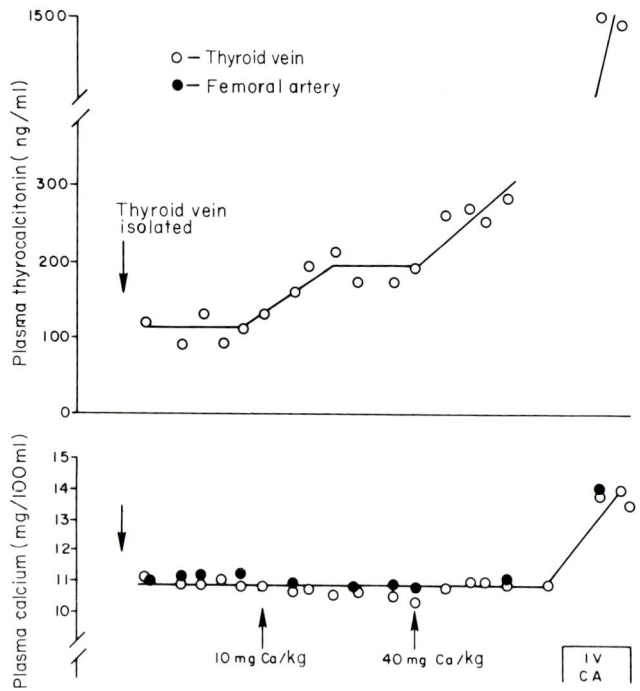

FIG. 6. Increase in concentration of thyrocalcitonin in thyroid venous plasma of a fasted pig after rapid intragastric administration of calcium at two dose levels (Cooper et al., 1971b).

TABLE I

Effect of Presence of Thyroid Gland[a] on Change in Calcium-45 Concentration[b] in Serum

Group	Calcium gavage	Mean paired Δ cpm/ml[c] ($\pm$ S.E.)
Intact thyroid (4)	no	$+563 \pm 185$
Thyrex (4)	no	$+602 \pm 185$
Intact thyroid (7)	yes	$-394^d \pm 150$
Thyrex (7)	yes	$+416 \pm 150$

[a] In prelabeled rats with parathyroid transplants.
[b] During 60 minute period after gavage.
[c] Observed cpm/ml serum $\sim$12,000.
[d] Significant at $P < 0.01$.

We now returned to the rat to test another aspect of the hypothesis—that release of a small amount of thyrocalcitonin would prevent hypercalcemia produced by calcium gavage. In this experiment (Fig. 8), acutely thyroparathyroidectomized rats were given 4 mg of calcium and injected with small doses of thyrocalcitonin intravenously. When no thyrocalcitonin was injected there was the usual hypercalcemia as expected whereas as little as 1 mU of thyrocalcitonin completely prevented hypercalcemia.

The next experiment (Table I), utilizing rats with parathyroid transplants, was designed to determine if bone resorption was inhibited during

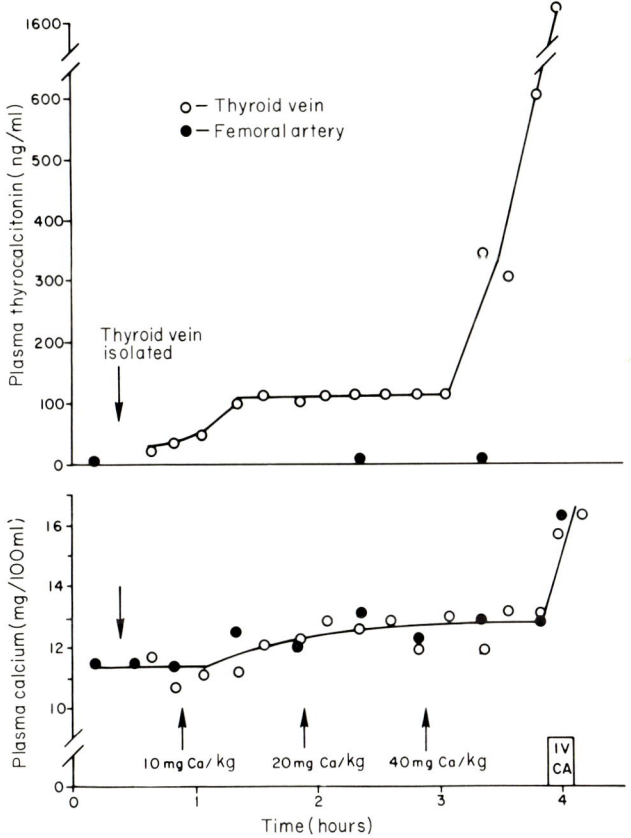

FIG. 7. Increase in concentration of thyrocalcitonin in thyroid venous plasma of a fasted pig after rapid intragastric administration of calcium sequentially at three increasing dose levels (Cooper et al., 1971b).

blood, increased, perhaps because the plasma calcium rose slightly although undetectably. We are continuing to challenge this part of our hypothesis in various ways and do not wish to overlook possible alternative mechanisms.

An attractive possibility explored by Gray and Cooper is that an in-intestinal hormone, capable (like pancreatic glucagon) of stimulating thyrocalcitonin secretion by direct action on the thyroid gland, is released when calcium is introduced into the intestine. This was first suggested to us by Dr. John Potts and has also been investigated by Care (1970). Gray and Cooper (1970) prepared various types of intestinal extracts and injected them into pigs. On some occasions there was an apparent increase in thyrocalcitonin release, but in general the results have been inconclusive. We are not yet in a position either to support or to rule out this explanation for the rise in thyrocalcitonin output resulting from oral calcium.

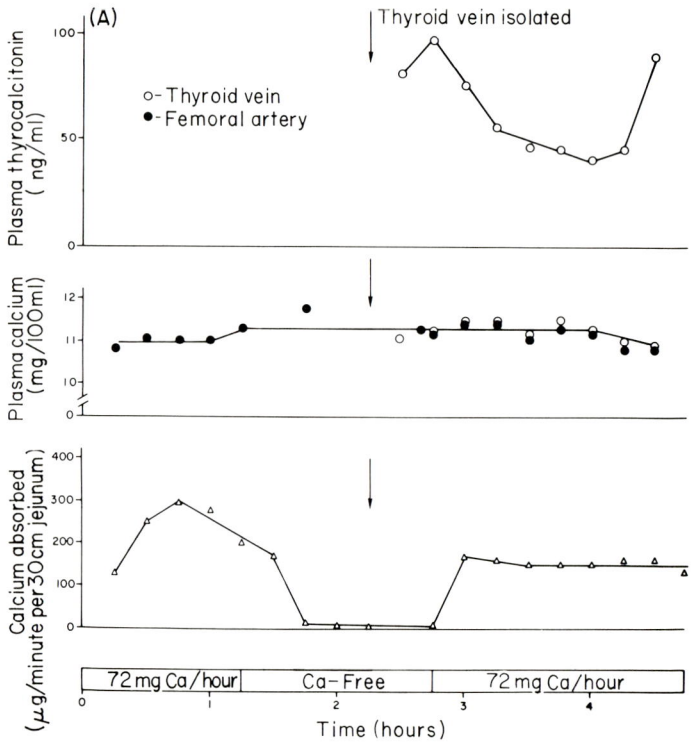

FIG. 10. Three experiments demonstrating increase in concentration of thyrocalcitonin in thyroid venous plasma during increased intestinal absorption of calcium from jejunal perfusion in female pigs (A) 14.3 kg, (B) 15.5 kg, (C) 26 kg. (Cooper et al., 1971b).

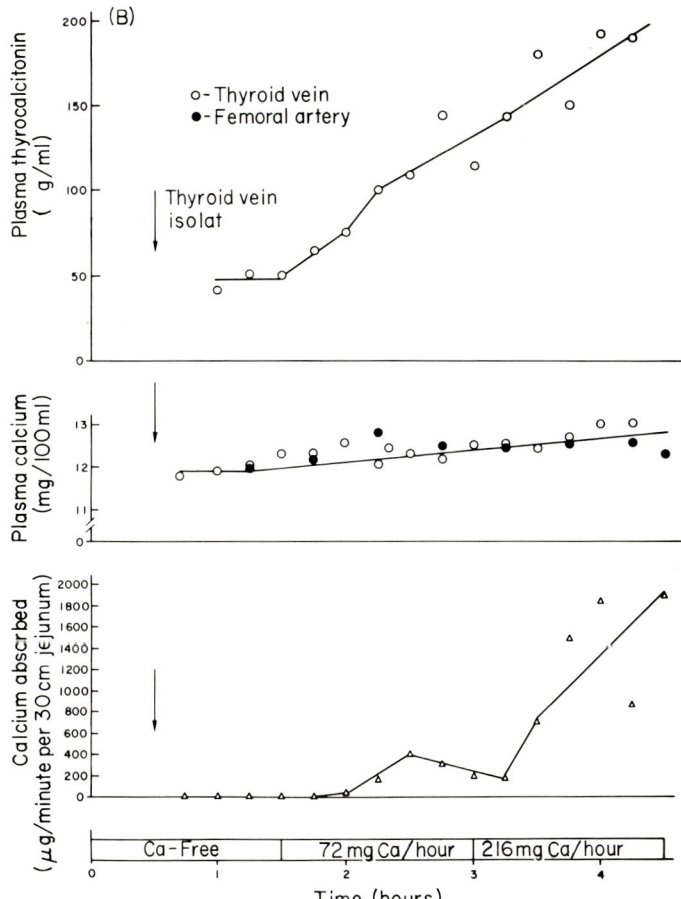

FIG. 10. (continued)

Most of our experiments have involved oral administration of calcium chloride, which is a rational model for the natural situation but not identical to it. However, similar results were obtained when rats consumed 55 mg of calcium in a 1% calcium laboratory diet over a period of 90 minutes (Gray and Munson, 1969). On the other hand, in another experiment (Gray and Munson, 1970), when the rats ate a different diet containing about the same amount of calcium but more phosphate, no hypercalcemia was seen in the thyroidectomized rats. Earlier, Bronner et al. (1967) had reported other dietary situations in which hypercalcemia did not occur in thyroidectomized rats after ingestion of calcium. We are studying this

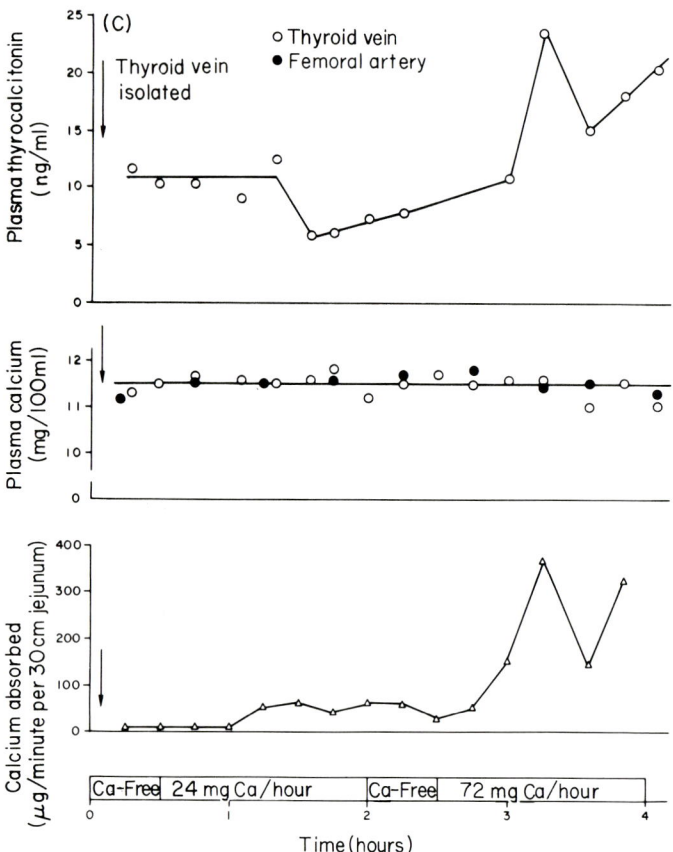

FIG. 10. (continued)

question further by varying the composition of the diet and the gavage fluid in our experiments in order to determine whether the protective action of the thyroid gland against hypercalcemia of dietary origin is the exception or the rule. Already, Dr. Schwesinger in our laboratory has demonstrated that calcium lactate, like calcium chloride, is more hypercalcemic in thyroidectomized rats than in thyroid-intact rats.

The weight of evidence appears to support the idea that the thyroid gland, through thyrocalcitonin, protects the animal against hypercalcemia of dietary origin. But there is still a further question before it can be concluded that we have identified a major physiological function for thyrocalcitonin. Is it of real importance to the animal to prevent transient hypercalcemia? We suggest that it is, but do not yet have conclusive evidence to support this belief. Preliminary experiments by Gray and Biddulph in our laboratory indicate that relatively brief episodes of hypercalcemia produce microscopic nephrocalcinosis in rats. In further investigation of this phenomenon, we will also look at the calcium content of the aorta, as suggested by Dr. Marshall Urist. When calcium is absorbed from the diet by the intestine, the amount lost in the urine (thus not available for deposition in bone) is largely dependent on the level of plasma calcium. The lower the plasma calcium, the less calcium is lost in the urine. Figure 11 illustrates the calcium-conserving action of endogenous and injected thyrocalcitonin following administration of calcium by stomach tube. Rats with intact thyroid glands excreted very little calcium, whereas thyroidectomized rats excreted a relatively tremendous amount—twenty times as much. If the thyroidectomized rats were given a small dose of thyrocalcitonin, loss of calcium was no greater than if the thyroid gland had been present. This mechanism for conservation of calcium for the skeleton may be of some significance, particularly during growth, pregnancy, and lactation.

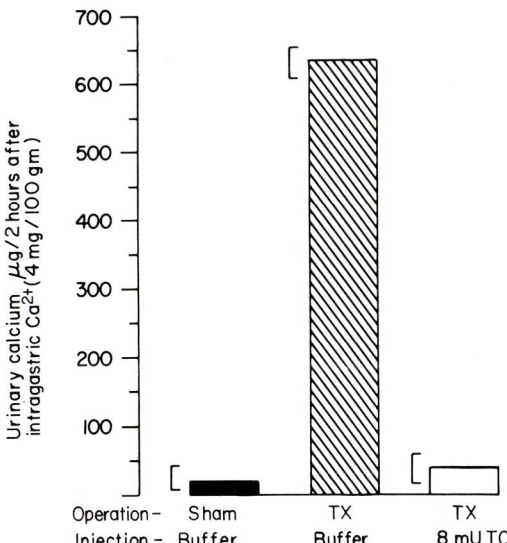

FIG. 11. Loss of calcium in urine of thyroidectomized rats (with parathyroid transplants) during 2 hour period after intragastric calcium as compared with sham-operated rats and thyroidectomized rats given a small dose of thyrocalcitonin subcutaneously at the time of gavage (Gray and Munson, 1970).

In summary, we have demonstrated that when ordinary amounts of calcium in certain forms are introduced into the intestine, there is little increase in blood calcium if the thyroid gland is present. If the thyroid gland is absent, hypercalcemia results. The forms of calcium that do and do not produce hypercalcemia have not yet been carefully defined.

Shortly after ingestion of calcium, the secretion of thyrocalcitonin increases, probably but not certainly because of a small, transient increase in circulating ionic calcium. Another possibility, not ruled out, is that a gastrointestinal hormone capable of stimulating thyrocalcitonin secretion is released when calcium is given by mouth.

A very small amount of thyrocalcitonin, consistent with the small increase in thyrocalcitonin secretion observed during calcium absorption, is sufficient to prevent hypercalcemia. Bone resorption is decreased during the period of calcium absorption and increased thyrocalcitonin secretion, which can account, at least in part, for the observed prevention of hypercalcemia. Prevention of hypercalcemia is accompanied by prevention of loss of calcium into the urine, thus conserving calcium for the skeleton. It is likely that prevention of hypercalcemia also protects against soft tissue calcification. Therefore, we suggest that prevention of hypercalcemia during absorption of calcium from the gut is an important physiological function of thyrocalcitonin. [Note added in proof: Cooper *et al.* (1971c) recently demonstrated that synthetic pentagastrin and native porcine gastrin are highly potent stimuli for secretion of thyrocalcitonin. We now hypothesize that gastrin or a related gastrointestinal peptide may be released by calcium in the gastrointestinal tract and thereby may contribute to protection against hypercalcemia after ingestion of calcium by stimulating secretion of thyrocalcitonin.]

ACKNOWLEDGMENT

We thank Mr. Robert T. James for expert technical assistance and Dr. Philip F. Hirsch for advice.

REFERENCES

Baghdiantz, A., Blanquet, P., Croizet, M., Moura, A. M., and Tayeau, F. (1965). *C. R. Acad. Sci.* **261**, 2779.
Bronner, F., Sammon, P. J., Stacey, R. E., and Shah, B. G. (1967). *Biochem. Med.* **1**, 261.
Bugnon, C., Maurat, J. P., Lenys, D., Moreau, N., and Rousselet, F. (1967). *C. R. Soc. Biol.* **161**, 2363.
Care, A. D. (1970). *Fed. Proc., Fed. Amer. Soc. Exp. Biol.* **29**, 253.
Care, A. D., Cooper, C. W., Duncan, T., and Orimo, H. (1968). *Endocrinology* **83**, 161.
Cooper, C. W., Hirsch, P. F., and Munson, P. L. (1970). *Endocrinology* **86**, 406.

Cooper, C. W., Deftos, L. J., and Potts, J. T., Jr. (1971a). *Endocrinology* **88,** 747.
Cooper, C. W., Gray, T. K., Hundley, J. D., and Mahgoub, A. M. (1971b). *Proc. Pan-Amer. Congr. Endocrinol.*, *7th*, 1970 (in press).
Cooper, C. W., Schwesinger, W. H., Mahgoub, A. M., and Ontjes, D. A. (1971c). *Science* **172,** 1238.
Deftos, L. J., Lee, M. R., and Potts, J. T., Jr. (1968). *Proc. Nat. Acad. Sci. U.S.* **60,** 293.
DeLuca, H. F., Morii, H., and Melancon, M. J., Jr. (1968). *In* "Parathyroid Hormone and Thyrocalcitonin (Calcitonin)" (R. V. Talmage and L. F. Belanger, eds.), p. 448. Excerpta Med. Found., Amsterdam.
Gittes, R. F., and Irvin, G. L. (1965). *Science* **148,** 1737.
Gray, T. K., and Cooper, C. W. (1970). Unpublished experiment.
Gray, T. K., and Munson, P. L. (1969). *Science* **166,** 512.
Gray, T. K., and Munson, P. L. (1970). Unpublished data.
Hirsch, P. F., and Munson, P. L. (1966). *Endocrinology* **79,** 655.
Hirsch, P. F., and Munson, P. L. (1969). *Physiol. Rev.* **49,** 548.
Munson, P. L., and Gray, T. K. (1970). *Fed. Proc., Fed. Amer. Soc. Exp. Biol.* **29,** 1206.
Talmage, R. V., Neuenschwander, J., and Kraintz, L. (1965). *Endocrinology* **76,** 103.

Discussion

Dr. Tashjian: I think, Paul, your demonstration of an acute protective effect of calcitonin in experimental animals is certainly the most convincing that any of us has seen to date. I thought it would be interesting to mention some information that we recently obtained in man using immunoassay for human calcitonin. In the acute situation, a positive direct correlation was found between the level of calcium and level of calcitonin after calcium infusions in man. However, in the chronic situation, this is not seen. We observe no increase above the normal level of hormone in patients with a variety of hypercalcemias from different causes nor in patients with hypocalcemia from various causes. And so I don't know whether this represents a species difference, or as Dr. Potts's studies have shown, that the homeostatic compensation which takes place in the chronic situation differs from that which takes place in the acute situation.

Dr. Munson: If I understand you correctly, you found that in pathological chronic hypercalcemia of various types the plasma thyrocalcitonin levels are not higher than normal. I don't think you meant to imply that repeated infusions of calcium in the same person failed to elicit a thyrocalcitonin response the second and third time, even though there was a normal response the first time.

Dr. Tashjian: The experiment wherein there were repeated infusions in the same patient within short periods of time has not been done. Repeated infusions at weekly intervals certainly don't lead to tachyphylaxis.

Dr. Copp: I am puzzled by the lack of significant increase in serum calcium following calcium loading in rats with intact thyroids. What stimulates calcitonin secretion? Have you investigated the possibility that the ionic calcium may be elevated even though the total calcium is normal?

Dr. Munson: We recognize this as an important question, but do not yet have the specific data to answer it. We have assumed, but are not sure, that the equilibrium between ionic and bound calcium in the plasma is so rapid that under normal circumstances during intestinal absorption of calcium, there would be no change in the proportion of ionic and bound calcium.

Dr. Mulrow: There is analogy in the adrenal gland between the potassium ions and secretion of aldosterone. Perfusion of the isolated sheep adrenal gland with blood having its potassium concentration increased by but a few tenths of a milliequivalent will stimulate aldosterone secretion. In more chronic studies in the rat, potassium loading results in an adaptation phenomenon so that the rat can dispose of the potassium load and has a high aldosterone secretion rate, yet the plasma potassium cannot be shown to be different from the rats receiving a normal diet. It seems likely that the adrenal gland of the rat on a high potassium diet senses a small change in ionic plasma potassium concentration.

Dr. Macintyre: Paul, if you did the experiments in adult animals with a slow bone turnover rate, I imagine that calcitonin would not be very effective in protecting them from hypercalcemia. If that is true, does that mean you think that calcitonin has a physiological role only in the young animal when bone turnover rate is high?

Dr. Munson: That is a very good point and we don't yet have all the data to answer your question fully. First, let me say that we are suggesting that protection against hypercalcemia during absorption of calcium from the gut is an important physiological function, but not necessarily the only one. With respect to the effect in older animals, Drs. Gutteridge and Toverud in our department recently found, as expected, that in older nonlactating female rats injection of thyrocalcitonin results in very little reduction in serum calcium, indicating a low rate of bone resorption. In contrast, lactating rats of the same age showed a strong hypocalcemic response to thyrocalcitonin, indicating a high rate of bone resorption. We plan to compare the response of lactating and nonlactating rats, intact and thyroidectomized, to calcium gavage. It may be that the protective effect of the thyroid gland against hypercalcemia during calcium absorption is as important in lactating rats as it appears to be in the young growing rat. We will also look for the phenomenon in pregnant rats. The effect may not be very prominent in older animals outside of pregnancy and lactation.

Dr. Talmage: Paul, it is your thesis that very minute changes in plasma calcium can change the secretory rate of thyrocalcitonin. If this is so, I wonder if you would try to explain some of the results we have reported over the past few years. Namely, that there are instances when the plasma calcium levels of thyroidectomized animals are lower rather than higher than those of thyroid-intact animals. To put this the other way, there appeared to be times when in the presence of intact thyroid glands rats maintained higher rather than lower plasma calcium levels. This appears to be related to the concurrent plasma phosphate concentration. Let me give three examples: If the plasma calcium level is followed over the 24 hours after nephrectomy, those animals with intact thyroids will maintain a statistically higher plasma calcium level than their thyroidectomized counterparts. A second example we can cite concerns the plasma calcium levels following parathyroidectomy from transplants. Also in this case, in the animals that have intact thyroids, the rate of fall in plasma calcium levels will be slower. And third, if the plasma calcium level is followed closely following phosphate administration, animals with intact thyroids will again have higher plasma calcium than thyroidectomized animals. Would you care to postulate on this phenomenon in the light of your theory?

Dr. Munson: It is a real challenge to attempt to interpret your very interesting results. I have no immediate explanation and only hope that your work will be carried further.

Dr. Spencer: I wonder about the hypocalcemia after thyroidectomy, namely, whether the high level of calcium in the blood is related to the high absorption of calcium from the intestine. We have noted that the absorption of calcium is very high in hypothyroid patients.

Dr. Munson: You pose an important question that our experiments really don't bear on. In our experiments, the time interval between removal of the thyroid gland and termination of the experiment, 65 to 125 minutes, was so short that the circulating levels of thyroxine and triiodothyronine were probably not significantly changed. We haven't yet attacked the question of how the whole situation might be affected by hypothyroidism or hyperthyroidism in the classic sense.

Dr. Bronner: Paul, with respect to your very elegant experiments, I would like to make two comments. One, it seems to me that the fact that you have a fairly rapid rise in measured thyrocalcitonin level without any obvious change in the plasma calcium would add to the likelihood that the acute release is like a derivative type of control. Moreover, the observation referred to earlier that there was no significant change in the measured thyrocalcitonin level in what appears to be a steady state would add support to this interpretation.

The other thought I had relates to the large increase in urinary calcium excretion you attribute to losses from bone. I suggest an alternate explanation, namely, that in the absence of thyrocalcitonin, the body responds with other available controls, including an increase in urinary calcium excretion. We know that the rat is capable of this, because in the rachitic state, its output of urinary calcium is very large, whereas it is not in the normal rat [S. Hurwitz, R. E. Stacey, and F. Bronner, *Am.r. J. Physiol.* **216**, 254 (1969)].

Normally, then, in the face of a rising plasma calcium load, thyrocalcitonin comes into play, but when this control is unavailable, the kidney takes on a larger role. It is because of this possibility that nephrocalcinosis might develop in a situation with extended stress. However, there is no reason to think that urinary calcium represents largely bone calcium. Rather, urinary calcium always represents a sampling of the plasma pool. Indeed, in your acute loading experiments, much of the calcium in the blood must have been derived from the load.

Dr. Hirsch: I would like to make a comment concerning Felix Bronner's explanation of the control mechanism. Dr. Bronner offers an attractive hypothesis, except that in most of the pig experiments that Paul Munson showed, the thyroid vein was isolated, and hence, no thyrocalcitonin was allowed to return to the pig. Yet, in all but one instance, the blood calcium did not rise despite the continuous absorption of calcium from the gut. It is difficult to explain why the calcium level does not rise when there is no thyrocalcitonin, especially if the physiological function of thyrocalcitonin is really to suppress an increase in blood calcium after its ingestion.

Dr. Perris: Dr. Munson, when you introduce calcium into the jejunum and then subsequently measure TCT, I presume there is a control, and that you have injected an equivalent concentration of sodium chloride into the jejunum. Have you also added other things, and do they have any effect on subsequent levels of TCT?

Dr. Munson: These experiments are recent enough that we have not yet adequately explored various control situations. In the few pigs in which Dr. Cooper administered isotonic sodium chloride intragastrically or intrajejunally, there was no change in thyrocalcitonin output by the gland. You may remember that in one of the experiments I showed (Fig. 12), during administration of a small amount of calcium accompanied by some calcium absorption, there was no change in thyrocalcitonin concentration in the thyroid venous plasma, indicating that the experimental procedure per se had no effect. Many other control situations should be investigated.

METABOLISM AND MECHANISM OF ACTION OF 25-HYDROXYCHOLECALCIFEROL*

H. F. DeLuca

Physiological Actions of Vitamin D

INTRODUCTION

It is now well accepted that there are two basic mechanisms whereby vitamin D elevates the plasma calcium and phosphate concentration to supersaturation levels with regard to bone mineral. These levels of plasma calcium and phosphate concentration are in turn necessary for the normal mineralization of bone (DeLuca, 1967, 1969). In the disease rickets, which we all recognize as a deficiency of vitamin D, the plasma levels of calcium and phosphate are undersaturated (Neumann, 1958). Clearly, then, the disease results by and large from a deficient supply of calcium and phosphate to the bone.

INTESTINAL ABSORPTION

The best known mechanism for the elevation of plasma calcium and phosphate in response to vitamin D is the markedly increased intestinal calcium and, secondarily, phosphate absorption. Although this phenome-

---

* Supported by USPHS Grant Number AMO-5800, AEC contract AT(11-1)-1668, and the Harry Steenbock Research Fund.

non was discovered as early as 1923 (Orr et al., 1923), it was not until the work of Nicolaysen and his collaborators (Nicolaysen and Eeg-Larsen, 1953) in the 1930's that it was established on a firm experimental basis. As has already been discussed in great detail in other sections of this book and elsewhere, calcium is absorbed by an active cation-oriented transport process (DeLuca, 1967; Schachter, 1963; Harrison and Harrison, 1963). It is some component of this process that is formed in response to vitamin D. The formation of this substance involves DNA transcription and protein synthesis (Zull et al., 1965, 1966; Norman, 1965). There is considerable disagreement as to how the vitamin D-induced substance participates in the transport reaction. Harrison and Harrison (1963, 1965) believe that the vitamin D-induced material is responsible for increased intestinal permeability to calcium. On the other hand, others believe that the vitamin D-induced substance participates in some way in the active transport process (Schachter, 1963; DeLuca, 1969). Wasserman and collaborators have advanced evidence that the vitamin D-induced substance is the calcium-binding protein which is presumably secreted by the goblet cells and which appears on the surface of the intestinal mucosa (Wasserman, 1970). DeLuca and his associates on the other hand discovered a calcium-stimulated ATPase in the brush borders which they feel participates in the transfer of calcium from the lumen of intestine to the cytoplasm (Martin et al., 1969; Melancon and DeLuca, 1970). Undoubtedly, all of these are partially right and only continued investigation will bring about a unification of these concepts.

Bone Mineral Mobilization

Besides the intestinal calcium transport mechanism, vitamin D participates or plays a very basic role in the mobilization of mineral from previously formed bone. This process, which was unknown until it was brought into focus by Bauer et al. (1955), appears to be a paradoxical effect of the vitamin in that it results in the demineralization of bone rather than its calcification. However, the mobilization of bone must be put into the context of contributing calcium and phosphate to the plasma which is in turn necessary for calcification of new organic matrix of bone. In any case, this is a cellularly-mediated process in which vitamin D plays a very basic role and is further augmented by the parathyroid hormone and is presumably inhibited by calcitonin (DeLuca et al., 1968). Thus, the bone mobilization mechanism and the intestinal absorption mechanism operate in concert to maintain the plasma calcium and phosphate concentration at supersaturation levels.

Renal Effects

Whether vitamin D is involved in the renal exchange of calcium and phosphate is unknown at the present time. However, current evidence suggests that if vitamin D does play a role in calcium reabsorption in the renal tubules, this effect is quantitatively small and contributes very little to the overall mineralization of bone.

Metabolism of Vitamin D

Isolation and Identification of 25-Hydroxycholecalciferol (25-HCC) and 25-Hydroxyergocalciferol (25-HEC)

In order to put the metabolism of vitamin D in its correct context in regard to its mechanism of action, it is essential to recall that an important characteristic of vitamin D action is its lag in inducing its characteristic physiological effect (DeLuca, 1967; Carlsson and Hollunger, 1954). The calcium transport mechanism of intestine does not appear immediately upon injection of vitamin D to vitamin D-deficient animals, but rather appears some 10–12 hours following a physiological dose of 10 IU of vitamin D_3. A somewhat longer lag period is required as might be expected when the route is by oral administration. As already discussed, part of this lag is due to the necessity for RNA and protein synthesis, presumably in the formation of the calcium transport substance. However, a good share of the lag is on the other hand required for the metabolism of vitamin D to metabolically active metabolites. With the synthesis of very high specific activity vitamin D_3 labeled in the 1,2 position by Neville and DeLuca (1966), it was possible to examine the fate of the vitamin D molecule during the lag period between its administration and its initiation of the calcium transport mechanism.

Following injection of the radioactive vitamin D_3, it was possible by means of methanol–chloroform extraction and silicic acid column chromatography to demonstrate the existence of at least three metabolite fractions as shown in Fig. 1 (Lund and DeLuca, 1966; Norman et al., 1964). The first of these was readily identified as an ester of vitamin D and long-chain fatty acids (Lund et al., 1967) and has been extensively examined by Fraser and Kodicek (1965, 1966). Fraction II is as yet unidentified although biologically active. Fraction III is unchanged vitamin D_3, but of greatest interest was the polar fraction IV. Lund and DeLuca (1966) demonstrated quite convincingly that this fraction was at least as biologically active as the parent vitamin and that it mimicked the effect of

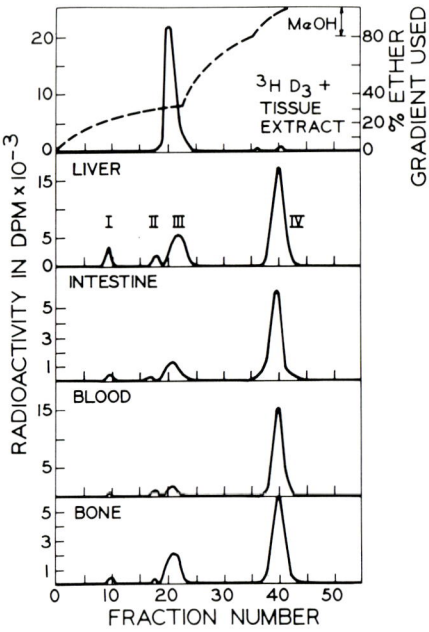

Fig. 1. Silicic acid column chromatographic profile of chloroform extracts of tissue from rats given 10 IU vitamin D_3 12 hours before. Solid line = radioactivity; broken line = solvent gradient; peak III represents unchanged vitamin D_3 (DeLuca, 1969).

vitamin D not only in the cure of rickets in rats, but also in inducing the intestinal calcium transport mechanism and in stimulating bone mineral mobilization. Most important, however, is the fact that this metabolite fraction acted more rapidly than the parent vitamin in inducing intestinal calcium transport (Morii et al., 1967). As one examined the dose–response relationship, it became evident that as the dose was decreased to physiological levels, the major radioactive component of the tissues became the peak IV metabolite fraction even before the onset of increased intestinal calcium transport. Peaks I and II, on the other hand, remained small in amount regardless of dose or time after dose. Thus, they were assigned little biological importance. However, with these data it was evident that fraction IV was or contained a possible candidate as the metabolically active form of vitamin D. This evidence was sufficient for the initiation of a concentrated attempt to isolate sufficient quantities of the metabolite for chemical identification. This was accomplished when Blunt et al. (1968ab) were able to isolate from the plasma of four pigs fed large doses of vitamin D for 26 days, 1.3 mg of the metabolite in pure form. It was identified by mass spectrometry, nuclear magnetic resonance, ultraviolet absorption spectrophotometry, and behavior on gas–liquid chromatography as 25-HCC (Fig. 2). In a similar fashion the biologically active metabolite of vitamin D_2 was isolated and identified as 25-HEC (Suda et al., 1969ab).

BIOLOGICAL ACTIVITY OF 25-HCC

25-HCC is one and one-half times more effective than cholecalciferol in the prevention or cure of rickets in rats and chickens (Blunt et al., 1968c). More important, however, is that 25-HCC is not only more effective in inducing intestinal calcium transport and inducing bone mineral mobilization, but it acts much more rapidly in both systems. Although these results provided very strong evidence that the 25-HCC is the circulating or hormonal form of vitamin D, final proof came with experiments dealing with isolated target organs of vitamin D action.

It has long been known that despite the fact that vitamin D is effective in vivo as a bone mineral mobilization agent, when added in vitro to organ cultures it was essentially without effect. This puzzling phenomenon defied tissue culturists until 25-HCC was highly purified in our laboratory. We submitted this sample to Drs. Raisz and Trummel at the University of Rochester to perform the necessary experiments. As shown in Fig. 3, 25-HCC is extremely effective in inducing bone mineral mobilization in organ cultures, whereas 320 IU/per milliliter of vitamin D_3 was without effect in the same system. 25-HCC worked synergistically with the parathyroid hormone to induce bone mineral mobilization (Trummel et al., 1969).

In our laboratory, a vascularly perfused intestine was developed which could carry out intestinal calcium transport for some 4–6 hours (Olson and

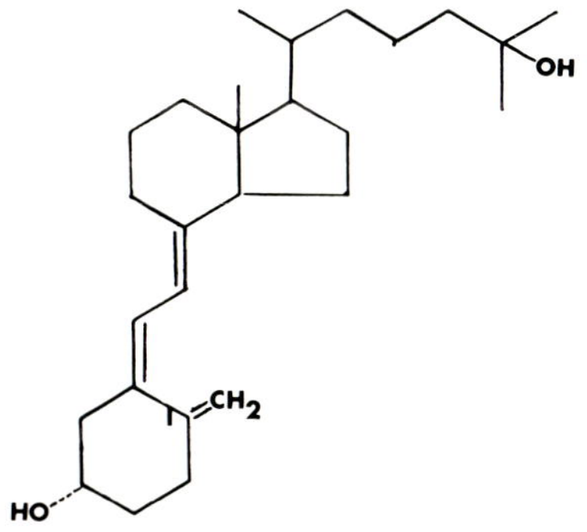

FIG. 2. 25-Hydroxycholecalciferol (25-HCC).

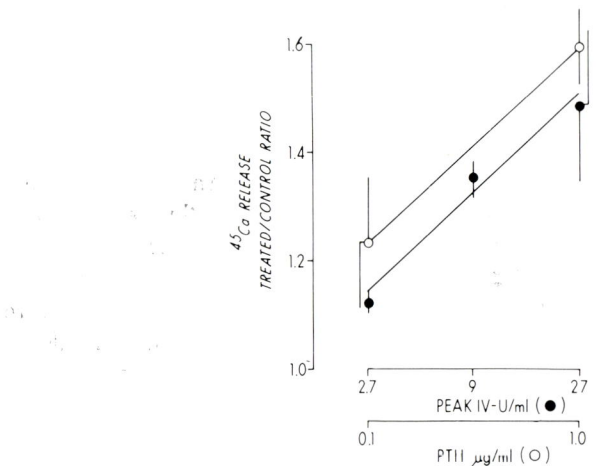

FIG. 3. Bone mineral mobilization response of limb bone organ cultures to 25-HCC (peak IV) *in vitro*, 320 IU vitamin D_3 per milliliter was without effect (Trummel et al., 1969).

DeLuca, 1969). As shown in Fig. 4, intestines taken from vitamin D-deficient animals have a very low rate of calcium transport. However, if the intestines are isolated from the same animals given a dose of vitamin D_3 12 hours before, clearly the classic effect of vitamin D on intestinal calcium transport can be observed. When 10,000 IU of vitamin D are perfused in the vascular system of these preparations, no response in intestinal calcium transport can be observed over the entire length of the experiment. However, if 2.5 µg of 25-HCC is infused, about 1½ hours later, the intestinal calcium transport system begins to rise to levels even beyond that of animals given vitamin D_3. Thus, in two targets of vitamin D action, 25-HCC is very effective in inducing the classic actions of vitamin D, whereas vitamin D_3 itself is not, illustrating convincingly that vitamin D_3 must be hydroxylated in the 25 position before it is effective in its two targets of action. These results establish that 25-HCC is at least a hormonal or circulating active form of the vitamin.

Vitamin D 25-Hydroxylase of Liver

If the vitamin D_3 is unable to exert its action in isolated intestine and bone, it seems reasonable to assume that these organs are unable to make sufficient quantities of the 25-hydroxy derivative. We next turned to the question as to where in the body is the 25-HCC synthesized. Evidence for this came in an indirect fashion. It has been observed by Avioli et al. (1967) and by Ponchon and DeLuca (1969a) that following intravenous injection of radioactive vitamin D, there is an initial fall in plasma radioactivity, as one might expect, as the tissues began to take up the radioactive cholecalciferol from the blood and as it became diluted in extracellular fluid. Ponchon and DeLuca (1969a) showed that at these early times when the plasma radioactivity is disappearing very rapidly, the liver takes up as much as 30–60% of the injected radioactivity. The plasma radioactivity curve at an hour and a half post injection reveals a curious rebound phenomenon in which the plasma radioactivity begins to rise before settling into an expected decay pattern. This rise in plasma radioactivity exactly correlates with the loss of radioactivity from the liver. The nature of the radioactivity which is lost from the liver is 25-HCC as demonstrated by chromatography of the blood plasma extracts. Thus, it was concluded that the liver is a major organ involved in the conversion of vitamin D_3 to the 25-hydroxy derivative. Confirmation of this was obtained by Ponchon et al. (1969) when it could be shown that animals

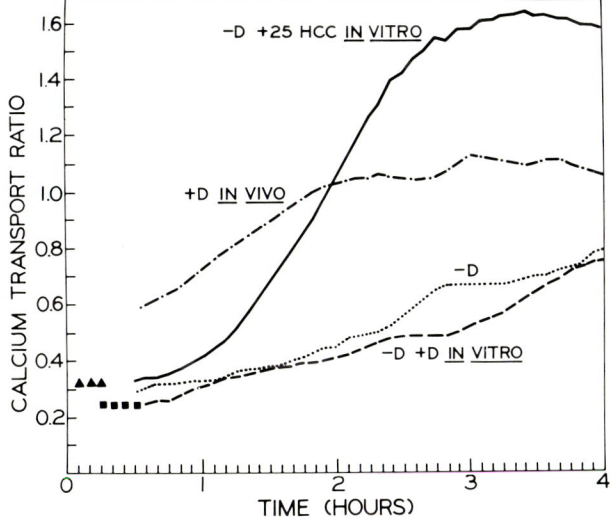

FIG. 4. Intestinal calcium transport response to 25-HCC *in vitro* in vascularly perfused intestine. (· · · · ·) = vitamin D-deficient intestine only; (·—·—·—) = intestine from a vitamin D-deficient rat given vitamin D_3 12 hours before; (– – – – –) = vitamin D-deficient intestine and 10,000 IU vitamin D_3 injected at ■■■; (———) = vitamin D-deficient intestine plus 2.5 μg 25-HCC injected at ▲▲▲ (DeLuca, 1969).

in which the liver is isolated by means of surgical manipulation are unable within 4 hours to convert vitamin D_3 to either 25-HCC or any of the further metabolites, while controls are perfectly able to carry out this conversion. Final proof that the liver is the site of 25-hydroxylation of vitamin D was obtained by Horsting and DeLuca (1969), who could demonstrate that homogenates of liver fortified with reduced pyridine nucleotide, oxygen, and magnesium ions are able to carry out the conversion of vitamin D_3 to the 25-hydroxy derivative. The results in Table I show quite clearly that in the homogenate reaction, reduced pyridine nucleotides are stimulatory, whereas molecular oxygen is essential for the 25-hydroxylation. At first sight it might be assumed that this hydroxylation is one of the standard hydroxylation systems found in liver. However, the inhibitor study indicates that this reaction is somewhat different from lipid peroxidation or steroid hydroxylation of the liver. Table II shows that none of the respiratory enzyme inhibitors is able to inhibit the reaction and in fact actualy stimulate the 25-hydroxylation reaction. This is understandable, since perhaps the respiratory systems compete with the hydroxylation reaction for the available oxygen. More surprising, however, is the fact that diphenylparaphenylenediamine is without effect on this hydroxylation, and further, a 3:1 mixture of carbon monoxide to oxygen had little or no effect on the hydroxylation. These two inhibitor studies suggest that this hydroxylation is unlike the standard steroid hydroxylation reactions and is unlike the lipid peroxidation

TABLE I

REQUIREMENT FOR OXYGEN AND REDUCED PYRIDINE NUCLEOTIDE BY VITAMIN D 25-HYDROXYLASE OF LIVER HOMOGENATE[a]

Medium	25-HCC produced/2 hours (dpm)
Experiment 1	
−TPN	9,200
+TPNH (generating system)	12,700
+DPNH (0.1 mM)	15,500
Experiment 2	
+Air	6,000
+Oxygen	10,800
+Nitrogen	0

[a] The reaction was continued for 2 hr as described by Horsting and DeLuca (1969). Whole rat liver homogenate was used.

TABLE II

Inhibitor Study of Vitamin D 25-Hydroxylase System of Rat Liver Mitochondria[a]

Inhibitor	25-HCC produced (dpm)
None	4700
Antimycin A (0.2 μmoles/gm protein)	6500
Rotenone (30 nmoles/gm protein)	9600
Sodium cyanide (1.3 mM)	7800
Sodium azide (1.3 mM)	5100
Diphenyl-p-phenylenediamine (3.8×10^{-6} M)	5100
$N_2:O_2$ (3:1)	4200
$CO:O_2$ (3:1)	3400

[a] Incubations were carried out as described by Horsting and DeLuca (1969), but liver mitochondria plus liver supernate served as the enzyme system.

systems heretofore studied in liver. It might also be mentioned that feeding of phenobarbital to rats did not change the level of the vitamin D 25-hydroxylase activity in liver, which agrees with the carbon monoxide–oxygen experiment. Almost as surprising is the finding (Table III) that at least two cell fractions are required for the 25-hydroxylation of vitamin

TABLE III

Subcellular Localization of Vitamin D 25-Hydroxylase of Liver[a]

Fraction	25-HCC produced (dpm)
Whole homogenate	9200
Crude nuclei	0
Crude mitochondria	0
Crude microsomes	0
Cytoplasm	0
Pure nuclei (2.3 M sucrose method) + cytoplasm	0
Pure mitochondria (0.44 M sucrose) + cytoplasm	8800
Microsomes + cytoplasm	4400
Crude nuclei + cytoplasm	4500
Mitochondria + kidney cytoplasm	0

[a] The reaction was carried out as described by Horsting and DeLuca (1969) except cell fractions isolated from equivalent weights of tissue were used as the source of the enzyme.

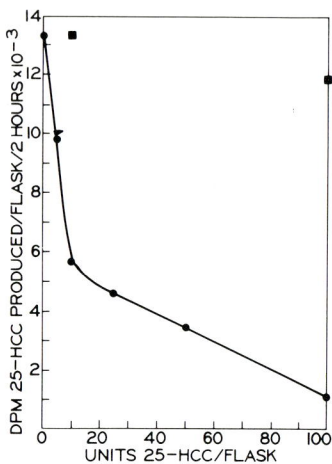

FIG. 5. Inhibition of 25-hydroxylation of vitamin D_3 by 25-HCC (circle) but not 25-hydroxydihydrotachysterol$_3$ (square). The hydroxylation reaction was carried out with liver homogenates as described by Horsting and DeLuca (1969).

D by liver. Clearly, a cytoplasmic fraction is required, and most probably the mitochondrial fraction carries out the hydroxylation. Certainly, pure nuclei plus cytoplasm and pure cytoplasm do not carry out the hydroxylation. However, pure mitochondria and microsomes are without hydroxylation activity by themselves. However, a combination of either mitochondria and cytoplasm, or less effectively, microsomes plus cytoplasm are able to carry out the hydroxylation. Most likely this represents a mitochondrial hydroxylation system in which fragments of mitochondria appearing in the microsomal fraction carry out the hydroxylation. Only additional experiments will be able to make this determination a certainty. The liver cytoplasmic fraction is very specific for liver, since kidney cytoplasm is without effect in the substitution for liver cytoplasm in the support of the 25-hydroxylase reaction.

INHIBITION OF VITAMIN D 25-HYDROXYLASE BY 25-HCC

Perhaps most interesting from a physiological point of view is the marked product inhibition of the 25-hydroxylase reaction. As shown in Fig. 5, it is evident that very small amounts of 25-HCC strongly inhibit the conversion of vitamin D_3 to the 25-hydroxy product. Of special note is the fact that 25-hydroxydihydrotachysterol, a very close analog of 25-hydroxy vitamin D, has no inhibitory effect on the vitamin D hydroxylase system. Thus, it is clear that the product inhibition is very compound specific. It is most likely that the product inhibition exhibited by 25-HCC is competitive with substrate. Hence, it is expected that large amounts of vitamin D would overcome the inhibition by 25-HCC. Should this inhibition occurs *in vivo*, it would provide an important control mechanism for the feed-in of active vitamin D into the plasma. This reaction would serve two purposes: (1) it would conserve vitamin D from times when the organism is exposed to large amounts of ultraviolet light or exposed to large dietary intakes of vitamin D and would tend to conserve the vitamin D for periods when the intake was minimal or essentially zero; (2) it would prevent vitamin D intoxication at relatively low levels of vitamin D. After a certain amount of 25-hydroxy vitamin D is produced, very strong product inhibition would prevent further conversion. However, if large amounts of vitamin D are administered, certainly this inhibition would be overcome and toxicity would be observed, but it would require very much higher levels of vitamin D_3 for this effect. Should this inhibition be important *in vivo*, then perhaps it would also explain the marked effectiveness of large amounts of dihydrotachysterol as compared to vitamin D_3, whereas the dihydrotachysterols are much less effective at low dosages. At the low dosages, most of the vitamin D would be converted to the 25-hydroxy analog unaffected by product inhibition. Similarly, the 25-hydroxydihydrotachysterol would be formed but the 25-hydroxy vitamin D_3 would be much more effective on a weight basis than would the 25-hydroxydihydrotachysterol. However, at the high doses, the production of 25-hydroxy vitamin D would be limited by product inhibition, whereas the production of 25-hydroxydihydrotachysterol would be relatively unaffected by product inhibition. It is clear, therefore, should this prove to be the case, the the dihydrotachysterol would be very much more effective at the high doses than would vitamin D_3. However, 25-hydroxy vitamin D_3 would nevertheless be more effective than 25-hydroxydihydrotachysterol, as shown by Suda *et al.* (1970a).

Prior administration of vitamin D_3 to rats will markedly reduce the ability of the liver preparations to hydroxylate the vitamin D_3 both *in vivo* and *in vitro*. However, if 25-HCC is given intravenously it elicits only slight inhibition. These results suggest that the blood level of 25-HCC cannot exhibit an inhibitory effect on the 25-hydroxylase enzyme. Thus, it is the liver level of 25-HCC that must play an important role in the regulation of 25-HCC production. It is furthermore obvious that the transfer of 25-HCC from the liver cells to the plasma must be an important reaction. In any case, it is evident that *in vivo* product inhibition is an important control mechanism in the production of the 25-hydroxy derivatives.

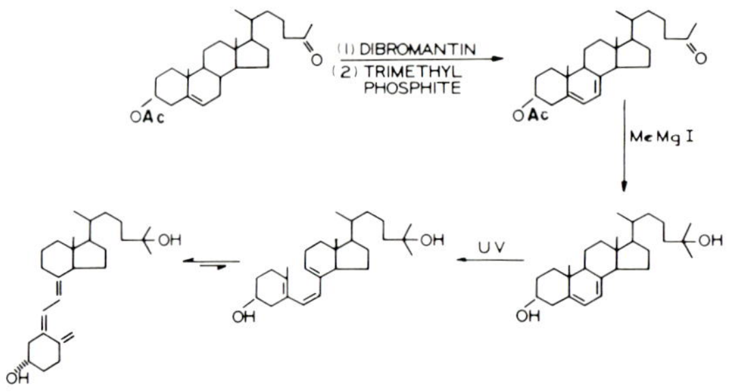

FIG. 6. Synthesis of 25-HCC starting with 3-acetoxynorcholesta-5-ene-25-one.

Metabolism of 25-HCC

METABOLITES OF 25-HCC

To establish with finality the structure of 25-HCC, to provide large amounts of 25-HCC for clinical investigation, and to provide radioactive 25-HCC, this compound was synthesized by three different routes, one of which is shown in Fig. 6, and one which provided the basis for the synthesis of radioactive 25-HCC. Using these radioactive preparations of the 25-HCC, it was possible to examine further the end-organ metabolism of the 25-HCC, especially in regard to the biological function of vitamin D. Prior to this, Stohs and DeLuca (1967) had demonstrated that the radioactivity derived from vitamin D in intestinal nuclei was predominantly in the form of polar metabolites. Haussler et al. (1968), Lawson et al. (1969), and Ponchon and DeLuca (1969b) showed that the radioactivity of intestinal nuclei was predominantly in the form of a metabolite more polar than 25-HCC. Cousins et al. (1970a) using tritium-labeled 25-HCC demonstrated that 25-HCC is converted rapidly to a metabolite, more polar than that described by any of the three previous groups (Fig. 7), which was called peak VI. This metabolite then decreases as the peak V metabolite appears. The peak V metabolite by our notation is identical with the peak p of Lawson et al. (1969) and 4B of Haussler et al. 1968). The rapidity of formation of the very polar metabolites of 25-HCC suggests that they may play a role at the tissue level in carrying out the function of vitamin D. Note that these conversions do not take place in the cytoplasmic fraction of the intestine. Continued examination has shown that bone, kidney, liver, and other tissues are capable of producing peak V metabolites (Cousins et al., 1970b). By means of liquid–liquid partition chromatography and other newer methods of

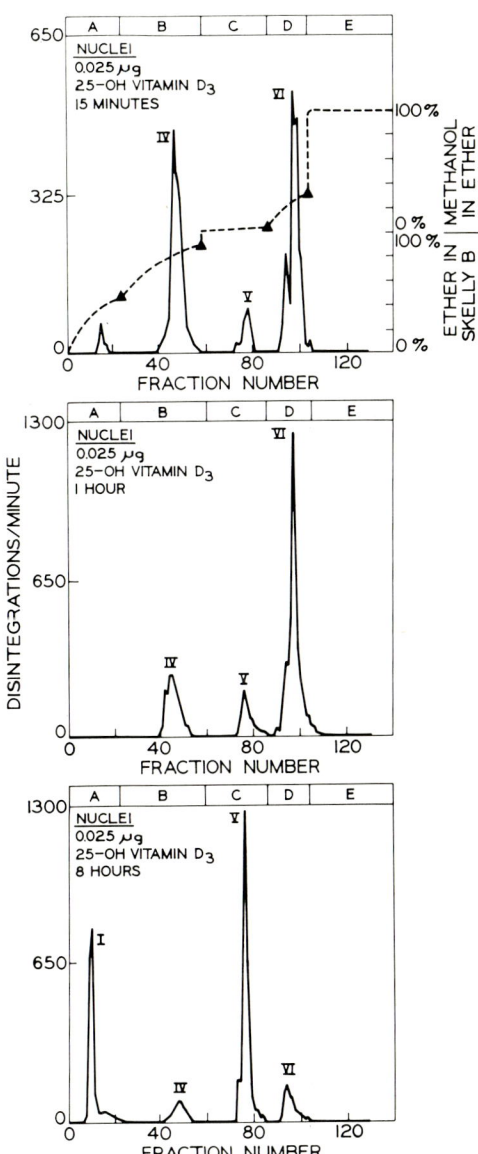

Fig. 7. Silicic acid column profiles of intestinal nuclear extracts from rats given 0.25 μg 25-HCC-26,27-^{3}H (Cousins et al., 1970a).

chromatographic examination in our laboratory, it has been demonstrated that there are several peak V metabolites. Most of these then appear in small amounts in the plasma, making feasible their isolation and identification from this source—a definite technical advantage. We have, therefore, initiated a large-scale program for the isolation and identification of all peak V metabolites of which there are approximately eight.

21, 25-Dihydroxycholecalciferol

By means of high resolution silicic acid column chromatography (Fig. 8), it became readily apparent that the peak V materials in the blood contain at least three components. The first of these, Va, was isolated in pure form by a combination of liquid–liquid partition chromatography and Sephadex LH20 chromatography (Suda et al., 1970b). A total of 200 μg was isolated from the plasma of eight pigs given large doses of vitamin D_3. Under the same conditions, 2.6 mg of 25-HCC would have been present in the plasma, demonstrating that Va is a minor metabolite of vitamin D in the plasma. The LH20 column was used to exclude a 426 molecular weight contaminant. This metabolite has an ultraviolet spectrum exactly that of vitamin D_3, indicating that the cis-triene structure is unchanged from the parent 25-HCC. The fragmentation pattern showed it to contain one additional hydroxyl (molecular weight 416) above 25-HCC. Two of the hydroxyls are found in the side chain, since Va, vitamin D_3, and 25-HCC give the characteristic 271 and 253 fragments. A mass of 59 fragment in the nonsilylated derivative and a mass of 131 in the silylated

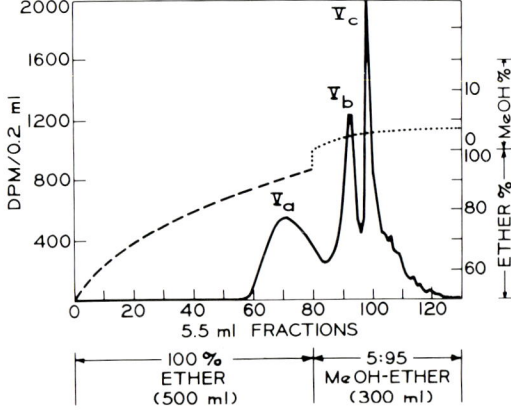

Fig. 8. High resolution silicic acid column profile of peak V (5% methanol–95% ether eluent of silicic acid) from the combined plasma extracts from pigs given 250,000 IU vitamin D_3 per day and chicks given 100 IU vitamin D_3-1,2-^{3}H 24 hours before sacrifice (Suda et al., 1970b).

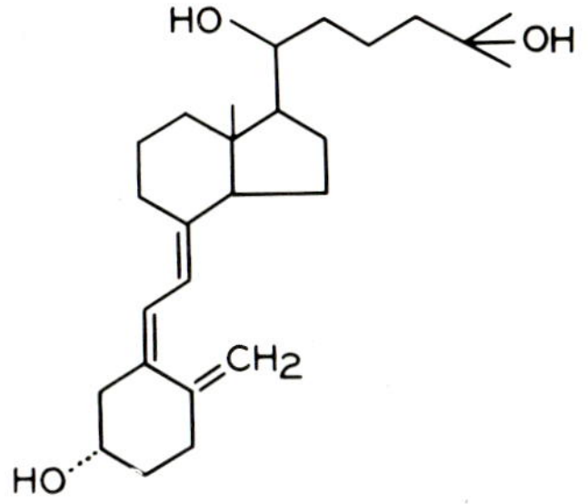

FIG. 9. 21,25-Dihydroxycholecalciferol (Suda et al., 1970b).

derivative showed one hydroxyl to be retained in the 25 position. Because no other side chain cleavages were observed, it was suggested that the added hydroxyl must be on the 21 position. By means of acetylation studies it was possible to demonstrate that the added alcohol is a primary alcohol, confirming this belief, and because periodate cleavage had no effect on the mass spectrum of the Va metabolite and because of the 131 fragment from the silylated derivative indicate that the 26 and 27 hydroxylations are quite impossible, it was concluded that this compound represented 21, 25-dihydroxycholecalciferol (Fig. 9). This metabolite, which is the second most plentiful vitamin D metabolite in the plasma, is formed with physiological doses of vitamin D. This metabolite has preferential activity in inducing bone mineral mobilization, whereas it has very slight activity on the intestinal transport system (Suda et al., 1970b). It is also approximately one-half as effective as vitamin D_3 in the cure of rickets in rats. This compound, then, might well represent the bone mobilization active form of 25-HCC. Obviously further experiments are necessary to confirm this belief.

25, 26-DIHYDROXYCHOLECALCIFEROL

The second metabolite in the peak V zone to be identified is that shown as Vc on the silicic acid chromatogram (Fig. 8). This Vc, when purified on liquid–liquid partition chromatography and LH20 chromatography, also shows an ultraviolet absorption spectrum identical with vitamin D and a mass spectrum showing a molecular weight of 416 or a trihydroxy compound. A mass fragment at 271 and 253 revealed this hydroxylation to be on the side chain as well. Acetylation studies revealed one primary hydroxyl and one tertiary hydroxyl on the side chain. Periodate treatment yielded a mass fragment of 384 which indicated that these hydroxyls were vicinal, and all other fragmentations were consistent with 25,26-dihydroxycholecalciferol (Suda et al., 1971). This metabolite is the third most plentiful metabolite in the plasma and appears to be formed in the liver.

Its biological activity reveals it to have essentially no effect on bone mobilization, very little effect if any on the prevention or cure of rickets in rats, and has a small but significant effect on intestinal transport. Exactly what the function of this metabolite might be is unknown at the present time and might be revealed upon further experimentation. The third major metabolite in the peak V region in the plasma has been highly purified, but has not yet been identified. It is biologically inactive in all systems tested. At the present time we are concentrating our effects on the isolation and identification of the peak V metabolite of intestine and kidney. The present results, then, suggest that the vitamin D_3 may be the storage form, the 25-HCC a circulating or hormonal form, and that the tissues produce specific metabolically active forms.

[Note added in proof: The metabolically active form of intestine has now been isolated in pure form and identified as 1,25-dihydroxycholecalciferol.]

ACTINOMYCIN D INHIBITION OF 25-HCC METABOLISM

A most exciting recent finding in our laboratory is that the prior treatment of both rats and chicks (Fig. 10) with actinomycin D markedly inhibits or prevents the conversion of 25-HCC to the peak V metabolite of intestine (Tanaka and DeLuca, 1971). If the radioactive 25-HCC is given prior to the injection of actinomycin D, the inhibition is no longer observed. These results tell us that the 25-HCC must initiate at least the unmasking or transcription of the gene which codes for a factor that

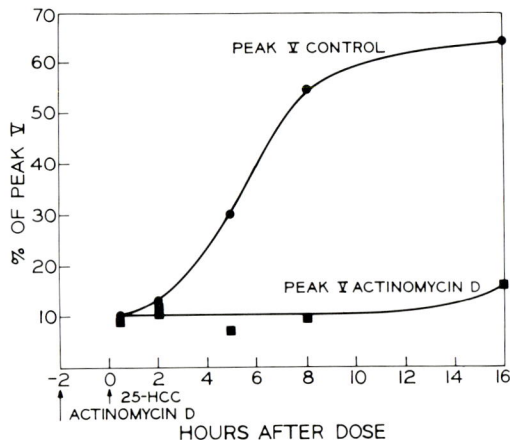

FIG. 10. Actinomycin D inhibition of 25-HCC-26,27-^{3}H metabolism in intestine to peak V.

is involved in the conversion of 25-HCC to the peak V metabolite. It is then the peak V metabolite that carries out the function of vitamin D on intestinal calcium transport.

Mechanism of Action of Vitamin D

Because actinomycin D blocks all vitamin D responses (Zull et al., 1965, 1966; Norman, 1965), because pulse-labeling of nuclear RNA has been shown in response to vitamin D (Stohs et al., 1967), and because unmasking of chromatin in response to vitamin D and 25-hydroxy vitamin D has been shown (Hallick and DeLuca, 1969), it is likely that vitamin D induces its intestinal and bone mobilization effects by causing the synthesis of a specific protein or proteins which participate in a calcium transport system. In the intestine, these proteins are either a calcium-dependent adenosine triphosphatase discovered in our laboratory (Martin et al., 1969; Melancon and DeLuca, 1970) or the calcium binding protein discovered in Wasserman's laboratory (Wasserman, 1970) or both. Without going into any additional detail, Fig. 11 demonstrates our current working hypothesis of how vitamin D might work in the intestine. 25-HCC induces the formation of an enzyme which converts 25-HCC further to the peak V metabolite which then is responsible for the formation of a calcium transport protein. This makes its appearance in the brush border as part of

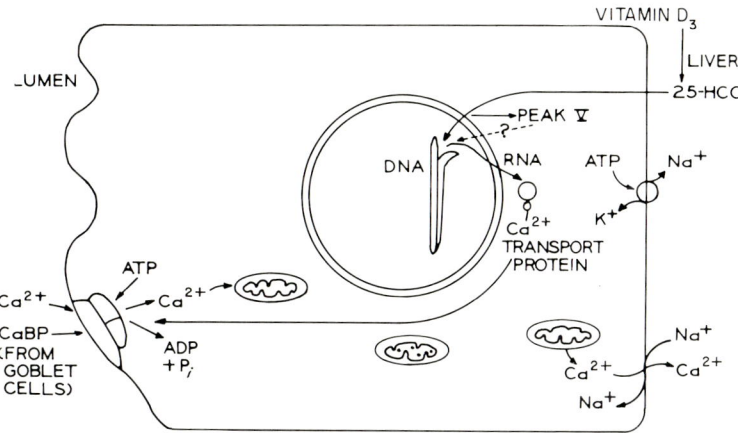

Fig. 11. Diagrammatic representation of our current working hypothesis of the mechanism of vitamin D action on intestinal mucosa.

the calcium-dependent ATPase system. This reaction is facilitated further by the secretion of calcium binding protein from the goblet cells onto the surface of the mucosa. Calcium entering by means of the ATP-dependent transfer process is immediately bound by organelles such as mitochondria which act as a shuttle system. The mitochondria release calcium in the low calcium gradient at the basal side of the cell where a downhill sodium gradient elicits an expulsion of calcium into the serosal fluid. This downhill sodium gradient then provides a final energy push for the calcium transport process. The sodium gradient is maintained by the well known Na^+/K^+ transport system.

It is evident that much has been learned in the last few years concerning vitamin D metabolism and its function which would have most certainly been a delight to Dr. Franklin McLean. I am sure, however, that he would be even more exicited about the future possibilities which have become evident in the examination of the vitamin D mechanism.

References

Avioli, L., McDonald, J., Lund, J., and DeLuca, H. F. (1967). *J. Clin. Invest.* **46**, 983.
Bauer, G. C. H., Carlsson, A., and Linquist, B. (1955). *Kgl. Fysiogra. Saellsk. Lund, Foerh.* **25**, 3.
Blunt, J. W., DeLuca, H. F., and Schnoes, H. K. (1968a). *Biochemistry* **7**, 3317.
Blunt, J. W., DeLuca, H. F., and Schnoes, H. K. (1968b). *Chem. Commun.* **14**, 801.
Blunt, J. W., Tanaka, Y., and DeLuca, H. F. (1968c). *Proc. Nat. Acad. Sci. U.S.* **61**, 1503.
Carlsson, A., and Hollunger, G. (1954). *Acta Physiol. Scand.* **31**, 301.
Cousins, R. J., DeLuca, H. F., Suda, T., Chen, T., and Tanaka, Y. (1970a). *Biochemistry* **9**, 1453.
Cousins, R. J., DeLuca, H. F., and Gray, R. (1970b). *Biochemistry* **9**, 3649.
DeLuca, H. F. (1967). *Vitam. Horm. (New York)* **25**, 315.
DeLuca, H. F. (1969). *Fed. Proc., Fed. Amer. Soc. Exp. Biol.* **28**, 1678.
DeLuca, H. F., Morii, H., and Melancon, M. J. (1968). *In* "Parathyroid Hormone and Thyrocalcitonin (Calcitonin)" (R. V. Talmage and L. F. Bélanger, eds.), pp. 448–454. Excerpta Med. Founda., Amsterdam.
Fraser, D. R., and Kodicek, E. (1965). *Biochem. J.* **96**, 59.
Fraser, D. R., and Kodicek, E. (1966). *Biochem. J.* **100**, 67.
Hallick, R. B., and DeLuca, H. F. (1969). *Proc. Nat. Acad. Sci. U.S.* **63**, 528.
Harrison, H. E., and Harrison, H. C. (1963). *In* "The Transfer of Calcium and Strontium Across Biological Membranes" (R. H. Wasserman, ed.), pp. 229–235. Academic Press, New York.
Harrison, H. E., and Harrison, H. C. (1965). *Amer. J. Physiol.* **208**, 370.
Haussler, M. R., Myrtle, J. F., and Norman, A. W. (1969). *J. Biol. Chem.* **243**, 4055.
Horsting, M., and DeLuca, H. F. (1969). *Biochem. Biophys, Res. Commun.* **36**, 251.
Lawson, D. E. M., Wilson, P. W., and Kodicek, E. (1969). *Biochem. J.* **115**, 269.
Lund, J., and DeLuca, H. F. (1966). J. Lipid. Res. **7**, 739.
Lund, J., DeLuca, H. F., and Horsting, M. (1967). *Arch. Biochem. Biophys.* **120**, 513 (1967).

Martin, D. L., Melancon, M. J., and DeLuca, H. F. (1969). *Biochem. Biophys. Res. Commun.* **35,** 819.
Melancon, M. J., and DeLuca, H. F. (1970). *Biochemistry* **9, 1658.**
Morii, H., Lund, J., Neville, P., and DeLuca, H. F. (1967). *Arch. Biochem. Biophys.* **120,** 508.
Neumann, W. F. (1958). *AMA Arch. Pathol.* **66,** 204.
Neville, P., and DeLuca, H. F. (1966). *Biochemistry* **5,** 2201.
Nicolaysen, R., and Eeg-Larsen, N. (1953). *Vitam. Horm. (New York)* **11,** 29.
Norman, A. W. (1965). *Science* **149,** 185.
Norman, A. W., Lund, J., and DeLuca, H. F. (1964). *Arch. Biochem. Biophys.* **108,** 12.
Olson, E. B., and DeLuca, H. F. (1969). *Science* **165,** 405.
Orr, W. J., Holt, L. E., Jr., Wilkens, L., and Boone, F. H. (1923). *Amer. J. Dis. Child.* **26,** 362.
Ponchon, G., and DeLuca, H. F. (1969a). *J. Clin. Invest.* **48,** 1273.
Ponchon, G., and DeLuca, H. F. (1969b). *J. Nutr.* **99,** 157.
Ponchon, G., Kennan, A. L., and DeLuca, H. F. (1969). *J. Clin. Invest.* **48,** 2032.
Schachter, D. (1963). *In* "The Transfer of Calcium and Strontium Across Biological Membranes" (R. H. Wasserman, ed.), pp. 197–210. Academic Press, New York.
Stohs, S. J., and DeLuca, H. F. (1967). *Biochemistry* **6,** 3338.
Stohs, S. J., Zull, J. E., and DeLuca, H. F. (1967). *Biochemistry* **6,** 1304.
Suda, T., DeLuca, H. F., Schnoes, H. K., and Blunt, J. W. (1969a). *Biochem. Biophys. Res. Commun.* **35,** 182.
Suda, T., DeLuca, H. F., Schnoes, H. K., and Blunt, J. W. (1969b). *Biochemistry* **8,** 3515.
Suda, T., Hallick, R. B., DeLuca, H. F., and Schnoes, H. K. (1970a). *Biochemistry* **9,** 1651.
Suda, T., DeLuca, H. F., Schnoes, H. K., Ponchon, G., Tanaka, Y., and Holick, M. F. (1970b). *Biochemistry* **9,** 2917.
Suda, T., DeLuca, H. F., Schnoes, H., Tanaka, Y., and Holick, M. F. (1970). *Biochemistry* **9,** 4776.
Tanaka, Y., and DeLuca, H. F. (1971). *Proc. Nat. Acad. Sci. U.S.* **68,** 605.
Trummel, C., Raisz, L. G., Blunt, J. W., and DeLuca, H. F. (1969). *Science* **163,** 1450.
Wasserman, R. H. (1970). *In* "The Fat Soluble Vitamins" (H. F. DeLuca and J. W. Suttie, eds.), p. 21. Univ. of Wisconsin Press, Madison.
Zull, J. E., Czarnowska-Misztal, E., and DeLuca, H. F. (1965). *Science* **149,** 182.
Zull, J. E., Czarnowska-Misztal, E., and DeLuca, H. F. (1966). *Proc. Nat. Acad. Sci. U.S.* **55,** 177.

Discussion

Dr. Urist: Before vitamin D was produced by irradiation of ergosterol, vitamin D was obtained from the livers mostly of tuna and cod fish. What is the chemical biology of vitamin D in marine Teleostei? Have you done studies on the liver of fishes that store these enormous quantities of vitamin D, and is threr a hydroxylase system missing in the liver of these species?

Dr. DeLuca: We have done only the following experiment. We have assayed fish liver oils to determine if they contain 25-HCC, and they do not. That activity is due to both vitamin D esters and nonhydroxylated vitamin D compounds. I want to make a slight correction to your statement; another source of vitamin D is ultraviolet radiation of skin.

Dr. Mechanic: On the chromotography separation subsequent to the second silicic acid column, I noticed that you did not show the contaminating peak of the 21,25-dihydroxycholecalciferol which was on the first column. I would venture to say there was no contaminant because, on silicic acid, you probably had an isotope effect. Tritium does give an isotope effect on silicic acid columns.

Dr. DeLuca: We did have a contaminant. We can show it readily by mass spectrometry. My guess is that it came out in the forewash, which wasn't shown in the figure.

Dr. Potts: Hector, do you think, on the basis of present evidence, that the lower activity of the intestinal and bone peak V metabolites relates more to difficulty in penetrating the cells, or do you think there is also some problem in effective transport in blood?

Dr. DeLuca: I think possibly both are true. For example, the peak V from intestine, which we are working on now, seems to be, at least in one experiment, more active when you give it orally than when you give it by intravenous injection. This would suggest that maybe there is a problem in transporting it in the blood. We just do not have adequate information.

Dr. Nichols: Hector, I wasn't quite clear whether you were able to put 25-hydroxy with a homogenate of bone or gut and get out the ultimate metabolite, or whether you were actually getting these out of blood. It is from blood, isn't it?

Dr. DeLuca: These were isolated from the blood of pigs given large amounts of vitamin D, just as we isolated the 25-hydroxy vitamin D originally. The difference is that these are one order of magnitude smaller in concentration in blood. We have done *in vitro* experiments, but they are rather young to talk about. Suffice it to say that we can get some of these conversions to take place *in vitro*, also.

Dr. Raisz: You described a cytoplasmic enzyme that requires mitochondria. Do the mitochondria have to come from the liver or can high energy intermediates or other substrates be substituted?

Dr. DeLuca: It cannot be substituted by mitochondria from any other source. It is a liver enzyme system. We haven't done experiments that exclude all the possibilities, but there is no evidence that the high energy compounds only are involved.

Dr. MacGregor: In the time course study, you showed that the metabolites associated with peak VI appeared before those in peak V. Do you have information on what is represented by peak VI?

Dr. DeLuca: We don't see peak VI generated in any other tissue but the intestine. We don't have any information on the nature of peak VI. The appearance of it seems to vary with the species. For example, the chicken shows very little peak VI metabolite, whereas the rat under these conditions showed very much of it. Our approach is to identify the peak V and, if we know this, we might be able to deduce the nature of peak VI.

Dr. Minkin: Dr. DeLuca, do you know enough about the sequence of metabolite formation to determine whether the peak V activity associated with 21,25-dihydroxycholecalciferol can be obtained from vitamin D_3 without going through 25-hydroxycholecalciferol?

Dr. DeLuca: We don't know that, of course. In the case of 21,25-dihydroxycholecalciferol, the isolation was from pigs given vitamin D_3. The 21,25 compound is formed from 25-hydroxy vitamin D_3, but we do not have an *in vitro* system that gives us the 21,25 compound.

INDUCTION OF BONE RESORPTION IN TISSUE CULTURE: INTERACTION OF HUMORAL AGENTS AND IONS*

Lawrence G. Raisz and Clarence L. Trummel

Parathyroid hormone (PTH) and 25-hydroxycholecalciferol (25-HCC), the active metabolite of vitamin D, can stimulate the resorption of mineral and matrix from fetal rat long bones in organ culture. Even with maximally effective doses, resorption begins slowly. The rate gradually increases reaching a maximum in about 2 days, so that in 3–4 days, the bone is usually completely resorbed (Raisz and Trummel, 1971; Raisz et al., 1969; Trummel et al., 1969). The response to PTH and 25-HCC also develops slowly *in vivo* (Bingham et al., 1969; Blunt et al., 1968; Zull et al., 1966). This slow response could occur either because the target cells gradually accumulate these agents which remain in or on the cell and progressively stimulate them to resorbing activity or because the target cells can produce so-called second messengers, which can continue to act independent of the continued presence of the stimulator. The latter possibility appears particularly likely for PTH, since its half life in the circulation is so short compared to the duration of its effect. Using an organ culture system, we found that relatively brief application of either PTH or 25-HCC could lead to the same progressive, and ultimately complete, stimulation of

---

* Supported in part by the USPHS Grants AM-06205 and 2TI-DE-00003-14.

resorption that was obtained with continuous application of these stimulators of bone resorption (Raisz and Trummel, 1971; Raisz et al., 1970). We have termed this response "induction" to indicate that these agents are stimulating the development of new cells and cell machinery for resorption. Since cells differentiated for bone resorption exist in control cultures, the term induction is not being used to indicate *de novo* morphogenesis, but only increased cell transformation.

Induction Model

The culture methods employed for these studies have been described previously (Raisz and Niemann, 1969). A chemically defined medium which supports bone resorption in organ culture is used, and bone resorption is measured as the release of previously incorporated ^{45}Ca into the medium from treated and control paired bones from opposite limbs of the same fetus. In early experiments, the bones were immediately exposed to PTH or 25-HCC upon explantation. After various periods, bones were washed and transferred to fresh control medium and cumulative ^{45}Ca release from treated and control bones was compared (Table I). In later experiments, the bones were precultured for 18–24 hours. This removed some of the exchangeable surface ^{45}Ca and permitted more precise exposures to various conditions during and after induction. With this model, the application of large doses of PTH or 25-HCC to the cultures for 2

TABLE I

48-Hour Response to Brief Versus Continuous Exposure to PTH (1 μg/ml)[a]

Exposure to PTH (hours)	No. of experiments	Cumulative 48-hour ^{45}Ca release (treated/control ratio)[b]
3	4	1.42 ± .12
6	6	1.61 ± .12
48	6	1.74 ± .17

[a] Bone shafts of radius or ulna of 19-day fetal rats were obtained from mothers which had been injected with ^{45}Ca on the previous day. Paired bones were cultured with and without purified bovine PTH (1–2000 U/mg) in a chemically defined medium (BGJ with bovine serum albumin fraction V, 1 mg/ml). Bones were washed and transferred at 3 or 6 hours either to control medium (brief exposure) or in a medium containing the same concentration of PTH (continuous exposure).

[b] Values are mean ±SE of indicated number of experiments with four paired cultures in each experiment.

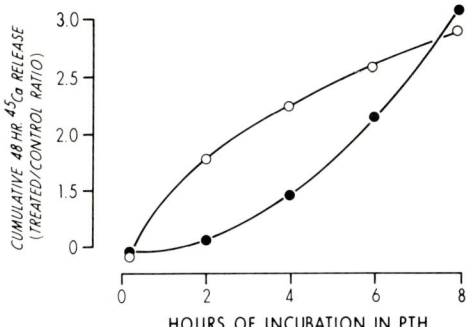

FIG. 1. Responses to varying periods of incubation with bovine PTH (3.2 μg/ml) followed by a wash and 2 hour incubation with normal guinea pig serum or anti-bovine PTH guinea pig serum (1:10 dilution), and then cultured in control medium for a total of 48 hours. Procedure otherwise similar to that of Table II. Values are means of treated/control ratios for cumulative 48 hour ^{45}Ca release for four paired cultures. Incubation with anti-PTH serum significantly decreased ($p < .05$) response after 2 or 4 hours of PTH, but not after 6 or 8 hours. Open circle indicates normal serum; solid circle indicates anti-PTH serum.

hours regularly lead to marked bone resorption. This did not mean that these agents were active only during the induction period. 25-HCC can enter the nucleus, and its metabolic transformation there has been described (DeLuca, 1971). Evidence that some of the effect of PTH was due to hormone bound reversibly to the bone after the initial induction was obtained using an antibody to PTH (Fig. 1). Bones exposed for 2 or 4 hours to PTH and then washed with anti-bovine PTH serum showed a diminished subsequent resorptive response when compared with bones treated with PTH for similar periods but washed for 2 hours with normal guinea pig serum. However, by 6–8 hours after application of PTH, the antibody no longer had any effect, suggesting that the hormone had become irreversibly bound, or, more likely, that the subsequent resorptive response no longer depended on its presence.

Role of RNA Synthesis

There is considerable evidence that the prolonged resorptive response of bone to brief applications of PTH or 25-HCC depends on new RNA synthesis. RNA synthesis is probably increased by treatment with PTH, but the changes are relatively small and show great variability under different experimental conditions. This may be because the major effect is in osteoclasts and their precursors, while osteoblasts are actually in-

TABLE II

Effect of Actinomycin D on the Induction of Bone Resorption by Parathyroid Hormone or 25-Hydroxycholecalciferol[a]

Length of Actinomycin D (0.04 μg/ml) treatment (hours)	48 hours ^{45}Ca release treated/control ratio[b]	
	PTH (3 μg/ml)	25-HCC (2–3 μg/ml)
No actinomycin D	3.00 ± .32[c]	2.31 ± .31[c]
−2 to 2	1.15 ± .06	0.99 ± .07
0–4	1.08 ± .06	1.27 ± .11
4–8	1.84 ± .24[c]	1.58 ± .19[c]

[a] Procedure was similar to that of Table I, except that bones were precultured for 18–24 hours; one of each pair of bones was then treated for 2 hours with PTH or 25-HCC and the other served as a control. Actinomycin D was added to both treated and control cultures at the indicated times. Bones were washed and transferred to control medium after treatment. From Raisz (1971).

[b] Values are mean ±SE for 4–16 paired cultures.

[c] Values significantly greater than 1.0, $p < .05$.

hibited (Bingham et al., 1969). Interpretation is also complicated by the finding that the uptake of labeled nucleosides as well as incorporation into RNA is affected, so that increased labeling does not necessarily mean increased net synthesis. Studies with inhibitors of DNA-dependent RNA synthesis and protein synthesis have shown that the hypercalcemic responses in vivo and the resorptive responses in vitro to both PTH and 25-HCC can be abolished by such agents (Raisz and Trummel, 1971; Tashjian, 1965; Zull et al., 1966). The use of Dactinomycin, an inhibitor of DNA-dependent RNA synthesis, in the induction model has given some indication of the time when the initial change in RNA synthesis must take place. Dactinomycin can inhibit induction when given before or simultaneously with the high concentrations of PTH and 25-HCC, but has less effect when applied 2 hours after the initial exposure to PTH or 25-HCC (Table II). If Dactinomycin acts on RNA synthesis in this model, then effects of PTH and 25-HCC on RNA synthesis must occur within the first 4 hours, which is sufficient to induce a subsequent resorptive response.

Role of Cyclic Adenosine 3′,5′-Monophosphate (cAMP)

Although PTH and 25-HCC are remarkably similar in their effects on bone resorption, they differ in two important respects: 25-HCC can enter the cell, and is probably transformed in the nucleus to a different metabolite, which may directly affect nuclear transcription (DeLuca, 1971); PTH probably does not enter the cell, although no direct data on this point are available, and it does produce a secondary response in bone cells consisting of activation of adenyl cyclase with production of increased concentrations of cAMP (Chase and Aurbach, 1970). This effect on cAMP concentration has not been observed in bones treated with 25-HCC. Aurbach and Chase (1970) have postulated that this effect on cAMP, which is rapid, represents the second messenger by which PTH causes subsequent cell transformation for resorption. This concept was supported by the observations that the dibutyryl derivative of cAMP can stimulate bone resorption both *in vivo* and *in vitro* (Raisz et al., 1969; Rasmussen et al., 1968; Vaes, 1968). Further exploration of this response in tissue culture, however, indicated some important differences between the effect of dibutyryl cAMP and the effects of PTH or 25-HCC (Raisz and Klein, 1969). The maximally effective concentration of dibutyryl cAMP does not produce as great an increase in the rate of bone resorption as that observed with maximal doses of PTH or 25-HCC; moreover, when the dose is increased, the stimulatory effect on bone resorption is actually lost. One possible explanation for this "autoinhibition" is that dibutyryl cAMP activates a second adenyl cyclase system in bone which is inhibitory. Thyrocalcitonin, an inhibitor of bone resorption, can produce a

TABLE III

Failure of Dibutyryl Cyclic Adenosine 3′, 5′-Monophosphate to Induce Resorption or Synergize with 25-Hydroxycholecalciferol or Parathyroid Hormone[a]

Treatment	Cumulative 48 hour ^{45}Ca release treated/control ratio[b]
25-HCC (0.3 µg/ml)	1.04 ± .07
25-HCC (1.0 µg/ml)	1.69 ± .31[c]
PTH (1 µg/ml)	1.08 ± .08
25-HCC (0.3 µg/ml) and PTH (1.0 µg/ml)	1.22 ± .06[c]
Dibutyryl cAMP (10^{-4} M)	1.02 ± .08
PTH (1.0 µg/ml) and dibutyryl cAMP (10^{-4} M)	1.12 ± .08
25-HCC (0.3 µg/ml) and dibutyryl cAMP (10^{-4} M)	0.94 ± .03
25-HCC (1.0 µg/ml) and dibutyryl cAMP (10^{-4} M)	0.96 ± .03

[a] Procedure as in Table II. Bones were precultured, and then one of each pair was treated as indicated for 2 hours, washed, and transferred to control medium.

[b] Values are mean ±SE of 4–8 paired cultures.

[c] Underlined values significantly greater than 1.0, $p < .05$.

modest but consistent increase in cAMP content of bone *in vitro* (Chase and Aurbach, 1970; Murad *et al.*, 1970).

We have attempted to examine the role of cAMP further in the induction model. Dibutyryl cAMP was found to be ineffective as an inducer over a range of 2–6 hour periods of application and at concentrations of 10^{-4}–10^{-3} M. Moreover, dibutyryl cAMP did not enhance the inductive response to ineffective doses of PTH or 25-HCC and actually inhibited the induction in response to larger doses of 25-HCC (Table III). In other experiments, theophylline and cAMP itself, alone or in combination with PTH, also failed to produce induction. These negative results could simply indicate that adding these agents to the medium did not alter cAMP concentration at the PTH-specific sites. However, there is direct evidence that these agents can enter cells, and in prolonged culture we have observed enhancement of PTH response with theophylline and direct stimulation of resorption with dibutyryl cAMP (Raisz and Klein, 1969). Hence, our repeated failure to affect induction response after brief exposure to agents affecting cAMP concentration could mean that the rapid transcriptional effect is mediated through some different second messenger.

Synergism between PTH and 25-HCC

Minimally effective or ineffective doses of 25-HCC and PTH can produce apparent synergism when given together either continuously or in induction (Table III). Synergism in induction can be produced when the agents are given sequentially. In the experiment shown in Table IV

TABLE IV

Synergistic Response to Sequential 2 hour Exposure to 25-Hydroxycholecalciferol and Parathyroid Hormone[a]

Treatment	Cumulative 48 hour ^{45}Ca release treated/control ratio[b]
PTH alone	$1.04 \pm .11$
25-HCC alone	$1.13 \pm .02$[c]
PTH and 25-HCC together	$1.11 \pm .06$[c]
PTH followed by 25-HCC	$1.14 \pm .06$[c]
25-HCC followed by PTH	$1.41 \pm .11$[c,d]

[a] Procedure as in Table II; 0.15 µg/ml 25-HCC, 0.3 µg/ml PTH.
[b] Values are mean ±SE for 4 paired cultures.
[c] Underlined values significantly greater than 1.0, $p < .05$.
[d] Significantly different from other groups, $p < .05$.

TABLE V

EFFECT OF 2 HOURS' EXPOSURE TO PARATHYROID HORMONE WITH OR
WITHOUT THYROCALCITONIN ON SUBSEQUENT RELEASE OF CALCIUM
FROM FETAL BONES IN CULTURE[a]

Treatment	Release of previously incorporated ^{45}Ca—cumulative treated/control ratio		
	12 hours	24 hours	48 hours[b]
PTH 0–2 hours	1.79 ± .20	2.48 ± .29	2.90 ± .40
TCT and PTH 0–2 hours	1.05 ± .03	1.75 ± .23	2.40 ± .33
TCT 0–2 hours PTH 2–4 hours	0.89 ± .06	1.54 ± .19	2.28 ± .43
PTH 0–2 hours TCT 2–4 hours	0.95 ± .04	1.52 ± .13	2.36 ± .36

[a] Procedure as in Table II. Partially purified rat thyroid calcitonin (5–10 MRC units/mg) was used; 1 µg/ml PTH, 1 µg/ml TCT.

[b] Values are mean ± SE for 4 paired cultures.

25-HCC followed by PTH was the most effective inducer. Further, studies are required to determine whether this is generally the case.

Effect of Thyrocalcitonin

If a second cAMP system in bone is responsible for the inhibitory effect of dibutyryl cAMP on induction and is also the mediator of calcitonin inhibition of bone resorption, then we might expect that rat thyroid calcitonin (TCT) can also inhibit induction. However, when TCT was applied briefly either before, during, or after a 2-hour induction with PTH (Table V), PTH-stimulated ^{45}Ca release was delayed for at least 12 hours, but the ultimate effect of PTH on bone resorption was not decreased. Even when TCT was given continuously after PTH induction, the inhibition of ^{45}Ca release was not maintained indefinitely, and the bones began to show accelerated resorption after 2 days despite addition of fresh TCT every 12 hours.

Effect of Calcium on Induction

It has been suggested that calcium translocations mediate the response to PTH in the kidney and 25-HCC in the intestine (Rasmussen et al.,

TABLE VI

Effect of Changing Medium Calcium Concentration on Response to 6 Hour or Continuous Exposure to Parathyroid Hormone[a]

Medium calcium concentration (mM)	Cumulative 48 hour ^{45}Ca release—treated/control ratio[b]	
	PTH—6 hours	PTH—48 hours
0.4	1.86 ± .21[c]	2.61 ± .13
1.5	2.71 ± .30	2.82 ± .31

[a] Procedure as in Table II. Bones treated for 6 hours at indicated calcium concentrations were then washed and transferred to control medium at normal calcium concentration. PTH, 3 μg/ml.

[b] Values are mean ±SE for 4 paired cultures. Values are significantly greater than 1.0, p <.05.

[c] Significantly less than response in normal (1.5 mM) calcium, p <.05.

1970; Zull et al., 1966). This possibility is difficult to test in bone, since it is so difficult to measure cell calcium when there is a large amount of calcified matrix immediately adjacent. The effects of varying medium calcium concentration during induction on the subsequent response have provided indirect support for a role of calcium ions in the induction process (Raisz, 1970). These effects are quite different from those of calcium on resorption itself (Raisz and Niemann, 1969). Resorption is little altered by a low medium calcium concentration when PTH is applied continu-

TABLE VII

Effect of Changing Medium Calcium Concentration During Induction on Response to 2 Hour Exposure to Low and Intermediate Doses of Parathyroid Hormone[a]

Medium calcium concentration (mM)	Cumulative 48 hour ^{45}Ca release—treated/control ratio[b]	
	PTH—0.1 μg/ml	PTH—0.3 μg/ml
0.4	1.16 ± .20[c]	1.68 ± .30[c,d]
1.5	1.60 ± .20[d]	2.18 ± .24[d]
3.0	1.51 ± .11[d]	2.34 ± .59[d]

[a] Procedure as in Table VI.

[b] Values are mean ±SE of 4 paired cultures.

[c] Significantly less than response to induction in normal (1.5 mM) calcium, p <.05.

[d] Values significantly greater than 1.0, p <.05.

TABLE VIII

Effect of Changing Medium Phosphate or Magnesium Concentration on Response to 2 Hour Exposure to Parathyroid Hormone[a]

Medium concentration		Cumulative 48 hour ^{45}Ca release—treated/control ratio[b]
Magnesium (mM)	Phosphate (mM)	
0.8	0.5	1.19 ± .13
0.8	1.0	1.55 ± .16[c]
0.8	2.0	1.82 ± .22[c]
0.4	1.0	1.70 ± .30[c]
1.6	1.0	1.82 ± .23[c]

[a] Procedures as in Table VI. All bones cultured at 0.8 mM magnesium and 1.0 mM phosphate before and after induction. PTH, 1.8 μg/ml.
[b] Values are mean ±SE for 4 paired cultures.
[c] Values significantly greater than 1.0, $p < .05$.

ously; however, if the calcium concentration is reduced only during the induction period and the bones are then returned to a medium of normal calcium concentration, the amount of bone resorption is generally reduced (Table VI). It was apparent that a low calcium concentration could impair induction by both PTH and 25-HCC (Raisz and Trummel, 1971). However, we have not been able to enhance induction with a submaximal dose of PTH by raising the medium calcium concentration above normal (Table VII).

The effect of other ions has not been examined extensively. In one experiment, changing magnesium concentration was ineffective, while changes in phosphate concentration had a paradoxical effect (Table VIII). Previous studies showed that the rate of bone resorption is inversely proportional to the phosphate concentration (Raisz and Niemann, 1969). This can be demonstrated after the initial stimulation of bone resorption by PTH or 25-HCC is well underway (Raisz et al., 1969). In contrast, the inductive response appears to be directly proportional to the phosphate concentration used during the period of application of PTH.

Conclusion

These results support the concept that PTH and 25-HCC stimulate bone resorption by initiating a cell transformation which does not require the continuous presence of either agent in the bathing medium. Induction may depend on the binding of these agents to the cell membrane or nucleus and the subsequent production of a second messenger which alters nuclear transcription. Attempts to identify cAMP as the mediator of this induction were unsuccessful. Induction was unaffected by the hormonal inhibitor of bone resorption, TCT. This provides further evidence for separate sites of action of PTH and TCT. A requirement for calcium ions in induction was demonstrated, but exposures to high calcium concentration did not enhance induction. This can be explained if calcium ions act in bone cells to couple excitation to response as they do in many other systems. Perhaps the amount of calcium bound to some specific cell constituent determines the mobility or reactivity and thence its function as the second messenger in the system. Evidence was also obtained for enhancement of induction by phosphate. This could be due simply to the ability of increased phosphate concentration to enhance the entry of calcium into cells (Stern and Austin, 1971), although other explanations must be considered.

While these observations do not yet permit us to choose between the wide array of cellular models currently proposed, they do show that induction in tissue culture may be a good system in which to test future hypotheses concerning the mechanism by which various agents stimulate or inhibit bone resorption, and indicate some of the characteristics which second messenger(s) as yet undiscovered should have if they are to mediate a transcriptional response to these agents.

REFERENCES

Aurbach, G. D., and Chase, L. R. (1970). *Fed. Proc., Fed. Amer. Soc. Exp. Biol.* 1179.
Bingham, P. J., Brazell, I. A., and Owen, M. (1969). *J. Endocrinol.* **45**, 387.
Blunt, J. S., Tanaka, Y., and DeLuca, H. (1968). *Proc. Nat. Acad. Sci. U.S.* **61**, 1503.
Chase, L. R., and Aurbach, G. D. (1970). *J. Biol. Chem.* **425**, 1524.
DeLuca, H. F. (1971). In "Cellular Mechanisms for Calcium Transfer and Homeostasis" (G. Nichols and R. Wasserman, eds.). pp. 421–440. Academic Press, New York.
Murad, F., Brewer, H. B., Jr., and Vaughan, M. (1970). *Proc. Nat. Acad. Sci. U.S.* **65**, 446.
Raisz, L. G. (1970). *Fed. Proc., Fed. Amer. Soc. Exp. Biol.* **29**, 1176.
Raisz, L.G. (1970). *Arch. Intern. Med.* **126**, 887.
Raisz, L. G., and Klein, D.C. (1969). *Fed. Proc., Fed. Amer. Soc. Exp. Biol.* **28**, 320.
Raisz, L. G., and Niemann, I. (1969). *Endocrinology* **85**, 446
Raisz, L. G., and Trummel, (1971). *In* "The Fat Soluble Vitamins" (H. F. Deluca and J. W. Suttie, eds.). Univ. of Wisconsin Press, Madison pp. 93–99.
Raisz, L. G., Brand, J. S., Klein, D. C., and Au, W.Y.W. (1969). *In* "Progress in Endocrinology" (E. Gual and F. J. G. Ebling, eds.), pp. 696–703. Excerpta Med. Found., Amsterdam.
Raisz, L. G., Klein, D. C., Trummel, C. L., and Brand, J. S. (1970). *In* "Hormone Regulation" (M. Hamburgh, ed.), pp. 525–536, Appleton, New York.
Rasmussen, H., Pechet, M., and Fast, D. (1968). *J. Clin. Invest.* **47**, 1843.

Rasmussen, H., Feinblatt, J., Nagata, N., and Pechet, M. (1970). *Fed. Proc., Fed. Amer. Soc. Exp. Biol.* **29**, 1190.
Stern, P. H., and Austin, J. (1970). *Fed. Proc., Fed. Amer. Soc. Exp. Biol.* **29**, 566.
Tashjian, A. H., Jr. (1965). *Endocrinology* **77**, 375.
Trummel, C. L., Raisz, L. G., Blunt, J. S., and DeLuca, H. (1969). *Science* **163**, 1450.
Vaes, G. (1968). *Nature (London)* **219**, 939.
Zull, J. E., Dzarnowska-Misztal, E., and DeLuca, H. F. (1966). *Proc. Nat. Acad. Sci. U.S.* **55**, 177.

Discussion

Dr. Urist: In his opening remarks, Dr. Raisz warned that people get "up tight" about use of the word "induction." Let us consider the population of cells in a bone tissue culture and note that the osteoprogenitor cells, osteoblasts, osteoclasts, and osteocytes in the system are already differentiated. These cells have all the enzyme systems of bone cells actively in operation, either for bone formation or for bone resorption. Changes in cell specialization, such as in bone formation and resorption, are reversible and, therefore, described by the term "modulation." The term "induction," as used by the biochemists to mean "initiate" or "activate," is not applicable here. The calcium ion in a purified enzyme system *in vitro* is referred to as an activator. While some people dismiss this kind of terminology as a matter of semantics, the question is whether it is justifiable. Scientists in fields lying between biochemistry and cell biology eventually must employ a common terminology. As a skillful scientist should, Dr. Raisz began by defining his terms, but then substituted the terms "activator," and "initiator," and ended with references to calcium ion as an inducer.

Dr. Raisz: You are right. "Induction" is a messy word. One reason I used induction is because we previously used the term "stimulation." There is a difference because here we are looking at the steps involving initiation of a cell transformation. While the bone cells are, in fact, differentiated, and these are osteoclasts in control bone, the "inducers" are transforming some cells, and are making new osteoclasts. This is what endocrinologists call "induction." I would be glad if this were settled by a conference on nomenclature somewhere else.

Dr. Belanger: Dr. Raisz, what is the evidence that resorption in your system is mediated by osteoclasts, and if so, where do the osteoclasts come from?

Dr. Raisz: Our evidence is histological. We see osteoclasts on the surfaces of the bone, where they seem to be resorbing bone. Of course, the evidence of Goldhaber [P. Goldhaber, *in* "The Parathyroid Glands" (P. J. Gaillard, R. V. Talmage, and A. Budy, eds.), pp. 152–169. Univ. of Chicago Press, Chicago, 1965] and Gaillard [P. J. Gaillard, *in* "The Parathyroids" (R. O. Greep and R. V. Talmage, eds.), pp. 20–45. Thomas, Springfield, Illinois, 1961] is cinematic. It looks convincing in their movies. Our system does not show osteocytic resorption. There may have been osteocytic resorption, but by the time we look at it, we can't see enlarged osteocytic lacuna, because there isn't any more trabeculum.

Dr. Belanger: I would like to make reference to the long-term experiments of Gaillard [P. J. Gaillard, *Proc. Kon. Ned. Akad. Wetensch.*, Ser C **63**, 25–37 (1960)] and Goldhaber [P. Goldhaber, *in* "Calcification in Biological Systems," Publ. No. 64, pp. 349–372. Amer. Ass. Advance. Sci., Washington, D.C., 1960]. The formation of new osteoclasts requires a fairly long time. I was wondering about your short-term experiments where osteocytes are already available.

Dr. Raisz: I assume that the osteoclasts that are already there are being stimulated. Bingham, Brazell, and Owen [P. J. Bingham, I. A. Brazell, and M. Owen, *J. Endocrinol.* **45,** 387 (1969)] showed an increased uridine uptake in existing osteoclasts in their system. We can see an increase in the number of osteoclasts as early as 12 hours. We don't see a clear cut increase in hydroxyproline release from the bone until about 12 hours.

One other point; under maximum stimulation, less than 10% of the bone mineral and matrix are resorbed at 24 hours. The next day, 25–30% gets resorbed. This continues until the bone disappears.

Dr. MacGregor: I wanted to ask about the actinomycin D experiment. Did you say that the level you used inhibited RNA synthesis by only 15% and the response to 25-HCC completely?

Dr. Raisz: Yes. RNA synthesis was measured by labeled uridine incorporation.

Dr. MacGregor: I think perhaps one would be led to the conclusion that actinomycin D is acting by a pathway not involving RNA synthesis, that is, by a side effect of the drug.

Dr. Raisz: There are data to show that low concentrations of actinomycin D can have a selective effect [W. K. Roberts and J. F. G. Neuman, *J. Mol. Biol.* **20,** 63 (1966)]. The usual finding is that ribosomal RNA is more inhibited at low concentrations. The problem here is that using sucrose gradients, we saw a change in messenger RNA. But if the new messenger RNA was polycystronic, as it should be to induce the many enzymes identified in the bone resorption process, I would assume that a very large area of the DNA must be opened up to initiate RNA synthesis to induce bone resorption. Therefore, a low dose of actinomycin D might inhibit. However, I must agree that no one can say that actinomycin D is not acting on something else in any given system.

Dr. MacGregor: The reason I bring out the point is that actinomycin D and RNA synthesis are so closely connected in a lot of people's minds, and naturally so; but it has been shown to have anomalous effects in many systems [E. O. Bransome, Jr., *Endocrinology* **85,** 1114 (1969); M. F. Singer and P. Leder, *Annu. Rev. Biochem.* **35,** 195 (1966); J. R. Tate, *Progr. Nucl. Acid Res. Mol. Biol.* **5,** 191 (1966); U. Clever and I. Sterbeck, *Biochim. Biophys. Acta* **217,** 108 (1970)].

Dr. Tashjian: You seemed to have shown that the incubation of PTH with its antiserum inhibits the effect of the hormone. Because of the rapidity of the stimulation of adenyl cyclase activity by PTH both *in vivo* and *in vitro*, does this shed any light on the fact that cAMP may or may not be involved in resorption, rather than on induction alone?

Dr. Raisz: That was one of the additional doubting pieces of evidence which makes me question the cAMP hypothesis. If our bones are producing cAMP as soon as Aurbach and Chase's bones are, and that causes induction, then we shouldn't be able to stop anything with a 2 hour removal. However, accumulation may have to take place.

Another problem is that, when we take away the PTH with the antibody, we may have a cell that can leak out something else necessary for induction. You can often turn around these arguments, but I am impressed with the number of experiments we have that do not support the cAMP hypothesis.

Dr. Rich: How sure are you that the 25-HCC and PTH had been removed by changing the medium in which the tissues were incubated?

Dr. Raisz: That is why we did the antibody experiment.

Dr. Rich: That would not exclude the possibility of 25-HCC having entered and become equilibrated within some component of the cells.

Dr. Raisz: We have some studies which haven't been fully analyzed yet. There is radioactivity in washed bones after the brief application of 25-HCC. I think it is reasonable to assume that the hormone is getting into the nucleus, and when we wash, we only remove it from the medium.

In the case of PTH, the alternative hypotheses remain that the PTH is brought into the cell irreversibly bound to the cell, or that the second messenger is formed. With 25-HCC, there is no evidence for a second messenger such as cAMP at the moment. No cAMP is formed in bone in response to 25-HCC, according to Chase and Aurbach (cited in text).

Dr. Borle: I was interested to see your lack of success with dibutyryl cAMP, because as you know, in our isolated kidney cell system PTH stimulates the formation of cAMP, but neither cAMP nor dibutyryl cAMP stimulates calcium transport. It does not increase the cellular pool of exchangeable calcium either. Can you explain to me how you reconcile these facts with the direct stimulation obtained by Klein with dibutyryl cAMP?

Dr. Raisz: We have a long list of stimulators of bone resorption which don't induce, by my definition here. Bacterial endotoxins [E. Hausmann, L. G. Raisz, and W. A. Miller, *Science* **168,** 862–865 (1970)] have prolonged stimulatory effects on bone resorption, but so far, none of them has shown a long-term response after brief exposure. One possible reason is that all of the agents act by a different mechanism from 25-HCC or PTH. A most attractive mechanism, on the basis of Dingle and Fell's [H. B. Fell and J. T. Dingle, *Biochem. J.* **87,** 403 (1963)] extensive work with vitamin A, is that lysosomal enzyme activation and release are involved. These processes might take a good deal of time to develop.

Dr. Goldhaber: I was interested in the data you didn't show, which had to do with the release of the proline-labeled collagen. This is a key experiment; we have all been looking forward to the double labeling of calcium and proline in a bone resorbing system. When you labeled with proline and calcium, was this a one-shot procedure, or did you label continuously so that the entire bone was uniformly labeled?

Dr. Raisz: In the work that John Brand and I have done, the tritiated proline is given in multiple injections to the pregnant rat on the day before sacrifice. Autoradiography of the bone shows that the label is distributed uniformly, except for an occasional bit of endosteal bone, which is not labeled at all. Presumably its formation preceded our labeling period.

The time course of calcium-45 release and tritiated hydroxyproline release under stimulation by PTH are parallel. There is a slightly greater amount of calcium-45 that is released, particularly on the first day. However, we don't know what the net calcium loss is, and more measurements have to be made. It looks as though 2 or 3% of the bone calcium comes out first and then the hydroxyproline comes out.

Dr. Goldhaber: Did you say that it took 12 hours before any of the hydroxyproline came out?

Dr. Raisz: That's right. At that time, only 1 to 2% of the calcium is released.

Dr. Goldhaber: What do you call that period where the calcium is coming out and the collagen remains in bone? Can this be the important process of exchange in which there are rapid alterations back and forth? Is this resorption? Is it not resorption? Is this halisteresis?

Dr. Raisz: I don't know. It is likely that the effects we see in the first 6 hours and that John Reynolds sees within 2 hours could be due to exchange. The only thing that bothers me about this is that in Reynolds' system, vitamin A is just as good as PTH in causing resorption.

Certainly, exchange might increase to yield the observed increase in calcium-45 going from bone to medium without net resorption. We are now trying to get enough bones and good enough analytic methods to be able to determine this.

Dr. Minkin: Dr. Raisz, have you tried altering calcium concentration during the induction period with the so-called noninducing resorbing agents? Also, have you incubated the tissue in the cold during an induction period and then incubated under normal conditions at 37°C?

Dr. Raisz: The answer to the first question is no. The answer to the second one is yes, but we only used a 1 hour period. We didn't dare use a 6 hour period. We felt we might damage the bones. We got some induction at 37°C and not at 0°C. This does not prove you have to have energy for induction. Low temperatures might slow uptake of PTH. It will be important to look at calcium effects on these agents. Calcium might increase their penetration into the cells and thus could induce, but we haven't done this yet.

Dr. Cohn: Are you concerned about the level of 25-HCC that you have been using in relation to physiological levels that might normally be circulating in the serum. Although you use less than a microgram, it is very potent material; 20 units of vitamin D, and certainly a smaller amount 25-HCC can cause a remarkable effect on calcium transport in a whole animal.

Dr. Raisz: We use high concentrations, but I am more concerned about PTH than 25-HCC, because in long-term experiments, we can get a significant effect from 0.9 IU/ml of the latter, a level which is found in blood after a loading dose of vitamin D. With PTH, the lowest effective concentration is .01 IU/ml, which is still an order of magnitude greater than blood levels. PTH may not work as well in tissue culture because it also requires something extraosseous that we aren't supplying. Maybe we have been misled by the good response to high doses of PTH and have not looked whether, like vitamin D, there is activation which makes PTH more effective in bone *in vivo*.

Dr. DeLuca: In our hands, the normal level of 25-hydroxy vitamin D that we see in human plasma is about 0.5 IU of antirachitic activity per milliliter. I would like to also remind Dr. Cohn that, in contrast to the intestinal transport response, if one plots dose of vitamin D versus bone mobilization, there is a dose relationship. I think this is why extensive mobilization of bone is obtained when really toxic amounts of vitamin D are given. This was pointed out quite a while ago by Carlsson, Bauer, and Lindquist. (*Acta Physiol. Scand.* **26**, 212. (1952)).

Abstracts of Submitted Papers

I. Calcification

TIME STUDY OF *IN VIVO* INCORPORATION OF ^{32}P-ORTHOPHOSPHATE INTO PHOSPHOLIPIDS OF CHICKEN EPIPHYSEAL TISSUES

E. Eisenberg and R. Wuthier

Nine 8-week-old chicks were given ^{32}P-orthophosphate, 1 mCi, intraperitonally and were killed 2, 14, 38, 86, and 169 hours after injection. Long-bone epiphyses were dissected and separated into zones. Lipids were extracted from each zone, each tissue was demineralized, and lipids were extracted again. The extracts were analyzed for total lipid and phospholipid content, types of phospholipids, and relative specific activity.

Total lipid content varied from 1.35 to 4.52% of dry demineralized weight; phospholipid was about half. In zones with higher calcium content, more phospholipid was extracted after demineralization than before. Neutral phospholipids were 80–90% of the total in predemineralization extracts and 48–65% in extracts after demineralization. The amount and types of phospholipid and their relation to degree of calcification corroborated data previously reported for the calf. Relative specific activity curves revealed a sluggish metabolic pattern in resting cartilage and very active phospholipid turnover in the other three epiphyseal zones. The different types of phospholipids had markedly different metabolic patterns from each other. Special features of the turnover patterns in proliferating and calcifying cartilage suggest that serine phospholipids and possibly phosphatidylethanolamine and inositol are "protectively" transporting calcium during the growth or calcification process.

METABOLIC ACTIVITY AT THE CEMENT LINE OF BONE

Josef Eschberger

So far, the cement line has been considered to be a relatively inactive zone that plays but a small role in bone metabolism. Resorption of bone at the cement line near fatigue fractures of long bones, however, suggests a high turnover of fluids with an increased surface activity in these zones. Microradiography in such cases shows concentric demineralization and collapse of the osteons. Different kinds of staining, the study of phosphatase reactions, and microradiography reveal a cavernous system at the cement line. Cytoplasmic processes of osteocytes extend into this cavernous system. Autonomic osteocytes in this system connect the adjoining osteons. The structural appearance of this system is best shown by alkaline phosphatase reaction in the fast growing juvenile bone.

CALCIFICATION OF THE CARTILAGE FORMED ON AVIAN BONES*

Brian K. Hall

Many of the membrane bones of the embryonic chick are characterized by the presence of prominent nodules of adventitious (secondary) cartilage, which cartilage shows the typical cartilage differentiation sequence: fibroblast→chondroblast→chondrocyte→hypertrophic chondrocyte. The matrix of the hypertrophic phase of the cartilage undergoes calcification, accompanied by onset of alkaline phosphatase activity, loss of glycogen activity, deposition of lipid, and enhancement of acid mucopolysaccharide (chondroitin sulphate) synthesis. Electron microscopic analysis indicates that calcification commences either as aggregation of needlelike inorganic phosphate crystals over osmiophilic round bodies (2000–2800 Å and

4800–4900 Å in diameter), or as deposition of crystals on collagen fibers. Disintegration of the chondrocytes accompanies calcification. The endoplasmic reticulum and cytoplasmic vacuoles first disintegrate, then the cytoplasmic membrane breaks down, mitochondria break down, and finally the nucleus becomes pyknotic. The calcification of this adventitious cartilage has many parallels to calcification of hypertrophic cartilage in endochondral ossification.

Areas where adventitious cartilage and primary nonhypertrophic cartilage are adjacent, as on the pterygoid–parasphenoid articulation, facilitate comparison of a calcifying with a noncalcifying cartilage. Comparative histochemical analysis of hypertrophic versus nonhypertrophic cartilage indicates that nonhypertrophic cartilage contains no lipid, alkaline phosphatse, or glycogen, whereas calcifying hypertrophic cartilage contains all three. Cellular hypertrophy is essential to calcification, and cellular mechanisms controlling synthesis of these three substances are obviously important in determining whether a cartilage shall undergo hypertrophy and calcify.

Injections of cortisone acetate, vitamin C and β-aminopropionitrile were used to suppress chondroitin sulfate synthesis, enhance collagen synthesis, and inhibit collagen cross linking, respectively. The first and third treatments inhibited calcification, the second enhanced calcification. It was concluded that the histochemical changes in collagen and chondroitin sulfate activity associated with calcification were not just parallel events but were causally related to the onset of calcification.

* This study was aided by Canadian National Research Council Grant A5056.

EVIDENCES OF A DIRECT EFFECT OF VITAMIN D_3 OR 25-HYDROXYCHOLECALCIFEROL UPON HUMAN ADULT BONE MINERALIZATION

P. Bordier, L. Miravet, S. Tun Chot, and D. Hioco

In the absence of vitamin D, a relative lack of the physiological process of mineralization of osteoid is found, although partial mineralization randomly located in osteoid develops. Hypophosphatemia, also present in vitamin D deficiency, results from a renal loss of phosphate. Within 6 days of its administration, vitamin D, by increasing tubular reabsorption of phosphate, normalizes serum phosphate concentration, a phenomenon which is associated with a consistent decrease in the circulating parathyroid hormone level. Serum calcium remains unchanged, although the effect of vitamin D upon mineralization has been claimed to be the consequence of the increased plasma phosphate that results from the vitamin D administration; oral supplements, given to vitamin D-deficient patients, were found to normalize phosphatemia and induce a marked increase in the partial calcification of osteoid. However, the amount of calcification front remained unchanged. Intravenous administration of a single dose of 40,000 IU of vitamin D_3 to these same patients induced a similar rise in serum phosphate but also caused a marked increase in the calcification front returning the values toward normal. 25-Hydroxycholecaliferol given orally or intravenously had the same effect on serum phosphate and on the calcification front.

From these results it is concluded that vitamin D, or more likely its metabolite, 25-hydroxycholecalciferol, has a direct effect upon the mineralization of osteoid which is not related to an increase in the systemic phosphate concentration. Since this effect is specifically upon the development of the calcification front rather than upon the random distribution of mineral in the osteoid, it is suggested that vitamin D participates in some fashion in the transport of calcium into the depths of the calcified osteoid.

ROLE OF PROTEIN–POLYSACCHARIDE AGGREGATES AS A BIOLOGICAL INHIBITOR OF MINERAL GROWTH

David S. Howell, Julio C. Pita, Juan F. Madruga, and Francisco J. Muller

In previous reports we demonstrated that solid tissue samples and micropuncture fluids from various nasal, articular, and growth plate cartilages contained a potent macromolecular inhibitor of mineral seeding *in vitro*, identified as an R2 fraction of protein–polysaccharides. Micropuncture fluid obtained from the already calcified sites lacked the R2 fraction. This R2 fraction had similar properties to PPL5 of Rosenberg and 1 mole ($10^6 g$ molecular weight fragment) bound 40,000 moles of dicalcium phosphate. In the current study with a new method of ultramicroanalytical ultracentrifugation, a fast PPC component was found in naturally occurring cartilage fluids with $s^5{}_{20}$ similar to purified PPL5 of Rosenberg. The supernates from ultracentrifugation of C_{fl} lacked the aggregate and were unable to inhibit mineral growth *in vitro*.

Highly purified PPL5 and PPL3 obtained from Dr. L. Rosenberg prepared in the same manner as for his Kleinschmidt monolayer electron microphotographs were studied in micro double-diffusion chambers under oil with constant pH and bicarbonate-buffered synthetic lymph resembling micropuncture cartilage fluid. Calcium, phosphorus, and ^{45}Ca measurements, as well as circular dichroism studies were made in relation to several variables. Comparisons of the fast and slow PPC moving components of Franek and Dunstone and those of Hascall and Sajdera indicated that the aggregate PPC forms inhibited mineral precipitation and growth at the stage of fine mineral particle formation.

Physical forces, including adjacency of like molecules but not viscosity, were indicated to be responsible for this effect. This phenomenon is conjectured to represent a homeostatic protective mechanism to lower chemical reactivity of mineral and perhaps other particulate extraneous materials which inadvertently form or appear in interstitial matrices.

CALCIFICATION OF CARTILAGE BY MEANS OF MINERALIZED SPHERULES

Herbert K. Kashiwa

The glyoxal bis (2-hydroxyanil) (GBHA) and the dilute silver acetate methods revealed calcium phosphate (carbonate) spherules in chondrocytes and matrices of calcifying cartilages in tibias from newborn rats and mice and in occipital bones from chick embryos. The fact that cellular minerals were present in a labile state and as spherules suggested that the minerals were perhaps complexed to a labile organic compound. Further investigations revealed lipids complexed to the minerals in the cytoplasm of chondrocytes, as well as in the matrix.

The mineralized spherules in the matrix at the zone of provisional calcification were smaller than those found distally in the spicules of calcified cartilage. After decalcification with Na_2EDTA, the spherical organic matrix stained with toluidine blue (metachromatic) and with aldehyde fuchsin, suggesting acid mucopolysaccharide as another possible constituent of the mineralized spherules. In all of the calcified cartilages examined, mineralized spherules were the major component of the trabeculae.

The sequence of cartilage calcification appeared to proceed by formation of labile lipid–calcium phosphate (carbonate) spherules within the chondrocytes, secretion of the spherules into the matrix, and fusion of the secreted spherules with incorporation of acid mucopolysaccharide to form the larger mineralized spherules.

DECALCIFIED BONE IMPLANTS UNDER HORMONAL INFLUENCE

Erkki V. S. Koskinen, Soini A. Ryöppy, and T. Sam Lindholm

One of the known drawbacks of bank bone, its inability to contribute directly to osteogenesis, might be compensated if it were possible to achieve sufficient increase of the implants' ability to induce osteogenesis. Previous work done on the formation of callus has demonstrated the effect of various hormones on this phenomenon. The present study concerned hormonal influence on decalcified bone implants and comparison of the effects with those seen in respect of the callus in experimental fractures.

Growth hormone (STH), thyrotropine (TSH), and cortisone were subjected to study of their influence upon decalcified, lyophilized bone homografts consisting of pieces of rat cortical bone, implanted in muscle and followed for 14 weeks. Examinations were made after various periods by radiological, histoquantitative, ^{45}Ca and tetracycline labeling, and microradiographic techniques. The changes observed in the implants were compared to those noted in the course of repair of experimental fractures of the rat tibia examined by the same techniques.

I. Calcification

Somatotropic and thyroid-stimulating hormone, administered in combination, accelerated the maturation of fracture callus, especially at the early phase of repair, while cortisone retarded the reparative process. In decalcified bone implants, the same hormones elicited effects resembling the foregoing. Histoquantitative analysis revealed somewhat stronger new bone formation by autoinduction under STH and TSH influence, and the proportion of other active components, such as hypertrophic mesenchyme, was higher. Under cortisone, there was less new bone formation than in the controls, but quite intense formation of new cartilage tissue was seen.

The changes seen in the matrix of the implant and the remodeling of the graft were different and delayed, compared to the formation of callus tissue. The difference seemed to become more strongly evident at the later stage in the graft. The slow rate of change, in comparison with maturation in fracture repair, is obviously due to the time needed to establish contact between implant and host bed. The activity of mesenchymal cells, absorption of the old matrix and ingrowth of sprouting capillaries, production of new bone, and finally formation of an ossicle constitute a chain of events which takes time to accomplish. Successful completion of the process is furthermore influenced by immunobiological and antigen factors, which have no effect upon callus formation which is a physiological process.

The total ^{45}Ca activity of the implants during the observation period was higher in the STH + TSH group and lower in the cortisone group than in the controls. This was corroborated by densitometric recordings made of the autoradiographs.

The findings suggest that the process of new bone formation by autoinduction in decalcified, lyophilized bone implants transplanted as homografts into skeletal muscle is subject to modification by the above-mentioned hormones.

MECHANISM OF CALCIFICATION

Fred Leonard, Clarence W. R. Wade, and Andrew F. Hegyeli

In a recent communication from this laboratory, a cyclic process for the calcification of skeletal tissue had been postulated in which ATP present at the mineralizing site first complexes calcium. The calcium complex is subsequently hydrolyzed to calcium acid pyrophosphate and then to hydroxyapatite. During the process, adenosine and orthophosphoric acid are formed which react to regenerate ATP.

In an experimental test of the mechanism, a study of the hydrolysis of ATP-^{14}C in the presence of calcium ion and 14-day-old chick embryo femurs was undertaken. The various hydrolysis products were separated using ion exchange thin-layer chromatography and were radioassayed. The results obtained indicated that adenosine formed and that it could be phosphorylated in the presence of orthophosphate and chick embryo bone.

The question as to why calcification does not normally occur in noncalcifying soft tissue, even though ATP, calcium, and phosphatases are present, was examined. Based on the facts that these tissues contain a high magnesium-to-calcium ratio, that the formation constant ratio (R) for $MgATP^{2-}/CaATP^{2-}$ is 2.95 and that magnesium inhibits ATP hydrolysis, it was possible to calculate "noncalcification indices" for various tissues and to predict the propensity for various soft tissues to calcify.

BIOLOGICAL ROLE OF HETEROLOGOUS ANTIBODIES AGAINST CARTILAGE PROTEIN POLYSACCHARIDE COMPLEX LIGHT FRACTION (PP-L)*

Tawfik Y. Sabet and Charles E. Hawley

PP-L was extracted from cartilage of calf scapula and was used to immunize rabbits. Hyperimmune sera were pooled and their IgG separated.

* This study was supported in part by a research grant no. 03036 from NIDR and a project grant no. 02201 from NIDR.

Immunodiffusion of purified antibodies gave two precipitation lines against calf PP-L and cross reacted with mouse epiphyseal cartilage. The effect of this antibody on newborn mouse femurs was studied in organ cultures for 2 weeks. Standardized gross photographs of explants after 1 and 2 weeks showed that all explants maintained their morphological characteristics. Histologically variable degrees of reduced width of hypertrophic zone and general absence of calcified zone of both epiphyseal plates were noted in antibody-treated cultures. In addition, the formation of a very fragile junction between bone and cartilage was also observed. It is concluded that PP-L is associated with the role of maintaining the orderly progress of chondrocyte differentiation through the zones of endochondral ossification and specific antibodies can disrupt this orderly process.

ISOLATION OF MEMBRANE-BOUNDED EXTRACELLULAR PARTICLES ASSOCIATED WITH CALCIFICATION IN CARTILAGE MATRIX

Stanley W. Sajdera, Margaret Whelan, H. Clarke Anderson, and S. Yousuf Ali

Matrix vesicles are extracellular, membrane-bounded particles which are associated with mineralization of cartilage matrix. Matrix vesicles were isolated from bovine fetal epiphyseal cartilage in the following way. Slices of epiphyseal cartilage were digested with collagenase (but not homogenized) and then partitioned into seven fractions by differential centrifugation. The cellular fractions, which sedimented at 1000–5000 g, contained 80% of the DNA in the digest. The fraction sedimenting at 150,000 g consisted largely of matrix vesicles, which often enclosed needles of apatite (identified by electron microscopy). This fraction also displayed the highest activity of alkaline phosphatase, pyrophosphatase, and ATPase. Over half the total activity of each of these enzymes was found in particulate form in the extracellular fractions, but most of the acid phosphatase activity was found in the cellular fractions, suggesting that matrix vesicles are not lysosomes. This appears to be the first instance of isolation of extracellular, membrane-bounded particles from any normal tissue.

The alkaline phosphatase activity of isolated vesicles is much more heat-labile than the pyrophosphatase and ATPase activities. The kinetics of thermal inactivation are not simple and suggest that several enzymes may be responsible for each of the phosphatase activities.

The presence of high activities of alkaline phosphatase, pyrophosphatase, and ATPase in mineralizing cartilage (but not in nonmineralizing reserve zone cartilage) and the association of these activities with the matrix vesicles suggest that phosphatases are essential for endochondral ossification. Three possible mechanisms by which these phosphatases could bring about mineralization follow. First, any phosphatase activity could increase the local concentration of orthophosphate by hydrolysis of ester phosphates. Second, pyrophosphatase could hydrolyze endogenous pyrophosphate which is known to inhibit formation of apatite. Third, ATPase may be part of an active transport process for increasing the concentration of calcium and/or phosphate inside the vesicles, where the first crystals of apatite are seen.

ELECTRON MICROSCOPE MEASUREMENTS OF ALKALINE EARTH TRANSPORT

Elizabeth Lloyd

The transport of calcium in the calcification process has been studied at the periosteal surface of the femur in a rapidly growing mouse using the electron microscope and electron microscope autoradiography with ^{133}Ba as a tracer. Our findings can be summarized as follows:

I. Calcification

1. Small centers of calcification are found close to the main body of bone, which has already been laid down with a decreasing gradient of bone mineral as we move away from the bone surface.

2. The main body of the osteoblasts is in general removed a considerable distance away from the bone surface (approx. $5\,\mu$). Only the extremities of a few cell processes are visible in the areas of active calcification.

3. There is no preponderance of mitochondria in the sites adjacent to bone calcification.

4. These mitochondria appear to contain only a few granules of the type found by Matthews in the cartilage plate area.

5. Preliminary results with ^{133}Ba as a tracer, given 10 minutes after injection of the isotope, show little or no radioactivity over the bone cells, but a much greater deposition in bone mineral.

From these results, therefore, it appears unlikely that mitochondrial granules are important in the normal calcification process in bone formation at the site studied. The mechanism of calcification at this site is still a matter for conjecture.

CALCIUM TRANSPORT AND CALCIFICATION STUDIES BY MICROPERFUSION

Marshall R. Urist, H. Peter Meyer, and Karen S. Merickel

Normal vascular and connective tissues resist influx or promote efflux of concentrations of Ca^{2+} and HPO_4^{2-}, ten times greater than the concentrations of normal blood plasma. Normally, the quantity of soft tissue calcium in the ear is 10 mmoles/kg. Transformation of noncalcifiable intercellular substances into calcifiable matrix occurs in a viable ear after a tenfold increase in uptake of calcium by residual tissue proteins of skin and arterial walls and a sixfold increase by matrix of cartilage. Perfusion of phosphate buffer produces calcification only in cartilage matrix where the level of protein-bound calcium (45 mmoles/kg) is normally higher—five times that in skin and subcutaneous tissue. Thus, the apatite mineral is correlated directly with the quantity of protein–calcium–phosphate complex in the tissue, not the ion products of the Ca^{2+} and HPO_4^{2-} in the perfusion solution. Hypoxia and injury, which lower tissue viability, increase Ca^{2+} ion penetration and enhance pathological calcification. Papain-induced dissociation of protein polysaccharides of cartilage matrix does not increase Ca^{2+} ion penetration or promote calcification. Diphosphonates inhibit calcification in all tissues of rabbit ear. ATP–calcium complexes, by mechanisms now unknown, produce mineral deposits limited strictly to subcutis.

II. Calcitonin: Calcium Ion Activity and Pharmacological Action: Tooth Formation

^{47}Ca TURNOVER OF A READILY EXCHANGEABLE CALCIUM POOL IN PREGNANT AND LACTATING COWS*

J. J. B. Anderson and W. C. Crackel

In studies designed to characterize bovine parturient hypocalcemia and paresis, parameters of ^{47}Ca kinetics were calculated in pregnant and lactating cows from the measured plasma specific activity curve. Size (E), half-life ($T_{\frac{1}{2}}$) and transfer rate ($TR = E \times 0.693/T_{\frac{1}{2}}$) of the pool were obtained by reverse extrapolation of a fairly linear portion of the curve arbitrarily selected between 20 and 64 hours post injection from semilog plots and fitted to a regression line by computer. Results were as follows: (1) during pregnancy (3 cows): E increased almost twofold, $T_{\frac{1}{2}}$ increased slightly, and TR increased moderately only within the last month of gestation; (2) at parturition and the onset of lactation (2 cows): E remained elevated, $T_{\frac{1}{2}}$ fell to about two-thirds, and TR increased to about one and one-half times prepartal values; and (3) during lactation (2 moderate to heavy lactating cows): E remained high (or continued to increase), and $T_{\frac{1}{2}}$ stayed depressed, and TR elevated (or continued to increase) as milk production rose to a maximum, whereas in 1 lightly lactating cow values of E, $T_{\frac{1}{2}}$, and TR were only slightly changed during production. One nonpregnant, nonlactating cow of the same age and breed served as a comparator and her measured mean values over a 1 year period were: $E = 46.6$ gm, $T_{\frac{1}{2}} = 24.4$ hours, and $TR = 1.30$ gm/hour.

* This study was supported by AEC Grant AT (11-1)-1339.

METABOLIC CLEARANCE RATE OF RADIOIODINATED HUMAN CALCITONIN IN MAN

Raymond Ardaillou, Pierre Sizonenko, Alain Meyrier, and Gabreil Vallèe

The characteristics of the disappearance of radioiodinated human synthetic calcitonin (HCT ^{125}I) from plasma have been studied in two groups—control subjects and end stage renal failure patients treated by hemodialysis. Constant infusion studies of HCT-^{125}I were performed in two similar groups. Concentration of HCT-^{125}I in plasma was estimated by chromatoelectrophoresis. Metabolic clearance rate was determined both from single injection and constant infusion studies, with fast initial distribution volume from the former. After single injection, the disappearance curve was multiexponential. The number of exponentials of the theoretical curve fitting the best with the experimental data varied individually but more often was three. Metabolic clearance rate values in normal man calculated from constant infusion studies were 82.3 ± 3.4 ml/minute/m². Values derived from single injection studies were similar, 77.0 ± 4.7 ml/minute/m². Fast initial distribution volumes were larger than plasma volumes, 70.7 ± 3.8 ml/kg. These results were compared to those obtained in end stage renal failure patients. Metabolic clearance rates were considerably lower, 33.2 ± 2.7 ml/minute/m² in constant infusion studies and 25.4 ± 3.5 ml/minute/m² in single injection studies. Fast initial distribution volumes were slightly higher, 91.7 ± 6.3, in that group. This fact emphasizes the important role of kidneys in the utilization and/or the degradation of human calcitonin.

EXTRAOSSEOUS ACTIONS OF CALCITONIN*

Gerard A. Charbon and Elisabeth E. M. Pieper

In earlier papers it was shown that parathyroid hormone given to anaesthetized dogs augments selectively the arterial hepatic and renal flows. The effect of parathyroid hormone was log-dose dependent; its maximum was reached within 1 minute after intravenous injection. A dose–response curve could be repeated on the same dog after $1\frac{1}{2}$ hours, when the effect was assessed on coeliac blood flow. The second dose–response curve could be shifted to the right by giving precedingly porcine calcitonin extract.

Since then this study was repeated with synthetic porcine calcitonin, salmon calcitonin extract, and fractions of synthetic porcine calcitonin containing the amino acids 1–9 (30 µg/kg) and 10–32 (70 µg/kg), respectively. Synthetic porcine calcitonin (10 and 20 µg/kg) and salmon calcitonin extract (1 MRC unit/kg), like porcine calcitonin extract, antagonized the parathyroid hormone-induced augmentation of coeliac flow, but only salmon calcitonin extract had at this dose level a similar action on the parathyroid hormone-induced augmentation of renal blood flow. Synthetic porcine calcitonin amino acids 1 to 9 had no influence, while amino acids 10–32 seemed to have the same effect as 10 µg synthetic porcine calcitonin but additional experiments are needed for a final conclusion.

An additional study was conducted with parathyroid extract and salmon calcitonin extract on pentagastrin and insulin-induced gastric secretion in trained dogs. No effect of parathyroid extract was seen, but salmon calcitonin extract decreased consistently the pepsin output after pentagastrin stimulation, without a similar alteration of volume, acid, sodium, potassium, calcium, magnesium, or chlorine output. No definite effect on insulin-induced secretion was observed.

A survey of these extraosseous actions of calcitonin leads to the working hypothesis that calcitonin acts on a number of tissues at the cellular membrane level and in particular changes its permeability to both extra- and intracellular compounds.

* This study was supported by the Netherlands Organization for Advancement of Pure Research (Z.W.O).

CRYSTAL-MATRIX RELATIONSHIP IN AMELOGENESIS*

Jay D. Decker

Enamel is a unique, natural composite material consisting of a biochemically well defined organic matrix and single-crystal filaments of hydroxyapatite. The crystals may be termed "whiskers" because of their large length diameter ratios. Crystals of hydroxyapatite examined from 4 to 6 day rat molar enamel are 40 Å thick, 150–200 Å wide, and indeterminately long, i.e., the length is not included within typical section thickness. The crystals present 180° axial twists at random intervals along their length and are organized into prisms. The crystals within a particular prism are organized with their long axis parallel to one another. Prisms are oriented at varying angles to one another, reflecting a laminated arrangement. Early in amelogenesis, enamel organic matrix appears amorphous. Prior to crystal nucleation, the organic matrix is organized to form elliptical tubules within which the newly forming crystals appear. Near the ameloblast, few tubules contain crystals. At progressively greater distances from the cell, the relative number of tubules containing crystals increases until all tubules seen contain them. A positive periodic acid–Schiff reaction on undecalcified sections accompanies the crystal nucleation and is limited to the area of prism development. In decalcified sections, elliptical tubules, homologous in size and distribution to those found in undecalcified sections, contain no crystals.

* This study was supported in part by NIH Grant FR-05346-09.

DIFFERENT ISOZYMES OF ACID PHOSPHATASE IN BONE AND DEVELOPING TEETH*

Lars E. Hammarstrom, Jacob S. Hanker, and Svein U. Toverud

Very favorable conditions for the demonstration of acid phosphatase isozymes, which are widely distributed in animal tissues, were devised. Unfixed freeze-dried 10 μ thick whole-body sections through the jaws and developing teeth of young rats were incubated in histochemical media containing about one-tenth the amount of hexazotized pararosaniline ordinarily employed. A high activity of acid phosphatase was found in osteoclasts, matrix secreting ameloblasts, in stratum intermedium of the enamel organ, and odontoblasts. The enzyme activity in osteoblasts, and post-secretory ameloblasts was considerably less. Incubation with sodium fluoride or copper sulfate selectively inhibited the acid phosphatase activity in the osteoclasts and reduced the enzyme activity in odontoblasts and secretory ameloblasts very little. Incubation with sodium tartrate inhibited the acid phosphatase in ameloblasts and odontoblasts, while there was little or no effect on osteoclastic acid phosphatase. Incubation with sodium molybdate inhibited the acid phosphatase in osteoclasts and secretory ameloblasts, while the enzyme activity was much less reduced in odontoblasts, stratum intermedium, and osteoblasts. It is suggested that the difference in sensitivity to the inhibitors used indicates different isozymes of acid phosphatase with tissue specific variations. The lability of osteoclastic acid phosphatase to fluoride may suggest a possible mechanism of action for fluoride in the treatment of osteoporosis.

* This study was supported by NIH DE02668 and a grant from the Swedish Medical Research Council to Dr. Hammarstrom (Project No. B71-24P-3261-01A).

PROVISIONAL CALCIFICATION OF CARTILAGE IN TISSUE CULTURE

Uriel S. Barzel

Work previously reported from this laboratory demonstrated that the chronic ingestion of alkali increased bone formation, and the chronic ingestion of acid increased bone resorption in normal adult rats. The suggestion was made that cellular mechanisms involved with bone formation are responsive to acid–base balance. This hypothesis was subjected to examination in a tissue culture system. Sixteen- and seventeen-day-old rat embryo femora were incubated at pH 7.4–7.5. Normal provisional calcification of the diaphysis associated with increase in length and weight was observed. At pH 6.8 there was increase in length and weight, but no observeable calcification in 16 day bones, and minimal calcification in 17 day bones. The growth and calcification seen at pH 7.5 were completely suppressed by the addition of arsenate to the incubation medium. Actinomycin D and cycloheximide also prevented an increase in size and weight of bone primordia grown at pH 7.5, but caused calcification to exceed that of the controls. This study demonstrated (1) that endochondral calcification may be pH-dependent, (2) that it is an energy requiring process, and (3) that its control is related to cellular protein synthesis activity.

BONE CELL RESPONSE TO SERUM CALCIUM-ALTERING DRUGS

Barbara G. Mills,* P. Holst, A. Haroutinian, and L. A. Bavetta

Recently, the role of cyclic 3′,5′-adenosine monophosphate (cAMP) as a mediator of hormone action has been found to be intimately involved

* Supported by Career Award (LAB) and USPH Research Grant AM-12702-01, National Institute of Arthritis and Metabolic Diseases.

in Ca^{2+} ion transport. Parathyroid extract causes an elevation of cAMP within target tissue such as renal or bone tissue. The mechanism of action is believed to depend on stimulation of cAMP production or inhibition of its destruction by cyclic phosphodiesterase. In spite of much evidence for the role of cAMP as the mediator of parathormone action, not all the physiological effects of parathyroid extract can be reproduced by cAMP. We compared the effect of dibutyryl-3′,5′-cyclic adenosine monophosphate (dibutyryl cAMP) with Ca^{2+}, EDTA, and parathyroid extract on bone cells of the costochondral junction in young rabbits. Although light microscopy showed similar effects after 2 hours of dibutyryl cAMP or 8 hours parathyroid extract, ultrastructural details showed dissimilarities, especially in the endoplasmic reticulum and the mitochondria. It was possible to correlate these changes with biochemical changes in an EDTA-soluble component of the bone matrix. Serum calcium levels were changed at the time of maximum histological and biochemical change. This work confirms the importance of the calcium ion as a determinant of cellular response to changes in extracellular fluid at the membrane level.

CALCIUM ION ACTIVITY IN PLASMA: EFFECTS OF METABOLIC AND RESPIRATORY ACID–BASE CHANGES

I. C. Radde, B. Hoeffken, and D. K. Parkinson

We have previously shown that rapid changes of calcium ion activity occur in neonates. It became obvious during the course of this work that variations in blood pH have contributed to the rapid swings in Ca^{2+} activity. We now confirm the direct correlation between pH and Ca^{2+} activity in experimental animals subjected to metabolic and respiratory acid–base changes. Acute metabolic acidosis and alkalosis were produced by sodium bicarbonate (I.V.) and hydrochloric acid (by stomach tube) administration, respectively. The expected inverse relationship between pH and Ca^{2+} activity was observed. Hyper- and hypo-ventilation in rats on a Byrd respirator was used to cause respiratory acid–base alterations. The changes in pH and Ca^{2+} were qualitatively and quantitatively similar to those produced by metabolic means. This suggests that pH, and not changes in the bicarbonate buffer system, is probably the major factor determining the Ca^{2+} activity/total Ca ratio in neonates and in other conditions associated with acid–base abnormalities.

A CALCIUM CONCENTRATION DEPENDENT HYPOCALCEMIC EFFECT OF CALCITONIN IN THE PERFUSED DOG LIMB

G. A. Rodan, U. A. Liberman, and M. Anbar

Addition of calcium to the perfusate (whole blood) of an isolated perfused dog limb is followed by a translocation of calcium from the perfusate, which observes first order kinetics relative to calcium concentration, [Ca]. Eventually [Ca] stabilizes at an elevated level, the elevation being proportional to the amount of calcium added. This enabled the study of the dependency of thyrocalcitonin (TCT) action on increased [Ca] not caused by changes in the rate of bone resorption.

The TCT induced hypocalcemia was linearly related to [Ca] at the time of TCT addition. The effect of age on TCT action was confirmed, a larger drop in [Ca] being observed in the young animals, under similar conditions. Administration of TCT before calcium addition showed that not only was the amount of translocated calcium increased by TCT, but also the rate of calcium transfer. Labeling the added calcium with ^{47}Ca revealed that the destination of translocated calcium was bone, a larger proportion of radioactivity being found in the bone of the TCT-treated limb, compared with the contralateral controls. These findings indicate that TCT facilitated a passive transfer of calcium from blood to some bone constituent (presumably cells) and increased the calcium capacity of the latter.

NATRIURIC EFFECT OF CALCITONIN IN MAN

Olav Bijvoet and Jaap van der Sluys Veer

In eight (8) patients porcine calcitonin was given by continuous infusion for 6–39 days (63 MRC units/24 hours). During the first 3 infusion days urinary sodium increased and body weight decreased by 0.5–1.6 kg. α-Amino nitrogen excretion increased, suggesting proximal tubular action. After 3 days and until the end of infusion, there was a new steady state with low body weight and normal sodium excretion. Aldosterone secretion rate and plasma renin activity were increased throughout infusion. When calcitonin was discontinued, there was sodium retention for 2 days and 0.3–1.6 kg weight gain. In short-term studies, porcine calcitonin and synthetic human calcitonin had identical effects excluding contribution of species difference or contamination. Cyclic AMP excretion was not increased; this excluded secondary stimulation of parathyroid hormone as a factor. Assuming a metabolic clearance rate of 140 ml/minute plasma calcitonin concentration was 0.300 MRC units/liter, a concentration observed in healthy persons given the stress of calcium infusion. The results suggest that calcitonin in physiological amounts causes a loss of sodium and water which is sufficient to strain volume homeostasis. It may have a function in sodium control in fish alternating between freshwater and the sea.

REMISSIONS IN PAGET'S DISEASE PRODUCED BY HUMAN SYNTHETIC CALCITONIN (CALCITONIN M)

N. J. Y. Woodhouse, M. Reiner, D. N. Kalu, L. Galante, G. F. Joplin, and I. MacIntyre

Paget's disease of bone is common and sometimes associated with severe pain and deformities. The abnormal bone is metabolically overactive; there is an increased skeletal uptake of calcium isotopes, an elevated excretion of urinary hydroxyproline, and a raised serum alkaline phosphatase level. These parameters correlate well with each other and the extent of the disease. As calcitonin lowers the rate of the bone resorption acutely, the long-term effects of the human hormone have been investigated in Paget's disease in an attempt to produce a clinical and biochemical improvement.

In view of the many differences in sequence between human and other calcitonins, it was thought advisable to use only the human synthetic hormone in a prolonged study so as to minimize both the risk of antibody formation and reactions from impurities. Five Pagetic patients were studied, four with severe bone pain, for periods of 4–9 months. Large doses were used (0.5 mg twice daily intramuscularly) to produce a rapid response, but it is possible that much smaller or less frequent doses would have been equally effective.

The results were the following:

1. A reduction in the uptake of calcium isotope into affected bone.
2. An immediate and progressive fall in urine hydroxyproline excretion indicating a sustained fall in bone resorption.
3. An improvement in positivity of the calcium balance which continued throughout the study.
4. A gradual reduction in serum alkaline phosphatase levels. Urine hydroxyproline and the serum alkaline phosphatase levels eventually returned to within the normal range.

Clinically, the involved limbs became much cooler, and dramatic relief of bone pain was claimed by three patients. These changes are very striking and strongly suggest that human calcitonin may prove useful in treating Paget's disease.

ACKNOWLEDGMENT

We are grateful to Ciba Limited of Basle, Switzerland, for providing us with the human synthetic calcitonin necessary to make this study.

RELATIONSHIP BETWEEN ALKALINE PHOSPHATASE, INORGANIC PYROPHOSPHATASE, AND L-ASCORBIC ACID IN CALCIFYING HAMSTER MOLARS

J. H. M. Wöltgens, S. L. Bonting, and Olav Bijvoet

Inorganic pyrophosphate (PP_i) in very low concentrations inhibits mineralization in bone and tooth. L-Ascorbic acid is known to have a similar action *in vitro*. An inorganic pyrophosphatase (PP_iase) has been demonstrated in homogenates of 3-day-old hamster molars. Five arguments favoring identity of this PP_iase with the alkaline phosphatase (p-NPPase) in these molars were obtained by mutual substrate cross inhibition, similarities in temperature–activity curves, ratio activities in stratum intermedium and ameloblasts, ratio activities in sediment and supernate, and equal distribution patterns in high voltage free-flowing electrophoresis.

A difference in inhibition of the two enzyme activities by 1 mM L-ascorbic acid at pH 8.9 (7% p-NPPase and 75% of PP_iase activity) could be explained from studies of the absorption of 1 mM L-ascorbic acid at 266 nm in the presence and absence of p-nitrophenyl phosphate (p-NPP) and PP_i under assay conditions. A spontaneous decrease in the absorption was obtained, which was influenced by PP_i, pH, and temperature (but not be p-NPP) which paralleled the degree of inhibition of both enzyme activities. This can explain the difference in inhibition of the p-NPPase and the PP_iase by L-ascorbic acid. From the Lineweaver–Burke plot it was concluded that the inhibition of PP_iase by ascorbic acid is of the non-competitive type. It is suggested that a redox reaction takes place between L-ascorbic acid and the enzyme which is influenced by PP_i and which leads to the enzyme inhibition.

III. Diphosphonates; Bone Resorption; Osteoporosis

MECHANICAL EFFECTS ON CELL MECHANISMS IN BONE

Göran C. H. Bauer and Tomihisa Koshino

In the nineteenth century, Wolff conceived what has since been accepted as a law of nature—remodeling of bone is guided by functional demands in accordance with mathematical laws. By roentgenography or histology, the clinician has daily opportunities to observe the structural aspects of this phenomenon. Lately, Bassett and others have observed that electric signals are elicited in bone subjected to mechanical stress. Direct quantification of cell action, as triggered by mechanical demands on bone, can now be recorded by radionuclide scintimetry *in vivo*.

In primary osteoarthritis of the knee in man, the attrition of articular cartilage occurs asymmetrically, causing an imbalance in the axial load of the joint. On weightbearing, the subchondral bone is therefore subjected to increased load on one side and decreased load on the other side of the joint, resulting in hypertrophy (sclerosis) and atrophy (osteopenia), respectively. A corresponding asymmetric metabolic pattern was recorded by ^{85}Sr scintimetry. The axial load on the knee joint was changed by osteotomy of the tibia in some of these knees. The ^{85}Sr scintimetry pattern recorded over subchondral bone was changed accordingly. When the osteotomy failed to achieve its mechanical purpose, the scintimetry pattern remained unchanged.

CANALICULAR AND INTERSTITIAL CHANGES IN OSTEOCYTIC OSTEOLYSIS*

Leonard F. Bélanger, S. S. Jande, and J. D. Cipera

Current electron microscopic observations on the rat jaw and chick tibia have revealed that the osteocyte's life cycle can be divided into three main episodes—the formative, resorptive, and degenerative phases. These phases are characterized by the changes occurring within the cells and also the response of their immediate environment. Measurements of the size of canaliculi in the tibia of normal and calcium-deprived young chicks have revealed a progressive and very significant increase ($P < 0.001$) of the size of the canaliculi and also a greater variation among individual units during the resorptive phase, but no further significant alteration during the degenerative phase. On the other hand, light microscope studies following impregnation of demineralized paraffin sections with iodinated starch have revealed that marked differences in the size of these channels could be recognized. Prominently large canaliculi were present in young bone, in magnesium-deficient rats, and in humans suffering from osteogenesis imperfecta and Paget's disease.

The increase in diameter related to osteocytic osteolysis demonstrated by electron microscopy was not obvious by this procedure. However, in the area of osteocytic resorption, the bone matrix became more heavily impregnated with the iodinated starch. These observations confirm the change in matrix density previously demonstrated by alpharadiography as a result of the lysosomal activity of the osteocyte.

* This study was supported by the Canadian Medical Research Council (MT 799 and MA 3083) and the Canada Department of Agriculture (EMR 116).

EFFECT OF CALCIUM DEFICIENCY ON HEALING OF EXPERIMENTAL FRACTURES IN THE AVIAN TARSUS AS DETERMINED BY THE FRACTURE REPAIR RATIO

John R. Beljan

The fracture repair ratio (FRR) has been found to be a convenient quantitative measurement of fracture repair in a standardized experimentally induced osseous injury. The *FRR* compares bone mineral content in a healing lesion with that in adjacent intact bone utilizing ^{125}I photon beam attenuation. In lieu of determining actual bone mineral content, the ratio of bone mineral in an osteotomy and adjacent normal bone is obtained from the formula

$$FRR = \frac{\ln(I_0/I_\alpha)}{\ln(I_0/I_\beta)};$$

where I_0 = unattenuated transmission (air beam), and I_α and I_β = transmission through osteotomy and normal bone, respectively.

When plotted as a function of time, *FRR* assumes a specific form, resembling a damped sinusoidal wave, which is characteristic of the avian bone under study (tibia and tarsus). Originally developed as an *in vitro* technique, the *FRR* has been nondestructively employed *in vivo* to precisely assess fracture repair in skeletally mature single-comb White Leghorn avians fed normal and calcium-deficient diets (calcium in synthetic diet 0.002% by weight).

The early *FRR* waveform is similar to normal in the calcium deficiency state, but is of lesser amplitude, suggesting reduction in quality of bone repair. After approximately 3 weeks, the repairing cortical defect shares

---

* Study supported by NASA Contract NAS2-5245.

the demineralizing response of the total skeletal mass in response to calcium deficiency. This implies that early bone repair is a relatively localized process, but once a critical temporal point in recalcification has been attained, the healing defect reflects the systemic skeletal response to inadequate calcium intake.

EFFECT OF PHOSPHONATES ON BONE TISSUE: STUDIES IN MAN AND ANIMALS

M. E. Cabanela and J. Jowsey

The following studies were designed to evaluate the effect of phosphonates on osteoporosis.

1. Twenty rats were given EHDP daily. Surgical immobilization of one hind limb was produced in these and twenty controls. The weight of the tibias and femurs and their calcium and phosphorus content were compared.

2. Cortisone-induced osteoporosis was studied in rats given EHDP. A consistant finding was an increase in the width of osteoid tissue ($p < .003$) in the treated animals. Bone loss appeared not to be affected.

3. Growing dogs were given EHDP by mouth. Serum and bone changes were compared with a control group and a group fed a rachitogenic diet. There were no significant differences in serum calcium or phosphorus, however, the rachitogenic-fed group developed elevated alkaline phosphatase levels. The width of osteoid in this group was slightly increased while the EHDP-fed group showed no elevation in alkaline phosphatase but a clear increase in osteoid width ($p < .01$).

4. Adult cats were given oral EHDP at levels ranging from 1 to 500 mg/kg/day. At the highest level, the animals died with hyperphosphatemia and renal damage. At both high and low dose levels an increase in osteoid width was found.

5. In four osteoporotic humans, EHDP was given orally at levels between 25 and 2.5 mg/kg/day for 3 months. All patients developed hyperphosphatemia and there was a tendency toward hypercalcemia in two patients. There was an increase in osteoid width. Bone resorption levels in these patients are at present being evaluated.

SITES AND MODES OF AN ESTROGEN–GESTAGEN COMBINATION ON CALCIUM AND PHOSPHATE METABOLISM IN SENILE OSTEOPOROSIS

Angelo Caniggia and Carlo Gennari

In thirty institutionalized women aged 50–66, we have studied the calcium and phosphate metabolism (calcemia, phosphatemia, calciuria, phosphaturia, hydroxyprolinuria, serum alkaline phosphatase, phosphate, and creatinine clearances; intestinal absorption of radiocalcium (^{47}Ca); intestinal absorption of radiophosphate (^{32}P); ^{47}Ca kinetics) before and after a 6 month treatment with an oral estrogen–gestagen combination (ethynilestradiol (0.10 mg) + vynilestronolone (2.50 mg) daily). These patients were affected by senile osteoporosis, demonstrated by clinical and laboratory features, X-ray, and needle biopsy of iliac crest. The patients have been randomized with a double blind technique (fifteen patients treated with the estrogen–gestagen combination, fifteen patients submitted to an identical treatment with placebo). We have carried out a statistical evaluation of all the results:

1. After the treatment, the response of patients who received the drug or the placebo are not statistically very different with respect to phosphatemia, serum alkaline phosphatase, calciuria, hydroxyprolinuria and creatinine clearance.

2. Significant difference in the estrogen–gestagen group have been found regarding: calcemia ($t = -2.739$, $P < 0.05$); phosphaturia ($t = 2.175$; $P < 0.05$); phosphate clearance ($t = 2.282$, $P < 0.05$).

3. Discriminative analysis of intestinal absorption of radiocalcium, evaluated with the ^{47}Ca oral test, demonstrated a statistically very different and significant response in the estrogen–gestagen-treated patients ($F = 14.470$, $P < 0.01$). These results are compatible with a net improvement of intestinal absorption of calcium.

4. Discriminative analysis of intestinal absorption of radiophosphate, evaluated with the ^{32}P oral test, demonstrated a significant response in the estrogen–gestagen-treated patients ($F = 9.866$, $P < 0.01$). These results are compatible with an improvement of intestinal absorption of phosphate.

5. The ^{47}Ca kinetics parameters A, α, and β (according to Anderson *et al.*) have been evaluated. After the treatment, the discriminative analysis showed $F = 7.73$, $P < 0.0001$. The contribution of the parameter β to the discriminative analysis was highly significant.

RESORPTION OF BONE COLLAGEN BY MULTINUCLEATED GIANT CELLS

James T. Irving and John D. Heeley

Young donor rats of an isogenously related strain were injected with proline-^{3}H (1μCi/gm) and killed from 6 hours to 28 days later. The scapulae were removed, decalcified with EDTA, and implanted subcutaneously into the backs of recipient rats. They were removed 14 days later with the surrounding tissue, sectioned, processed for autoradiography and stained with H & E. In all cases there was a giant cell response around the bone. In bones removed from the donor animals, 6 hours after proline injections, the label was on the edge of the appositional side of the bone and the giant cells did not remove it. By 28 days after proline administration when, due to apposition and resorption, the label was on the other side of the bone, giant cells were seen removing the label, which, however, they did not ingest. It thus appears, as has been suggested in the literature, that recently formed bone collagen is removed with difficulty, but older collagen can be resorbed.

EFFECT OF DISODIUM ETHANE-1-HYDROXY-1,-1-DIPHOSPHONATE ON BONE FORMATION IN ANIMALS

W. R. King, M. D. Francis, and W. R. Michael

The effect of disodium ethane-1-hydroxy-1,1-diphosphonate (Na_2EHDP) on bone formation in the rat and dog has been investigated. Osteoid seam width was increased in long bones of dogs given subcutaneous doses of 4 mg Na_2EHDP/kg/day for 4 weeks, and although the bones appeared to be osteomalacic histologically, total bone mineral was normal. Similar tissue changes occurred in rats given Na_2EHDP at doses of 2.5–7.5 mg/kg/day for 2 weeks. However, significant but small increases in bone mineral over control values were observed in this dose range. The data in total indicate that the histologically determined changes probably did not represent true osteomalacia. In rats given doses of 10 mg Na_2EHDP/kg/day and greater subcutaneously for 2 weeks, similar tissue changes concomitant with significant loss of bone mineral were found. These effects together are indicative of osteomalacia, but they are reversible as determined by histology, electron microprobe, and chemical analyses. Increased osteoid in bones with normal or slightly elevated mineral content may be due to increased osteoblastic and/or decreased resorptive activity. The mechanism of action in both formation of increased osteoid and subsequent mineralization may be related to diffusion gradients of EHDP in the bones.

EFFECTIVENESS OF DIPHOSPHONATES IN PREVENTING OSTEOPOROSIS OF DISUSE IN THE RAT

W. R. Michael, W. R. King, and M. D. Francis

The effectiveness of two diphosphonates, disodium dichloromethane-diphosphonate (Cl_2MDP) and disodium ethane-1-hydroxy-1,1-diphosphonate (EHDP) in preventing or reducing osteoporosis of disuse in rats has been studied. Each compound was administered orally to groups of ten adult male Sprague–Dawley rats at doses of 0.25, 2.5, and 5.0 mg phosphorus per kilogram of body weight per day. The left hind leg of each animal was immobilized by resecting 0.5–1.0 cm of the sciatic nerve on the fourth day of diphosphonate administration. Control animals of the same age and weight were subjected to an identical procedure except that distilled water was administered daily in place of the diphosphonate. The study was terminated 28 days after limb immobilization.

Total bone mineral content of the femurs and tibias from the diphosphonate treated animals was compared with corresponding data from the control animals. Cl_2MDP and EHDP were both shown to be effective in preventing or inhibiting bone loss resulting from the limb immobilization. Bones from the immobilized leg of rats treated with Cl_2MDP contained more total mineral and a greater mineral density than the corresponding bones from control rats. Bones from both the mobile and immobilized legs of animals administered EHDP revealed dose-related increases in total mineral without changes in mineral density, when compared to corresponding bones of control animals. The data for EHDP suggest that the compound may be capable of stimulating increased bone formation.

OSTEOPOROSIS AND PARATHYROID GLANDS: THE EFFECT OF PROLONGED CALCIUM DEFICIENCY ON THYROPARATHYROID-ECTOMIZED ADULT RATS

J. A. Sevastikoglou

Earlier investigations carried out in this laboratory showed that adult male rats maintained on a low calcium, normal phosphorus diet with adequate amounts of vitamin D develop characteristic osteoporotic changes. It has also been found that a significant hyperplasy of the parathyroids occurs in these rats, which was considered to indicate the importance of the parathyroids in the pathomechanism of this form of osteoporosis.

In a new experiment, adult male thyroparathyroidectomized rats were, 2 months after surgery, given the earlier used low calcium diet for 6 months. These rats developed clear signs of osteoporosis recognized in plain radiograms by microradiography, and by a significant decrease of "femur score," as compared with the control animals. Bone and serum specific activities were significantly higher in the treated than the control rats, these changes corresponding to the earlier observations. In six out of the eight osteoporotic rats, a significant fall of the serum calcium level persisted 2 months after surgery, indicating that the developed osteoporotic changes were not due to the presence of accessory parathyroids.

These results show that low calcium intake induces osteoporosis in thyroparathyroidectomized rats, which might indicate that the characteristic skeletal changes may develop independently of the parathyroids. The results of the present study take exception to the observations reported in adult parathyroidectomized cats, in which no signs of osteoporosis could be detected despite maintainance on a low calcium diet for 12 months.

ROLE OF A LIPOPROTEIN IN THE INTRACELLULAR HYDROXYAPATITE FORMATION IN BACTERIONEMA MATRUCHOTII

J. J. Vogel* and J. Ennever

Bacterionema matruchotii is an oral microorganism which when grown in a calcium-enriched medium can acquire hydroxyapatite intracellularly. The initial event in this process is the intracellular binding of calcium. Chemical separation of the cells has shown that a crude phospholipid fraction is largely responsible for calcium binding and the subsequent apatite nucleation. Our current research indicates that the nucleating moiety is a lipoprotein complex involving a basic protein and certain acidic phospholipids. It is likely that the lipoprotein is associated with the mesosomes, intracytoplasmic membranes. A correlation can be drawn between the phenomenon seen in *B. matruchotii* and the recent evidence for the involvement of lipids and membranous structures in the early stages of vertebrate calcification.

* Supported in part by USPHS Grant DE 02232.

HORMONAL EFFECTS ON CALCIUM TRANSPORT IN LIVER

S. Wallach, A. B. Chausmer, and B. S. Sherman

In vivo and *in vitro* studies indicate that mammalian liver cells transport calcium by a facilitated diffusion process Techniques for the simultaneous quantitation of the rates of influx and efflux of calcium in liver slices have been developed and applied to studies of the hormonal control of calcium transport. Parathyroid hormone administered for 6 hours to 3 days induced a biphasic 50% increase in calcium influx into liver cells without affecting calcium efflux. The transmembrane nature of the parathyroid hormone stimulation of calcium transport was verified by cryostatic radioautography. Parathyroid hormone stimulation was not reversed by the coadministration of calcitonin. Parathyroid hormone stimulation of transport was accompanied by a parallel increase in the ability of 75,000 g supernates of liver homogenates to bind calcium competitively against Chelex-100 resin. The calcium-binding principle (s) eluted from Sephadex G-75 and G-25 columns in a retarded position. The administration of l-thyroxine (T_4) for 1 day to 3 weeks induced a 30–60% increase in calcium influx, and also caused a 15–30% increase in calcium efflux. T_4 stimulation was not accompanied by an increase in calcium binding by 75,000 g liver homogenates. The addition of glucagon *in vitro* caused a 20% increase in the influx and efflux of calcium. The addition of cyclic AMP, dibutyryl cyclic AMP, and prostaglandin E_1, but not prostaglandins E_2, A_1, and F_1, yielded effects identical to that of glucagon, indicating that adenyl cyclase activation can influence calcium transport in liver. However, the accumulated data suggest that parathyroid hormone and T_4 exert their effects by other mechanisms, possibly involving protein synthetic activity.

IV. Intestinal Absorption of Calcium and Bone Metabolism

OSTEOCYTE AS A BONE PUMP

James S. Arnold and Harold M. Frost

A model of osteocyte function makes these proposals:

1. Osteocytes pump water from the periosteocyte space, down the canalicular network to an exposed bone surface, and thence to the extravascular fluid.

2. Most of this water originally enters bone at histologically distant bone surfaces and percolates through the mineralized bone intervening between them and osteocyte lacunae to reach the periosteocyte space.

3. The percolate carries dissolved calcium, a minor fraction of which exchanges during its transit through the percolation bed with the calcium in the bone mineral.

4. Osmotic pressure could drive this pump, for osteocytes eject into the periosteocyte spaces a variety of water-binding metabolic biochemical products, and the water–product aggregates have large molecular size relative to water molecules. The molecular sieve property of bone would make such aggregates traverse canalicular bores more readily than the surrounding mineralized bony substance.

25-HYDROXYCHOLECALCIFEROL (25-HCC): EFFECTS IN DEFICIENCY RICKETS AND VITAMIN D-RESISTANT RICKETS

Sonia Balsan

The effects of 25-HCC were investigated in deficiency rickets, hereditary hypophosphatemia, pseudodeficiency rickets, and resistant rickets secondary to cystinosis or tyrosinosis. Three protocols were used:

1. Eight days after a single oral dose (16,000 iu), in the three deficiency rickets cases studied, serum calcium, phosphorus, and alkaline phosphatase were normalized, citratemia increased. No significant biological effects were observed in the different types of resistant rickets.

2. Administration of 2600 iu per day for 2 months were done in four deficiency rickets and ten hereditary hypophosphatemia cases. Complete biological recovery, healing of skeletal lesions and "catch-up" growth were obtained in deficiency rickets. In contrast, all hereditary hypophosphatemia cases maintained their abnormally low serum phosphorus concentrations.

3. Effects of increasing doses of 25-HCC (6000–30,000 iu per day) were studied in four pseudodeficiency rickets and thirteen hereditary phosphatemia cases. In all four patients with pseudodeficiency rickets correction of the biological abnormalities, skeletal lesions, and "catch-up" growth were obtained. In patients with hereditary hypophosphatemia, sensitivity to 25-HCC was variable. In five patients it was possible to obtain and maintain a serum $P \geq 30$ mg/liter with daily doses of 25-HCC varying from 6000 to 12,000 iu. In the remaining eight children, 18,000–30,000 iu per day were insufficient. The only side effect observed during this investigation was an increase in the urinary output of calcium in four children. Hypercalciuria was easily controlled by oral phosphate supplementation.

Conclusions: (1) 25-HCC has antirachitic activity in children; (2) patients with rickets resistant to vitamin D were also resistant to 25-HCC. Therefore a defect in the conversion of vitamin D to 25-HCC is not the metabolic defect in these patients.

INDUCTION OF CALCIUM-BINDING PROTEIN (CaBP) BIOSYNTHESIS BY VITAMIN D_3 AND 25-HYDROXYCHOLECALCIFEROL (25-HCC)*

Ronal R. MacGregor, David V. Cohn, and James W. Hamilton

Vitamin D (20 iu) was administered to frankly rachitic chicks followed by leucine-^{3}H. ^{45}Ca transport was measured in parallel groups of chicks. The vitamin at this dose caused calcium transport to double by 24 hours and led to an increase in incorporation of leucine into CaBP but not into total tissue proteins. In contrast, 500 iu of vitamin D increased the incorporation of leucine-^{3}H into all tissue proteins. In a second type of experiment, marginally deficient birds were used. Twenty iu of vitamin D doubled the incorporation of leucine-^{3}H into CaBP by 9 hours, but there was no change in calcium transport at this time. By 12–16 hours, the rate of synthesis of CaBP approached maximum and calcium transport increased by 30–50%. When 25-HCC was administered instead of vitamin D_3, similar results were obtained, except that the effects on biosynthesis and calcium transport occurred at 3–5 hours. Following administration of either vitamin D or 25-HCC, the amount of CaBP (determined by calcium-binding activity) increased in parallel with calcium transport. These data show that (a) appearance of CaBP induced by vitamin D is due to *de novo* biosynthesis, and (b) the net increase in biosynthetic rate of CaBP precedes an actual increase in calcium transport.

* This study was supported in part by grant from NIDR.

EFFECT OF CORTISOL ON CALCIUM-BINDING PROTEIN IN RAT DUODENUM

G. Eilon, E. Mor, H. Karaman, and J. Menczel

Active absorption of calcium is inhibited by corticosteroids. A calcium-binding protein (CaBP) was found in the epithelial cells of the duodenum, and there is evidence that the active transport of calcium is correlated with CaBP.

Male rats, Sabra strain, weighing 80–100 gm were injected ip with 10 mg hydrocortisone. They were sacrificed at intervals of 1–70 hours. The specific activity of CaBP of the duodenal mucosa was determined. High specific activities of CaBP were found in the animals treated with hydrocortisone as compared to the control animals. Hydrocortisone was found to be most effective 4 hours after administration. ^{45}Ca was given by intragastric intubation, and a twofold decrease in ^{45}Ca serum levels was found 4 hours after cortisol administration as compared to control animals. The cortisol-induced CaBP was analyzed by acrylamide gel electrophoresis, as well as by immunodiffusion techniques, and was found to be identical to normal or vitamin D-induced CaBP in rat duodenum.

Active calcium transport in duodenum is a complex phenomenon and does not only depend on the calcium-binding protein.

A STUDY OF NEPHRON PERMEABILITY TO CALCIUM BY MICROINJECTION TECHNIQUE

M. Gagnan-Brunette and M. Aras

The nephron permeability to calcium has been studied by intracapillary (ICI) and intratubular injections (ITI) of ^{45}Ca and ^{3}H Inulin in saline diuretic and calcium-loaded rats (PCa = 7.93 ± 1 mEq/liter). After each injection, ureteral urine was collected bilaterally by serial fractions. After 18 ICI in saline-loaded rats, the ^{3}H In excretion was equal (18.4 ± 4.8% and 16.9 ± 4.4%) and simultaneous (183 ± 70 and 197 ± 57 seconds) in both kidneys. The low excretion of ^{45}Ca did not provide any evidence of peak excretion on either side. After calcium loading, the peak of ^{45}Ca excretion appears slightly prior to the ^{3}H In peak. The fraction of ^{45}Ca excreted was equal in both kidneys. After 22 ITI performed in saline- and calcium-loaded rats, the ^{3}H In was recovered, almost quantitatively, whereas the proportion of ^{45}Ca excreted was $6.3 \pm 5.1\%$ and $12.9 \pm 12.6\%$, respectively. The simultaneous fractional excretion of cold calcium was lower ($1.6 \pm 0.6\%$ and $9.9 \pm 4\%$). In saline rats, the appearance time of ^{3}H In and ^{45}Ca is identical, whereas the peak excretion of ^{45}Ca preceeds slightly (12 seconds) the Inulin peak ($P < 0.02$). After calcium loading, both appearance time and peak excretion of ^{45}Ca were detected prior the corresponding values for Inulin, suggesting a more direct pathway in calcium-loaded rats. There is a correlation between the TF/P Inulin and the proportion of ^{45}Ca excreted. In conclusion, the slight precession of ^{45}Ca over ^{3}H In output in ICI and ITI suggests a certain nephron permeability for calcium, in contrast to the total impermeability found previously for magnesium.

A STUDY OF CALCIUM-BINDING PROTEINS IN HUMAN ANIMAL SMALL BOWEL MUCOSA*

A. J. W. Hitchman, J. M. Finlay, and Joan E. Harrison

Human small bowel mucosa was examined for calcium-binding protein similar to the Vitamin D-dependent calcium-binding protein reported by Wasserman *et al.* in chicks and other animals. A quantitative estimate of Vitamin D-dependent calcium-binding protein in humans might provide a useful measure of Vitamin D activity at the tissue level. Calcium-binding proteins from human and animal duodenal mucosa have been partially separated and characterized by gel filtration, electrophoresis, and the Chelex 100 radio-calcium binding test. Problems have been encountered related to availability of suitable tissue and sensitivity of procedures. The calcium-binding proteins show species differences. The chick has only one such protein, molecular weight 24,000–28,000, while both the human and rat

* This study was supported by M.R.C. Grant No. MA 3114.

have two such proteins. In the normal rat one has a molecular weight of about 12,000 and is probably the previously reported calcium-binding protein. The human has a similar protein which also has a molecular weight of about 12,000. Both human and rat have a more prominent calcium-binding protein, molecular weight > 50,000, whose vitamin D dependency is not established. A strongly anionic protein similar to chick calcium-binding protein was demonstrated by electrophoresis in some human studies.

A METHOD FOR STUDYING THE CONFIGURATION, DIMENSIONS, AND DISTRIBUTION OF REMODELING CENTERS ON THE ENDOSTEAL, CORTICAL, AND TRABECULAR SURFACES

Z. F. Jaworski and H. M. Frost

The morphology and dynamics of haversian remodeling are known (osteons run parallel to the long axis of long bones), but although turnover rate of the spongiosa exceeds that of the cortex the configuration, dimensions, and distribution of remodeling centers on endosteal surfaces are practically unknown. Acquaintance with these features is a prerequisite for (1) proper interpretation of thin, decalcified and undecalcified section of bone (e.g., the estimate of osteoid seam thickness or trabecular remodeling based on tetracycline labeling) and (2) elucidation of the mechanism of bone loss (or gain) with aging and osteoporosis.

We report a new method of studying remodeling on endosteal surface which consists of (1) removing the bone marrow from thick (200–300 μ) undecalcified section of the vertebrae, rib, or iliac crest, (2) surface staining with Tetrachrome, and (3) inspection of endosteal surfaces under the stereomicroscope combined with microphotography. Bone-forming centers are identified because of a green color taken by the nonmineralized osteoid. Thus, in conjunction with the study of thick (50–70 μ) undecalcified cross sections similarly stained, a three dimensional picture of remodeling centers on endosteal surfaces can be reconstructed.

The typical remodeling center on endosteal centers in three sites studied measures approximately 4–500 μ by 500–2000 μ (surface) by 60–80 μ (thickness). Interestingly, although the configuration of haversian and endosteal remodeling centers differ, they turn over approximately the same volume of lamellar bone, i.e., 0.05 mm^3 per center. Preliminary observations indicate that distribution and density (number per unit surface area) of the remodeling centers vary with the location in a given bone, the age, and the disease.

TRANSPORT OF IODOANTIPYRINE-^{125}I (I-Ap) IN CORTICAL BONE

P. J. Kelly, Tada Yipintsoi, and James B. Bassingthwaighte

Cortical bone partition coefficient for I-Ap was determined when venous isotope activity was changing and also in the steady state. The partition coefficient λ was 0.15 ± 0.027. The cellular–osteocyte water space of this bone was 0.15 ± 0.03. Serial elutions of this cortical bone indicated that 96.4 ± 1.4% of I-Ap moved into water. These three observations suggest that the volume distribution of I-Ap is identical to the cellular–osteocyte water space of bone, since in most tissues I-Ap can be considered as a tracer for water. Further experiments indicate that I-Ap removal from bone is not diffusion limited but blood flow limited. Exponential analysis of washout curves of I-Ap from bone suggest 22% of the indicator traverses a high flow region (mean, 0.265 ml/ml bone/minute) and the remainder a slow flow region 0.012 ml/ml bone/minute. Total blood flow was 0.0152 ± 0.003 ml/ml bone/minute determined by the residue function method and was 0.0145 ± 0.003 by the two exponential method.

Ca^{2+} SENSITIVE ATPase IN DUODENAL MUCOSA: LOCALIZATION IN BASAL MEMBRANES

D. K. Parkinson and I. C. Radde

A calcium-sensitive ATPase has been delineated in duodenal mucosa of the rat. A brush border fraction was prepared by the method of Forstner et al., and the homogenate was further fractionated according to Quigley as described for Na$^+$K$^+$-ATPase. Specimens (0.1 ml) of homogenate were incubated with varying Ca^{2+} concentrations in 20 mM tris buffer (pH 7.6) and 70 mM sodium chloride and 5 mM Na$_2$ATP and P$_i$ production measured and expressed as micromoles P$_i$ per milligram enzyme protein per 30 minutes as indicator for ATP hydrolysis. A Ca^{2+}-sensitive ATPase was found which was also sensitive to, but did not require, Mg^{2+} for activation. The ionic requirements of Ca^{2+}-sensitive ATPase in whole mucosa were similar to those described for Ca^{2+}-sensitive ATPase of renal cortical membrane. The enzyme also hydrolyzed GTP and ITP, but not ADP. Only 8–10% of the total enzyme activity was localized in the brush border fraction, whereas approximately 80% was recovered from fractions consisting of mitochondrial and cell membranes from lateral and antiluminal surfaces. Localization of the bulk of Ca^{2+}-sensitive ATPase activity in the cell fractions other than brush border is in accord with Schachter's hypothesis on Ca^{2+} transport across the intestinal mucosal cell with Ca^{2+} entering the cell from the luminal surface passively, being transported across the cell in combination with calcium-binding protein and being actively extruded at the antiluminal surface.

REFRACTIVE INDEX OF NEWLY FORMING BONE TISSUE

W. L. Past

The purpose of this investigation was to obtain significant information about the mineral portion of newly forming bone tissue. Microscopic interferometric measurements of specific bone foci were made in femurs from 14–21 mm mouse fetuses. The femurs had been frozen, sectioned at 6 μm, and dehydrated. The mean refractive index (n) was generally between 1.500 and 1.530. By histochemical fractionation of some of the bone sections prior to microinterferometry it was possible to calculate the n and effective thickness (t) of each of the three major compartments of the bone: the mineral (M), collagen (C), and glycoprotein (GP). The M compartment was removed by exposure to 25 mM/liter calcium chloride, and the M and GP compartments by exposure to a solution with no calcium.

Results of preliminary experiments: n_C was 1.530 and n_{GP} 1.538; n_M was generally less than the n for the whole (dehydrated) bone; and t_M was about two-thirds the thickness of the whole bone. The observed values for n_M were low in comparison to the indices of refraction of various calcium phosphates in pure form. It was postulated that the low values resulted from a hydration layer on the bone crystals and water contained within unit particles of amorphous calcium phosphate.

BOVINE SERUM ALBUMIN (BSA) CALCIUM-BINDING STUDIES WITH A CALCIUM-SELECTIVE LIQUID MEMBRANE ELECTRODE

C. E. Sachs and A. M. Bourdeau

Dialysis equilibria in a thermostated system were performed dipping cellophane bags, containing concentrations of BSA, in a bathing fluid. The bathing fluid was a 150 mM NaCl solution with concentrations of calcium chloride varying from 0.5 to 2.5. mM, and a few drops of triethanolamine to stabilize the solution to the desired pH. The solutions inside the bags were made of a dilution with the bathing fluid of commercially available BSA solution to the approximate desired concentrations (0.3–1.8 mM). Equilibrium for calcium exchanges was obtained in 12–16 hours at 27°C. Bathing fluid and bag solutions were analysed for pH, sodium, chlorine, total and ionized Ca^{2+}, and total protein. Ca^{2+} was measured electrometrically with the flow-through Orion liquid membrane electrode. Different equilibria were studied varying pH and pCa in the bathing fluid.

The mean number of calcium moles bound per BSA mole was calculated from the slope of a total calcium versus total albumin plot. For lower BSA concentrations (0.3–1 mM) the mean number is constant. For a 1 mM pCa, the mean number increased with pH. For a constant pH at 7.0, the mean number, increased with pCa. At higher BSA concentration an abrupt change in the slope of the plot was observed. For a 1 mM pCa, the abcissa of the breaking point was independent of pH. For a constant pH at 7.0, this abcissa increased with pCa.

The deviation from linearity of the considered plot suggests that the calcium-binding capacity of BSA depends on a multiple equilibria system without interference of sites affected beyond a given concentration by an activity coefficient type factor due to electrostatic and/or steric hindrance.

PASSAGE OF CALCIUM AND STRONTIUM ACROSS THE INTESTINE IN MAN

Herta Spencer, Janet Warren, and Joseph Samachson

The difference in the intestinal absorption of calcium and strontium and the marked Ca/Sr discrimination against strontium is well known. The Ca/Sr discrimination ratio of the intestinal absorption determined in this research unit in man averaged 2.6. Studies were then performed of the passage of strontium and calcium in the opposite direction, i.e., from the bloodstream into the intestine. ^{85}Sr and ^{47}Ca were given intravenously and the plasma levels and the fecal and urinary excretions of the radioisotopes were determined. In contrast to the marked discrimination against the passage of strontium from the intestine into the bloodstream, the excretions of ^{85}Sr and ^{47}Ca into the intestine were almost equal, and the ^{85}Sr/^{47}Ca excretion ratio averaged 1.2. The data indicate that the differences in the passage of calcium and strontium from the intestine into the plasma are related to the presence or absence of food in the stomach and intestine and that the intestinal Ca/Sr discrimination can be abolished by the ingestion of certain minerals.

CONCEPT OF ELECTROPOSITIVE CRYSTAL BOND BASED ON OSSIFICATION AND OTHER PHENOMENA

Tomasz Cieszyński

On the basis of bone formation studies, the author proposes the concept of a new crystal bond assuming that there are positrons oscillating in the crystal lattice able to attract the outer electronic covers of the surrounding atoms. The number of positrons in the lattice unit and their kinetic energy are related to the temperature of the system.

This concept finds further support in other physical phenomena, e.g., in silver crystallization from silver nitrate solutions near the positively polarized electrode, in ^{22}Na decay with emission of positrons unchangeable into radiation, in Hall's effect occuring in p-type semiconductors, in X-ray diffraction analysis when ascribing a physical meaning to the negative electron densities rejected generally in this procedure, as well as in another biophysical effect, the electrosynthesis of melanin.

SUBJECT INDEX

A

ATPase, calcium-sensitive, 136–141, 148, 149
 inhibition of, 141–144, 148
 significance of, 144–146

B

Bone apatite, 9–12
Bone cells and calcium transport, 211–237
 calcium content of, 213–219
 calcium fluxes in, 226–231, 236
 hormone effects on, 228–231, 233, 235
 identity of, 220–225, 236, 237
 ion effects on, 230–231, 237
 location of calcium in, 218–219
 model for calcium transport in, 231–235
 separation of, 213–218, 220–223
 tetracycline labeling of, 223–225
Bone formation rate, 198–200
Bone "membrane," 200–205, 209
 anatomy of, 201–202, 206, 207
 "bone fluid" composition, 202–204, 207, 208
 function of, 202–205
Bone mineral solubility, 197–198
Bone resorption
 rate, 198–200
 in tissue culture, 441–454
  bone cells involved in, 451–452
  effect of calcitonin on, 447
   of calcium on, 447–449, 454
   of 25-HCC on, 446–447
   of PTH on, 446–447, 452, 453
  role of cyclic nucleotide in, 444–446, 452–453

  of RNA synthesis in, 443–444, 452
Bone sialoprotein, 63–73
 binding of calcium to, 69–70
  of radioelements to, 68–69, 73
 composition of, 65–67
 concentration as function of age, 72
 functions of, 70–71
 isolation of, 64–65, 73
 physical properties of, 68

C

Calcified tissues, development of, 25–40
 in bone, 32–34
 bone and dental tissue at Molecular level, 30–32
 at phenomenological level, 32
 cytodifferentiation, 27, 40
 in dental tissue, 34–36
 general process, 26–30
 limitations imposed by experiment, 29–30
  by models, 29
 theoretical limitations of, 27–30
Calcitonin, 403–419
 control of hypercalcemia by, 403–407
 mechanism of release, 410–412, 419
 protective role of, 412–418
 secretion in response to calcium, 407–410, 417, 418
Calcium
 absorption from GI tract, 293–312
  active transport in, 293–294, 311
  calcium binding protein in, 294, 305–308, 310, 311, 312
  adaptation in, 298–305
  calcium sensitive ATPase in, 307, 312
  diffusion in, 293

511

vitamin D in, 293–298, 300–303, 305, 307, 310
binding, 41–62
  ion competition for binding, 44, 55, 59–60
  to nucleic acids, 42–51
    DNA, 43–48, 62
    RNA, 48–51
  to phospholipids, 51–58, 61, 62
    phospholipid protein complexes, 55–58, 62
    purified preparations, 52–55
in biosphere, 3–4
in erythrocytes, 135–149
  concentration gradiets, 136, 140–141
  content of, 136
  effects of glycosides on, 135–136 141–142
  influx, 136
  transport of, 136–146
reservoir in mammary cells, 344
transfer across avian shell gland, 351–370
  anatomy of, 352–357
  localization of calcium in, 357–358
  role of mitochondria in, 363–370
  studies of, 358–363, 369, 370
transport
  across chick chorioallantoic membrane, 371–389
    bioenergetics of, 379–382, 385–387
    calcium location in, 375–379, 386, 387
    calcium transporting cells in, 375–379, 385, 386
    control of, 388–389
    effects of age on, 375
    of inhibitors on, 375
    by membrane, 374–375, 388
    mitochondria in, 387
    preparation of membrane, 373–374
    structure of membrane, 371–373
    sulfhydryl groups and, 382–385
  in kidney cells, 151–174
    calcium fluxes in, 151–153, 162–170, 172–174
    cell calcium pools, 151, 153–162, 170–172
    effects of external ions on fluxes 154, 162–172, 174

  on pools, 152–162, 171
  model for cell calcium transport, 170–171
  role of mitochondria in, 156–162, 164, 170–171, 173
across mammary gland, 339, 344–347, 349
across placenta, 339–343, 348
in sarcoplasmic membranes, 175–193
  ATPase, 175–176, 183
  phospholipase, 180–183, 193
  phospholipids, 176–183
  phosphoprotein, 176, 191
  across sarcoplasmic reticulum membranes, 175–176, 183, 192
    isolation of phosphopeptide, 188–192
  protein composition of sarcoplasmic reticulum membranes, 183–188
uptake in gut mucosal cells, 313–337
  calcium binding in, 325–330
  cell integrity, 321–327
  comparison with other systems, 332–334
  effect of inhibitors on, 320–321
  nature of calcium binder, 330–332, 336–337
  preparation of cells, 317
  specificity of binding, 330
  stability of cells in, 317, 321–327, 334, 336–337
  time course of, 327–329
Calcium phosphate, amorphous, 12–15 23, 24
Carbonate apatites, 8–9

E

Extracellular calcium concentration, relation of, 101–131
  to cell mitosis, 102–105, 126, 130, 131
  to erythropoiesis, 110–118, 120, 128, 130
  to growth of animals, 105–107, 127
  to lymphopoiesis and structure in thymus, 107–110, 120–122, 128, 130
  to mechanisms involved in, 103–105, 122–124, 127–129

Subject Index

Extracellular fluid (ECF) Ca × P ion products, 197–198
   acid prodution and calcium release, 198
   lysosomes, 198
   nucleation, 198

H

Human parathyroid hormone, 393–401
   activity of, 397–399
   amino acid sequence of, 395–396, 401
   immunology of, 398–399
   isolation of, 394–395, 400
   potency of, 398
   potential uses of, 398–399
   relation of vitamin D to, 399–400
   synthesis of active fragment of, 397
Hydroxyapatite, 5–8, 24, 39, 40

M

Mitochondrial granules and cell calcium regulation, 239–255
   analyses of, 242–243
   in bone, 245–247
   in calciphylactic skin, 247
   in cartilage, 243–245, 254
   chemical composition of, 247–251, 253
   distribution of, 243–247, 255
   effects of vitamin D, 251
   electromicroscopy of, 241, 254
   in gut, 243–245
   isolation of, 241
   methods for identification, 241–243
   numbers of, 243

O

Osteocytes, 257–289
   bone formation by, 257–285
      measurement of, 258, 260–264, 287
   bone resorption measurement of, 264
   calcium homeostasis, 284–285
   canaliculi measurement of, 265–266, 275
   general functions of, 257–258, 284–285
   osteoblastic bone formation, 282–284
   osteocytic bone formation, 266–272, 282–284, 286, 288, 289
   osteocytic bone resorption, 273, 280–281, 283, 289

P

Porcine parathyroid hormone, 400–401

S

Serum calcium homeostasis, 198–199, 205
Skeletal calcium fluxes, 198–199
Squid giant axon, 77–100
   biionic action potential of, 80–88
   effects of calcium inside and outside of, 79–80, 84–86
      of univalent cations inside and outside of, 86–88, 99
   intracellular perfusion of, 78–79
   ion exchange in nerve excitation, 88–89
   ionic mechanism of nerve excitation, 88–89, 96
   membrane change during nerve excitation, 77, 88–96, 98, 99

T

Tissue mineralization, 15–20, 40
Tissues, calcified, see Calcified tissues

V

Vitamin D, 421–440
   mechanism of action of, 437–438
   metabolism of, 423–432, 439
      of 25-hydroxy derivative of, 432–437, 440
   physiological actions of, 421–423

X

X-ray diffraction, 5, 9, 12, 23

QP
535
C2
W6
1970

AUG 8 1973